MW01004311

Care of the
Geriatric Patient

SERIES EDITOR

Fred F. Ferri, MD, FACP

Clinical Associate Professor
Brown University School of Medicine
Chief, Division of Internal Medicine
St. Joseph's Hospital and Fatima Hospital
Providence, Rhode Island

OTHER HANDBOOKS IN THE
"PRACTICAL GUIDE TO THE CARE OF" SERIES

Ambulatory Patient
Critically Ill Patient
Gynecologic/Obstetric Patient
Medical Patient
Pediatric Patient
Psychiatric Patient
Surgical Patient

Practical Guide to the
Care of the
Geriatric Patient

Second Edition

Fred F. Ferri, MD, FACP

Clinical Associate Professor of Medicine
Department of Community Health, Brown University
Chief, Division of Internal Medicine
St. Joseph's Hospital and Fatima Hospital, Providence, Rhode Island

Marsha D. Fretwell, MD

Clinical Associate Professor of Medicine
University of North Carolina
Chapel Hill, North Carolina

Tom J. Wachtel, MD

Physician-in-charge, Division of Geriatrics
Rhode Island Hospital
Professor of Community Health and Medicine
Brown University School of Medicine
Providence, Rhode Island

with 66 illustrations

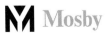

St. Louis   Baltimore   Boston   Carlsbad   Chicago   Naples   New York
Philadelphia   Portland   London   Madrid   Mexico City   Singapore
Sydney   Tokyo   Toronto   Wiesbaden

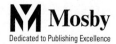

Mosby
Dedicated to Publishing Excellence

Vice-President and Publisher: Anne S. Patterson
Editor: Emma D. Underdown
Developmental Editor: Christy Wells
Project Manager: John Rogers
Senior Production Editor: Lavon Wirch Peters
Manuscript Editor: Mary Wright
Design Coordinator: Yael Kats
Manufacturing Manager: Theresa Fuchs
Cover Illustration: David Zielinski

SECOND EDITION

Printed in the United States of America
Composition by The Clarinda Company
Printing/binding by R.R. Donnelley & Sons Company

Mosby–Year Book, Inc.
11830 Westline Industrial Drive
St. Louis, Missouri 63146

International Standard Book Number 0-8151-3194-1

96 97 98 99 00 / 9 8 7 6 5 4 3 2 1

Contributors

Bruce Bialor, M.D.

Fellow, Division of General
  Internal Medicine
Rhode Island Hospital
Providence, Rhode Island

Michele G. Cyr, M.D.

Director, Division of General
  Internal Medicine
Rhode Island Hospital
Associate Professor of Medicine
Brown University School of
  Medicine
Providence, Rhode Island

Mark J. Fagan, M.D.

Director, Medical Primary Care
  Unit
Rhode Island Hospital
Assistant Professor of Medicine
Brown University School of
  Medicine
Providence, Rhode Island

James Grant, M.D.

Associate Clinical Professor of
  Medicine
Yale University School of
  Medicine
New Haven, Connecticut

Jennifer Jeremiah, M.D.

Assistant Physician
Division of General Medicine
Rhode Island Hospital
Clinical Assistant Professor of
  Medicine
Brown University School of
  Medicine
Providence, Rhode Island

Peter S. Margolis, M.D.

Clinical Gastroenterologist
Division of Gastroenterology
Rhode Island Hospital
Clinical Assistant Professor of
  Medicine
Brown University School of
  Medicine
Providence, Rhode Island

Dennis J. Mikolich, M.D.

Chief, Division of Infectious
  Diseases
Providence Veterans Affairs
  Medical Center
Clinical Associate Professor of
  Medicine
Brown University School of
  Medicine
Providence, Rhode Island

Thomas A. Parrino, M.D.

Professor of Medicine
Brown University
Providence, Rhode Island
Assistant Chief of Staff
VA New England HealthCare
   Network
Boston, Massachusetts

Jack L. Schwartzwald, M.D.

Assistant Physician
Division of General Internal
   Medicine
Rhode Island Hospital
Clinical Instructor of Medicine
Brown University School of
   Medicine
Providence, Rhode Island

Michael D. Stein, M.D.

Associate Physician
Division of General Medicine
Rhode Island Hospital
Associate Professor of Medicine
Brown University School of
   Medicine
Providence, Rhode Island

Raymond H. Stone, Jr.

Manager, Health Promotions
   Department
Columbia Cape Fear Memorial
   Hospital
Wilmington, North Carolina

Dominick Tammaro, M.D.

Associate Physician
Division of General Internal
   Medicine
Assistant Professor of Medicine
Brown University School of
   Medicine
Providence, Rhode Island

Lynn Wachtel, F.N.P., M.S.N.

Family Nurse Practitioner
Healthy Kids Initiative
Providence, Rhode Island

Preface

The coexistence of biologic and behavioral changes associated with aging and the common presence of multiple acute and chronic diseases make the practice of geriatrics both challenging and time intensive. This manual is intended to be a concise guide for all clinicians involved in the care of elderly patients. In keeping with the style of the *Practical Guides* series, this pocket-size manual provides a compressed yet comprehensive overview of geriatric medicine. Geriatric syndromes such as dementia, delirium, incontinence, pressure ulcers, osteoporosis, and prostatic disease are presented together with internal medicine as applied to the elderly. In particular, the coverage of functional syndromes and system abnormalities has been vastly expanded in this second edition. Furthermore, specific care issues related to the various settings of geriatrics practice, such as nursing homes or home care, are presented as well. Numerous tables and illustrations are used extensively throughout the text to simplify complex issues and enhance recollection of principal points.

This book's practical approach, with its emphasis on clinical correlations, should make it a useful reference for both students and clinicians who are actively involved in the care of the geriatric patient and help these caregivers find answers to most clinical questions at the bedside without having to consult another reference.

Fred F. Ferri, MD
Marsha D. Fretwell, MD
Tom J. Wachtel, MD

What Do You See, Nurse?

What do you see, nurse, what do you see?
What are you thinking when you look at me?
A crabbit old woman, not very wise,
Uncertain of habit, with far away eyes,
Who dribbles her food, and makes not reply,
When you say in a loud voice, "I do wish you'd try!"
Who seems not to notice the things that you do,
And forever is losing a stocking or shoe.
Who unresisting or not, lets you do as you will
With bathing and feeding, the long day to fill.
Is that what you're thinking, is that what you see?
Then open your eyes, you're not looking at me.
I'll tell you who I am as I sit here so still,
As I move at your bidding, as I eat at your will.
I am a small child of ten with a father and mother,
Brothers and sisters who love one another.
A young girl of sixteen with wings at her feet
Dreaming that soon now, a lover she'll meet.
A bride soon at twenty, my heart gives a leap,
Remembering the vows that I promised to keep.
At twenty-five now I have young of my own
Who need me to build a secure happy home.
A woman of thirty, my young now grow fast,
Bound to each other with ties that should last.
At forty my young soon will be gone,
But my man stays beside me to see I don't mourn.
At 50 once more babies play around my knee,
Again we know children, my loved one and me.
Dark days are upon me, my husband is dead,
I look to the future, I shudder with dread,
For my young are all busy rearing young of their own
And I think of the years and the love I have known.
I'm an old lady now and nature is cruel,
'Tis her jest to make old age look like a fool.
The body it crumbles, grace and vigor depart,
And now there is a stone where I once had a heart.
But inside this old carcass a young girl still dwells.
And now and again my battered heart swells.
I remember the joys, I remember the pain,
And I am loving and living life over again.
I think of the years all too few, gone so fast,
And accept the stark fact that nothing can last.
So open your eyes, nurse, open and see,
Not a crabbit old woman, look closer, see me.

Poem found in the belongings of an elderly woman who died in a nursing home in Ireland. Reproduced from Christiansen JL, Grzybowski JM, editors: *Biology of aging,* St Louis, 1993, Mosby.

To our families

Their constant support
and encouragement made
this book a reality

Contents

Biology, Epidemiology, and Demographics of Aging

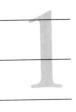

PHYSIOLOGY OF AGING
Fred F. Ferri, MD

1. General comments
   a. Definitions: **aging** describes the temporal process of growing old. The World Health Organization (WHO) characterizes a population between 65 and 75 as **elderly**. The term **old** is used for between 76 and 90 and **very old** for over age 90
   b. Aging is associated with a progressive decline in homeostatic control and the ability to respond to stress and/or change
   c. Elderly individuals are heterogeneous with respect to their physiologic function, their burden of illness, and any associated disability
   d. Normal aging can be subdivided into **successful** and **usual** aging[1] (Figure 1-1)
      (1) **Successful aging** (also known as **optimal aging**) describes individuals who demonstrate minimal physiologic decline from aging alone. Healthful strategies such as exercise, modification of diet, social and intellectual stimulation, and cessation of smoking enhance a person's quality of life and promote successful aging
      (2) **Usual aging** refers to the more common mode of aging. It is associated, e.g., with the observed decline in renal, immune, visual, and hearing function
2. Rate of age-associated decline in normal function varies with each organ system
   a. Digestive system is less affected than other organ systems
   b. Diaphragm and cardiac muscle are not significantly affected by age
   c. Table 1-1 summarizes physiologic changes associated with aging and their clinical implications
      (1) Body weight increases in middle age and subsequently decreases in the elderly, especially after 74 years of age
      (2) Lean body mass decreases (decreased muscle mass)
      (3) The percentage of body fat does not appear to increase significantly after age 40. The major reason for the increase in body fat

Text continued on p. 8.

Table 1-1 Comparison of physiologic changes in various organ systems and their clinical implications

	Physiologic Changes with Aging	Clinical Implications
Cardiovascular System	Impaired • Myocardial diastolic function Increased • Response to sympathetic nervous stimulation • Total peripheral vascular resistance • Plasma volume • Stiffness of aorta and other major arteries Decreased • Stroke volume • Interstitial volume • Ventricular filling time • Vascular compliance • Baroreflex sensitivity • Number of pacemaker cells	Decreased • Cardiac output • Reflex tachycardia • Heart rate Increased • Afterload • Susceptibility to hypotensive effect of diuretics • Risk of orthostatic hypotension • Systolic blood pressure Myocardial hypertrophy Limited efficacy of direct-acting vasodilators High prevalence of sick sinus syndrome and other atrial arrhythmias
Respiratory System	Alteration of collagen and elastin Collapse of small airways No change in total lung capacity (TLC) Ventilation-perfusion imbalance Increased • Diameter of trachea and central airways • Residual lung volume (RV) • Alveolar dead space	Decreased • Lung elasticity • Arterial saturation • Maximal oxygen uptake (VO_{2max}) Increased risk of infection

Continued

	Decreased	
	• Forced vital capacity (FVC)	
	• Expiratory flow rate	
	• Forced expiratory volume in 1 sec (FEV_1)	
	• Ratio of FEV_1 to FVC	
	• Carbon monoxide diffusion	
	• Respiratory muscle strength and endurance	
Gastrointestinal System	Pancreatic acinar atrophy	Increased
	Decreased	• Half-life of lipid-soluble drugs
	• Hepatic mass	• Constipation
	• Hepatic blood flow	
	• Microsomal enzyme activity	
	• Amplitude of esophageal contraction during peristalsis	
	• Colonic transit time	
	• Gastric acid production	
Nervous System (Including Ophthalmic and Auditory)	Decreased	Increased risk of syncope
	• Brain weight (5%–7%)	Decreased
	• Blood flow to brain (15%–20%)	• Pressure and light touch sensation
	• Number of neurons in putamen and locus ceruleus	• Olfaction
	• Purkinje cells in cerebellar cortex	
	• Pacinian and Meissner's corpuscles	
	• Binding sites for dopamine	

Table 1-1 Comparison of physiologic changes in various organ systems and their clinical implications—cont'd

	Physiologic Changes with Aging	Clinical Implications
Nervous System—cont'd	Increased lipofuscin pigment accumulation (particularly in hippocampus and frontal cortex) Altered baroreflex sensitivity Increased • Rigidity of iris • Accumulation of yellow substance in lens Decreased • Size of anterior chamber • Elasticity of lens Loss of cochlear neurons	Decreased size of pupils Alteration of color perception (e.g., blue appears green-blue) Increased risk of glaucoma Presbyopia Impaired adaptation to darkness Significant impairment of vision in presence of glare Hearing loss for pure tones (higher frequencies > lower frequencies)
Skin and Connective Tissue	Decreased • Vascularity of dermis • Epidermal turnover time • Melanocytes • Function of eccrine sweat glands • Dermis density Flattened dermoepidermal junction Cytoarchitectural disarray	Dry skin Decreased sweating response Prolonged wound healing Poor insulation Uneven tanning Hair graying (graying of axillary hair is one of most reliable signs of aging) Increased blistering

Skin and Connective Tissue—cont'd	Loss of collagen Increased glycosaminoglycans (photoaging secondary to sun exposure)	Tendency to neoplasia Wrinkled yellowed leathery skin (photoaging)
Musculoskeletal System	Decreased • Bone mass • Muscle mass • Lean body mass • Elasticity of collagen matrix of bone • Repair of microfractures • Osteoblastic activity > osteoclastic activity • Trabecular bone > cortical bone • Number of muscle fibers • Intervertebral disk space • Joint space in trunk and extremities • Compliance of chest wall Flattening of arch of feet	Osteoporosis Decreased muscle strength Loss of height Increased • Curvature of spine • Muscular work for breathing Gait impairment
Renal and Urologic System	Decreased • Renal mass • GFR • Renal tubular secretion and concentrating ability • Exchangeable potassium • Bladder capacity	Decreased drug clearance (e.g., digoxin, pro-cainamide, quinidine) Facilitation of incontinence Decreased creatinine clearance (8 ml/min/1.73 m^2/decade after 30 yr of age) Decreased renal blood flow Decreased maximum urine osmolality

Continued

Table 1-1 Comparison of physiologic changes in various organ systems and their clinical implications—cont'd

	Physiologic Changes with Aging	Clinical Implications
Renal and Urologic System—cont'd	Increased • Bladder residual volume • Uninhibited bladder contractions • Nocturnal sodium and fluid excretion	
Endocrine System	Increased • Norepinephrine levels • Vasopressin secretion • Insulin and pancreatic polypeptide • Atrial natriuretic peptide • Parathormone Decreased • Plasma renin activity • Aldosterone concentration • Growth hormone response to GHRH • Metabolism of thyroxine • Conversion of thyroxine to triiodothyronine • Secretion of estrogens, androgens, and androgen precursors Resistance to insulin-stimulated glucose uptake	Impaired • Extracellular volume regulation • Sodium homeostasis • Glucose tolerance Impaired • Response to catecholamine stimulation
Reproductive System	Decreased • Vaginal secretions • Estrogen levels	Increased susceptibility to urinary tract infections Alteration in vaginal flora

Reproductive System—cont'd	• Bactericidal prostatic secretions Increased • Vaginal pH • Chromosomal abnormalities in germ cells • Prostatic hypertrophy	Impaired micturition
Hematopoietic System	Increased • Marrow fat • RBC mass in females (secondary to end of menstrual loss) Decreased amount of active bone marrow	Decreased functional reserve for hematopoiesis
Immune System	Involution of thymus • Decreased number of newly formed T lymphocytes • Decreased capability of T lymphocytes to proliferate in response to mitogens or antigens Increased helper T lymphocytes (OKT4) Decreased • Suppressor T lymphocytes (OKT5, OKT8) • Secretion of interleukin-2 • Humoral immunity (decreased antibody response to new antigens)	Anergy to various skin tests Inadequate response to extrinsic antigens (e.g., pneumococcal vaccine) Decreased killing of intracellular pathogens by microphages Decreased T-cell function Decreased antibody response

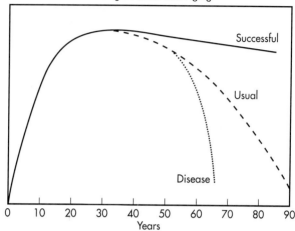

Figure 1-1
Successful and usual patterns of normal aging. Incremental growth (physiologic, functional, or reserve capacities) peaks at age 30; thereafter, there is a variable decline with successful aging showing minimal decrements. (From Yoshikawa TT, Cobbs EL, Brummel-Smith K, editors: *Ambulatory geriatric care,* St Louis, 1993, Mosby, p 171.)

in older persons appears to be weight gain rather than a true age-related increase in percentage body fat. Previous studies suggesting a marked increase in percentage body fat with advancing age did not correct for the presence of an increased body mass index that commonly occurs in middle age[2]

    (4) Plasma volume increases, interstitial volume decreases

    (5) Height decreases

  d. Selected age-related laboratory variations are described in Table 1-2

3. Theories on aging

  a. The search for the most likely causes of biologic aging has resulted in the following theories

    (1) **Free radical:** free radicals (obtained primarily via metabolism of oxygen) damage cellular protein, DNA, and enzymes, resulting in altered cellular metabolism and accumulation of lipofuscin and other substances. Senescence is caused by the accumulation of irreversible damage. Use of antioxidants such as vitamins E and C may be effective in limiting damage from free radicals and extending life

    (2) **Error and somatic mutation:** somatic mutations and errors in DNA and/or RNA synthesis result in abnormal protein synthesis and impaired cellular function. As people age, environmental exposure results in a progressive increase of destructive mutations

Table 1-2   Selected age-related laboratory variations

Laboratory Test	Age-Associated Change
TSH T3 Vasopressin FBS	? Increased
FSH LH PTH Aldosterone Androgens Angiotensin II	Decreased
WBC Hemoglobin/hematocrit MCV Platelets Free thyroxine index Calcium BUN Cortisol GH	No significant change

(3) **Wear and tear:** inability to continuously repair damage to crucial cellular components (e.g., DNA) results in declining cellular function and subsequent tissue destruction

(4) **Pacemaker:** life span patterns are specific for each animal species. Limitations on cell replication in various organs or organ systems result in cellular damage and death

(5) **Immunologic:** with increasing age, reduction occurs in immune system function and recognition of one's own cells. Aging results from active self-destruction mediated by the immune system

b. Each theory has its merits; unfortunately, no one theory accounts for all observed phenomena

c. It is important to note that life-style factors such as lack of exercise, smoking, alcohol, inadequate diet, and obesity can significantly affect the functional decline of older people (Figure 1-2)

References

1. Walsh J: Successful aging. In Yoshikawa TT, Cobbs EL, Brummel-Smith K: *Ambulatory geriatric care,* St Louis, 1993, Mosby.
2. Silver AJ et al: Effect of aging on body fat, *J Am Geriatr Soc* 41:211-213, 1993.

1.2   **EPIDEMIOLOGY AND DEMOGRAPHICS**[1]
Fred F. Ferri, MD

1. **Definitions**
   a. **Squaring of the pyramid:** term used to describe the changing de-

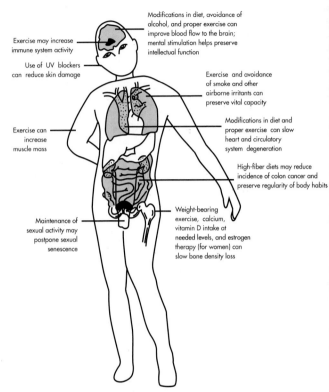

Figure 1-2
Life-style factors can affect aging process. (From Christiansen JL, Grzybowski JM, editors: *Biology of aging,* St Louis, 1993, Mosby.)

mography of the U.S. population. It refers to the increasing percentage of elderly coupled with the proportional decrease of the younger population
  b. **Age-dependency ratio:** ratio of elderly persons to remainder of population who are likely to be employed. It is currently 1:6 and considered high compared to other countries
2. **Sex**
  a. Elderly females outnumber elderly males 1.5:1 overall, 3:1 for those age 95 and over
3. **Race**
  a. Eighty-nine percent of U.S. elderly are Caucasian, 8% African-American, and 3% other races
  b. The proportion of non-Caucasians is increasing
  c. Caucasians outlive African-Americans by an average of 7 years

4. **Education**
   a. Fifty-five percent of elderly have completed high school, 10% have completed college
5. **Living arrangements**
   a. Nursing home residents account for 5% of the elderly (over 65) population
   b. Advanced age is associated with increased chance of residing in institutions. Only 1% of persons aged 65 to 74 reside in long-term–care institutions compared to over 20% of those aged 85 or older
   c. For every disabled elderly person residing in a nursing home there are two others in the community requiring equal levels of assistance
   d. Sixty-seven percent of the elderly live in a family setting (80% of males and 55% of females)
   e. Forty percent of females live alone, compared to only 15% of males
   f. Eighty percent of home owners do not have a mortgage on their home
6. **Marital status**
   a. Widows outnumber widowers 5:1
   b. Fifty-two percent of older females are widows
   c. Males over 65 are twice as likely to be married compared to females of the same age-group (80% vs. 40%)
7. **Employment**
   a. Twelve percent of elderly continue to work (18% of males and 8% of females)
   b. Twenty-five percent are self-employed compared to 10% of the population
8. **Health dollar expenditure**
   a. The elderly represent 12% of the population yet account for 32% of the total health care expenditure
   b. Twenty percent of the elderly account for 80% of the older population expenditure
   c. Most elderly spend the bulk of their lifetime expenditures during the final 5 years of life
9. **Elderly abuse**
   a. Four percent of the nation's elderly (1 million persons) are victims of abuse or neglect
   b. Only 15% of elder abuse comes to the attention of authorities
   c. Family members or significant caretakers are the most frequent perpetrators of abuse
10. **Mortality**
    a. The major cause of death (45%) in the elderly is cardiovascular disease. Its incidence is declining
    b. Malignant neoplasms represent the second most common cause of death (20%). The incidence of neoplasms has slightly increased
    c. Cardiovascular disease (stroke) is the third leading cause of death. Mortality for strokes has declined
    d. Chronic obstructive pulmonary disease represents the fourth leading cause of death between ages 55 and 74, whereas pneumonia is the fourth leading cause in patients over age 75
    e. Other major causes of death are accidents and diabetes. Mortality from these has declined

Table 1-3   Leading causes of death in United States

Rank	Age 55-74		Age 75+	
	Male	Female	Male	Female
1	Heart disease	Cancer	Heart disease	Heart disease
2	Cancer	Heart disease	Cancer	Cancer
3	COPD	Cerebrovascular disease	Cerebrovascular disease	Cerebrovascular disease
4	Cerebrovascular disease	COPD	Pneumonia, influenza	Pneumonia, influenza
5	Accidents	Diabetes	COPD	Arteriosclerosis

From Silverberg E, Lubera JA: CA 39(1):9, 1989.

Table 1-4   Major causes of morbidity in the elderly

Rank	Chronic Condition	Approximate Frequency in 65+ Age-Group (%)
1	Arthritis	55
2	Hypertension	45
3	Hearing impairment	40
4	Heart disease	35
5	Visual impairment	25

   f. Overall mortality is decreasing in the United States. More individuals are surviving to advanced age; however, the maximum life expectancy has changed little
   g. The five leading causes of death by age-group and sex are described in Table 1-3
11. **Morbidity**
   a. The major causes of morbidity are described in Table 1-4

References

1. Bock JC: *Geriatric review syllabus,* New York, 1991, American Geriatric Society.

    LIFE EXPECTANCY
      Tom J. Wachtel, MD

1. Definitions and concepts
   a. Life expectancy is defined as the average length of life expected for a population of individuals of a given age. Life expectancy, not otherwise specified, is calculated from birth. Age-specific life expectancy is calculated for a group of individuals of a specific age
   b. U.S. life expectancies based on the 1990 census are presented in Table 1-5
   c. The calculation of life expectancy is based on the age configuration of the population at the time that a census is taken; therefore life expectancies are calculated as though an individual were able to live every year of his or her life in the present year. This, of course, is not true; the younger a person is, the more likely to benefit from advances in community health and medical progress or be penalized by epidemics of new diseases (e.g., AIDS) or other social calamities such as war
   d. As people age, the differences between women and men or between African-Americans and Caucasians attenuate so that little difference in life expectancy remains at age 85
   e. Maximum life span is defined as the length of the longest-lived members of a species. The longest recorded human life is 117 years (a French woman). Current research suggests that average human life span in the absence of premature death from disease or trauma approximates 85 years with a standard deviation of 4 to 5 years

Table 1-5 Life expectancy by race, sex, and age: 1991

Age in 1990 (yr)	Caucasian		African-American	
	Male	Female	Male	Female
At birth	72.7	79.4	64.5	73.6
20	54.0	60.3	46.7	55.3
40	35.6	41.0	30.1	36.8
50	26.7	31.6	22.5	22.5
55	22.5	27.2	19.0	24.2
60	18.7	23.0	15.9	20.5
65	15.2	19.1	13.2	17.2
70	12.1	15.4	10.7	14.1
75	9.4	12.0	8.6	11.2
80	7.1	9.0	6.7	8.6
85 and over	5.2	6.4	5.0	6.3

   f. Life span is species specific and is believed to be genetically determined; an almost perfect correlation exists between maximum cell doublings in tissue culture for a given species and the life span for that species. Therefore it should not be surprising to find longevity running in certain families. However, the mechanism of aging (senescence) has not been identified; and although theories abound (e.g., accumulation of oxygen free radicals, growth hormone deficit), most interventions to correct them (e.g., antioxidants, growth hormone) have not been proven to be effective fountains of youth. The only promising means to increase longevity to date are food restriction (works in rats) and lowering body temperature (works in hamsters)

   g. Current thinking attributes the limit on life span to a progressive decline in organ reserve that begins for humans at age 20 to 30. Reserve function is needed to respond to lifetime stress. When reserve function has declined to about 20% above basal levels, routine daily perturbations cannot be overcome and death will occur with minor illnesses or trauma that would be trivial for vigorous individuals

2. Compression of mortality (and morbidity) and the rectangularization of the population survival curve

   a. Although human life span has not varied over the past millenary, human life expectancy has increased dramatically. For example, life expectancy from birth in the United States in 1900 was 47 years; and in 1990 it was 75.4 years. This gain can be attributed to improvement in infant mortality and primary preventive measures such as sanitation and immunization. Progress in and increased access to medical care can also take some credit for the gains in life expectancy

   b. The combination of a finite limit on life span and an increase in life expectancy results in more individuals achieving their maximum life potential of 85 ± 5 years in the population. This trend is demonstrated graphically by a narrowing bell-shaped curve of the number of deaths

that occur in the population or by the rectangularization of the population survival (Figure 1-3)
3. Future trends
   a. The rectangularization of population survival, the compression of morbidity, and the compression of senescence are predicated on the hy-

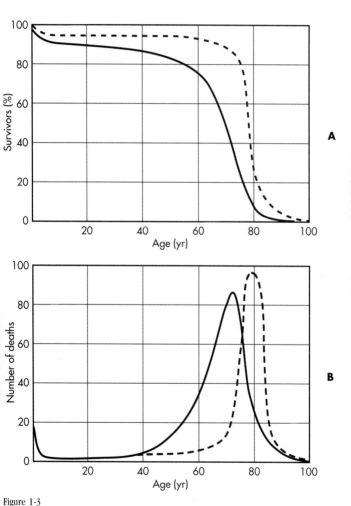

Figure 1-3
A, Proportion of survivors in the population (Y axis) by age (X axis). **B,** Number of deaths per year in each 1-year age bracket. *Solid line,* present; *dotted line,* future.

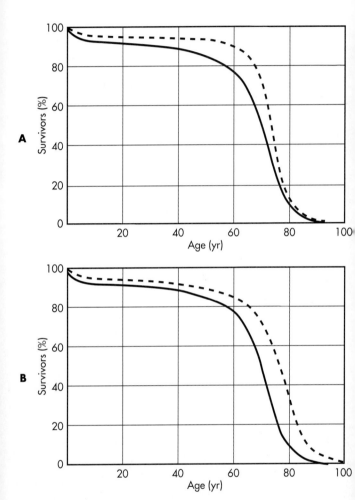

Figure 1-4
A, Rectangularization of population survival curve as a result of disease prevention
and mortality compression (*solid line:* population survival curve, circa 1970; *broken
line:* conceptual future survival curve). **B,** Prolongation of life expectancy without
mortality/morbidity compression in a model where clinical disease is not prevented
but only postponed and treated aggressively and successfully in older people (*solid
line:* population survival curve, circa 1970; *broken line:* conceptual future survival
curve).

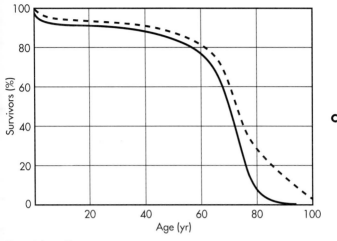

Figure 1-4, cont'd.

C, Change in a population survival curve where oldest segment of population is experiencing greatest decline in mortality (*solid line:* population survival curve, circa 1970; *broken line:* conceptual future survival curve).

pothesis of a finite limit of organ reserve (Figure 1-4, *A*). As stated by Fries, "As the organ reserve decreases so does the ability to restore homeostasis, and eventually even the smallest perturbation prevents homeostasis to be restored. The inevitable result is natural death, even without disease" or after a short acute illness (e.g., pneumonia)

b. Alternately, progress in medical technology (e.g., artificial organs) could conceivably halt the trend toward rectangularization and simply move the entire survival curve to the right (Figure 1-4, *B*)

c. The secular trend toward rectangularization of population survival curves is not inconsistent with a (transient) contemporary widening of the period of morbidity and mortality associated with recent data that indicate that the elderly citizens of our population are enjoying the greatest decline in mortality (Figure 1-4, *C*)

d. Possible reasons for the recent downturn in cardiovascular disease and related deaths can be attributed to reduced dietary saturated fat and cholesterol levels, positive developments in medical care for coronary heart disease and stroke, better treatment of hypertension, and improved access to health care for the elderly since 1965 because of the Medicare program

Suggested readings

Fries JF: Aging, natural death, and the compression of morbidity, *N Engl J Med* 303:130-135, 1980.

Fries JF: Life expectancy. Life span. In Maddox GL, editor: *The encyclopedia of aging,* New York, 1987, Springer Publishing Co.

Gibbons A: Gerontology research comes of age, *Science* 250:622-625, 1990.

Manton KG, Vaupel JW: Survival after the age of 80 in the US, Sweden, France, England and Japan, *N Engl J Med* 333:1232-1235, 1995.

Masoro EJ: Life-extension. In Maddox GL, editor: *The encyclopedia of aging,* New York, 1987, Springer Publishing Co.

Olshansky SJ, Carnes BA, Cassel C: In search of Methuselah: estimating the upper limits to human longevity, *Science* 250:634-640, 1990.

Rosenwaike I, Yaffe N, Sage PC: The recent decline in mortality of the extreme aged: an analysis of statistical data, *Am J Public Health* 70:1074-1080, 1980.

Statistical abstract of the United States, 1994. U.S. Department of Commerce, Bureau of the Census.

Wachtel TJ: The connection between health promotion and health care costs. Does it matter? *Am J Med* 94:451-454, 1993.

Comprehensive
Geriatric Assessment

Marsha D. Fretwell, MD

BACKGROUND

1. **Definition of comprehensive geriatric assessment (CGA):** comprehensive geriatric assessment is a systematic approach to the collection of patient data that allows evaluation of the patient's health status and functional impairments in multiple areas or domains
2. **Why is CGA needed?**
   a. Older patients often seek or are brought to medical attention because of a nonspecific loss in either physical or mental function
   b. Although the traditional goal of the physician is to diagnose and treat the medical illness or illnesses underlying the loss of function, regaining lost function and maintaining independence are often the primary goals of the older patient and family members
3. **Does CGA work?**
   a. Comprehensive and functionally based assessments integrate the functional and medical goals of older patients and their physicians
   b. CGA acknowledges that frail older persons are subject to multiple physical and mental diseases that interact in complex ways to complicate efforts to achieve satisfactory outcomes
   c. Comprehensive assessments that specifically address functional impairments in older patients have been shown to improve their health care outcomes (Table 2-1)

2.2 **STEPS IN COMPREHENSIVE GERIATRIC ASSESSMENT**

Like the traditional SOAP approach to organizing patient information, in CGA, one first collects the *S*ubjective and *O*bjective data base, second integrates that information into an *A*ssessment, and finally creates a care *P*lan.

Step 1. Subjective and objective data base

1. **Chief complaint.** The reason for seeking medical attention should be stated in both the older patient's and the family's or caretaker's words, when possible. It should address the specific functional losses that the

19

Table 2-1 Significant benefits of geriatric assessment programs

Type of Benefit	Form of Benefits
Process of care	New diagnoses/problems uncovered
	Reduced medications
Patient outcomes	Improved scores on functional status tests
	Improved scores on affective or cognitive function tests
	Prolonged survival
Nursing home use	Improved placement
	Reduction in mean days in nursing homes
Health care use/costs	Increased use of home health care
	Reduced use of hospital services (mean days or hospitalization rates)
	Reduced medical care costs

From Rubenstein LZ et al: *J Am Geriatr Soc* 39(suppl):85, 1991.

patient may be experiencing as well as the more traditional medical complaints
2. **Initial screen of vision, hearing, and cognition.** Before beginning, it is important that the older patient be able to see and hear the examiner, pay attention to questions, and give an accurate history. A brief check of vision (using the Rosenbaum chart while the patient wears corrective lenses [Figure 2-1]), of hearing (whispering in the patient's ear or placing a watch against the patient's ear), and of cognitive function (asking the patient to repeat the names of three objects [pencil, apple, book] after they are said and again in 3 minutes) is suggested
3. **Biomedical data**
   a. Medical diagnosis, present and past, with a statement of duration and impact on patient's physical and mental function
   b. Nutritional data, including any changes in weight and appetite
   c. Medications
      (1) Include duration of use and any adverse drug reactions
      (2) Estimate creatinine clearance to evaluate appropriate dosing
      (3) Review impact of each medication on patient's physical and mental functions, i.e., appetite, gait, mood, memory, sexual performance, constipation, and incontinence
4. **Psychologic data** (see Appendix VI for examples of functional assessment instruments)
   a. Cognitive function, including any episodes of acute confusion following medications, hospitalizations, surgery, or change in living situation
   b. Emotional function screen for depression, paranoia, anxiety, hallucinations, personality, and coping styles
   c. Perceptive function, including vision, hearing, and speech
5. **Social data**
   a. Individual social skills, including marital history, issues of physical and emotional intimacy, acceptance of help, presence of a confidante

ROSENBAUM POCKET VISION SCREENER

			distance equivalent
95			$\frac{20}{800}$
874			$\frac{20}{400}$

		Point	Jaeger	distance equivalent
2843		26	16	$\frac{20}{200}$
6 3 8 E Ш Э X O O		14	10	$\frac{20}{100}$
8 7 4 5 Э M Ш O X O		10	7	$\frac{20}{70}$
6 3 9 2 5 M E Э X O X		8	5	$\frac{20}{50}$
4 2 8 3 6 5 Ш E M O X O		6	3	$\frac{20}{40}$
3 7 4 2 5 8 Э Ш Э X X O		5	2	$\frac{20}{30}$
9 3 7 8 2 6 Ш M E X O O		4	1	$\frac{20}{25}$
4 2 8 7 3 9 E Ш M O O X		3	1+	$\frac{20}{20}$

Card is held in good light 14 inches from eye. Record vision for each eye separately with and without glasses. Presbyopic patients should read thru bifocal segment. Check myopes with glasses only.

DESIGN COURTESY J. G. ROSENBAUM, M.D.

PUPIL GAUGE (mm.)

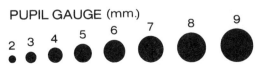

2   3   4   5   6   7   8   9

Figure 2-1

Rosenbaum chart for testing near vision. (From Ferri FF: *Practical guide to the care of the medical patient,* ed 2, St Louis, 1991, Mosby, p 16.)

      b. Family support system, including numbers and relationships between potential caretakers, use of existing community resources

      c. Values about medical treatments such as surgery, feeding tubes, ventilators, cardiopulmonary resuscitation. Document existence of prior directives such as durable power of attorney or living will

6. **Summary scales for function** (see Appendix VI for examples of functional assessment instruments)

      a. Basic activities of daily living (ADLs), such as dressing, bathing, getting out of bed, toileting, and feeding independently

      b. Instrumental ADLs, such as shopping, using transportation, management of medications and one's finances independently

7. **Physical examination**

      a. General

          (1) Routine evaluation for orthostatic changes in pulse and blood pressure

          (2) Examination of skin for malignant changes

          (3) Actual observation of gait, mobility, and balance as patient enters room and gets in and out of chair

          (4) Actual observation of patient performing the basic or instrumental ADLs

      b. Head, ears, eyes, nose, and throat

          (1) Evaluation for evidence of recent trauma or fall

          (2) Presence of cerumen in ear canals

          (3) Any focal changes in extraocular or facial muscles

          (4) Cataracts

          (5) Presence of lower lid ectropion

          (6) Thyroid nodules

          (7) Carotid bruits

          (8) Intraoral dryness or lesions

          (9) Salivary gland obstruction

      c. Upper body

          (1) Full range of motion of the arms

          (2) Full breast examination as well as routine cardiopulmonary, carotid, and peripheral vascular evaluation

      d. Abdominal, rectal, and genital examination

          (1) Evaluation for bladder or rectal prolapse

          (2) Leakage of urine

          (3) Femoral and inguinal hernias

          (4) Full range of motion of the hips

          (5) Routine palpation of abdomen

      e. Neurologic

          (1) Folstein Mini-Mental State Exam, recording the subcategories of orientation, registration of short-term memory, attention, and language

          (2) Any focal changes in muscle strength and reflexes

          (3) Balance

          (4) Vibratory sensation

8. **Laboratory evaluation**

      a. General

          (1) CBC

          (2) Electrolytes

    (3) BUN
    (4) Creatinine
    (5) Glucose
    (6) Urinalysis
    (7) Sedimentation rate
  b. Nutrition
    (1) Albumin
    (2) Cholesterol profile
  c. Cognition
    (1) Calcium
    (2) T_4 and TSH
    (3) Vitamin B_{12}
    (4) Transaminase, alkaline phosphatase
    (5) Blood levels of relevant medications

Step 2. Assessment: integrating patient data and organizing the problem list

Nine areas of concern or attributes of the older patient, if systematically reviewed in preparation of the care plan, lead to improved health outcomes and satisfaction with care. The areas of concern can be used as a problem checklist to identify areas relevant to the individual patient. Then they can be used as the goals of care and the means by which one can efficiently monitor the progress of care.

    The areas of concern have been chosen because they are the critical variables that influence health outcomes in older patients. They not only provide a comprehensive view of the complexly ill patient but also assist the physician in providing accurate prognostic information to older patients and their families.

1. **Areas of concern**
  a. Diagnosis
    (1) List diagnoses
    (2) Categorize each by severity, degree of reversibility, and impact on the function (nutrition, defecation, continence, cognition, emotion, and mobility)
  b. Medications
    (1) List all medications, including over-the-counter drugs
    (2) Categorize each by site of excretion (liver or kidney) and impact on function
    (3) Evaluate dosage; check blood levels when available
  c. Nutrition
    (1) Establish baseline for oral intake, weight, and albumin
    (2) If baseline is abnormal, list etiologic factors (diseases, medications, depression, impaction, etc.)
    (3) Categorize etiologic factors by degree of reversibility
  d. Continence
    (1) Establish baseline for accidents
    (2) If applicable, list etiologic factors (diseases, medications, change in location, impaction)
    (3) Categorize etiologic factors by degree of reversibility
  e. Defecation
    (1) Establish baseline for constipation, impaction

      (2) If applicable, list etiologic factors (diseases, medications, immobility, depression, etc.)

      (3) Categorize etiologic factors by degree of reversibility

  f. Cognition

      (1) Establish baseline for short-term memory impairment, impairment of attention (delirium), hallucinations

      (2) If applicable, list etiologic factors (disease, medications, change in location, depression, impaction, etc.)

      (3) Categorize etiologic factors by degree of reversibility

  g. Emotion

      (1) Establish baseline for anxiety, agitation, depression, failure to thrive (sleep, appetite disturbance, energy disorder)

      (2) If applicable, list etiologic factors (disease, medications, change in location, delirium, impaction, etc.)

      (3) Categorize etiologic factors by degree of reversibility

  h. Mobility

      (1) Establish baseline for dependence in bed transfers, walking within and outside house, use of transportation

      (2) If applicable, list etiologic factors (disease, medications, depression, incontinence, life-style)

      (3) Categorize etiologic factors by degree of reversibility

  i. Cooperation with care plan

      (1) Establish baseline for active or passive lack of cooperation with care plan

      (2) If applicable, list etiologic factors (inappropriate care plan, impaired caretaker, disease, medications, depression, personality disorder, etc.)

      (3) Categorize etiologic factors by degree of reversibility

  j. Advance directives

2. **Giving accurate prognosis.** This process, which focuses on both medical and functional information, provides the physician with a data base that allows formulation of accurate prognostic statements for the patient and family. This in turn allows patients and families to participate meaningfully in making decisions about medical care

Step 3. Care plan: reconciliation between standards of medical practice and patient preference

1. Reconciliation between the existing or usual standards of medical practice and those that each older patient prefers for treatment is the most critical step in creating an appropriate and successful care plan for older patients

2. Within each area of concern, assess and identify reversible or potentially treatable etiologic factors

3. Make treatment recommendations consistent with the standard of medical practice for each problem listed in the areas of concern

4. Reconcile or check the recommendation against the patient's preference for treatment. Any older patients may request no surgery, no feeding tubes, no nursing home placement, no chemotherapy, for example, but it is important to consider individual preferences in each area of concern

Table 2-2   Outcomes of care checklist

Areas of Concern	Evaluation
1. Diagnosis 2. Medications	Are diagnoses accurate and treatments appropriate?
3. Nutrition 4. Continence 5. Defecation	Are intake and output appropriate?
6. Cognition 7. Emotion 8. Mobility	How is patient thinking, feeling, and doing?
9. Cooperation with care plan	Are all persons involved working together?

5. Once recommendations have been reconciled with the patient preferences, patient and physician have common goals and treatment can proceed

Step 4. Checklist: monitoring outcomes of care

1. The nine areas of concern (Table 2-2) offer a comprehensive and convenient checklist by which the physician can monitor
   a. Outcomes of care plan recommendations
   b. Reevaluation of the patient's current medical and functional status
   c. Creation of up-to-date care plans that reflect new findings
2. Performance of the CGA provides a systematic approach to patient care and a framework for ongoing and objective inquiry into the human characteristics and behaviors influencing health outcomes
3. By applying a comprehensive assessment, the multiple, complex biopsychosocial variables become predictable patterns rather than isolated events
4. By focusing the care plan on everyday functions that are so important to older patients and their families, greater patient and physician satisfaction with care is achieved

Suggested readings

Applegate WB, Blass JP, Williams TF: Instruments for the functional assessment of older patients, *N Engl J Med* 322:1207, 1990.
Fretwell MD: Comprehensive functional assessment. In Abrams WB, Berkow R, editors: *The Merck manual of geriatrics,* Rahway, NJ, 1990, Merck Sharp & Dohme.
Lachs MS et al: A simple procedure for general screening for functional disability in elderly patients, *Ann Intern Med* 112:699, 1990.
Sui AL, Reuben DB, Moore AA: Comprehensive geriatric assessment. In Hassard WR et al: *Principles of geriatric medicine and gerontology,* New York, 1994, McGraw-Hill.

Health Maintenance in the Elderly

PREVENTIVE MEDICINE AND HEALTH MAINTENANCE
Tom J. Wachtel, MD

Definition

Prevention refers to measures taken to avoid or postpone the occurrence of diseases and their complications.

1. Primary prevention: avoid or postpone occurrence of disease
2. Secondary prevention: early detection (e.g., screening) of disease to enhance the treatment outcomes
3. Tertiary prevention: treatment of chronic conditions (e.g., hypertension, diabetes mellitus, hyperlipidemia) to avoid or postpone complications
4. The impact of preventive health measures should be judged by their effect on health status (quality or quantity of life) not by the potential to save health care costs because life prolongation may actually come with a price tag rather than savings. Nevertheless, if a limit of human life span exists, a strategy of postponement may lead to actual prevention (and cost savings), with people dying of "old age" without ever being ill or disabled (see Chapter 1). Much of the progress in life expectancy achieved for humanity during the twentieth century can be attributed to community health interventions. The practicing physician also can provide substantial benefits to patients

Primary prevention

1. Cardiovascular disease prevention
   a. Smoking cessation
   b. Reduction of serum cholesterol (also tertiary prevention)
   c. Treatment of hypertension (also tertiary prevention)
   d. Exercise (aerobic)
   e. Maintenance of ideal body weight
   f. Prophylactic low-dose aspirin
   g. Postmenopausal estrogen replacement therapy
   h. Stress management or reduction
2. Cancer prevention
   a. Smoking cessation

    b. Avoidance of occupational and environmental exposures (e.g., asbestos, radon, benzene)

    c. Avoidance of sun exposure

    d. Diet (high fiber, low fat)

    e. Certain cancer screening programs may provide primary prevention (e.g., detection and treatment of premalignant cervical conditions or colon polyps)

3. Injury prevention

    a. Alcohol avoidance

    b. Seat belt use

    c. Motorcycle and bicycle helmet use

    d. Occupational and home safety enhancing actions (see Chapter 8)

    e. Fall prevention in the elderly

    f. Firearm avoidance and gun legislation and enforcement

    g. Domestic violence education and legislation and enforcement

4. Chronic lung disease prevention: smoking cessation

5. Osteoporosis prevention

    a. Dietary calcium

    b. Calcium supplements (1500 mg calcium per day in postmenopausal women)

    c. Weight-bearing exercise (resistive not aerobic)

    d. Postmenopausal estrogen replacement therapy

       (1) Posthysterectomy patients: Premarin 0.625 mg qd

       (2) Intact uterus patients: Premarin 0.625 mg qd and Provera 2.5 mg qd to prevent endometrial cancer risk increased by unopposed estrogen

6. Infectious disease prevention

    a. Safer sex

    b. Immunizations

       (1) Routine immunization in adults

          (a) Tetanus

             • Primary—tetanus toxoid, 0.5 ml three times (first and second 1 to 2 months apart, third 6 to 12 months later)

             • Booster every 10 years or at 65 years and stop

          (b) Influenza: annual for adults over age 65, especially important in people with high-risk conditions (e.g., diabetes mellitus, chronic lung disease)

          (c) Pneumococcal polysaccharide, 0.5 ml once; same indications as influenza

             • NOTE: Vaccinate those whose previous vaccination status is unknown

             • Booster every 10 years

       (2) Special recommendations for travelers: travel plan dependent; check with experts

    c. Tuberculosis

       (1) Purified protein derivative (PPD)

          (a) Yearly for institutionalized elderly, alcoholics, recent immigrants from high-prevalence countries

          (b) Every 3 to 5 years for general population

(c) Close contacts of infectious TB cases who share the same
household or other enclosed environment

A skin test reaction to tuberculin can be detected 2 to 10 weeks after the
initial infection and persists indefinitely unless anergy develops. The
Mantoux test rather than a multiple puncture test should be used for PPD
testing. The Mantoux test is performed by injecting 0.1 ml of PPD
tuberculin containing 5 tuberculin units (TU) intradermally on the forearm. The injection should be made just beneath the surface of the skin,
with the needle level facing upward to produce a discrete wheal. The test
should be ready for evaluation 48 to 72 hours later, but positive reactions
may be read up to 1 week after testing. The diameter of induration (not
erythema) should be measured transversely to the long axis of the forearm. The result should be recorded as the number of millimeters of
induration and not simply as positive or negative. Control skin test
antigens may be used to test for anergy in patients with immunosuppressive disorders.

1. The classification of tuberculin skin test results depends on the group
   being tested. The CDC has adopted the following classification system
   a. A tuberculin reaction >5 mm is classified as positive in the following
      groups
      (1) Persons who have had recent close contact with a patient with
          infectious tuberculosis
      (2) Persons who have chest radiographs with fibrotic lesions likely to
          represent old healed tuberculosis
   b. A tuberculin reaction ≥10 mm is classified as positive in persons who
      do not meet the above criteria but have other risk factors for tubercu-
      losis
      (1) Persons with medical risk factors
      (2) Foreign-born persons from high-prevalence areas
      (3) Medically underserved, low-income populations, including high-
          risk minorities
   c. A tuberculin reaction ≥15 mm is classified as positive in all other
      persons
2. **All persons with a positive PPD test result should have a chest x-ray
   study to evaluate for active tuberculosis before considering preventive therapy**
3. Beware
   a. A negative tuberculin skin test result does not rule out the diagnosis
      of tuberculosis or tuberculous infection
   b. There is a common misconception that the "booster phenomenon"
      indicates a false-positive tuberculin test result caused by sensitiza-
      tion from repeated tuberculin testing. In fact, repeated tuberculin
      testing of uninfected persons does not sensitize to tuberculin, and
      a positive test result "caused by" the booster phenomenon is truly
      positive. In two-step testing (recommended for elderly debilitated
      persons), a second PPD test is placed 1 week after a first negative
      test result
   c. Positive tuberculin reactions in bacille Calmette-Guérin (BCG)–
      vaccinated persons usually indicate true infection with *Mycobacterium
      tuberculosis*

PREVENTIVE THERAPY

The goal of preventive therapy is to reduce the risk of developing active tuberculosis in persons who are infected. In considering a course of preventive therapy, one must weigh the known efficacy of this treatment against the toxicity of the medication isoniazid (INH), 300 mg per day, the drug of choice. Because the risk of drug-induced hepatitis increases with age, chemoprophylaxis in the elderly is recommended only in the following groups

- Recent skin conversion
- Recent contact with infectious person
- Abnormal chest x-ray consistent with past TB
- Diabetes
- Long-term corticosteroid therapy

Twelve months of continuous preventive therapy is recommended for persons with stable abnormal chest radiographs consistent with past tuberculosis. Other groups should receive a minimum of 6 continuous months of preventive therapy. Isoniazid can be given twice weekly in a dose of 15 mg/kg (up to 900 mg) when therapy must be directly observed and resources are inadequate for daily observed therapy.

Persons receiving preventive therapy should be monitored for

- Symptoms of neurotoxicity such as paresthesias of the hand and feet (high risk: persons with diabetes, alcoholism); pyridoxine (50 mg/day) reduces the incidence
- Signs consistent with hepatitis such as anorexia, nausea, vomiting, dark urine, jaundice, unexplained fever, right upper quadrant tenderness
- Abnormalities of liver transaminases (10% to 20%), with higher risk for hepatotoxicity occurring among persons older than 35 years; if the ALT level is greater than three to five times the upper limit of normal, preventive therapy should be reconsidered
- The emergence of multidrug–resistant TB is leading to new chemoprophylaxis regimens (e.g., rifampin). Please keep informed.

Persons with positive PPDs who do not receive chemoprophylaxis or who cannot complete a full course of it should have a chest x-ray every 1 to 2 years.

Secondary prevention

1. Cancer
   a. Cervical cancer: Pap smear every 1 to 3 years. Controversial in low-risk women over 65 previously screened or over 75 not previously screened. However, a pelvic exam should still be performed after those age thresholds to screen for endometrial and ovarian cancer. Not doing a Pap smear as part of a routine pelvic exam is difficult to justify except on the basis of its cost
   b. Breast cancer: breast self-examination, monthly after menses; annual breast examination by physician after age 40 years; mammography (see Chapter 6) every 1 to 2 years after age 40
   c. Colorectal cancer
      (1) Rectal examination yearly in all adults after age 40
      (2) Testing for fecal occult blood yearly (three pairs of specimens) or during rectal exam in all adults after age 50 and in high-risk persons (i.e., family history of adenocarcinomas, inflammatory bowel disease, or history of colorectal polyps) after age 40

(3) Endoscopy (sigmoidoscopy or colonoscopy) or double air contrast barium enema study in all adults after age 50 (every 5 years) or preferentially in high-risk adults

d. Lung cancer: chest x-ray study and sputum cytology have marginal effectiveness even in high-risk people (e.g., smokers, asbestos exposure)

e. Endometrial cancer: use of endometrial biopsy is controversial without symptoms

f. Prostate cancer: annual digital rectal exam in men over 40 years; prostate-specific antigen (PSA) (recommended by the American Cancer Society) annually between ages 50 and 70 (see Chapter 6)

g. Urologic cancers (renal cell and transitional): urinalysis for blood and urinary cytology not proved effective

h. Ovarian cancer: annual pelvic exam after age 40, Ca 1-25 antigen not proved effective

i. Testicular
   (1) Monthly self-examination
   (2) Tumor markers (HCG, alpha-fetoprotein) not indicated for screening

j. Hepatoma: alpha-fetoprotein not proven effective but may be considered in patient with chronic active hepatitis B infection, cirrhosis, or hemochromatosis

k. Skin cancer: monthly skin self-examination with special attention to pigmented lesions

l. All other cancers: physical examination with special attention to nasopharyngeal region, thyroid, liver, spleen, pelvic and genital organs, lymph node areas, and skin

2. Total cholesterol every 3 to 5 years

3. Routine use of blood chemistries, CBC, and urinalysis: no specific indication; usual recommendation—one baseline set of CBC, urinalysis, fasting blood glucose, bun, creatinine, calcium, AST, alkaline, phosphatase, total T_4

4. Baseline ECG (give copy to patient to help decision making in an emergency care setting in the event of chest pain)

5. Blood pressure measurement every 3 years before age 40 and yearly thereafter

6. Visual acuity and glaucoma screening every 1 to 3 years after age 50

7. Hearing evaluation every 3 years after age 50

8. Physical and mental function (cognitive and affective) assessment as needed in geriatric patients

Tertiary prevention

The treatment of many chronic illnesses often has tertiary prevention as the single therapeutic goal (e.g., management of hypercholesterolemia) or as an added benefit to symptom relief (e.g., management of heart failure with ACE inhibitors).

Prevention implementation

1. Add "Health maintenance" to the problem list in the medical record
2. Use a prevention flowchart (Figure 3-1). Without a flowchart (paper or

RHODE ISLAND HOSPITAL
Health Maintenance - Flow Sheet MPCU

Date:																	
Assessment																	
Height	× 1																
Weight	q visit																
Blood pressure	q visit																
Pulse	q visit																
Exams																	
Breast self-exam	q month																
Pelvic exam	q 1–3 years																
Digital rectal exam	q year after 40																
Visual acuity	q year																
Hearing assessment	q year																
Testicular self-exam																	
Intraocular pressure (over 65)	q year																
Dental exam by dentist	q year																
Health Risk (Yes or No)																	
Smoking																	
Alcohol/drugs																	
Seat belts																	
Safe sex																	
Exercise																	
Diet																	

Figure 3-1
Health maintenance flowchart for the medical record.   *Continued*

computerized) compliance within health maintenance schedules is unlikely
3. Physician reminders
4. Patient reminders (by mail)
5. Educate patients so they request preventive services when they are
   due

Laboratory

Stool guaiac	q year after 40												
Pap smear	q 3 years												
Mammography q 1-2 yrs after 40													
Cholesterol	q 3-5 yrs												

Immunization-check if up to date

Flu vaccine	(over 65) q year												
Pneumovax	(over 65) × 1												
Tetanus booster	q 10 years												

Figure 3-1, cont'd.

Suggested readings

Eddy DM, editor: *Common screening tests,* Philadelphia, 1991, American College of Physicians.

Gardner P, Schaffner W: Immunization of adults, *N Engl J Med* 328:1252-1258, 1993.

Hayward RSA et al: Preventive care guidelines: 1991, *Ann Intern Med* 114:758-783, 1991.

Manson JE et al: The primary prevention of myocardial infarction, *N Engl J Med* 326:1406-1416, 1992.

Preventive Services Task Force: *Guide to clinical preventive services: report of the US Preventive Services Task Force,* Baltimore, 1989, Williams & Wilkins.

Riggs BL, Melton LJ: The prevention and treatment of osteoporosis, *N Engl J Med* 327:620-627, 1992.

Sox HC Jr: Preventive health services in adults, *N Engl J Med* 330:1589-1595, 1994.

3.2   PREOPERATIVE MEDICAL CONSULTATION
Dominick Tammaro, MD

Goals of the consultant

1. Identify medical conditions that place the patient at high risk for perioperative morbidity and mortality
2. Recommend and, if necessary, implement measures aimed at reducing the risks of medical morbidity and mortality

3. Monitor the patient's condition while hospitalized, along with surgical colleagues, to respond to and treat medical morbid events as they occur
4. The consultant should
   a. Have a clear idea of the questions posed by the surgeons
   b. Be focused and specific in the recommendations made
   c. Be concise and clear
   d. Keep the surgeon fully informed of your assessment and recommendations; this is especially true if your recommendations will delay or cancel plans for surgery
   e. Not attempt to direct decisions that are the responsibility of the anesthesiologist or surgeon, such as type of anesthetic agents or surgical approach

General epidemiology

Cardiac and pulmonary adverse events comprise the bulk of perioperative complications. Approximately 50% of postoperative deaths are due to pulmonary complications. Of these complications, atelectasis and pneumonia are most common, followed by respiratory failure and prolonged ventilatory dependence.

Age as a risk factor for surgery

Several studies have indicated that a higher rate of perioperative mortality exists in the elderly population although the exact basis for that increased risk remains controversial and is likely multifactorial. In 1977 Goldman[1] identified age as a predictor of cardiac morbidity and mortality in the perioperative period. Some authors have suggested that age greater than 60 years predicts a fourfold to fivefold increase in perioperative mortality over younger patients, with even higher risk in emergency situations.

   The cause of the increased surgical risk in elderly patients is not clear. There are physiologic changes that limit the ability to increase cardiac output under stress such as hypotension or fever. In addition, a well-described decline in vital capacity begins before age 60 and is accelerated by smoking. Airways are less elastic and may undergo premature closure, resulting in air trapping. Glomerular filtration declines with age, and the kidney is less able to respond to a salt or volume load accordingly. Elderly patients may be more prone to deep venous thrombosis (DVT) and may have longer periods of postoperative immobilization. Last, elderly patients have high rates of comorbid disease that may have a significant bearing on perioperative morbidity and mortality. This last factor makes it difficult to identify whether age is an independent predictor of risk or rather a marker for other independent variables.

   Once it is determined that a surgical procedure will be of benefit to an elderly patient, steps can be taken to minimize perioperative risk. The status of comorbid diseases should be optimized in the preoperative period, especially with respect to volume status and cardiac and pulmonary diseases. Emergency operations carry a higher risk than routine, elective procedures; therefore the timing of surgery may present an easily modifiable risk factor. Every effort should be made to plan routine operations at a time when the condition in question (e.g., inguinal hernia, cholelithiasis) is relatively stable.

Pulmonary Considerations

WHAT ARE THE MAJOR PULMONARY RISK FACTORS?

1. **COPD:** the most important pulmonary determinant of perioperative pulmonary risk is **airway flow rate.** Obstructive lung disease is therefore the major risk factor for perioperative pulmonary complications. A definite risk exists if the patient has evidence of bronchospasm on exam. Other measures to assess pulmonary risk are based on pulmonary function testing
   a. FEV > 2 L: low risk
      FEV 1 to 2 L: moderate risk
      FEV < 1 L: high risk
   b. FEV_1/FVC < 75%: increased risk
   c. Postoperative FEV can decrease by 60% after upper abdominal or thoracic surgery. If postoperative predicted FEV < 1 L, high risk
   d. MVV < 50% predicts increased risk
2. **Smoking:** increased risk of postoperative atelectasis, twofold increased risk of postoperative pneumonia
3. **Site:** upper abdominal and thoracic surgery increases risk of postoperative pneumonia tenfold
4. **Age >60:** independent risk factor or may be due to normal decreased FEV_1 with aging
5. **Obesity:** moderate obesity poses no increased surgical risk. Massive obesity or weight more than 250 lb is associated with increased surgical mortality; it causes decreased chest wall compliance because of increased intraabdominal resistance resulting in increased atelectasis risk and work of breathing. Increased gastric residual volume may lead to aspiration
6. **Duration of anesthesia >3 hours:** a risk because of prolonged effects on ciliary clearance
7. **Type of anesthesia:** spinal anesthesia can pose as great a risk for pulmonary complications of surgery as can general anesthesia
8. **Upper respiratory infections:** can increase risk of perioperative pneumonia and hypoxia because of increase in sputum production and decreased ciliary clearance

WHO SHOULD HAVE PREOPERATIVE PULMONARY FUNCTION TESTS?

1. All upper abdominal and thoracic surgery patients if risks are present
2. Patients with respiratory symptoms
3. Long-standing smokers, even without symptoms
4. Patients with a history of COPD
5. Elderly patients
6. Patients undergoing pulmonary resection

Indications for preoperative arterial blood gas sampling are roughly same as for pulmonary function tests. If there is no suspicion of CO_2 retention, however, hypoxia can easily be excluded by pulse oximetry.

INTERVENTIONS TO REDUCE PULMONARY RISK

Ideally the consultant will have enough time before the surgery is planned to recommend or implement interventions designed to minimize perioperative pulmonary risk. These interventions are aimed at increasing airway flow rates.

1. Patient should stop smoking 2 months before surgery (cessation at least 1 week preoperatively has been shown to confer some benefit)
2. If the patient is wheezing on exam or if airway flow rates improve by at least 15% on pulmonary function tests with bronchodilator therapy, begin treatment with theophylline or inhaled bronchodilators
3. Eliminate purulent sputum with antibiotic therapy and consider a short course of steroid therapy
4. Although not shown to provide a statistically significant benefit when ordered preoperatively, incentive spirometry in high-risk patients or for high-risk surgery may be of benefit in selected patients during the postoperative period. Patient education on the use of postoperative incentive spirometry should be carried out in the preoperative period
5. Weight loss for obese patients
6. Treatment of congestive heart failure

Cardiac risk factor assessment

Coronary artery disease (CAD), congestive heart failure, and arrhythmias are the leading causes of perioperative cardiac morbidity and mortality. Of the 27 million patients who undergo surgery each year in the United States, 8 million have CAD or risk factors for CAD and 1 million have perioperative complications related to cardiac disease. The consultant must identify patients at high risk for cardiac complications in the perioperative period and attempt to minimize that risk.

1. **Recent myocardial infarction** (<3 months) increases the risk of perioperative MI by over 30%. This risk declines to and remains at about 5% 6 months after MI. Recent MI is one of the most important predictors of perioperative cardiac morbidity and mortality. Unstable angina or new ischemic ECG changes are also of concern and warrant evaluation and treatment preoperatively. The following guidelines can be applied
   a. Patients who have had an MI less than 6 months before an elective surgical procedure should have the procedure delayed. Note that "elective" can be a relative term, such as when applied to a colectomy for colon cancer; therefore some judgment must be exercised in recommending a specific postponement
   b. ECG: patients with documented or suspected CAD should have a preoperative ECG and follow-up ECGs on the second and third postoperative day
   c. Exercise stress testing: patients with suspected active CAD should have preoperative exercise stress testing although its value in this setting is still unclear
   d. Echo: Preoperative clinical evidence of LV dysfunction, valvular heart disease, and prior MI are predictive of an increased risk of adverse cardiac events in patients undergoing surgical procedures. There are no "hard" data that use of echo as a preoperative screening tool adds any benefit to outcome. The echo should be used for the same indications in preoperative patients as in nonpreoperative patients; that is, it should be used to quantify valvular function in a patient with a new or suspicious murmur or to evaluate the cause of CHF. Since these

situations may affect the outcome of surgery, it may be necessary to delay the procedure until data are obtained. Recent data support the value of finding a new wall-motion abnormality by stress echo or dobutamine echo as a predictor of adverse cardiac events

e. Dipyridamole thallium stress testing is very sensitive (89% to 100%) and reasonably specific (53% to 80%) in predicting adverse cardiac events, especially in patients who will have vascular surgery procedures. Specificity can be increased by application of this modality to the subgroup of patients with coronary risk factors. This type of testing in unselected patients may not be helpful or cost effective

2. **Congestive heart failure (CHF)** is a risk factor for perioperative pulmonary edema. Patients with no history of CHF have a risk of about 2% to 6% of this complication in the perioperative period compared to 6% in patients with a history of CHF and 30% in patients actually in CHF preoperatively. The two periods of greatest risk for CHF in the postoperative period are immediately after surgery (after fluid administration while the myocardial depressant effects of anesthetic agents are still observed) and about 48 hours postoperatively (when third-space fluids are mobilized)

   a. Patients who have an S3 gallop or jugular venous distention and have mild to moderate symptoms should be treated to resolve CHF before surgery

   b. Patients with severe LV dysfunction and clinically uncompensated CHF may benefit from intraoperative Swan-Ganz catheter monitoring of pulmonary capillary wedge pressure

3. **Valvular heart disease** raises the risk of postoperative pulmonary edema. Patients with severe aortic stenosis are at greatest risk and have a fourteenfold greater incidence of cardiac death in the postoperative period. In addition, SBE prophylaxis may be indicated

4. **Hypertension** with a diastolic blood pressure less than 110 mm Hg does not confer additional perioperative risk to the surgical patient. Antihypertensive medications should be continued until surgery and then converted to a parenteral form if the patient will be unable to take oral medications

5. **Arrhythmias** should be approached in a manner similar to nonsurgical patients

   Table 3-1 summarizes the major cardiac risk factors. Figure 3-2 displays an algorithm for assessing patients with cardiac disease.

DVT prophylaxis

DVT prophylaxis is a common problem for the consultant. Patient-related risk factors include

- Age <40
- Predisposition to clotting, e.g., hypercoagulable state
- Prior history of DVT
- Medical conditions predisposing to venous stasis (RV failure, pregnancy)
- Estrogen?

Surgical risk factors include

- Duration of surgery, especially >30 minutes
- Postoperative immobilization

Table 3-1 Cardiac risk factors

Factor	Risk
Coronary artery disease	
Myocardial infarction within 6 mo	xx
Myocardial infarction more than 6 mo ago	x
Disabling angina	xxx
Unstable angina within 6 mo	xx
Alveolar pulmonary edema	
Within 1 wk	xx
Ever	x
Valvular disease	
Suspected critical aortic stenosis	xxx
Arrhythmias	
Rhythm other than sinus or sinus plus APBs* on last preoperative ECG	x
More than five premature ventricular contractions at any time before surgery	x
Poor general medical status	x
Age >70 yr	x
Emergency operation	xx

x, Slight ↑ risk; *xx*, moderate ↑ risk; *xxx*, high ↑ risk.
*Atrial premature beats.

- Orthopedic or pelvic/GU procedures

The benefit of DVT prophylaxis must always be considered along with risk.

Other organ systems

1. **Hematologic:** many surgeons and anesthesiologists recommend a hematocrit above 30 preoperatively, although there is little evidence to support this position. Thrombocytopenia, in the case of normally functioning platelets, does not prolong bleeding time until the platelet count drops below 100,000 and does not usually impair surgical hemostasis until the count drops below 50,000

2. **Renal:** patients with a GFR greater than 50 ml/min generally have no increased risk of surgical morbidity if their renal disease is chronic. Patients with a GFR less than 50 should have careful monitoring of fluid balance, electrolytes, drug dosages, and hemostasis

3. **Liver:** patients with long-term liver disease and minimal impairment (no ascites; normal bilirubin, albumin, and prothrombin time) are at no increased risk of surgery. Surgical risk increases with degree of liver impairment, and patient's condition should be optimized preoperatively to correct coagulation disorders, electrolyte abnormalities, and fluid status

4. **Endocrine**
   a. Patients with severe **hypothyroidism** should have at least partial thyroxine replacement preoperatively
   b. Surgery in patients with **hyperthyroidism** may precipitate thyroid storm, and therefore these patients should receive antithyroid medica-

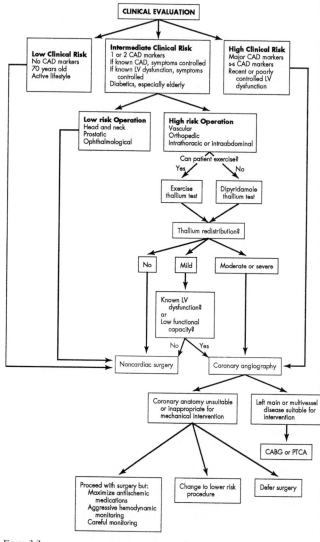

Figure 3-2
For legend see opposite page.

Figure 3-2

Suggested algorithm for estimation of preoperative coronary risk of elective or semielective surgery. Most important considerations are patient's clinical risk profile, nature of the surgical procedure, and results of noninvasive testing or coronary angiography or both if indicated. Urgent surgery may preempt risk stratification. CAD markers: age ≥70 years, prior angina, prior MI, previous congestive heart failure or ventricular arrhythmias or both, diabetes mellitus, and Q waves on resting ECG. Major CAD markers: recent MI complicated by angina, congestive heart failure, or positive stress test result; unstable or new onset angina; recent non–Q wave anterior MI; more than two CAD markers in selected patients. Moderate or severe thallium redistribution: thallium redistribution in more than one planar view, more than one coronary arterial territory, or four or more myocardial segments. (From Abramson SA et al: *Prog Cardiovasc Dis* 34:205, 1991.)

---

tion and beta blockade preoperatively

c. Patients with **diabetes mellitus** should have glucose levels well controlled preoperatively. Patients on oral hypoglycemic agents may have the drug held on the morning of surgery and have serum glucose "covered" with regular insulin until they are eating again. Patients on insulin may receive half of the usual dose of AM insulin preoperatively and be given a 5% dextrose solution IV throughout the day of surgery with ongoing glucose monitoring

d. Patients in whom **adrenal suppression** is suspected should be given hydrocortisone sodium succinate IV 100 mg every 6 to 8 hours with adequate fluid and electrolyte repletion. Treatment should continue through the period of stress

STRATEGIES FOR OVERALL RISK ASSESSMENT

Preoperative laboratory testing should be applied selectively to patients for whom there are particular concerns based on history and physical examination in the office. Table 3-2 provides a reasonable approach to such testing as an adjunct to history and physical examination in selected patients.

Reference

1. Goldman L et al: Multifactorial index of cardiac risk in noncardiac surgical procedures, *N Engl J Med* 297(16):845-850, 1977.

Suggested readings

Abraham SA et al: Coronary risk of non-cardiac surgery, *Prog Cardiovasc Dis* 34(3):205-234, 1991.

Caputo GM, Gross RJ: Medical consultation on surgical services: an annotated bibliography, *Annals Intern Med* 118:290-297, 1993.

Collins R et al: Reduction in fatal pulmonary embolism and venous thrombosis by perioperative administration of SQ heparin, *N Engl J Med* 318(18):1162-1173, 1988.

Cygan R, Wartakin H: Stopping and restarting medications in the preoperative period, *J Gen Intern Med* 2:270-283, 1987.

Detsky AS et al: Predicting cardiac complications in patients undergoing non-cardiac surgery, *J Gen Intern Med* 1:211-219, 1986.

Eagle A et al: Dipyridamole thallium screening in patients undergoing vascular surgery, *JAMA* 257(16):1285-1289, 1987.

Gass GD et al: Preoperative pulmonary function testing to predict postoperative morbidity and mortality, *Chest* 89(1):127, 1986.

Table 3-2 Simplified strategy for preoperative testing*

Preoperative Condition	Hemoglobin M	Hemoglobin F	WBC	PT/PTT	PLT/BT
Procedure with blood loss	Obtain	Obtain			
Procedure without blood loss					
Neonates	Obtain	Obtain			
Age <40 yr		Obtain			
Age 40-49 yr		Obtain			
Age 50-64 yr		Obtain			
Age ≥65 yr	Obtain	Obtain			
Cardiovascular disease					
Pulmonary disease					
Malignancy	Obtain	Obtain	Obtain for leukemias only	Obtain for leukemias only	
Radiation therapy			Obtain		
Hepatic disease				Obtain	
Exposure to hepatitis					
Renal disease	Obtain	Obtain			
Bleeding disorder				Obtain	Obtain
Diabetes					
Smoking ≥20 cigarettes/day	Obtain	Obtain			
Possible pregnancy					
Diuretic use					
Digoxin use					
Steroid use					
Anticoagulant use	Obtain	Obtain		Obtain	
Central nervous system disease			Obtain		

Data from Roizen MF: Routine preoperative evaluation. In Miller RD, editor: *Anesthesia,* New York, 1982, Churchill Livingstone; and Blery C, Chastang CI, Gaudy JH: Critical assessment of routine preoperative investigations, *Effective Health Care* 1:111, 1983.

WBC, White blood cell count; *PT/PTT,* prothrombin time and partial thromboplastin time; *PLT/BT,* platelet count and bleeding time; *elect,* electrolytes (i.e., sodium, potassium, chloride, carbon dioxide, and proteins); *Creat/BUN,* creatinine or blood urea nitrogen; *AST/ALP,* aspartate aminotransferase and alkaline phosphatase; *T/S,* blood typing and screening for unexpected antibodies.

*Not all diseases are included in this table. The physician's judgment is needed regarding patients with diseases not listed.

Elect	Creat/BUN	Blood Glucose	AST/ALP	Roentgenogram	ECG	Pregnancy	T/S
							Obtain
					Men only Obtain		
				Perhaps obtain	Obtain		
	Obtain			Obtain	Obtain		
				Obtain	Obtain		
				Obtain			
				Obtain	Obtain		
			Obtain				
			Obtain				
Obtain	Obtain						
Obtain	Obtain	Obtain			Obtain		
				Obtain			
						Obtain	
Obtain	Obtain						
Obtain	Obtain				Obtain		
Obtain		Obtain					
Obtain	Obtain	Obtain			Obtain		

Kroenke K: Preoperative evaluation, *J Gen Intern Med* 2:257, July/August 1987.

Lubin MF: Is age a risk factor for surgery? *Med Clin North Am* 77(2):327, 1993.

Merli GJ, Weitz HH: The medical consultant, *Med Clin North Am* 71:353-354, 1987.

Merli GJ et al: Prophylaxis for deep vein thrombosis and pulmonary embolism in the surgical patient, *Med Clin North Am* 71(3):377, 1987.

Mohr DN, Jett JR: Preoperative evaluation of pulmonary risk factors, *J Gen Intern Med* 3:277-285, 1988.

NIH Consensus Conference: prevention of venous thrombosis and pulmonary embolism, *JAMA* 256(6):744, 1986.

Preoperative pulmonary function testing: American College of Physicians position paper, *Ann Intern Med* 112(10):793-794, 1990.

3.3   **MENOPAUSE**
Michele G. Cyr, MD

Definition

Menopause is defined as the permanent cessation of menstruation that results from loss of ovarian function. Typically menopause occurs after the age of 40 years. *Natural menopause* refers to the gradual deterioration of ovarian function, whereas *surgical menopause* refers to bilateral oophorectomy.

Epidemiology

By the year 2000 there will be approximately 30 million women in the United States who are postmenopausal.

Diagnosis

Menopause can be diagnosed retrospectively after 6 to 12 months of amenorrhea in women more than 55 years of age. It may be diagnosed earlier or in patients who have had a hysterectomy without oophorectomy with a follicle-stimulating hormone (FSH) level ≥ 40 mIU/ml.

Symptoms

1. Hot flashes: approximately 75% of U.S. women experience hot flashes, but they are severe in only 10% to 15% of women; hot flashes persist for more than 4 years in 85% of these women and for 5 years in 20% to 50% of women
2. Vaginal dryness: usually begins several years after menopause and may worsen with time; approximately 25% of women experience this effect by 5 years after menopause
3. Psychologic symptoms: mood changes may occur at menopause; no evidence suggests that a true "menopausal depression" exists, although depression is common among women
4. Incontinence: stress type is related to relaxation of pelvic ligaments
5. Miscellaneous symptoms: reported by some women at menopause; may or may not be related to estrogen deficiency
   a. Memory changes: may be related to problems concentrating
   b. Formication: feeling of insects crawling on skin
   c. Headaches
   d. Fatigue: may be related to insomnia from nighttime hot flashes

Associated conditions

1. Osteoporosis
2. Coronary artery disease

Management goals

1. Symptom treatment: both hormonal and nonhormonal treatments are available; the nonhormonal therapies have been less well studied
2. Prevention of long-term conditions of osteoporosis and coronary artery disease: behavioral changes and hormonal therapy

Management

1. Nonhormonal treatment of symptoms
   a. Hot flashes
      (1) Vitamin E, ≤400 IU/day
      (2) Paced breathing exercises
      (3) Avoidance of precipitants (e.g., hot spicy foods, hot drinks, hot rooms, stress)
   b. Vaginal dryness: vaginal lubricants; some are used as needed for intercourse, and others are effective for several days
   c. Urinary incontinence: Kegel exercises
2. Nonhormonal prevention of associated conditions
   a. Osteoporosis
      (1) Calcium: 1000 to 1500 mg daily (dietary or supplements or both)
      (2) Vitamin D: 15-minute sun exposure daily or 400 to 500 U/day if housebound
      (3) Weight-bearing exercises
   b. Heart disease
      (1) Low-fat diet
      (2) Exercise to achieve cardiovascular fitness
      (3) Smoking cessation
      (4) Treatment of hypertension

Hormonal treatment

1. Symptoms
   a. Patients with hysterectomy: estrogen therapy alone, with taper in 2 to 5 years if treating hot flashes
   b. Patients with uterus: estrogen and progesterone, with taper in 2 to 5 years if treating hot flashes
2. Prevention of osteoporosis and heart disease
   a. Patients with hysterectomy: estrogen therapy alone
   b. Patients with uterus who have
      (1) Heart disease: progesterone and estrogen
      (2) Risk factors for heart disease: progesterone and estrogen
      (3) Risk factors for hip fracture: progesterone and estrogen
      (4) Breast cancer risk: use no hormonal therapy

Hormonal replacement regimens

1. Unopposed estrogen: for women who have had hysterectomy or who submit to pretreatment and yearly endometrial biopsies

2. Cyclic combined: for woman with uterus
   a. Conjugated estrogen: 0.625 mg PO or equivalent daily (patch, 0.05 to 0.1 mg twice weekly), plus progesterone: 5 to 10 mg PO 12 days/mo
   b. Continuous combined: for woman with uterus who does not tolerate side effects of higher progesterone dose or does not want to have bleeding withdrawal associated with cyclic combined
      (1) Estrogen: 0.625 mg PO daily (patch, 0.05 to 0.1 mg twice weekly)
      (2) Progesterone: 2.5 mg PO daily

Side effects of hormonal therapy

1. Estrogen: bloating, breast tenderness, headache, nausea
2. Progesterone: bloating, breast tenderness, PMS symptoms
3. Cyclic combined: bleeding—85% to 95% after progestin, 15% to 25% before progestin
4. Combined continuous: 30% to 50% irregular bleeding for first year

Evaluation

1. Annual breast exam and pelvic exam
2. Annual mammogram and Pap smears
3. Endometrial biopsies
   a. For patients treated with
      (1) Unopposed estrogen: pretreatment and yearly examination
      (2) Cyclic estrogen and progesterone: no pretreatment; biopsy if irregular bleeding occurs before day 6 of progesterone therapy
      (3) Continuous combined: no pretreatment; biopsy if prolonged bleeding >10 days or bleeding beyond 6 months of treatment
   b. Anyone with postmenopausal bleeding not receiving hormone replacement therapy
   c. RBC or histiocytes on Pap smear
4. Bone densitometry: not routinely recommended but may be helpful for women deciding about hormone replacement therapy

Suggested readings

American College of Physicians: Guidelines for counseling postmenopausal women about preventive hormone therapy, *Ann Intern Med* 117:1038-1041, 1992.

Belchetz PE: Hormonal treatment of postmenopausal women, *N Engl J Med* 15:1062-1071, 1994.

Gorsky RD et al: Relative risks and benefits of long-term estrogen replacement therapy: a decision analysis, *Obstet Gynecol* 2:162-166, 1994.

Grady D et al: Hormone therapy to prevent disease and prolong life in postmenopausal women, *Ann Intern Med* 117:1016-1037, 1991.

Landau C, Cyr MG, Moulton AW: *The complete book of menopause: every woman's guide to good health,* New York, 1994, Putnam & Son.

| 3.4 | **EXERCISE AND AGING** |

Raymond H. Stone, Jr., PhD, and Marsha D. Fretwell, MD

Background

1. **Aging, disease, and disuse**
   a. It is now clear that some of the physical and mental decline and loss

of functional reserve usually blamed on aging alone can be more accurately attributed to a complex interaction among genetic aging, disease, and disuse
   b. Societal norms about aging reduce expectations of both mental and physical performance and promote inactivity and disuse
   c. In turn, disuse exacerbates the decline in endurance, strength, and flexibility related to the true changes of aging and/or disease
2. **Epidemiology**
   a. Less than one third of older adults do any type of regular exercise
   b. Twenty percent reductions in endurance (aerobic) exercise capacity, fifty percent reductions in muscle strength, and twenty-three percent reductions in lean body or muscle mass are routinely noted in cross-sectional and longitudinal studies including individuals between the ages of 20 and 90 years
   c. Approximately 50% of individuals over 60 years have signs of osteoarthritis on knee films and 20% of older adults are using a nonsteroidal antiinflammatory prescription, suggesting that joint pain and stiffness are significant problems
3. **Documented benefits of regular exercise**
   a. Improvement in functional capacities
      (1) Increased gait velocity
      (2) Increased stair-climbing power
      (3) Reduced time rising up from the kneeling position on the floor at a normal pace
      (4) Increased distance stepping up on a box
   b. Improvement in cardiorespiratory function
      (1) Increase in maximal oxygen uptake
      (2) Lower heart rate and blood at a given intensity (submaximal)
      (3) Lower myocardial oxygen cost at a given absolute intensity (submaximal)
      (4) Increased exercise threshold and reserve for the onset of disease symptoms, i.e., angina pectoris
      (5) Increased exercise threshold for accumulation of serum lactate
   c. Reduction in coronary artery disease risk factors
      (1) Reduced resting systolic and diastolic pressures in hypertensives
      (2) Reduced body fat and increased lean body mass
      (3) Increased HDL cholesterol and decreased serum triglycerides
      (4) Improved sensitivity to insulin, decline in serum insulin levels; improved glucose tolerance in non–insulin dependent diabetes
   d. Reduction in mortality from CAD
      (1) Primary prevention: higher activity and fitness levels are associated with lower mortality from CAD
      (2) Secondary prevention: comprehensive cardiac rehabilitation programs reduce premature cardiovascular death but not nonfatal events
   e. Improvement (6% to 9%) in bone density in postmenopausal women
   f. Improvement (10% to 25%) in functional status of arthritis patients
      (1) Faster gait velocity
      (2) Improvement in physical activity
      (3) Lower depression scores

(4) Less pain and less pain medications

(5) **Exercise does not increase pain!**

Deliberate exercise prescriptions

1. **Definition:** planned exercise programs that are designed to
   a. Improve endurance (aerobic) exercise capacity, muscle strength, joint flexibility, and overall functional ability
   b. Reduce cardiovascular risk factors such as weight, dyslipidemias, hypertension, and elevated pulse rates
2. **Target patients with**
   a. Increased cardiovascular risk factors
   b. Arthritis or decrease in joint range of motion
   c. A history of falls
   d. Loss of muscle mass, strength, and endurance
   e. Gait disorders
   f. Decreased aerobic capacity
   g. Osteoporosis
3. **Deliberate exercise as a treatment plan**
   a. Any increase in activity level (even very small) is better than a continuance of the downward spiral of functional status
   b. Each prescription should address
      (1) Muscular strength
      (2) Muscular endurance
      (3) Cardiorespiratory endurance
      (4) Flexibility and coordination
      (5) Prevention of relapse
   c. The starting point for deliberate exercise is an activity that is both tolerated well and enjoyed by the older adult. Most people quit exercise within the first 6 weeks because it is too intense. Walking is an appropriate start-up activity
   d. Consider the following factors to determine the appropriate level of intensity
      (1) Is patient on medications that influence heart rate?
      (2) Is patient at risk for cardiovascular or orthopedic injury?
      (3) What is patient's current level of fitness?
      (4) What is patient's recent exercise experience?
      (5) What are patient's preferences for exercise modality?
      (6) What are targeted goals or objectives of patient and physician?
   e. After the patient has demonstrated an understanding of the activity and a tolerance for regular activity, other components can be slowly added but never to the point where past consistency or gains are compromised. *This is to be a lifetime program;* do not do too much too soon
   f. Relapse prevention
      (1) Regular follow-up and modification are critical to the long-term success of any exercise program
      (2) The physician should understand and emphasize the specific benefits to the patient
      (3) The physician should outline clearly the commitment required of the patient
      (4) The physician should provide both group and individual support

Prescription principles and suggestions

1. **Prescription principles:** every exercise program should include a warm-up period, an activity phase, and then a cool-down period
   a. Warm-up period: this is usually a 5 to 10-minute period. The warm-up period can consist of gentle stretching, light calisthenics, or an activity done at low intensity (i.e., walking or stationary bicycling at less than target heart rate). This is an important transition phase that allows the musculoskeletal and cardiorespiratory systems to prepare for physical activity
   b. Activity phase: this is the cardiorespiratory or aerobic part of the workout. The basic recommendations for a cardiorespiratory program are easily recalled through use of mnemonic *FITT*
      (1) F = Frequency
         (a) At least 3 days/wk
         (b) Encourage patient to make this a habit, similar to brushing teeth
         (c) Choose a time of day that is convenient
         (d) Schedule exercise as any appointment
         (e) When weight reduction is a major goal, daily exercise can be extremely helpful
      (2) I = Intensity
         (a) The intensity depends on the age of the individual, the presence or absence of cardiovascular disease or risk factors
         (b) Light to moderate intensity (<70% of maximum heart rate for age)
         (c) Vigorous intensity (>70% of maximum heart rate for age)
         (d) Moderate intensity allows the participant to comfortably carry on a conversation
      (3) T = Type (mode) of physical activity
         (a) Aerobic activity is a sustained, rhythmic activity using large muscle groups
         (b) Ask the patient to chose an activity that is enjoyable. This increases success in making this life-style change
         (c) Suggest several different types of exercise to increase enjoyment and improve compliance
         (d) Discourage patient from beginning an unrealistic activity, i.e., one that is too strenuous or incompatible with life-style
      (4) T = Time (duration) of physical activity
         (a) The goal of 20 to 60 minutes per session is recommended
         (b) For weight reduction, recommend low-intensity exercise for a longer duration, at least 30 minutes
         (c) Sedentary patient may need to start slowly with 5- to 10-minute sessions
         (d) Some patients may prefer/tolerate two or three brief sessions per day rather than a single session. This builds self-confidence and compliance
   c. Cool-down period: this is usually 5 to 10 minutes. As with the warm-up period, a low-intensity activity, e.g., walking or stretching, should be performed. This period is important to prevent hypotension that may occur at the sudden cessation of exercise

2. **Prescription for healthy older adults**
   a. For aerobic exercise capacity
      (1) Overload gradually by increasing duration of the exercise modality until the patient can complete 20 minutes of continuous cardiorespiratory activity
      (2) At this point, add to intensity
   b. For muscular strength
      (1) Begin with a resistance that allows completion of 8 to 10 reps with moderate exertion for one set only, using all the major muscle groups. Do this at least two times per week with at least 48 hours of rest between sessions
      (2) Add one set after 3 or 4 weeks as opposed to adding weight. After completion of 10 reps on the second set, the individual can add 5% weight to increase intensity every 3 weeks
   c. For muscular endurance
      (1) Use the same progression principles but with half the resistance that is used for muscular strength
      (2) Sets should include 15 reps and can add one session per week to the muscle-strengthening program
   d. For resistance training (to preserve bone mass)
      (1) Form in resistance training means moving the weight both in the concentric and eccentric contraction in a slow controlled manner without use of jerking or momentum
      (2) In general, it is safer to use weight machines as opposed to free weights
      (3) Proper form for resistance training allows for normal breathing (no breath holding allowed)
   e. For flexibility
      (1) Optimal functional ability requires an adequate range of motion in all joints
      (2) Flexibility in lower back, hamstring, and shoulder regions is critical
      (3) All exercise programs should emphasize proper stretching in the upper and lower trunk, neck, and hip regions
      (4) Static stretching is done by slowly stretching the muscle to a point of mild discomfort, taking and releasing a deep breath, and holding stretch for a period of time (begin with 10 seconds and gradually build up to 30 seconds)
      (5) This progression will slowly increase the range of motion over several weeks
      (6) For the very frail and deconditioned older adult, static stretching might be an appropriate start to an exercise program and be all the intensity that can be tolerated

3. **Prescription for cardiac patients**
   a. After a cardiac event, patients should exercise in an established cardiac rehabilitation program under a physician's supervision for phases 1 and 2
   b. Phase 3 exercise should remain under physician supervision but can use ACCN and *ACSM's Guidelines for Exercise Testing and Prescriptions* for individualized exercise prescriptions

   c. Resistance training should be held off until 4 to 6 weeks of super-
      vised cardiorespiratory endurance exercise have been completed

4. **Prescription for pulmonary patients**
   a. Exercise at 50% Vo_2 peak, or
   b. Exercise at near maximal intensity (drastically limits the duration of
      the exercise time), or
   c. Exercise at an intensity that is above the anaerobic threshold, or
   d. Use dyspnea ratings to set intensity, i.e., moderate intensity exercise
      corresponds to a 3 dyspnea rating (50% Vo_2 peak); vigorous intensity
      corresponds to a 6 dyspnea rating (85% Vo_2 peak)
   e. Frequent exercise sessions may be needed in the initial stages of the
      exercise program
   f. The goal remains to work up to 20 to 30 minutes of continuous car-
      diorespiratory activity
   g. **The patient should maintain Sao_2 >88%**

5. **Prescription for diabetic patients**
   a. This disease responds best to a program of a minimum of 5 days/wk
      with an endurance component on each day
   b. Blood glucose should be monitored before and after exercise
   c. Intensity should be very low at the beginning and build up gradually.
      This allow patients to adjust their diet to the exercise program and
      glucose stabilization
   d. Begin program with multiple short exercise time and work up to 20
      to 30 minutes of continuous activity. The last 15 minutes of continu-
      ous activity are the most beneficial in improving glucose tolerance

6. **Prescription for obese patients**
   a. Chose an activity that maximizes caloric expenditure (<70% Vo_2
      peak), minimizes stress on joints, and monitors orthopedic concerns
   b. At first, set daily caloric expenditure for exercise at 200 to 300 Kcal
   c. Cross training with some non–weight bearing activities should be in-
      cluded
   d. Posture and body mechanics should be emphasized. Proper attention
      to engaging the lower abdominal and gluteal muscles to stabilize the
      lower back are critical to safer functional activity and ADLs
   e. **This is a 24 hr/day exercise program**

Role of the physician

1. Physician plays a critical role in success of any exercise program
2. **The patient must truly believe that the physician's philosophy toward
   good health includes exercise as a major component equal to all other
   factors that determine good health**
3. **Physician must serve as an example, a role model, if the treatment
   plan is to achieve maximum outcomes**
4. **A positive attitude is critical to the success of the program**

Suggested readings

American College of Sports Medicine: *ACSM's resource manual for guidelines for
   exercise testing and prescription,* ed 2, Philadelphia, 1993, Lea & Febiger.
American College of Sports Medicine: *ACSM's guidelines for exercise testing and prescription,* ed 5, Philadelphia, 1995, Williams & Wilkins.

Dalsky GP: The role of exercise in the prevention of osteoporosis, *Compr Ther* 15:30, 1989.

Fiatarone MA et al: Exercise training and nutritional supplementation for physical frailty in very elderly people, *N Engl J Med* 330:1769, 1994.

Kovar PA et al: Supervised fitness walking in patients with osteoarthritis of the knee: a randomized controlled trial, *Ann Intern Med* 116:529, 1992.

Schwartz RS, Buchner DM: Exercise in the elderly: physiologic and functional effects. In Hazzard WR et al, editors: *Principles of geriatric medicine and gerontology,* ed 3, New York, 1994, McGraw-Hill.

Skelton DA et al: Effects of resistance training on strength, power, and selected functional abilities of women aged 75 and older, *J Am Geriatr Soc* 43:1081, 1995.

Cognitive Dysfunction

Marsha D. Fretwell, MD

DELIRIUM

Background

Delirium is both a common and a serious syndrome affecting the outcomes of hospitalized older patients. Delirium is often the cardinal symptom for the presentation of serious physical illness or drug intoxication. Patients with dementia are particularly susceptible to delirium. Early recognition and appropriate management of delirium will substantially improve the medical and functional outcomes of acute hospitalization in the frail older patient.

Definition and diagnostic criteria

1. Delirium is characterized by
   a. Global cognitive impairment
   b. Disturbances of attention
   c. Reduced level of consciousness
   d. Reduced or increased psychomotor activity
   e. Disorganized sleep-wake cycle
   f. Acute onset, fluctuating course, and a relatively brief duration
2. The American Psychiatric Association's diagnostic criteria for delirium are described in the box on pp. 52-54
3. The Confusion Assessment Method (CAM) Diagnostic Algorithm requires the presence of features 1 and 2 and either 3 or 4 for a diagnosis of delirium; see the box on p. 55

Frequency and importance

1. Delirium occurs in 15% to 55% of hospitalized older adults over age 70
2. Approximately 50% of delirious patients are delirious at admission, and 50% become delirious while in the hospital
3. Of delirious patients 32% to 67% go unrecognized by house staff and attending physicians
4. Delirium is often the presenting feature of a physical illness or adverse drug reaction. If it is unrecognized, the medical condition will also go unrecognized and untreated
5. Delirium has an associated mortality of 10% to 65%

Diagnostic Criteria for Delirium

Delirium Due to a General Medical Condition

A. Disturbance of consciousness (i.e., reduced clarity of awareness of the environment) with reduced ability to focus, sustain, or shift attention.

B. A change in cognition (e.g., memory deficit, disorientation, language disturbance) or the development of a perceptual disturbance that is not better accounted for by a preexisting, established, or evolving dementia.

C. The disturbance develops over a short period of time (usually hours to days) and tends to fluctuate during the course of the day.

D. There is evidence from the history, physical examination, or laboratory findings that the disturbance is caused by the direct physiologic consequences of a general medical condition.

Coding note: If delirium is superimposed on a preexisting dementia of the Alzheimer's type or vascular dementia, indicate the delirium by coding the appropriate subtype of the dementia, e.g., dementia of the Alzheimer's type, with late onset, with delirium.

Coding note: Include the name of the general medical condition on Axis I, e.g., delirium due to hepatic encephalopathy; also code the general medical condition on Axis III.

Delirium Due to Intoxication

A. Disturbance of consciousness (i.e., reduced clarity of awareness of the environment) with reduced ability to focus, sustain, or shift attention.

B. A change in cognition (e.g., memory deficit, disorientation, language disturbance) or the development of a perceptual disturbance that is not better accounted for by a preexisting, established, or evolving dementia.

C. The disturbance develops over a short period of time (usually hours to days) and tends to fluctuate during the course of the day.

D. There is evidence from the history, physical examination, or laboratory findings of either (1) or (2):

    (1) The symptoms in criteria A and B developed during substance intoxication.

    (2) Medication use is etiologically related to the disturbance.*

Note: This diagnosis should be made instead of a diagnosis of substance intoxication only when the cognitive symptoms are in excess of those usually associated with the intoxication syndrome and when the symptoms are sufficiently severe to warrant independent clinical attention.

Code (Specific substance) intoxication delirium: (Alcohol; amphetamine [or amphetamine-like substance]; cannabis; cocaine; hallucinogen; inhalant; opioid; phencyclidine [or phencyclidine-like substance]; sedative, hypnotic, or anxiolytic; other [or unknown] substance [e.g., cimetidine, digitalis, benztropine])

Delirium Due to Withdrawal

A. Disturbance of consciousness (i.e., reduced clarity of awareness of the environment) with reduced ability to focus, sustain, or shift attention.
B. A change in cognition (e.g., memory deficit, disorientation, language disturbance) or the development of a perceptual disturbance that is not better accounted for by a preexisting, established, or evolving dementia.
C. The disturbance develops over a short period of time (usually hours to days) and tends to fluctuate during the course of the day.
D. There is evidence from the history, physical examination, or laboratory findings that the symptoms in criteria A and B developed during, or shortly after, a withdrawal syndrome.

Note: This diagnosis should be made instead of a diagnosis of substance withdrawal only when the cognitive symptoms are in excess of those usually associated with the withdrawal syndrome and when the symptoms are sufficiently severe to warrant independent clinical attention.

Code (Specific substance) withdrawal delirium: (Alcohol; sedative, hypnotic, or anxiolytic; other [or unknown] substance)

Delirium Due to Multiple Etiologies

A. Disturbance of consciousness (i.e., reduced clarity of awareness of the environment) with reduced ability to focus, sustain, or shift attention.
B. A change in cognition (e.g., memory deficit, disorientation, language disturbance) or the development of a perceptual disturbance that is not better accounted for by a preexisting, established, or evolving dementia.
C. The disturbance develops over a short period of time (usually hours to days) and tends to fluctuate during the course of the day.
D. There is evidence from the history, physical examination, or laboratory findings that the delirium has more than one etiology (e.g., more than one etiological general medical condition, a general medical condition plus substance intoxication, or medication side effect).

Coding note: Use multiple codes reflecting specific delirium and specific etiologies, e.g., delirium due to viral encephalitis, alcohol withdrawal delirium.

Continued

Diagnostic Criteria for Delirium—cont'd

Delirium Not Otherwise Specified

This category should be used to diagnose a delirium that does not meet criteria for any of the specific types of delirium described in this section.

Examples include

1. A clinical presentation of delirium that is suspected to be due to general medical condition or substance use but for which there is insufficient evidence to establish a specific etiology
2. Delirium due to causes not listed in this section (e.g., sensory deprivation)

From DSM-IV, *Diagnostic and Statistical Manual of Mental Disorders,* ed 4. Copyright American Psychiatric Association, Washington, 1994. Used with permission.

*NOTE: The diagnosis should be recorded as substance-induced delirium if related to medication use.

Etiology and predictors

1. Delirium is caused by one or more organic factors that bring about widespread cerebral dysfunction
   a. Predisposing factors
      (1) Age over 65
      (2) Brain damage
      (3) Chronic cerebral diseases, e.g., Alzheimer's disease
   b. Facilitating factors
      (1) Psychologic stress, e.g., change in environment
      (2) Sleep loss
      (3) Sensory deprivation and overload
   c. Precipitating factors
      (1) Primary cerebral diseases
      (2) Systemic illnesses affecting the brain secondarily, e.g., metabolic encephalopathies, neoplasms, infections, and cardiovascular and collagen diseases
      (3) Intoxication with exogenous substances, including medical and recreational drugs, and poisons
      (4) Withdrawal from substances such as alcohol or sedative-hypnotics
2. In older patients, more than one factor is often present
3. Intoxication with medications, particularly anticholinergic, is probably the most common cause of delirium in the hospitalized older patient; see the box on p. 56
4. The metabolic abnormalities, medical diseases, and surgical procedures most frequently associated with delirium are
   a. Hyponatremia, hypokalemia, uremia, and hypoalbuminemia
   b. Congestive heart failure
   c. Infections such as urinary tract and pneumonia
   d. Fever or hypothermia
   e. Repair of hip fractures and open heart surgery

The Confusion Assessment Method (CAM)*
Diagnostic Algorithm

Feature 1.   Acute Onset and Fluctuating Course

This feature is usually obtained from a family member or nurse and is shown by positive responses to the following questions: Is there evidence of an acute change in mental status from the patient's baseline? Did the (abnormal) behavior fluctuate during the day, i.e., tend to come and go, or increase and decrease in severity?

Feature 2.   Inattention

This feature is shown by a positive response to the following question: Did the patient have difficulty focusing attention, e.g., being easily distractible, or having difficulty keeping track of what was being said?

Feature 3.   Disorganized Thinking

This feature is shown by a positive response to the following question: Was the patient's thinking disorganized or incoherent, e.g., rambling or irrelevant conversation, unclear or illogical flow of ideas, or unpredictable switching from subject to subject?

Feature 4.   Altered Level of Consciousness

This feature is shown by any answer other than "alert" to the following question: Overall, how would you rate this patient's level of consciousness? (alert [normal], vigilant [hyperalert] lethargic [drowsy, easily aroused], stupor [difficult to arouse] or coma [unarousable])

From Inouye SK: *Am J Med* 97:278, 1994.

*The diagnosis of delirium by CAM requires the presence of feature 1 and 2 and either 3 or 4.

Diagnosis

The diagnosis of delirium is made on clinical grounds and has two crucial steps: (1) the recognition of delirium on the basis of history from nurses and family members and the essential clinical features and (2) identification of its cause or causes. The comprehensive geriatric assessment process described in Chapter 2 is useful in guiding the diagnosis and identification of causes.

1. **Data base**
   a. Chief complaint
      (1) Families and caretakers bring patient to medical attention because of acute onset of confusion, restlessness, difficulty in thinking coherently, insomnia, disturbing dreams, or frank hallucinations. Information about time of onset and duration of symptoms is critical
      (2) Hallucinations are often the focus of concern to caretakers
      (3) Patients may appear either somnolent or hyperactive with delirium

Medications Associated With Delirium

Sedative-hypnotics
    Benzodiazepines (flurazepam, diazepam)
    Barbiturates
    Sleeping medications (chloral hydrate)
Narcotics
Anticholinergics
    Antihistamines (diphenhydramine, hydroxyzine)
    Antispasmodics (belladonna, diphenoxylate)
    Tricyclic antidepressants (amitriptyline, imipramine)
    Phenothiazines (haloperidol, thorazine, thioridazine)
    Antiparkinsonian agents (benztropine, trihexyphenidyl)
    Antiarrhythmics (quinidine, disopyramide)
Cardiac (digitalis, lidocaine, amiodarone)
Antihypertensives (propranolol, methyldopa, reserpine)
Antibiotics (aminoglycosides, penicillins, cephalosporins, sulfon-
    amides)
Miscellaneous

Cimetidine	Lithium
Steroids	Anticonvulsants
Metoclopramide	Nonsteroidal antiinflammatory drugs
Levodopa	Salicylates

From Inouye SK: *Am J Med* 97:278, 1994.

  b. Initial screen of vision, hearing, and cognition
    (1) Patient may either have difficulty remaining awake or be easily distracted
    (2) Patient is unable to count backward from 10 to 1 or to name days of the week in reverse order
    (3) Patients with very low scores on Folstein Mini-Mental State Examination should be evaluated for delirium *before* being given diagnosis of dementia (see Appendix XV)
  c. Biomedical, psychologic, social, and functional history should focus on etiologic factors discussed above
  d. Review medication list: discontinue all psychoactive medication (or substitute less toxic alternatives). Review side effects of all medications
  e. Physical examination
    (1) Fever, hypothermia, low cardiac output, dehydration, hyperthyroidism or hypothyroidism, signs of pneumonia, and/or urinary tract infection should be evaluated and corrected
    (2) Evaluation of cognitive function generally reveals an inability to attend, rambling thoughts, somnolence, or agitation
    (3) Usually there is an absence of new focal neurologic changes
  f. Targeted laboratory evaluation
    (1) Electrolytes
    (2) BUN, creatinine

     (3) CBC with differential
     (4) Glucose, calcium, and phosphate
     (5) Liver enzyme tests
     (6) Blood level of all medications
  g. Search for occult infections
     (1) Chest x-ray
     (2) Urine, sputum, and blood cultures
  h. When no obvious cause is identified by above history, physical examination, and laboratory evaluation, consider the following in selected patients
     (1) Laboratory tests: magnesium, thyroid function tests, vitamin B_{12} level, toxicology screen, ammonia level
     (2) Arterial blood gas: in patients with dyspnea, tachypnea, acute pulmonary process, or history of significant respiratory disease
     (3) Electrocardiogram: in patients with chest pain, shortness of breath, or cardiac disease history
     (4) Cerebrospinal fluid examination: in febrile patients where meningitis is suspected
     (5) CT or MRI brain imaging: in patients with new focal neurologic signs or history/signs of head injury
     (6) Electroencephalogram: in patients where occult seizure disorder is suspected and delirium must be differentiated from functional psychiatric disorders

2. **Assessment and management of delirium**
  a. Treatment of the underlying causes: the causative factors listed above should be pursued, treated, and/or reversed whenever possible (management of organ system abnormalities and medical diagnoses are covered in Chapter 6; issues relating to the optimal use of medications are outlined in Chapter 7)
  b. Symptomatic treatment: treat agitation with high-potency, low-anticholinergic antipsychotics, such as haloperidol orally or parenterally. Start 1.0 to 2.0 mg q2h until a moderate level of sedation is achieved. Then take the entire dose required to achieve sedation (usually no more than 4 to 6 mg) and divide into two equal doses for the next day. Reduce dose in half each day until patient is in a dose range of 0.5 mg po bid. Stop the haloperidol if patient remains sedated after first day. If the patient was not on haloperidol before hospitalization, it is unlikely that he or she will need to be discharged on it. Most toxicity associated with haloperidol is during long-term use, not in its use to control acute agitation
  c. New functional impairments that inevitably accompany delirium in older patients (e.g., malnutrition, incontinence, impactions, falling, and disruptive or uncooperative behaviors) should be anticipated and prevented, if possible (management of each is covered in detail in Chapter 5)

4.2   DEMENTIA

Definition

Dementia is a syndrome characterized by an impairment in two or more intellectual or cognitive functions despite a state of clear consciousness. The

persistent and stable nature of the impairment distinguishes dementia from
the altered consciousness and fluctuating deficits of delirium.

Epidemiology

The prevalence of dementia in the community-dwelling population over 65
years is between 10% and 50%. In the nursing home population, more than
50% of the patients carry the diagnosis of a dementing disorder. The most
common diseases causing dementia are Alzheimer's disease and cerebrovascular accidents, which together account for two thirds of the cases.

Classification of dementia syndromes

1. **Cortical/subcortical system:** initially, dementias were described as
   either cortical or subcortical depending on the clinical patterns demonstrated by the patients with various dementias. Neuropathologic and
   imaging studies now show that this system is not anatomically accurate.
   For instance, the so-called cortical dementias such as Alzheimer's are
   not restricted to the cortex. In this case the basic pathology is in
   the subcortical cholinergic fiber pathways, which then project to the
   cortex
   a. Cortical dementia
      (1) Characterized by prominent amnesia, aphasia, apraxia, and agno-
          sia
      (2) Includes Alzheimer's disease, Jakob-Creutzfeldt disease, Pick's
          disease, and cerebrovascular accidents
   b. Subcortical dementia
      (1) Characterized by amnesia, slowness of thought, and lack of ini-
          tiative in all cognitive function. Disorders of movement and gait
          and depression in mood are frequent
      (2) Includes Parkinson's disease, Huntington's disease, and hydro-
          cephalus
   c. Focal cognitive syndromes
      (1) Characterized by relatively isolated deficits of memory or
          language
      (2) Includes chronic alcohol toxicity, thiamine deficiency, posten-
          cephalitic syndrome, subdural hematoma, vitamin B_{12} deficiency
2. **DSM-IV,** *Diagnostic and Statistical Manual of Mental Disorders,* ed
   4: the complete diagnosis and clinical features of the DSM-IV classification system can be seen in the box on pp. 59-63. The 1994 clinical
   diagnostic criteria created by the American Psychiatric Association classify the dementias in the following schema
   a. Dementia of the Alzheimer's type
   b. Vascular dementia
   c. Dementia caused by other general medical conditions
      (1) HIV disease
      (2) Head trauma
      (3) Parkinson's disease
      (4) Huntington's disease
      (5) Pick's disease
      (6) Jakob-Creutzfeldt disease
      (7) Normal-pressure hydrocephalus

Text continued on p. 63.

Dementia

Dementia of the Alzheimer's Type

A. The development of multiple cognitive deficits manifested by both

   (1) Memory impairment (impaired ability to learn new information and to recall previously learned information)

   (2) One (or more) of the following cognitive disturbances:

      (a) Aphasia (language disturbance)

      (b) Apraxia (impaired ability to carry out motor activities despite intact motor function)

      (c) Agnosia (failure to recognize or identify objects despite intact sensory function)

      (d) Disturbance in executive functioning (i.e., planning, organizing, sequencing, abstracting)

B. The cognitive deficits in criteria A1 and A2 each cause significant impairment in social or occupational functioning and represent a significant decline from a previous level of functioning.

C. The course is characterized by gradual onset and continuing cognitive decline.

D. The cognitive deficits in criteria A1 and A2 are not due to any of the following:

   (1) Other central nervous system conditions that cause progressive deficits in memory and cognition (e.g., cerebrovascular disease, Parkinson's disease, Huntington's disease, subdural hematoma, normal-pressure hydrocephalus, brain tumor)

   (2) Systemic conditions that are known to cause dementia (e.g., hypothyroidism, vitamin B_{12} or folic acid deficiency, niacin deficiency, hypercalcemia, neurosyphilis, HIV infection)

   (3) Substance-induced conditions

E. The deficits do not occur exclusively during the course of a delirium.

F. The disturbance is not better accounted for by another Axis I disorder (e.g., major depressive disorder, schizophrenia).

Code based on type of onset and predominant features:

With early onset: if onset is at age 65 years or below

With delirium: if delirium is superimposed on the dementia

With delusions: if delusions are the predominant feature

With depressed mood: if depressed mood (including presentations that meet full symptom criteria for a major depressive episode) is the predominant feature. A separate diagnosis of mood disorder due to a general medical condition is not given.

Uncomplicated: if none of the above predominates in the current clinical presentation

With late onset: if onset is after age 65 years

Specify if:

With behavioral disturbance

Coding note: Also code Alzheimer's disease on Axis III.

Continued

Dementia—cont'd

Dementia Due to Vascular Disorders

A. The development of multiple cognitive deficits manifested by both
   (1) Memory impairment (impaired ability to learn new information or to recall previously learned information)
   (2) One (or more) of the following cognitive disturbances:
      (a) Aphasia (language disturbance)
      (b) Apraxia (impaired ability to carry out motor activities despite intact motor function)
      (c) Agnosia (failure to recognize or identify objects despite intact sensory function)
      (d) Disturbance in executive functioning (i.e., planning, organizing, sequencing, abstracting)
B. The cognitive deficits in criteria A1 and A2 each cause significant impairment in social or occupational functioning and represent a significant decline from a previous level of functioning.
C. Focal neurologic signs and symptoms (e.g., exaggeration of deep tendon reflexes, extensor plantar response, pseudobulbar palsy, gait abnormalities, weakness of an extremity) or laboratory evidence indicative of cerebrovascular disease (e.g., multiple infarctions involving cortex and underlying white matter) that are judged to be etiologically related to the disturbance.
D. The deficits do not occur exclusively during the course of a delirium.

Code based on predominant features:
   With delirium: if delirium is superimposed on the dementia
   With delusions: if delusions are the predominant feature
   With depressed mood: if depressed mood (including presentations that meet full symptom criteria for a major depressive episode) is the predominant feature. A separate diagnosis of mood disorder due to a general medical condition is not given.
   Uncomplicated: if none of the above predominates in the current clinical presentation
Specify if:
   With behavioral disturbance
   Coding note: Also code cerebrovascular condition on Axis III.

Dementia Due to Other General Medical Conditions

A. The development of multiple cognitive deficits manifested by both
  (1) Memory impairment (impaired ability to learn new information or to recall previously learned information)
  (2) One (or more) of the following cognitive disturbances:
    (a) Aphasia (language disturbance)
    (b) Apraxia (impaired ability to carry out motor activities despite intact motor function)
    (c) Agnosia (failure to recognize or identify objects despite intact sensory function)
    (d) Disturbance in executive functioning (i.e., planning, organizing, sequencing, abstracting)

B. The cognitive deficits in criteria A1 and A2 each cause significant impairment in social or occupational functioning and represent a significant decline from a previous level of functioning.

C. There is evidence from the history, physical examination, or laboratory findings that the disturbance is the direct physiologic consequence of one of the general medical conditions listed below.

D. The deficits do not occur exclusively during the course of a delirium.

Dementia due to HIV Disease
  Coding note: Also code HIV infection affecting central nervous system on Axis III.

Dementia due to Head Trauma
  Coding note: Also code head injury on Axis III.

Dementia due to Parkinson's Disease
  Coding note: Also code Parkinson's disease on Axis III.

Dementia due to Huntington's Disease
  Coding note: Also code Huntington's disease on Axis III.

Dementia due to Pick's Disease
  Coding note: Also code Pick's disease on Axis III.

Dementia due to Jakob-Creutzfeldt Disease
  Coding note: Also code Jakob-Creutzfeldt disease on Axis III.

Dementia due to . . . *[indicate the general medical condition not listed above]*
  For example, normal-pressure hydrocephalus, hypothyroidism, brain tumor, vitamin B_{12} deficiency, intracranial radiation
  Coding note: Also code the general medical condition on Axis III.

Continued

Dementia—cont'd

Substance-Induced Persisting Dementia

A. The development of multiple cognitive deficits manifested by both
   (1) Memory impairment (impaired ability to learn new information or to recall previously learned information)
   (2) One (or more) of the following cognitive disturbances:
      (a) Aphasia (language disturbance)
      (b) Apraxia (impaired ability to carry out motor activities despite intact motor function)
      (c) Agnosia (failure to recognize or identify objects despite intact sensory function)
      (d) Disturbance in executive functioning (i.e., planning, organizing, sequencing, abstracting)
B. The cognitive deficits in criteria A1 and A2 each cause significant impairment in social or occupational functioning and represent a significant decline from a previous level of functioning.
C. The deficits do not occur exclusively during the course of a delirium and persist beyond the usual duration of substance intoxication or withdrawal.
D. There is evidence from the history, physical examination, or laboratory findings that the deficits are etiologically related to the persisting effects of substance use (e.g., a drug of abuse, a medication).

Code (Specific substance)-induced persisting dementia: (Alcohol; inhalant; sedative, hypnotic, or anxiolytic; other [or unknown] substance)

Dementia Due to Multiple Etiologies

A. The development of multiple cognitive deficits manifested by both
   (1) Memory impairment (impaired ability to learn new information or to recall previously learned information)
   (2) One (or more) of the following cognitive disturbances:
      (a) Aphasia (language disturbance)
      (b) Apraxia (impaired ability to carry out motor activities despite intact motor function)
      (c) Agnosia (failure to recognize or identify objects despite intact sensory function)
      (d) Disturbance in executive functioning (i.e., planning, organizing, sequencing, abstracting)
B. The cognitive deficits in criteria A1 and A2 each cause significant impairment in social or occupational functioning and represent a significant decline from a previous level of functioning.
C. There is evidence from the history, physical examination, or laboratory findings that the disturbance has more than one etiology (e.g., head trauma plus chronic alcohol use, dementia of the Alzheimer's type with the subsequent development of vascular dementia).

> **Dementia Due to Multiple Etiologies—cont'd**
>
> D. The deficits do not occur exclusively during the course of a delirium.
>
> **Coding note:** Use multiple codes based on specific dementias and specific etiologies, e.g., dementia of the Alzheimer's type, with late onset, uncomplicated; vascular dementia, uncomplicated.
>
> **Dementia Not Otherwise Specified**
>
> This category should be used to diagnose a dementia that does not meet criteria for any of the specific types described in this section.
>
> An example is a clinical presentation of dementia for which there is insufficient evidence to establish a specific etiology.

Table from DSM-IV, *Diagnostic and statistical manual of mental disorders,* ed 4. Copyright American Psychiatric Association, Washington, 1994. Used with permission.

      (8) Hypothyroidism
      (9) Vitamin B_{12} deficiency
   d. Substance-induced persisting dementia
      (1) Alcohol
      (2) Inhalants
      (3) Sedative, hypnotic, or anxiolytic medications
   e. Dementia caused by multiple etiologies
      (1) Alzheimer's/vascular
      (2) Vascular/alcohol
      (3) Head trauma/alcohol
3. **Neuropathologic definitions**
   a. Alzheimer's disease: amyloid plaques and neurofibrillary tangles seen mostly in the postcentral and temporoparietal areas
   b. Vascular dementia: multiple areas of focal ischemic changes. Lacunas are tiny deep infarctions resulting from small arteries in subcortical structures, such as basal ganglia, thalamus, and internal capsule
   c. Pick's disease: swollen neurons (Pick's cells) and intraneuronal inclusions (Pick's bodies) seen mostly in frontal temporal lobes. May be accompanied by demyelination and gliosis of the frontal lobe white matter
   d. Frontal lobe dementia: no plaques or tangles, marked frontal gliosis and neuronal loss
   e. Parkinson's disease: predominant degeneration of dopaminergic cells in the substantia nigra, globus pallidus, putamen, and caudate
   f. Syphilis: diffuse degeneration with marked lymphocytic infiltration throughout
   g. Jakob-Creutzfeldt disease: spongiform neuronal degeneration and gliosis throughout the cortical and subcortical gray matter. White matter is spared
   h. Huntington's disease: disruption of the corticostriatothalamocortical relays

4. **Single–photon emission computed tomography definition:** another type of classification used single–photon emission computed tomography (SPECT), clinical evaluation, and autopsy diagnosis of 27 consecutive dementia patients seen at a university clinic.[1] Four different types of brain hypoperfusion were seen on SPECT
   a. Bilateral posterior temporal and parietal lobes (17/27)
      (1) Nine cases had Alzheimer's disease pathologic findings
      (2) One case had Alzheimer's and Parkinson's
      (3) One case had atypical Alzheimer's (diffuse)
      (4) Two cases had Lewy body variant of Alzheimer's
      (5) Two cases had Alzheimer's and ischemic foci
      (6) One case had Parkinson's disease pathologic findings
      (7) One case had diffuse cortical Lewy bodies
   b. Bilateral frontal lobes (7/27)
      (1) Four cases had frontal gliosis and neuronal loss
      (2) Three cases had Pick's bodies
   c. Mottled (2/27)
      (1) Two cases had Jakob-Creutzfeldt pathologic findings
   d. Focal (2/27)
      (1) One case had Alzheimer's and ischemic foci (noted above)
      (2) One case had focal laminar necrosis in right posterior region

Diagnosis

1. Chief complaint: families often bring patient to medical attention because of memory problems (e.g., repetitive questions, misplacement of items, missed appointments, getting lost away from home), hallucinations, disruptive behavior, insomnia, and anxiety/depression disorders
2. Initial screen of cognitive function: diagnosis requires a documentation of a decline in cognition from a previous level. Perform Folstein Mini-Mental State Exam (see Appendix XV)
   a. Orientation to time and space: based on intact registration and recall (short-term memory); orientation to space is preserved longer than orientation to time
   b. Registration: depends on hearing and paying attention; if patient unable to complete task, consider the diagnosis of delirium (see above)
   c. Attention and calculation: to avoid educational bias, use simple tasks such as saying the days of the week forward and backward or counting backward from 20 to 0; since this function is preserved very late in Alzheimer's disease, if patient unable to complete task, consider a frontal lobe dementia such as Pick's disease or delirium
   d. Recall: patients with early stages of dementia will make first errors in this function, often with no other errors in the examination. Errors in orientation follow next
   e. Language: patients with early stages of Alzheimer's disease will have specific difficulty drawing a clock showing a given time. This is a measure of the characteristic visual-spatial impairment
   f. Consider comprehensive neuropsychologic testing by a qualified neuropsychologist to confirm screening mental status testing. This testing

can help differentiate parietal-temporal dementias (AD or PD) from frontal-temporal dementias, such as Pick's, or focal dementias, such as vascular dementias

3. Medical history: review treatable causes of dementia
   a. Metabolic disorders (e.g., glucose, calcium, thyroid, renal, hypoxia)
   b. CNS infections (e.g., HIV, syphilis, viral encephalitis)
   c. Medication induced (see Chapter 7)
   d. Nutrition (vitamin B_{12}, folate, thiamine)
   e. Depression

4. Neurologic history: the onset and course of neurologic symptoms provide clues to the etiology
   a. Sudden onset suggests a stroke
   b. Subacute course over weeks and months suggests a tumor or Jakob-Creutzfeldt disease
   c. Early appearance of a spasticlike gait with urinary incontinence suggests hydrocephalus
   d. Rigidity, bradykinesis, etc. suggest Parkinson's disease
   e. A recent fall suggests subdural hematoma
   f. Insidious onset and progression in the absence of early motor signs suggest Alzheimer's disease
   g. Personality changes such as disinhibition, lack of insight, difficulty with concentration that outweighs memory problems suggest frontal lobe dementia

5. Physical examination: fever, atrial fibrillation, low cardiac output, dehydration, hyperthyroidism or hypothyroidism, and signs of infection are evaluated. Asymmetric motor signs, abnormal involuntary movements, bradykinesis, and gait disorders suggest a neurologic etiology

6. Laboratory evaluation
   a. Electrolytes, BUN, creatinine, calcium, glucose, magnesium, thyroid function tests, CBC with differential, vitamin B_{12}, folate, VDRL, blood levels of ethanol, any current medications
   b. CT scan and MRI may detect cerebrovascular accidents, hematomas, hydrocephalus, tumor, or other focal lesions
   c. PET (positron emission tomography) and SPECT (single–photon emission computed tomography) reveal specific location of hypometabolism in the different dementias. Currently they are available only as research instruments at large academic programs

Management of dementia syndromes

1. Establish cause of dementia (may be multifactorial)
   a. Alzheimer's disease
   b. Vascular dementia
   c. Parkinson's disease
   d. Thyroid disorders
   e. Subdural hematomas
   f. Hydrocephalus
   g. Depression
   h. Hyperglycemia, hypercalcemia
   i. Vitamin deficiency

2. Remove or replace all medications that may negatively influence cognitive function
   a. Acetaminophen 650 mg q4h while awake is an excellent strategy for primary pain management. For the short-term treatment of more serious pain (hip fracture and surgery, lower back muscle spasms), acetaminophen 1 g q4h while awake is well tolerated
   b. Nortriptyline 10 to 30 mg/day is an effective antianxiety agent. If the anticholinergic side effect is not tolerated, nefazodone (Serzone) at 50 mg po bid enhances both serotonergic and noradrenergic neurotransmitter function
3. Consider tacrine HCl (Cognex) therapy for patients with early stages of Alzheimer's disease. Tacrine HCl is a potent centrally acting anticholinesterase, which in theory improves cognitive function associated with Alzheimer's by replacing the known cholinergic deficiency. By blocking the enzyme responsible for breaking down choline, the patient experiences increased CNS cholinergic activity. There is uncertainty of the ability of tacrine therapy to make significant improvements in patient's cognitive function. It may be of limited benefit for a small group of Alzheimer's patients, those who are physically healthy with mild to moderate dementia
   a. Involve the patient and families in discussion about the possible risks and benefits of tacrine HCl. Your local Alzheimer's association has complete packages of literature for patients and families. Call 1-800-272-3900 for information
   b. Check baseline liver function tests
   c. Give initial dose of 40 mg/day q6wk and check liver function tests weekly for 3 months
   d. If liver function tests are within normal limits, increase to 80 mg/day for another 6 weeks and recheck liver function tests
   e. A reversible elevation of tranaminases occurs in at least 25% of patients. If this occurs, stop the tacrine HCl until they are normal and then restart medication at a lower dose
4. Treatment and prevention of vascular dementia[2]
   a. Brain-at-risk stage
      (1) At risk: hypertensives, smokers, diabetics, patients with atrial fibrillation, cardiac patients, and those with asymptomatic extracranial arterial disease
      (2) Therapeutic measures: smoking cessation, exercise, diet, potassium, estrogen replacement, antihypertensives, lipid-lowering drugs, anticoagulants for atrial fibrillation, and aspirin
   b. Predementia stage
      (1) History of TIAs, stroke, subtle cognitive impairments, and silent cerebral infarctions
      (2) Therapeutic measures: carotid endarterectomy for intracranial carotid stenosis, anticoagulants, aspirin, ticlopidine
   c. Dementia stage
      (1) Patients have atherosclerosis of extracranial arteries, cardiac embolism, intracranial small vessel disease
      (2) Therapeutic measures: antidepressants, antihypertensives, aspirin, and ticlopidine

5. For individuals with frontal lobe dementia, low doses of methylphenidate, such as 10 mg bid, are often useful to extend attention span
6. Educate patient and caretaker about increased susceptibility to
   a. Delirium from medications, changes in living situation, hospitalization, or stresses of any kind
   b. Anxiety, depression, paranoia, and hallucinations
7. Encourage family to create a calm, caretaking environment by structuring daily and weekly activities
8. Educate family about need to assist the patient in regular toileting every 2 to 3 hours to avoid incontinence. Easy on and off clothing is recommended
9. Educate patient and caretakers about the nature of amnesia, aphasia, apraxia, and agnosia and the disabilities they cause. Emphasize that the patient's feelings are quite intact despite loss of these cognitive functions. Help caretakers relate to the fear and/or frustration that the patient is experiencing
10. Encourage patient and family to discuss diagnosis openly, to make out durable power of attorney for health care and financial decision making
11. Encourage patient and family to take advantage of community resources for the care of those with dementing disorders
    a. Senior citizens and daycare centers
    b. Alzheimer's disease support groups (1-800-272-3900)
    c. Respite programs
    d. Geriatric assessment and care centers

References

1. Read SL et al: SPECT in dementia: clinical and pathological correlation, *J Am Geriatr Soc* 43:1243, 1995.
2. Hachinski V: Preventable senility: a call for action against the vascular dementias, *Lancet* 340:645, 1992.

Suggested readings

Caine ED, Grossman H, Lyness JM: Delirium, dementia, and amnestic and other cognitive disorders and mental disorders due to general medical conditions. In Kaplan HI, Sadock BJ, editors: *Comprehensive textbook of psychiatry,* ed 6, Baltimore, 1995, Williams & Wilkins.

Folstein MF et al: Mini-mental state: a practical method of grading the cognitive state of the patient for the physician, *J Psychiatr Rev* 12:189, 1975.

Francis J, Martin D, Kapoor WN: A prospective study of delirium in hospitalized elderly, *JAMA* 268:1097, 1990.

Inouye SK: The dilemma of delirium: clinical and research controversies regarding diagnosis and evaluation of delirium in hospitalized elderly medical patients, *Am J Med* 97:278, 1994.

Lipowski ZJ: Delirium (acute confusional states). In Hazzard WR et al, editors: *Principles of geriatric medicine and gerontology,* New York, 1994, McGraw-Hill.

Wolf-Klein GP: New Alzheimer's drug expands your options in symptom management, *Geriatrics* 48:30, 1993.

Selected Functiona
Syndrome

NUTRITION
Marsha D. Fretwell, MD

OBESITY

Definition

Obesity refers to an excess of body fat. Clinically useful measures of obesity include
- A body weight more than 30% above the age-, height-, and sex-specific population average
- A body-mass index (BMI), in kg weight/m height squared, that exceeds 27
- A waist/hip ratio of 1.0 for males and 0.85 for females

The two major types of obesity are central, or abdominal, and peripheral, or lower body.

Epidemiology

The prevalence of obesity depends on the definition used. In general, 10% of Americans are seriously obese, and 25% to 30% are overweight.

Significance

1. Central or abdominal type of obesity is highly associated with increased morbidity and mortality from atherosclerotic cardiovascular disease. Individuals with waist/hip ratios that exceed 1.0 for males and 0.85 for females are more likely to have the obesity-linked risk factors for atherosclerotic coronary artery disease, which include
   a. Hypertension
   b. Non–insulin-dependent diabetes mellitus
   c. Hyperinsulinemia
   d. Hypercholesterolemia
   e. Hypertriglyceridemia
   f. Reduced high-density lipoprotein cholesterol levels
2. All obesity is associated with increased morbidity from
   a. Cholelithiasis

   b. Endometrial cancer
   c. Osteoarthritis, especially of the knee

Diagnosis

1. Measurement of height and weight to calculate BMI

$$\frac{\text{Weight in kilograms}}{\text{Height in meters squared}} = \text{BMI}$$

2. Measurement of waist and hip to calculate waist/hip ratio

$$\frac{\text{Waist}}{\text{Hip}} = \text{Ratio}$$

3. Waist is measured at the narrowest point between the rib cage and iliac crests, and hip is measured at the maximal point for the buttocks

Causes of obesity

Weight gain requires an intake of energy that is greater than its expenditure. Once obtained, obesity is commonly maintained at a level of caloric intake insufficient to produce obesity, because the accompanying morbidity prevents physical activity. The cause of obesity is not fully understood. Potential explanations include

- A metabolic defect
- Abnormal regulation of satiety
- Fat cell size, number, and distribution
- Body image
- Diminished levels of physical activity
- Socioeconomic factors
- Genetics

Treatment of obesity

To date, obesity has resisted our best therapeutic efforts. In theory the treatment is simple: increase physical activity and reduce caloric intake. In reality, although many achieve short-term weight loss, over the years the results are dismal. Approaches include

- Diet
- Behavioral therapy
- Exercise
- Medications
- Surgery

Recently it has been suggested that obesity should be treated like hypertension or diabetes, as a chronic physiologically based disorder that requires ongoing medication therapy to reduce the excessive morbidity and mortality associated with the disorder. Programs of this type offer treatment with appetite suppressant drugs such as phentermine and fenfluramine or fluoxetine with interdisciplinary support by physicians, psychologists, nutritionists, and exercise physiologists.

PROTEIN-CALORIE MALNUTRITION

Definition

A serum albumin level less than 3.5 g/dl reflects visceral protein depletion.

Epidemiology

Twenty to sixty percent of older patients in hospitals and nursing homes suffer from inadequate nutrition and/or protein-calorie malnutrition.

Significance in medical care of older patients

1. Adequate protein nutrition is critical for maintenance of skin integrity, healing of surgical wounds, and effective functioning of the immune system for host defense against infections
2. The stress of acute illness and the use of glucose as the primary source of nutrition during the early stages of hospital care accelerate nitrogen wasting and protein malnutrition
3. Nourishing patients is perceived by caretakers as a central feature of excellent care; patients who become malnourished during the process of dying may be seen as a failure of caretaking

Diagnosis

1. History of weight loss
2. Measurement of height and weight
3. Serum albumin level (less than 3.5 g/dl equals visceral protein depletion). Appendix III describes other useful parameters

Treatable causes

REMEMBER: Older patients are likely to have multiple causes
1. Depression and failure-to-thrive syndromes
2. Drugs
3. Chronic obstructive pulmonary disease, CHF
4. Intestinal ischemia
5. Metabolic causes (hyperthyroidism)
6. Zinc deficiency (secondary to diuretics)
7. Malabsorption syndromes
8. Chronic impaction
9. Social factors (isolation, poverty, manipulation of caretaker to regain locus of control)

Treatment

All etiologic factors must be treated. Dietary consultation is useful to confirm diagnosis, plan appropriate diet supplementation, and educate the patient and family
1. Remove all offending drugs (see Chapter 7)
2. Remove impaction
3. Supplement intake of protein, vitamins, trace elements, fats, and carbohydrates
4. Treat depression and failure-to-thrive syndrome with low-dose tricyclic antidepressants, selective serotonin reuptake inhibitors (except fluoxetine HCl) or electroconvulsive therapy, if necessary

5. Maintain optimal pulmonary and cardiac function
6. Treat intestinal ischemia with nitrates or calcium channel blockers
7. Treat metabolic or malabsorption syndromes
8. Obtain social service consultation

WEIGHT LOSS

1. **Unexplained weight loss in ambulatory patients:** a review of unexplained weight loss in older ambulatory patients found these final diagnoses
   - Unknown etiology 24%
   - Depression 18%
   - Cancer (lung, colon, breast, pancreas, prostate) 16%
   - GI other than cancer (occult ulcers, achalasia, hepatitis) 11%
   - Hyperthyroidism 9%
   - Medications (e.g., procainamide, theophylline, thyroxine, nitrofurantoin) 9%
   - Neurologic abnormalities (Alzheimer's, CVA) 7%
   - Other (TB, poor intake, cholesterol phobia) 6%
2. **No obvious cause of weight loss:** a very gradual loss of weight is often noted over the last 6 months of life in individuals who have no observable medical illnesses. A number of age-associated changes might lead to a reduced caloric intake and weight loss in individuals over 85 years. These include
   a. Decreased demand (lower metabolic rate and reduced physical activity)
   b. Decreased sensory input (taste, smell, vision)
   c. Decreased feeding drive (neurotransmitters)
   d. Increased activity of satiety factors (cholecystokinin)

REFUSAL OF FOOD AND THE PLACEMENT OF FEEDING TUBES

1. The lowest level of function measured on Katz's Activities of Daily Living is the ability to feed oneself. Individuals who are unable to feed themselves because of cognitive or physical disabilities are usually hand fed by caretakers
2. When an older individual refuses food, one additional cause should be considered: preparation for death
3. Evaluation of this patient should include
   a. Comprehensive geriatric assessment to provide physician, patient, and family with complete and accurate prognostic information
   b. Careful focus on the treatable causes of weight loss and protein malnutrition, especially depression and impaction
   c. Respect for patient's preferences about tube feedings, both current and historic (see Chapter 10 for discussion of competency and proxy decision making)
   d. Continued support and care (including offerings of food) for those who refuse hand or tube feedings

DEHYDRATION

With aging, there is slow, chronic dehydration.

Risk factors

1. Age-associated changes such as decreased thirst perception, abnormal vasopressin responses to osmotic stimuli, and decreased ability of renal tubules to reabsorb water
2. Fear of urinary incontinence
3. Fear of dysphagia and aspiration
4. Administration of diuretics
5. Age-associated anorexia
6. Decreased water access as a result of immobility, poor visual acuity, and altered mental status
7. Acute medical illnesses with increased insensible losses from fever, diaphoresis, tachypnea, emesis, or diarrhea

Assessment

1. Weight loss, orthostatic BP, skin turgor, fever
2. Electrolytes, BUN, glucose, urinalysis
3. Charting of intake and output, including insensible loss

Treatment

1. Address underlying acute and chronic illness (e.g., infections)
2. Calculate free water deficit (FWD)

$$\text{FWD} = \text{Weight (kg)} \times 0.45 - (140/\text{serum Na}) \times \text{Weight (kg)} \times 0.45$$

3. Replace FWD at a rate of 25%/day
4. Monitor for signs of fluid overload
5. Monitor electrolytes and BUN
6. Address chronic risk factors (e.g., diuretics, fear of incontinence, immobility, confusion, dysphagia)

Suggested readings

Foster DW: Eating disorders: obesity, anorexia nervosa, and bulimia nervosa. In Wilson JD, Foster DW, editors: *Williams textbook of endocrinology,* ed 8, Philadelphia, 1992, WB Saunders.

Hoffman NB: Dehydration in the elderly: insidious and manageable, *Geriatrics* 42:35, 1991.

Morley JE: Nutrition and aging. In Hazzard WR et al, editors: *Principles of geriatric medicine and gerontology,* New York, 1990, McGraw-Hill.

Thompson MP, Morris LK: Unexplained weight loss in the ambulatory elderly, *J Am Geriatr Soc* 39:497, 1991.

Weintraub M et al: Long-term weight control: the National Heart, Lung, and Blood Institute funded multimodal intervention study, *Clin Pharmacol Ther* 51(5; suppl):581, 1992.

5.2   URINARY INCONTINENCE
Marsha D. Fretwell, MD

Epidemiology

1. The prevalence of urinary incontinence increases with age. It is 11% in men and 17% in women over 65 and increases to over 20% after age 80
2. The prevalence also varies with the general health of the patient. It is 25% in elderly living in the community, 35% in acute care hospitals, and over 50% in the institutionalized elderly

3. The economic cost of incontinence exceeded $10 billion in 1987. The average cost for supplies and laundry alone exceeds $1000/yr for each incontinent person living in the community. The cost in social terms is even more impressive (social isolation, interference with domestic life and ADLs, scorn and derision by society in general, institutionalization of the patient)

4. Physicians in general have a low awareness of incontinence. Less than one third of community physicians document incontinence on patient problem lists. A recent study revealed that 24% of incontinent patients believed that the physician or nurse with whom they had discussed their problem was either embarrassed or unsympathetic and nearly 40% of patients assumed that their urinary incontinence was a result of their age

Physiology of micturition

1. Understanding incontinence requires knowledge of the fundamentals of the complex physiology of micturition

2. Figure 5-1 illustrates the three major components involved in urine storage and release
   a. Central nervous system (CNS): inhibition from the cortical (frontal lobe) micturition center permits bladder relaxation and filling and sphincter closure to prevent leakage of urine. When cortical inhibition ceases (e.g., the patient wants to urinate), the brainstem (pontine) micturition center sends impulses down the spinal cord to the detrusor muscle, resulting in muscle contraction
   b. Bladder: increase in bladder volume stimulates proprioception receptors in the bladder wall and results in transmission of sensory impulses through the sacral nerves (S2-S4 roots) to trigger bladder contraction. This stimulus for bladder contraction is under inhibitory control by the central inhibitory center. Cholinergic stimulation (e.g., bethanechol, urecholine) results in bladder contraction
   c. Bladder outlet: the two major factors in maintaining urethral pressure are the internal and external urethral sphincters
      (1) Internal sphincter: alpha-adrenergic stimulation causes muscle contraction, preventing flow of urine
      (2) External sphincter: it consists of striated muscle under voluntary control. Contraction prevents flow of urine. Estrogen deficiency in women can result in decreased competence of the internal and external sphincters

Age-related changes in urologic function

Normal aging does not cause urinary incontinence. The following changes can, however, contribute to incontinence

1. Decreased bladder capacity
2. Increased residual urine
3. Increased uninhibited bladder contractions
4. Increased nocturnal sodium and fluid excretion
5. Decreased urethral resistance in women associated with decrease in estrogen
6. Increased urethral resistance in males associated with enlargement of prostate gland
7. Weakness of pelvic floor muscles in women

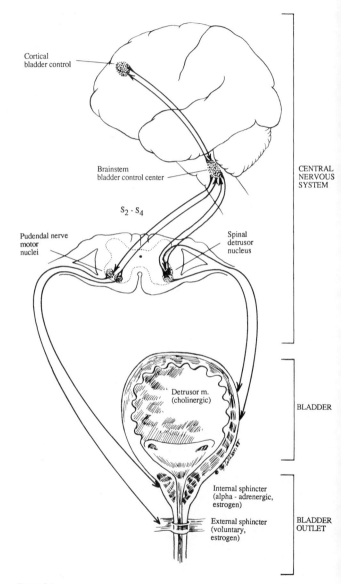

Figure 5-1

Simplified diagram of neurologic bladder control. (Redrawn from Lavizzo-Mourey SC et al: *Practicing prevention for the elderly,* Philadelphia, 1989, Hanley & Belfus.)

Types of incontinence

1. **Stress incontinence:** patient is aware but involuntarily loses small amounts of urine with increases in intraabdominal pressure (e.g., laughing, coughing, exercising)
2. **Urge incontinence:** patient is aware but leaks large volumes of urine because of inability to delay voiding after sensation of bladder fullness is perceived
3. **Overflow incontinence:** patient is not aware of small volumes of urine being continually leaked as a result of the mechanical forces on an overextended bladder

Clinical evaluation of the incontinent patient

1. History
   a. Type (stress, urge, overflow, or mixed)
   b. Timing (new onset, persistent)
   c. Flow pattern (large infrequent flow, small intermittent flow, time of day or night)
   d. Associated symptoms (straining to void, dripping, dysuria, incomplete emptying)
   e. Pertinent associated diagnoses (cancer, diabetes, acute illness, neurologic disease, lower urinary tract surgery)
   f. Medications, including over-the-counter drugs
2. Physical examination
   a. Stress test for urine leakage with full bladder
   b. Palpation for bladder distention after voiding
   c. Pelvic exam (atrophic vaginitis or urethritis; prolapse or pelvic mass)
   d. Rectal exam (resting tone and voluntary control of anal sphincter; prostate nodules; fecal impaction)
   e. Neurologic exam (cognitive function, sacral reflexes, perineal sensation)
3. Laboratory investigation
   a. Electrolytes, calcium, glucose, BUN
   b. Urine analysis and culture
   c. Chart of incontinence pattern
   d. Postvoid measurement of residual volume
   Figure 5-2 illustrates the suggested diagnostic flow diagram.

New onset of urinary incontinence

Many or most older patients are best described as "compensated incontinent," and any disruption of these carefully maintained compensation strategies (e.g., an acute illness, hospitalization, a change in location, introduction of new medications) may precipitate the acute onset of incontinence. Specific causes include

1. Diagnoses: acute symptomatic UTIs, polyuria associated with hyperglycemia and hypercalcemia, nocturia associated with occult CHF, atrophic vaginitis and urethritis
2. Medications
   a. Diuretics = polyuria, frequency, urgency
   b. Anticholinergics = urinary retention, overflow incontinence, impaction

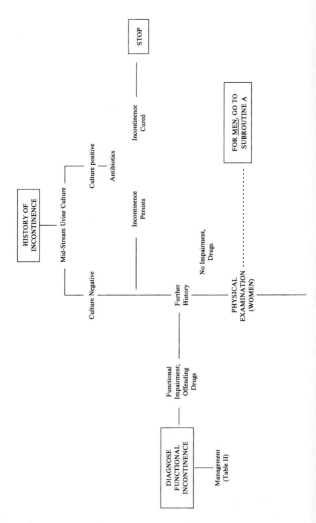

Figure 5-2
Flow diagram for evaluating urinary incontinence. (Redrawn from Lavizzo-Mourey SC
et al: *Practicing prevention for the elderly,* Philadelphia, 1989, Hanley & Belfus.)

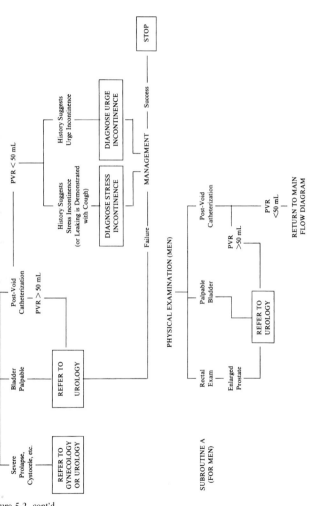

Figure 5-2, cont'd.
For legend see opposite page.

c. Psychotropics = anticholinergic actions, sedation, immobility, rigidity, delirium
d. Narcotic analgesics = urinary retention, fecal impaction, sedation, delirium
e. Alpha-adrenergic blockers = incompetent urethral sphincter
f. Alpha-adrenergic agonists = urinary retention
g. Beta-adrenergic agonists = urinary retention
h. Calcium channel blockers = urinary retention
i. Alcohol = polyuria, frequency, urgency, sedation, delirium, immobility

3. Nutrition: the use of 24-hour IV fluid therapy in immobilized older hospital patients may precipitate urgency, frequency, and nocturnal polyuria
4. Defecation: fecal impaction may lead to a mechanical obstruction of the bladder outlet and to urinary retention and overflow
5. Cognition: delirium disrupts the central cortical inhibiting influence over the sacral micturition center and leads to a restriction in mobility by physical or chemical restraints (see Chapter 4)
6. Emotion: depression and failure-to-thrive syndromes reduce motivation to be continent
7. Mobility: immobility of any and all etiologies disrupts appropriate toileting behavior
8. Cooperation with care plan: lack of information about nurse call bell or location of toilet, urinal, or bedpan reduces patient's ability to cooperate with continence care plan

Mnemonics and acronyms to evaluate most common causes of acute, reversible incontinence

1. Resnick's mnemonic "DIAPPERS"
   D = Delirium and dementia
   I = Infections
   A = Atrophic vaginitis, atrophic urethritis, atonic bladder
   P = Psychologic causes (e.g., depression), prostatism
   P = Pharmacologic agents
   E = Endocrine abnormalities (diabetes, hypercalcemia, hypothyroidism)
   R = Restricted mobility (severe degenerative joint disease, restraints, postural hypotension)
   S = Stool impaction (causes up to 10% of incontinence in nursing homes)
2. The acronym "DRIP"
   D = Delirium
   R = Restricted mobility, retention
   I = Infection, inflammation
   P = Polyuria, pharmaceuticals

The prognosis of new onset urinary incontinence in the setting of hospitalization for acute illness is very good if appropriate interventions of the causes of transient urinary incontinence are applied. Over 75% of these patients will be cured by this approach. If after discharge and resolution of the acute illness the patient has persistent incontinence, further evaluation and intervention are always indicated.

'ersistent urinary incontinence

. Neurologic causes: Normal micturition requires coordination of both the central and peripheral nervous systems
  a. Cerebral cortex exerts a predominantly inhibitory influence on the sacral spinal cord reflex. Diseases such as dementia, delirium, stroke, and parkinsonism lead to an *urge incontinence without awareness*
  b. Brainstem, cerebellum, and suprasacral spinal cord exert a predominantly facilitatory and coordinating influence. Diseases such as stroke and multiple sclerosis lead to an *overflow incontinence without awareness,* referred to as *neurogenic* or *detrusor-sphincter dyssynergy*
  c. Sacral spinal cord reflexly controls bladder filling and emptying. Local irritations in the bladder and outflow obstructions lead to *urge incontinence with awareness.* Injuries to the sacral cord, persistent outlet obstruction, and diabetes mellitus lead to an acontractile bladder and *overflow incontinence without awareness*
. Urologic causes: normal micturition requires that the bladder and lower genitourinary tract appropriately perform their storage and emptying functions
  a. Failure to store urine may be caused by
    (1) A hyperactive or poorly compliant bladder (secondary to cystitis, stones, tumor, or diverticuli) leading to *urge incontinence*
    (2) Diminished outflow tract resistance (secondary to laxity of pelvic floor muscles, bladder outlet, or sphincter weakness) leading to *stress incontinence*
  b. Failure to empty bladder may be caused by
    (1) A poorly contractile bladder (secondary to diabetes mellitus) leading to *overflow incontinence*
    (2) Increased outflow resistance (secondary to anatomic obstruction by prostate, stricture, or cystocele) leading to chronic urinary retention and *overflow incontinence*
. Mixed types of incontinence: often more than one type of incontinence is present simultaneously. The most common example is the development of urge incontinence in a woman with a typical history of stress incontinence. In all patients, the goal of the evaluation and treatment is continence; if that is not achieved by treatment of the most obvious cause of incontinence, multiple etiologic factors must be considered

1anagement of persistent incontinence

. Complete clinical evaluation
. Is this incontinence of *new onset* during acute hospitalization? If so, proceed with assessment and treatment of the causes of transient incontinence as outlined above
. Does patient have a *postvoid residual volume* of greater than 150 ml? If so (and this is most often seen in older men), urologic consultation is recommended
. Does the patient have a *urinary infection?* If so, sterilize the urine
. Does the patient have any of the following? If so, urologic, gynecologic, or urodynamic consultation is recommended
  a. Recent history of lower urinary tract or pelvic surgery or irradiation

      b. Recurrent urinary tract infections
      c. Marked pelvic prolapse
      d. Marked prostatic enlargement or nodules
      e. Severe hesitancy, straining, or interrupted stream
      f. Hematuria

6. Does the patient have *stress incontinence?* If so, one or more of the following treatments should be attempted
      a. Pelvic floor or Kegel exercises
      b. Alpha-adrenergic agonists (imipramine, pseudoephedrine, or phenylpropanolamine)
      c. Estrogen (oral or topical)
      d. Biofeedback, behavioral training
      e. Surgical bladder neck suspension

7. Does the patient have *urge incontinence?* If so, one or more of the following treatments should be attempted
      a. Bladder relaxants (oxybutynin, flavoxate, or imipramine)
      b. Estrogen (if vaginal cell atrophy is present)
      c. Biofeedback, behavioral training
      d. Surgical removal of bladder irritants or outlet obstruction

8. Does the patient have *overflow incontinence?*
      a. Attempt to decompress bladder with short-term (10 days) indwelling or intermittent catheterization
      b. Surgical removal of obstruction
      c. Alpha-adrenergic blocker (prazosin)
      d. Intermittent catheterization as maintenance
      e. Indwelling catheterization

9. Is the patient still incontinent?
      a. Consider mixed incontinence of multiple etiologies
      b. Consider referral to incontinence specialist (geriatric nurse or physician, urologist, or gynecologist)
      c. Train the caretaker(s)
      d. External collection devices and incontinence undergarments and pads

Indications for use of Foley catheters

1. Short term
      a. Monitoring volume status in acute illness (should not exceed 3 or 4 days)
      b. Bladder decompression in overflow incontinence (10 to 14 days)
      c. Skin breakdown and pressure sores (this patient group has highest risk of nosocomial UTIs; every effort should be made to improve nutrition and mobility and remove catheter)

2. Long term
      a. Care of terminally ill
      b. Urinary retention that cannot be managed medically or surgically and is causing renal disease, UTIs, or persistent overflow incontinence

Suggested readings

Ouslander JG: Urinary incontinence. In Hazzard WR et al, editors: *Principles of geriatric medicine and gerontology,* New York, 1994, McGraw-Hill.

Resnick NR, Yalla SV: Management of urinary incontinence in the elderly, *N Engl J Med* 313:800, 1985.

DEFECATION
Marsha D. Fretwell, MD

1. There are two types of colonic motility: shuttling and mass peristalsis
   a. Shuttling of the fecal bolus between the haustra of the bowel is continuous, although decreased at night and increased after meals. Its purpose is to promote absorption of water from the fecal bolus
   b. Mass peristalsis occurs two to three times/day and is stimulated by the gastrocolic reflex and physical mobility. It moves the fecal bolus from the transverse colon to the rectum and creates the urge to defecate
2. Frequency of defecation and transit time are unchanged in active, older persons
   a. The normal range of frequency of defecation is from three times/day to three times/wk
   b. Transit time is markedly slowed by sedentary life-styles and low-fiber diets

CONSTIPATION AND IMPACTION

Definitions

1. Constipation: a change in bowel function, with diminished frequency of defecation and often increased difficulty with defecation
2. Impaction: the end result of prolonged exposure of accumulated stool to the absorptive forces of the colon and rectum

Etiology in older persons

1. Decreased physical mobility and low-fiber diets leading to prolonged colon transit time
2. Systemic diseases (e.g., hypothyroidism, uremia, hypercalcemia, depression, or neurologic disorders such as parkinsonism, cerebrovascular accidents, and diabetes)
3. Hypokalemia, hypomagnesemia
4. Medications (e.g., anticholinergics, codeine, aluminum hydroxide, calcium channel blockers, nonsteroidal antiinflammatory drugs, iron)
5. Diseases of the colon (e.g., irritable bowel syndrome, diverticulitis)
6. Dyschezia or the failure of the defecation mechanism

Presentation

1. Complaints about a change in daily pattern
2. Secondary fecal incontinence
3. Refusal to eat
4. Urinary retention or incontinence
5. Refusal or resistance to taking new medication

Clinical evaluation

1. History: focus on patient's perception of change in daily bowel habits, symptoms relating to the etiologic factors (e.g., diseases, depression, new drugs) listed before, particularly those of localized abdominal pain or rectal bleeding

2. Physical examination: focus on possible underlying systemic diseases and careful abdominal and rectal exams, including a guaiac testing of the stool
   a. Rectum full of stool suggests dyschezia
   b. Rectum empty suggests decreased motility of the entire colon
3. Laboratory or special studies
   a. Glucose, thyroid function, calcium, electrolytes, magnesium, and BUN
   b. Sigmoidoscopy and colonoscopy as indicated

Management

1. Acute impaction
   a. Impaction must be reversed immediately, using local maneuvers such as
      (1) Manual removal of hard fecal masses
      (2) Stimulant suppositories
      (3) Enemas
   b. Work closely with the family or nursing staff, with the goal of resolving this within 48 hours
2. Constipation
   a. Treat all underlying systemic diseases, especially depression
   b. Replace potassium and magnesium
   c. Remove or replace all offending medication
   d. Train bowel by utilizing timing of the postprandial gastrocolic reflex along with glycerin suppositories
   e. Increase patient mobility
   f. Increase daily intake of fluids and dietary fiber
   g. Use laxatives as shown in Table 5-1
3. Prevention: once constipation or impaction has been successfully treated, steps should be taken to ensure that it does not recur
   a. Encourage continuation of exercise and increase in dietary fiber
   b. Encourage regular bowel pattern
   c. Anticipate constipation when initiating any additional medications by choosing less constipating alternative or by adding laxative
   d. Monitor bowel function at every visit
   e. Educate caretakers

Complications in hospitalized older patients

When very old or cognitively impaired patients are admitted to the hospital for the treatment of acute illnesses, they are often unable to give histories or volunteer other complaints. Because of chronic illnesses, ongoing medications, and immobility, many of these individuals are already constipated and have impending or existing fecal impactions. This state is usually not addressed until the fourth or fifth day of hospitalization and has serious consequences for the patient.

1. Refusal of food or feedings: it is normal to resist food or feedings when one is unable to evacuate the bowel
2. Aspiration of food or feedings: this is caused by the well-intended attempts of caretakers to nourish patients
3. Avoid aspiration pneumonia as a complication of hospitalization by evaluating and reversing all fecal impactions within the first 48 hours of care

Table 5-1   Laxatives

Class	Agent	Dosage
Bulk-forming agents	Calcium polycarbophil (Fibercon)	2 tab qd-qid with 8 oz of liquid after each dose
	High-fiber supplement (Fibermed)	2 biscuits qd
	Psyllium hydrophilic mucilloid (Metamucil)	1 tbsp or packet qd-tid with 8 oz of liquid with each dose
	Psyllium, senna (Perdiem)	1 tbsp qd-bid with 8 oz of liquid with each dose
Osmotic agents	Lactulose (Chronulac, Cephulac)	1-2 tbsp qd-bid
	Sorbitol (30%-70%)	30 ml qd
	Glycerin suppository	1-2 qd
Stimulants	Castor oil	30-60 ml qd
	Bisacodyl (Dulcolax)	5-15 mg PO qd
	Phenolphthalein (Ex-Lax)	10 mg PR qd / 1-2 qd
Emollients	Casanthranol docusate sodium (Pericolace)	100 mg PO bid
Salts	Milk of magnesia	30 ml qd
	Magnesium citrate	30 ml qd

From Ferri FF: *Practical guide to the care of the medical patient,* ed 3, St Louis, 1995, Mosby.

FECAL INCONTINENCE

Overflow incontinence

1. Secondary to the impact of a chronically distended rectum on anal sphincter tone. Semisolid feces (in constipation) and watery diarrhea (in impactions) tend to leak out many times each day
2. Treatment is the same as that described under constipation and impaction

Anorectal incontinence

1. Associated with damage to the external pudendal nerve and consequent weakness in the pelvic floor musculature, loss of anal reflex, and loss of sphincter tone. The individual is aware but leaks fecal material several time each day
2. Treatment includes pelvic floor exercises, biofeedback, and often surgery. Referral to a surgeon specializing in anorectal surgery is recommended

Neurogenic incontinence

1. Associated with injury to higher cortical inhibitory centers. It usually follows a postprandial gastrocolic reflex
2. Treatment is directed at training the caretaker to anticipate and structure a bowel evacuation pattern. Modifications in diet, exercise, and medica-

tions combined with a regular trip to the toilet after meals will usually lead to continence

Symptomatic incontinence

1. Caused by a variety of colorectal diseases that cause significant diarrhea
2. Evaluation and treatment are directed at specific etiologies such as viral gastroenteritis or antibiotic-induced colitis. This should be carefully considered if fecal incontinence persists after the treatment of constipation and impaction

Suggested readings

Brocklehurst JC: Disorders of the lower bowel. In Abrams WB, Berkow R, editors: *The Merck manual of geriatrics,* Rahway, NJ, 1990, Merck Sharp & Dohme.
Cheskin LJ, Shuster MM: Colonic disorders. In Hazzard WR et al, editors: *Principles of geriatric medicine and gerontology,* New York, 1994, McGraw-Hill.

5.4 COGNITION

The most common syndromes leading to cognitive impairment are delirium and the dementias (see Chapter 4).

5.5 EMOTION
Marsha D. Fretwell, MD

ANXIETY DISORDERS

Definition

Anxiety disorders are defined by persistence (>6 months) of the following symptoms
1. Motor tension (shakiness, jumpiness, trembling, inability to relax)
2. Autonomic hyperactivity (sweating, palpitations, dry mouth, dizziness, hot or cold spells, frequent urination, diarrhea)
3. Apprehensive expectation (constant worry or anticipation of personal/ family misfortune)
4. Vigilance and scanning (distractibility, poor concentration, insomnia, edginess)

Epidemiology

Anxiety disorders are common in later life, with more than 5% of community-dwelling older persons meeting the DSM-IV criteria. Because of the association of anxiety with many medical diseases, with adverse drug reactions, and with delirium and dementia, as many as half of the patients in physicians' offices, acute care hospitals, and nursing homes may have one or more of the above symptoms of anxiety.

Significance in medical care of older patients

1. Anxiety disorders often underlie recurrent episodes of acute medical illness that appear resistant to best therapeutic efforts. These include patients with
   a. Hypochondrias
   b. Recurrent episodes of shortness of breath and chest pain

   c. Hypertension
   d. Peptic ulcer symptoms
   e. Irritable bowel syndrome
   f. Somatization
   g. A discrepancy between functional capacity and actual performance of the ADLs
2. Other complications of anxiety disorders include
   a. Alcohol abuse
   b. Insomnia
   c. Increased mortality of cardiovascular origin
   d. Depression
   e. Suicide

DEPRESSION AND FAILURE-TO-THRIVE SYNDROMES

Definitions

Depression and failure-to-thrive syndromes are best seen as part of the same continuum as anxiety and delirium. Acute anxiety attacks and delirium represent a psychophysiologic response to an acute, overwhelming stress; chronic anxiety disorders, depression, and failure-to-thrive syndromes represent a psychophysiologic response to a chronic, seemingly unresolvable stress.

   There are two major types of stresses: psychologic (usually loss of a significant other or a job) and physical (usually acute physical illness or chronic impairment). In medical practice this translates into three major clinical presentations of depression in older patients.

1. *Community-dwelling individuals* who have recently experienced a significant loss and whose initial presentation is one of depressed mood and loss of pleasure, accompanied by vegetative symptoms
2. *Recently ill or hospitalized individuals* whose initial presentation is primarily a failure-to-thrive or vegetative state (loss of appetite, energy, and sleep-wake rhythm) without clear symptoms of depressed mood. This group is best identified by a decline in physical and cognitive function that is out of proportion to or unexplained by the recent episode of illness
3. *Individuals with recent onset of delusions, hallucinations, or disruptive behavior* may represent an initial presentation of depressed mood and/or a failure-to-thrive syndrome (see Hallucinations, Paranoia, and Disruptive behavior)

Epidemiology

The prevalence of depression and failure-to-thrive syndromes varies among the sites of care and residence. Between 25% and 30% of hospitalized older individuals, 20% of individuals in a skilled nursing facility, and 5% of community-dwelling individuals meet the criteria for major depression.

SUICIDE

Most older individuals who commit suicide have seen their primary care physicians in the preceding month and have expressed symptoms of anxiety and depression. Patient characteristics that help to identify those at risk for committing suicide include
1. Male sex

2. Presence of painful or disabling physical illness; think particularly of impotence and incontinence following prostate surgery
3. Solitary living situation
4. Depression, especially associated with agitation, excessive guilt, self-reproach, and insomnia
5. Bereavement
6. History of previous attempt or psychiatric illness

Significance in medical care

Depression and failure-to-thrive syndromes promote the loss of physical, cognitive, and social function in older patients and prevent older individuals from regaining their physical and cognitive function following treatment of acute medical illnesses. Despite appropriate treatment of medical and surgical diseases, undiagnosed and/or untreated depression leads to poor patient outcomes.

Diagnosis

A comprehensive geriatric assessment (see Chapter 2) is particularly useful in clarification of diagnosis and implementation of treatment in this difficult group of patients.
1. Data base
    a. Chief complaint
        (1) Primary: symptoms of anxiety or depressed mood, difficulty swallowing, sleep, appetite
        (2) Secondary: failure to resolve medical problem despite best efforts of primary care and specialty physicians
    b. Initial screen of vision, hearing, and cognition: mild impairments in short-term memory may be promoting anxiety and/or interfering with cooperation with care plan
    c. Biomedical history: consider symptoms of hypothyroidism and hyperthyroidism, occult pulmonary emboli or metastases, carcinoma of the pancreas (see the box below)

Symptoms of Depression

The Differential Diagnosis of Depressive Symptoms in Late Life (DSM-IV) lists the following symptoms as diagnostic criteria for major depression:
- Depressed mood and/or loss of interest or pleasure plus four of the following:
    - Weight loss or gain
    - Insomnia or hypersomnia
    - Psychomotor retardation or agitation
    - Loss of energy
    - Feelings of worthlessness
    - Difficulty concentrating
    - Recurrent thoughts of death or suicide

    d. Psychosocial history: focus on current and past history of anxiety, depression, use of drugs and alcohol, paranoia, hallucinations, social skills, support system, family history of anxiety and depression

    e. Physical examination: focus carefully on the areas of health and symptoms of greatest concern to the patient; evaluate for hypothyroidism or hyperthyroidism

    f. Laboratory and diagnostic evaluation: obtain and review all old records to update the laboratory and diagnostic data base. Repeat only those tests that are necessary, since anxious, depressed older patients often experience unintentional adverse effects from diagnostic workups (i.e., GI workups)

2. Assessment: patient data are integrated and organized in the problem list (Table 5-2)

3. Care plan

    a. Within each area of concern, assess and identify reversible or potentially treatable etiologic factors

    b. Make treatment recommendations consistent with standard medical practice for each problem listed

    c. Reconcile recommendations against patient's preference for treatment

Treatment issues

1. When an anxiety or depression disorder is documented as the etiologic factor underlying recalcitrant and recurrent physical symptoms or there is a decline in physical and cognitive function that cannot be explained by physical disease (a failure to thrive), it is appropriate to focus on the management of these disorders as the primary and most effective means of resolving the patient's problems. The requirements for effective management of anxiety, depression, and failure to thrive are shown in the box below and in the box on p. 89

Requirements for Effective Management of Anxiety and Depression

1. A trusting and comforting relationship between the patient and the physician
2. A sensitivity to emotional distress and its individualized and complex manifestations in older individuals
3. A careful diagnostic process that reassures both the physician and the older patient that the anxiety- or depression-associated physical symptoms or disability are not disease based
4. A knowledge of various treatment approaches
    a. Psychologic
    b. Pharmacologic
    c. Electroconvulsive therapy
5. An effective referral network for counseling and when symptoms persist despite appropriate primary care management
6. Careful follow-up, especially if medications are prescribed

Table 5-2 Evaluation for anxiety, depression, and failure to thrive

Areas of Concern	Focus of Evaluation	
Diagnosis	Acute:	Delirium, MI, PAT, anemia, hypoglycemia, hypercalcemia, hypothyroidism or hyperthyroidism, metastases to lung, CNS tumor or metastases, cerebrovascular event
	Chronic:	Dementia, pulmonary disease, mitral valve prolapse, irritable bowel syndrome, lower back or other intractable pain syndromes
Medications	Drug toxicity	
	Anticholinergic, digoxin, prednisone, antihypertensive side effects, over-the-counter cold drugs, theophylline	
	Withdrawal of sedative-hypnotics (Xanax) and alcohol	
Nutrition	Caffeine, vitamin deficiencies	
	Difficulty with swallowing	
Continence	Increased frequency; fear of urge incontinence may underlie nocturnal arousal and anxiety	
Defecation	May experience either constipation or diarrhea	
Cognition	Impairment in short-term memory often underlies emergence of anxiety or depressive disorder in a susceptible individual	
Emotion	Check for the mood and vegetative (e.g., sleep, energy, appetite) signs of depression, hallucinations, paranoia, and delusions	
	Ask about suicide	
Mobility	Check for a reduction in personal and social mobility. Review diagnoses carefully to rule out physical etiologies such as Parkinson's disease or a cerebrovascular accident	
	Look for fear of falling	
Cooperation with care plan	Consider anxiety, depression, or failure-to-thrive syndromes whenever physical symptoms or reduced physical function persists despite a careful review of history, physical exam, and laboratory evaluation	

2. Many older patients have experienced lifelong mild symptoms of anxiety ("I've always been a worrier") that have not seemed to interfere with their functioning
   a. Unexplained loss of functioning is the clue to the clinician that the patient's coping strategies have been overwhelmed and specific treatment is indicated

Management of Failure-to-Thrive Syndromes
at the End of Hospitalization

1. Establish diagnosis by ruling out all disease or medication etiologies that might underlie the unexplained loss of physical and cognitive function
2. Work with nurses, dietitian, social worker, physical therapist, and family to create integrated care plan that addresses the malnutrition, incontinence, constipation, confusion, immobility, and difficulty with discharge planning simultaneously
3. Initiate tricyclic antidepressants
   a. Patient with anxious affect: nortriptyline
   b. Patient with flat affect: desipramine
4. Start low and move to maximal dosage of tricyclic antidepressants over 4 days:
   a. 55-75 years: 25-75 mg/day
   b. 76-85 years: 10-50 mg/day
   c. 86 years and up: 10-30 mg/day
5. Initiate dietary supplements, laxatives, physical therapy, and bladder training programs
6. Discuss prognosis and discharge planning with patient and family
7. Monitor tricyclic antidepressant blood levels
   a. Therapeutic levels: 50 to 150 μg/dl
   b. Maintain patients at lower threshold: 50 to 60 μg/dl
8. Therapeutic response (improved energy, appetite, and sleep) seen within 3 days of achieving therapeutic level
9. Once patient stabilized back in community (4 to 6 weeks), medication may be discontinued

   b. Merely acknowledging the current specific stresses or the general stresses associated with aging can be an important first step in treatment
3. Educating patients about anxiety, depression, or a failure-to-thrive syndrome as the cause of their disabling symptoms must be done without invalidating their perceptions of the reality of these symptoms. Once the physician is confident about the source of anxiety- or depression-related symptoms, careful management of the anxiety and depression must be balanced by setting limits on further testing, referrals to specialists, and new medications
4. Anxiety disorders and depression may often be associated with impairments of short-term memory in older patients, a finding that alters traditional approaches to treatment
   a. Anxiolytic benzodiazepines, often the first-line medications in the treatment of anxiety, may further impair cognitive function
   b. For that reason, low doses of tricyclic antidepressants and/or antipsychotics are recommended as a safer long-term alternative. Table 5-3 shows recommended management for anxiety disorders

Table 5-3 Recommended treatments for anxiety and depression

Category	Treatment of Choice
Generalized anxiety disorder	Pharmacotherapy (nortriptyline, buspirone, thioridazine, benzodiazepines, beta blockers) Psychologic (counseling, psychotherapy)
Obsessive-compulsive disorder	Pharmacotherapy (clomipramine, fluoxetine) Psychologic (cognitive-behavior therapy, psychotherapy)
Panic disorder	Pharmacotherapy (imipramine, nortriptyline) Psychologic (cognitive-behavior therapy)
Posttraumatic stress disorder	Psychologic (psychotherapy) Pharmacotherapy (buspirone, benzodiazepines)
Depression	Psychologic (psychotherapy) Pharmacotherapy (nortriptyline, desipramine, trazodone, lithium, doxepin) Electroconvulsive therapy

5. Depression may often be associated with significant vegetative or failure-to-thrive symptoms (sleep disorder, decreased appetite, poor energy), a finding that alters the approach to treatment
   a. Fluoxetine, a newer medication classified as a selective serotonin reuptake inhibitor (SSRI), is very useful in younger depressed patients but may intensify anorexia and weight loss in older patients
   b. If an older patient displays a degree of agitation or anxiety with the symptoms of failure to thrive, desipramine or some of the SSRIs may further increase these symptoms
   c. Nortriptyline is recommended for the more agitated depressed patient, whereas desipramine or one of the SSRIs such as paroxetine or sertraline is useful for the more psychomotor-retarded individual
   d. In all medications, begin with the lowest possible dosage for 3 to 5 days to ascertain if the patient is going to tolerate that particular type of antidepressant, then begin to titrate upward
   e. Often, individuals will need long-term continuation and maintenance of treatment to maintain quality of life
6. If patients with failure to thrive are particularly sensitive to the anticholinergic effect of the tricyclic antidepressant, a trial of methylphenidate may be useful. Some patients with failure to thrive respond with an increase in physical function to being given an accurate prognostic statement. These patients often feel that they are dying and that they will never leave the hospital. Accurate prognosis and a concerted movement to discharge should always be attempted as the first therapy

Severe and pharmacologically resistant major depressive disorders

Two groups of patients may require additional therapy: those with psychotic symptoms accompanying their depression and those who remain pervasively psychomotor retarded, anorexic, and sleepless, despite appropriate pharmacologic therapy.

1. Psychotic symptoms associated with depression are treated by adding an antipsychotic medication (thioridazine 10 to 30 mg/day) to the antidepressant therapy. Using both medications at the lowest effective dosage will prevent the development of an additive anticholinergic effect
2. Referral to a geropsychiatrist, an in-patient psychiatric treatment unit, and use of electroconvulsive therapy are all appropriate next steps when counseling and antidepressant medications have not been effective in controlling symptoms. Patients who experience multiple adverse reactions to low doses of several types of antidepressants may also benefit from a referral

PARANOIA

Definition

Paranoia is a state in which there are systematic delusions or beliefs that are persecutory in nature. Several clinically distinct syndromes are described

1. Abnormal suspiciousness: a person may have vague complaints of external forces plotting against him or her. Under the perception of a loss of control, these beliefs become focal and are often directed at children over the issue of finances
2. Abnormal suspiciousness associated with memory loss and delirium or attention deficits: an inability to find one's personal belongings or way in a familiar setting is often the trigger for suspecting others of plotting against one
3. Paraphrenia (late-onset): syndrome in which an individual not only believes that individuals are plotting against him or her (delusional thinking) but also experiences hallucinations (e.g., hearing noises on the roof or in the basement or experiencing electric shocks)

Epidemiology

Between 2% and 5% of community-dwelling older persons exhibit abnormal suspiciousness; the prevalence of delusions and hallucinations in older persons is 4% to 5%. Paraphrenia is often associated with female sex, social isolation, and a past history of difficult social interactions.

Diagnosis

Individuals with paraphrenia or paranoid delusions are usually willing to discuss them with a sympathetic clinician. One question often serves to identify patients who are paranoid: "Is anyone trying to harm you?"

Assessment

Whenever an older person experiences persistent delusional thinking or hallucinations, an assessment for dementia, delirium (see Chapter 4), offending medications (see Chapter 7), depression, or an anxiety disorder (see above) should be completed.

Treatment

1. A trusting and supportive relationship: the clinician is willing to listen to complaints and fears but must not deceive the patient by pretending to agree with paranoid beliefs. Responding to and validating the emotional affect of the complaints and hallucinations are important
2. Antipsychotic drug therapy: initial dosages may range from 10 to 25 mg/day of thioridazine. Although haloperidol (1 to 3 mg/day) or risperidone (0.5 to 1.5 mg/day) is also effective, these patients often require long-term therapy and must be monitored carefully for extrapyramidal side effects
3. Cooperation with treatment depends on the level of trust; assuring the older patient that the medication will help improve sleep and decrease anxiety and working with the family will help ensure initial compliance

HALLUCINATIONS

1. The new onset of hallucinations occurs most frequently in older patients who are experiencing
   a. Delirium and dementia
   b. Anxiety and depression
   c. Loss of vision and hearing
   d. Extreme old age
   e. Social isolation
2. Hallucinations are perceptions in the visual, auditory, olfactory, or touch realms that are experienced as very real by the individual patient, yet are not experienced by the observer

Evaluation

1. Assessments for dementia and delirium (see Chapter 4)
2. Assessment for offending medications
3. Assessment for depression (see Table 5-2)
4. In cognitively intact individuals assess for social isolation, anxiety, extreme age, loss of vision and hearing
5. Ask about inadequate lighting
6. Given the multiple etiologies and the anxiety that hallucinations provoke in patients and caregivers, comprehensive geriatric assessment is suggested for individuals who present with hallucinations (see Chapter 2)

Management

1. Considerations
   a. Whenever hallucinations are frightening or lead to disruption in the behavior of the patient, treatment is indicated
   b. It is important to note that patients appear truly unable to discern any difference between their hallucinatory and real perceptions
   c. Reassurance should be focused on the experienced feeling (i.e., fear), not on the patient's distortion of time and space
   d. Particularly in nondelirious patients, failure to validate their reality often frustrates and angers them. In this situation, it is appropriate and helpful to validate feelings without correcting the time-space orientation
   e. Time-space orientation is more useful as a long-term environmental strategy to structure daily activities for cognitively impaired individuals

2. Delirium
  a. The hallucinations that accompany the agitation of delirium should resolve with
    (1) Appropriate treatment of the underlying systemic disorder
    (2) The removal of the offending medications
    (3) Short-term treatment with haloperidol
  b. If they do not, the patient should be carefully evaluated for more long-term causes of hallucinations (see below)
3. Dementia
  a. The most common hallucinatory syndrome of dementia is referred to as "sundowning" because of its onset between 4 and 6 PM
    (1) It is more common in the winter, in new and stressful situations, and in patients with concurrent anxiety and depression
    (2) It is important to note that a patient may be alert and reasonably coherent on morning rounds and completely out of control at sundown; trust the family and nurses
    (3) Patients are often unable to articulate the content of the hallucinations and often wander aimlessly or appear agitated
    (4) Regular treatment with low doses of antipsychotics (thioridazine 10 to 25 mg or haloperidol 0.5 to 1 mg) and antianxiety agents (nortriptyline 10 to 25 mg) is preferred to physical restraints
4. Loss of hearing and vision
  a. In otherwise healthy and cognitively intact individuals, these hallucinations are not frightening and do not have to be treated with medications
  b. Every attempt should be made to optimize vision and hearing, by both medical referrals and changes in the person's home environment (e.g., improved lighting and telephones with volume controls)
  c. Social isolation exacerbates these hallucinations
5. Extreme old age
  a. In otherwise healthy and cognitively intact individuals, hallucinations may occur, especially in times of stress or with social isolation
  b. These hallucinations may frequently involve visions of individuals who have already died, i.e., parents or spouse, and have the characteristics of a dream state, except the older individual feels that the visions are really happening
  c. These individuals are also particularly susceptible to drug-induced delirium with hallucinations
  d. Once all reversible causes have been considered and only if the hallucinations are frightening and affecting overall function, medication with methylphenidate 5 to 10 mg/day sometimes helps the individual be able to keep these dreamlike hallucinations from impinging on their waking state
6. Social isolation
  a. This often exacerbates hallucinations in individuals with other predisposing problems
  b. Individuals with cognitive, vision, or hearing impairments are often isolated from human interaction despite living in nursing homes or with others
  c. The stimulation of caring human interaction is often the safest and most effective therapy for hallucinations

SLEEP DISORDERS

Age-related changes

Age-related disturbances of the circadian sleep-wake cycle lead to changes in sleep patterns. Older people

1. Spend more time in bed
2. Spend less time asleep
3. Are more easily aroused from sleep
4. May experience daytime fatigue and napping
5. Are less tolerant of phase shifts of the sleep-wake schedule (e.g., jet lag)
   Many healthy older individuals experience these age-related changes in sleep, yet feel refreshed and energetic during the day.

Definition and estimated frequency

Table 5-4 outlines the Association of Sleep Disorders classification.

Table 5-4   Major sleep disorders of the elderly

ASD* Classification	Clinical Problem	Estimated Frequency
Disorders of initiating and maintaining sleep	Sleep apnea	16%-18%
	Nocturnal myoclonus	0%-33%
	Restless legs	5%
	Psychophysiologic problem	21%-31%
	Psychiatric problem	18%-47%
	Drugs/alcohol	21%
	Symptoms of organic disease (e.g., arthritic pain, nocturia, nocturnal dyspnea, chronic brain syndrome)	Common; exact frequency unknown
Disorders of excessive sleepiness	Sleep apnea	28%-71%
	Nocturnal myoclonus	16%
	Narcolepsy	11%-29%
	Drugs	Common
	Miscellaneous (e.g., postinfection fatigue, chronic brain syndrome)	?Common
Disrupted sleep-wake cycle	Early morning arousal, evening drowsiness	?Common
Parasomnias	Abnormal sleep behaviors (e.g., nocturnal confusion, wandering, seizures)	?Less common

*Association of Sleep Disorders.

Diagnosis (Table 5-5)

1. Data base
   a. Chief complaint: individuals have difficulty falling asleep, staying awake during the day, or staying asleep for the entire night. They complain that they do not feel refreshed by the hours that they do sleep. Demented patients are often brought by the family or nursing home caretakers. Sleep apnea patients are also most often identified by family
   b. Initial screen of hearing, vision, and cognitive function: short-term memory impairments often underlie sleep disorders
   c. Biomedical and psychosocial history: Table 5-5 outlines the many interacting biomedical and psychosocial factors that may underlie a sleep disorder in an older person (e.g., nocturia, leg twitches, shortness of breath, or nightmares may awaken; worrying may prevent initiation of sleep; early morning awakening or extended morning sleep suggests depression)

Table 5-5   Evaluation for sleep disorders

Area of Concern	Focus of Evaluation
Diagnosis	Primary
	Sleep apnea syndrome
	Periodic leg movements
	Secondary
	Arthritis and other pain syndromes
	Respiratory or cardiac diseases
Medications	Timing of medications such as sympathomimetics or diuretics
	Long-term use of alcohol or sedative-hypnotics
	Nightmares initiated by propranolol, levodopa, reserpine, or withdrawal of benzodiazepines or alcohol
Nutrition	Timing or excessive use of coffee, teas, and soft drinks containing caffeine before bedtime
Continence	Fear of or actual urge type incontinence in an aware individual
Defecation	Fear of or actual fecal incontinence
Cognition	Delirium
	Dementia
Emotion	Anxiety disorders with arousal
	Depression
	Paranoid ideations
	Nightmares (dream anxiety)
Mobility	Immobility secondary to illness or sedentary life-style
Cooperation with care plan	Learned behaviors incompatible with sleep
	Alcohol use

    d. Physical exam: focus on signs of the primary and secondary diseases that may underlie a sleep disorder (e.g., obesity and hypertension in sleep apnea or occult CHF)

    e. Laboratory and diagnostic evaluation
       (1) Blood alcohol levels
       (2) Blood levels of medications
       (3) Oxygen levels or degree of oxygen saturation
       (4) Electrolytes

2. Assessment: patient data are integrated and organized in the problem list (Table 5-6)

3. Care plan
    a. Within each area of concern listed in Table 5-5, assess and identify the reversible or potentially treatable etiologic factors underlying the sleep disorder
    b. Make treatment recommendations consistent with standard of medical practice for each problem listed
    c. Reconcile recommendations against the patient's preference for treatment

Treatment

The basic elements of therapy of sleep disturbances are summarized in Table 5-6.

Medications

If the etiologic factors are assessed and appropriately treated, most older patients will achieve an adequate amount of sleep to maintain their quality of life and ADLs. Anxiety disorders and/or depression is the most common cause of sleep disorders in older patients. If no clear-cut diagnostic factor is apparent and the older patient is still symptomatic, trials of low doses (10 to 30 mg) of a slightly sedating tricyclic antidepressant such as nortriptyline at bedtime are often effective in reestablishing a normal sleep-wake rhythm or cycle. Additionally, bright lighting (300 to 500 watts halogen) from 4 to 9 PM, especially from September to March, can help regulate the diurnal rhythm and improve nighttime sleep.

DISRUPTIVE BEHAVIOR

Definition

As individuals age and become dependent on their families and other caretakers, certain behaviors may emerge that are disruptive to the caretaking relationship. Disruptive behavior are activities of a patient perceived by nurses or family caretakers to be physically or emotionally harmful to the patient, other patients in proximity, or caretakers themselves. These behaviors may include

1. Disturbed physical behavior: striking out, physical abuse of others, self-destructive behavior, throwing objects around the room, restless agitation

2. Resistance to restriction: removes Foley catheter or IV lines, wanders out of house or off the unit, enters others' rooms

Table 5-6 Treatment of sleep disorders in older patients

Area of Concern	Recommendation
Diagnoses	
Primary sleep disorders	
Sleep apnea syndrome	Weight loss, nasal oxygen, tracheostomy, referral to sleep disorder center
Periodic leg movement	Muscle relaxants (short-acting benzodiazepines)
Secondary diseases	
Pain	Acetaminophen 650-1000 mg q4h regularly
Shortness of breath	Optimize respiratory and cardiac function
Medications	Discontinue or replace offending drugs; introduce others
	Initiate alcohol withdrawal and treatment program
Nutrition	Minimize or alter timing of stimulants (coffee, tea, soda)
	Initiate alcohol treatment program
Continence	Evaluate and treat urinary incontinence
Defecation	Evaluate and treat constipation, impaction, or fecal incontinence
Cognition	Evaluate and treat delirium
	Evaluate and treat dementia
Emotion	Treat anxiety, depression, and paranoia
Mobility	Advise patient that daytime activities such as social involvement and regular physical exercise can improve sleep
Cooperation with care plan	Encourage patient to regularize and curtail hours in bed and be physically and socially active during the daytime
	Encourage patient to create an optimal environment for sleep (reduced noise and light)

3. Resistance to physical care: spits out or refuses medications, spits out food, resists assistance with ADLs
4. Disturbed verbal behavior: screams/yells, verbally abusive or threatening, repetitive vocalizations
5. Disturbed social behavior: urinates/defecates in inappropriate places, takes others' belongings, hoards items, sexually inappropriate behavior

Factors influencing disruptive behaviors

1. Patient characteristics: cognitive impairment, hallucinations, delusions, physical health status, immobility, incontinence
2. Characteristics of the physical and social environment: noise level, inadequate lighting, relocation from familiar to unfamiliar places, physical restraints, family malfunctioning
3. Characteristics of caretakers: expectations or tolerance of certain behaviors, educational experience, ethnic background, stress or frustration tolerance levels

Epidemiology

The prevalence of disruptive behavior in nursing home patients is 25% to 30%. Eighty percent of patients who exhibit disruptive behavior have cognitive impairments. Those disruptive patients with cognitive impairments are more likely to also have hallucinations.

Significance in medical and long-term care

Disruptive behavior can become a major obstacle to both diagnosis and treatment of medical diseases and the provision of long-term care. Attempts to manage disruptive behaviors with physical and chemical restraints often lead to progressive declines in patients' physical, cognitive, and emotional function and an increased susceptibility to falls and infections.

Diagnosis

Disruptive behavior is not a diagnostic term, and many different factors can interact to promote it in each individual. Again, comprehensive geriatric assessment (review of all medical diagnoses; adverse effects of existing medications; impairments in sensory and auditory perceptions and communication; cognitive impairments such as delirium; dementia, and hallucinations; emotional symptoms such as anxiety, depression, delusions, and paranoia; and immobility) is useful in systematically documenting and treating the various etiologic factors.

Management

Table 5-7 outlines the steps in the management of disruptive patients.

Suggested readings

Billig N et al: Pharmacologic treatment of agitation in a nursing home, *J Am Geriatr Soc* 39:1002, 1991.

Blazer DG: Anxiety disorders. In Abrams WB, Berkow R, editors: *The Merck manual of geriatrics,* Rahway, NJ, 1990, Merck Sharp & Dohme.

Blazer DG: Schizophrenia and schizophreniform disorders. In Abrams WB, Berkow R, editors: *The Merck manual of geriatrics,* Rahway, NJ, 1990, Merck Sharp & Dohme.

Blazer DG: Depression. In Hazzard WR et al, editors: *Principles of geriatric medicine and gerontology,* New York, 1994, McGraw-Hill.

Costa PT, McCrae RR: Personality and aging. In Hazzard WR et al, editors: *Principles of geriatric medicine and gerontology,* New York, 1994, McGraw-Hill.

Fogel BS, Fretwell MD: Reclassification of depression in the medically ill elderly, *J Am Geriatr Soc* 33:446, 1985.

Ford DE, Kamerow DB: Epidemiologic study of sleep disturbances and psychiatric disorders: an opportunity for prevention? *JAMA* 262:1479, 1989.

Table 5-7 Management of the disruptive older patient

Area of Concern	Recommendation
Diagnosis	Treat all active medical diseases
Medications	Remove or replace medications that may adversely affect patient
Nutrition	Respect patient's preferences for types of food and eating site
Continence	Evaluate and treat incontinence
	Place commode near bed
Defecation	Initiate bowel program to structure appropriate behavior
Cognition	Evaluate and treat delirium and any hallucinations
	Document degree of cognitive impairment
Emotion	Target pharmacologic treatments to specific states
	Anxiety, agitation
	Depression
	Paranoia
	Delusions
Mobility	Optimize patient's mobility
Cooperation with care plan	Understand premorbid personality and family function and structure care appropriately

Haponik EF: Sleep problems. In Hazzard WR et al, editors: *Principles of geriatric medicine and gerontology,* New York, 1994, McGraw-Hill.

Herrera CO: Sleep disorders. In Abrams WB, Berkow R, editors: *The Merck manual of geriatrics,* Rahway, NJ, 1990, Merck Sharp & Dohme.

Holroyd S, Rabins PV. Personality disorders. In Hazzard WR et al, editors: *Principles of geriatric medicine and gerontology,* New York, 1994, McGraw-Hill.

Laitman LB, Davis KL: Paraphrenias and other psychosis. In Hazzard WR et al, editors: *Principles of geriatric medicine and gerontology,* New York, 1994, McGraw-Hill.

Prinz PN et al: Geriatric sleep disorders and aging, *N Engl J Med* 323:520, 1990.

Reynolds CF: Treatment of depression in late life, *Am J Med* 97(suppl 6A):39S, 1994.

Sheikh JI: Anxiety disorders in the elderly. In Blazer DG, Hazzard WR, editors: *Current problems in geriatrics,* St Louis, 1991, Mosby.

Sternberg J et al: Disruptive behavior in the elderly: nurses' perception, *Clin Gerontol* 8(3):43, 1989.

Wells KB et al: The functioning and well-being of depressed patients: results from the medical outcomes study, *JAMA* 262:914, 1989.

 5.6   **MOBILITY**

Marsha D. Fretwell, MD

The ability to move freely in either the home environment or the larger community environment is critical to the physical and emotional independence that is valued by many older patients. Older patients with profound slowness or an abnormal pattern of ambulation are said to have a gait disorder.

Gait disorders

The etiologic factors that underlie gait disorders in older patients include
1. Diagnoses
   a. Neurologic diseases
      (1) Cerebrovascular accidents
      (2) Parkinson's disease
      (3) Normal-pressure hydrocephalus
      (4) Peripheral neuropathy
      (5) Cerebellar ataxia
      (6) Subdural hematoma
      (7) Vitamin B_{12} deficiency
      (8) Cervical tumors and spondylosis
      (9) Progressive supranuclear palsy
   b. Other diseases
      (1) Hypothyroidism
      (2) Hyperthyroidism
      (3) Unsuspected fractures
      (4) Osteoarthritis
2. Medications: any medication causing hypotension, dopamine depletion, proximal muscle weakness, or oversedation (see Chapter 7)
3. Nutrition
   a. Folate, thiamine, pyridoxine, vitamin B_{12} deficiencies
   b. Protein malnutrition
   c. Alcohol abuse
4. Cognition
   a. Delirium
   b. Dementia
5. Emotion
   a. Fear of falling or physically expressed anxiety disorder
   b. Depression and failure-to-thrive syndromes at the end of hospitalization for acute illness
6. Cooperation with care plan
   a. Sedentary life-style
   b. Environmental and social barriers

Falls

Although most falls are not associated with fractures, over 90% of hip fractures are the result of a fall, and fear of falling causes as many as 50% of older patients to limit their activities in some way to avoid falls. The most common factors associated with falls as a cause of hip fracture include
1. Diagnoses
   a. Parkinson's disease
   b. Cerebrovascular accidents
   c. Visual impairments
   d. Lower limb dysfunctions
2. Medications
   a. Long-acting barbiturates
   b. Antidepressants

3. Nutrition
   a. Lower body mass
   b. Postprandial orthostatic hypotension

Diagnosis

1. Data base (see Table 5-8 for predisposing risk factors and potential intervention)
   a. Chief complaint: the history of a fall, problems with balance, a gradual reduction in mobility, or no complaints are the usual presentation for an older individual who has a gait disorder
   b. Initial screen of vision, hearing, and cognition: difficulty with distant vision and a mild impairment in short-term memory may be present
   c. Medical history: review the treatable causes of a gait disorder: delirium; hypothyroidism and hyperthyroidism; Parkinson's disease; a series of small CVAs; medications that may influence balance, blood pressure, and alertness; symptoms of vitamin deficiencies; and weight loss
   d. Psychosocial history: check for anxiety about ambulation, depression, dependent personality, physical and social barriers to ambulation outside of home
   e. Physical exam: to detect deficits in motor, balance, and/or skeletal/joint function—orthostatic hypotension, arrhythmia, carotid or vertebrobasilar artery involvement, decreased vision, loss of balance and increased sway, deforming arthritis, limitation of joint range of motion, bradykinesis, tremor, decreased vibratory sense, asymmetric motor signs (see Table 5-9 for performance-oriented evaluation of balance and gait)
   f. Laboratory evaluation
      (1) Electrolytes, BUN, calcium, glucose, thyroid function test, CBC, folate, vitamin B_{12}, blood levels of ethanol and current medications
      (2) CT or MRI for patients with motor signs, gait apraxia of frontal origins, or ataxia of cerebellar origin
      (3) Cervical spine films for those with bilateral long-tract signs
      (4) Neurophysiologic studies (electromyography, nerve-conduction studies, and testing of evoked potentials) in patients with sensory abnormalities

Management of gait disorders and prevention of falls

Establish cause of gait disorder and/or fall (may be multifactorial). Treat all reversible specific causes, for instance

1. Diagnoses
   a. Parkinson's disease
   b. Vitamin B_{12} deficiency
   c. Cervical spondylosis
   d. Control of arthritis pain
   e. Syncope (see Chapter 6)
2. Medications
   a. Remove or replace all medications that interfere with motor, balance, or joint functioning
   b. Acetaminophen 650 to 1000 mg q4-6h while awake is excellent strategy for pain management of arthritis

Table 5-8   Predisposing risk factors and potential interventions

Risk Factor	Potential Interventions
Sensory	
Vision: close-range and distance perception, dark adaptation	Appropriate refraction; surgery; medications; good lighting
Hearing	Cerumen removal; hearing aid
Vestibular	
Drugs, previous infections, surgery, benign positional vertigo	Avoidance of toxic drugs; surgery; balance exercises, good lighting
Proprioceptive	
Peripheral nerves, spinal cord	Treatment of underlying disease; good lighting; appropriate walking aid and footwear
Cervical: arthritis, spondylosis	Balance exercises; surgery
Central neurologic	
Any central nervous system disease impairing problem solving and judgment	Treatment of underlying disease; supervised, structured, safe environment
Musculoskeletal	
Arthritides, especially lower extremities	Medical and possibly surgical treatment of underlying disease
Muscle weakness, contractures	Strengthening exercises; balance and gait training; appropriate adaptive devices
Foot disorders: bunions, calluses, deformities	Podiatry; appropriate footwear
Systemic diseases	
Postural hypotension	Hydration; lowest effective dosage of necessary medications; reconditioning exercises; elevation of head of bed; stockings
Cardiac, respiratory, metabolic diseases	Treatment of underlying diseases
Depression	Careful consideration to risk/benefit ratio of antidepressant medication
Medications	
All—especially sedating medications	Lowest effective dosage of essential medications, starting low and increasing slowly
Environment	Environmental hazard checklist; appropriate adaptations and manipulations

From Tinetti ME: Falls. In Hazzard WR et al, editors: *Principles of geriatric medicine and gerontology*, New York, 1994, McGraw-Hill.

Table 5-9 Performance-oriented evaluation of balance and gait

Abnormal Maneuver	Possible Causes*	Possible Therapeutic or Rehabilitative Measures†	Possible Preventive or Adaptive Measures†
Difficulty arising from chair	Proximal muscle weakness (many causes) Arthritides (especially involving hip and knees) Parkinson's syndrome Hemiparesis or paraparesis Deconditioning	Treatment of specific disease states (e.g., with steroids, L-dopa) Hip and quadricep exercises Transfer training	High, firm chair with arms Raised toilet seats Ejection chairs
Instability on first standing	Postural hypotension Cerebellar disease Multisensory deficits Lower-extremity weakness or pain Foot pain causing reduced weight bearing	Treatment of specific diseases (e.g., adequate salt and fluid status, fluorticone) Jobst stockings Hip and knee exercises Foot problem correction	Slow rising Head of bed on blocks Supportive aid (e.g., walker, quadcane)
Instability with nudge on sternum or pull test	Parkinson's syndrome Back problems Normal-pressure hydrocephalus ? Peripheral neuropathy Deconditioning	Treatment of specific diseases (e.g., with L-dopa, shunt) ? Back exercises Analgesia ? Balance exercises (e.g., Frankel's)	Obstacle-free environment Appropriate walking aid (cane, walker) Night-lights (less likely to fall if bump into object) Close observation with acute illness (high risk of falling) Avoidance of slippers

Continued

Table 5-9 Performance-oriented evaluation of balance and gait—cont'd

Abnormal Maneuver	Possible Causes*	Possible Therapeutic or Rehabilitative Measures†	Possible Preventive or Adaptive Measures†
Instability with eyes closed (stable with eyes open)	Multisensory deficits Reduced proprioception, position sense (e.g., B_{12} deficiency, diabetes mellitus)	Treatment of specific diseases (e.g., B_{12} deficiency) Visual, hearing problem correction	Bright lights Night-lights Cane
Instability on neck turning or extension	Cervical arthritis Cervical spondylosis Vertebral-basilar insufficiency	? Balance exercises ? Antiarthritic medication ? Cervical collar ? Neck exercises	Avoidance of quick turns Turning of body, not just head Storage of objects in home low enough to avoid need to look up
Instability on turning	Cerebellar disease Hemiparesis Visual field cut Reduced proprioception Mild ataxia	Gait training ? Proprioceptive exercises	Appropriate walking aid Obstacle-free environment Properly fitting shoes
Unsafeness on sitting down (misjudges distance or falls into chair)	Reduced vision Proximal myopathies Apraxia	Treatment of specific diseases ? Coordination training Leg-strengthening exercises	High, firm chairs with arms, in good repair Transfer training

Selected Functional Syndromes 105

Decreased step height and length (bilateral)‡	Parkinson's syndrome	Treatment of specific diseases (e.g., with L-dopa)	Avoidance of throw rugs
	Pseudobulbar palsy	Vision correction	Good lighting
	Myelopathy (usually spastic gait)	Gait training (correct problems, suggest compensations, increase confidence)	Proper footwear (good fit, not too much friction or slipperiness)
	Normal-pressure hydrocephalus		Appropriate walking aid
	Advanced Alzheimer's disease (frontal lobe gait)		
	Compensation for reduced vision or proprioception		
	Fear of falling		
	Habit		

From Tinetti ME: Falls. In Hazzard WR et al, editors: *Principles of geriatric medicine and gerontology*, New York, 1994, McGraw-Hill.

*This is not an exhaustive list.

†Most of these measures have not been subjected to clinical trials; evidence for effectiveness is usually anecdotal at best.

‡There will often be a flexed posture with all of these conditions.

3. Nutrition: replete with vitamins and protein; instruct in rising slowly after meals
4. Continence
   a. Evaluate and modify bathroom with nonslip tiles, grab bars, elevated toilet seat
   b. Treat urge incontinence
5. Cognition: treat delirium or metabolic encephalopathy
6. Emotion
   a. Treat fear of falling as any other chronic and debilitating anxiety disorder (see Section 5.4)
   b. Treat failure-to-thrive syndromes at the end of acute hospitalization with low-dose nortriptyline or desipramine (see Section 5.4)
7. Mobility
   a. Physical therapy with gait training and recommendations for ongoing muscle-strengthening exercises
   b. Evaluation of the home environment to remove loose throw rugs, secure all handrails, clear clutter in stairways, and tack down loose carpet edges
8. Cooperation with care plan
   a. Educate patient and family on the importance of all factors leading to gait disorders, immobility, and falling
   b. Emphasize the importance of daily physical exercise, motivation to change long-standing health behaviors, and reorganization of the home

Suggested readings

Cunha UV: Differential diagnosis of gait disorders in the elderly, *Geriatrics* 43:33, 1988.

Grisso JA et al: Risk factors for falls as a cause of hip fracture in women, *N Engl J Med* 324:1326, 1991.

Sudarsky L: Geriatrics: gait disorders in the elderly, *N Engl J Med* 322:1441, 1990.

 SEXUALITY AND AGING
Tom J. Wachtel, MD

SEXUAL ACTIVITY IN OLDER ADULTS

Human sexual expression is a multifactorial end point, which to date has been studied inadequately in the aged. Lopsided demographics combined with older male spouses in the majority of married couples, societal norms and expectations (current and, perhaps more relevant, from three quarters of a century ago), environmental and functional limitations, comorbidities, and physiologic changes of sexual function may all interplay and contribute to decreased sexual activity in older adults.

1. Demographics
   a. Women outlive men in the U.S. population (1987) because they have a 7-year longer life expectancy

Age	65-74	75-84	85+
Men	7,824,000	3,489,000	806,000
Women	9,844,000	5,811,000	2,061,000

b. Elderly women are more likely to be widowed because they outlive men in terms of life expectancy and outlive their husbands because they are typically younger than them

	Married	Widowed	Other
Marital Status[1]			
Men			
65-74	79.5%	9.3%	11.2%
75+	68.6%	22.7%	8.7%
Women			
65-75	49.9%	38.9%	11.3%
75+	23.4%	67.7%	8.9%

2. Societal norms and expectations
   a. Religious beliefs: sex as a means to procreate only
   b. Linkage of sexual desirability to youthful appearance
   c. Less permissive sexuality among older cohorts, thereby linking sex to marriage at a time when widowhood increases exponentially
   d. Unwillingness by adult children to accept or support new intimate relationships for their widowed parent
   e. Societal attitudes regarding sex in general and sex in the elderly in particular
3. External barriers to sexual activity
   a. Social isolation related to living arrangements[1]

	Live Alone	Live With Spouse	Other
Men			
65-75	12.0%	78.9%	8.8%
75+	19.9%	67.4%	12.8%
Women			
65-75	35.0%	49.1%	15.9%
75+	49.9%	22.8%	27.3%

   b. Lack of opportunity for social interactions
   c. Lack of opportunity for intimacy in many institutional settings
4. Nonsexual personal barriers to sexual activity or performance
   a. Functional limitations
      (1) Physical
         (a) Instrumental ADLs: transportation or communication problems
         (b) ADLs
         (c) Continence
      (2) Mental (dementia)
   b. Debilitating illness
   c. Neuromusculoskeletal illness limiting movement or causing pain with movement

    d. Psychologic
       (1) Depression
       (2) Anxiety, stress
       (3) Body image self-perception
       (4) Performance anxiety (males)
    e. Medications
       (1) Antihypertensives
       (2) Antipsychotics
       (3) Antidepressants (tricyclics and serotonin receptor inhibitors)
       (4) Narcotics
       (5) Anticholinergics
       (6) Anxiolytics/sedatives
       (7) Antiandrogens and estrogens in males
       (8) Antiestrogens and progesterone in females
       (9) Other
    f. Alcohol and drug abuse

GENITAL/SEXUAL PROBLEMS ASSOCIATED WITH AGING

Female

Current evidence suggests an independent epidemiologic association between menopause and sexual decline, although the effects of menopause and estrogen deficiency are difficult to separate from other interacting factors. Our understanding of sexual physiology is further complicated by individual variation. Indeed, some women experience enhanced sexual activity or satisfaction after menopause.

Nevertheless, the impact of estrogen deficiency is genital atrophy, manifested by atrophic vaginitis (with irritation and dyspareunia), clitoral and labial atrophy, decreased vaginal lubrication, and decreased clitoral tumescence during intercourse.

These changes can be prevented or postponed by treatment with topical or oral estrogens, and once established, changes can be treated with estrogens. In addition (in particular in women who will not or cannot use estrogens), a water-based lubricating jelly (e.g., KY) should be recommended. Lubricating jelly will also help a male with borderline erectile function achieve penetration.

Male

Impotence is defined as the sustained inability to achieve or maintain an erection of sufficient quality to permit penetration and ejaculation. Loss of libido is not impotence but may accompany it. NOTE: Ejaculatory control "improves" with aging.

Etiology*

1. Arterial insufficiency (large or small vessel disease)
2. Neuropathy
    a. Autonomic neuropathy (e.g., in diabetes)
    b. Spinal cord injury or other cord pathologic condition
    c. Brain pathologic condition (vascular, neoplastic, multiple sclerosis)

*See relevant chapters for details.

3. Toxic
   a. Alcohol
   b. Opiates
   c. Prescription drugs (e.g., antihypertensives, tricyclic antidepressants)
4. Endocrine
   a. Pituitary tumors or pathologic conditions (secondary hypogonadism)
   b. Primary hypogonadism (surgical or medical castration, genetic, trauma, infection, metabolic [e.g., hemochromatosis], toxic [e.g., alcohol])
   c. Thyroid dysfunction
   d. Adrenal dysfunction
5. Pelvic surgery (e.g., cystectomy, abdominopelvic bowel resection, prostatectomy)
6. Abnormal penile anatomy
   a. Congenital (chordee)
   b. Acquired (Peyronie's disease)
7. Any condition that causes painful intercourse
   a. Urethritis, prostatitis, epididymitis
   b. Penile skin infections (herpes, *Candida*)
   c. Lower back and hip arthropathies
8. Chronic debilitating illness
9. Psychogenic
   a. Stressful life situations
   b. Depression
   c. Anxiety
   NOTE: Preoccupation about successful sexual performance may lead to loss of arousal.

Evaluation

1. History
   a. Duration
   b. Absolute vs. relative impotence
   c. Loss of libido suggests a psychogenic cause or contribution or an endocrine cause
   d. Presence of morning erection suggests psychogenic cause
2. Examination
   a. Vascular exam
   b. Neurologic exam
   c. Exam of genitalia
   d. Signs of endocrine disease
3. Diagnostic procedures
   a. Urinalysis
   b. Fasting blood glucose
   c. Testosterone, LH, FSH, prolactin levels
   d. Thyroid function tests
   e. Nocturnal penile tumescence test at home or in sleep lab
   f. Noninvasive vascular testing
   g. Nerve conduction velocity
   h. Cystometrics for autonomic neuropathy

Treatment

1. Treat any underlying reversible organic cause (e.g., vascular reconstructive surgery); eliminate impotence-causing drugs (intramuscular testosterone injections should be used only in documented hypogonadism)
2. Intra–corpus cavernosum papaverine injection (3% priapism as complication): to be prescribed and monitored by a urologist (sometimes combined with phentolamine or prostaglandin)
3. Negative-pressure suction devices
4. Implantable penile prosthesis; two types
   a. Inflatable
   b. Permanently stiff

COUPLES ISSUES/SEXUAL COUNSELING

Some older couples are no longer engaging in sexual activities and have no interest in discussing the issue. Nevertheless, before laying sexuality to rest, the physician should ascertain the lack of interest or the unwillingness to discuss it with each partner separately if both partners are the physician's patients. In addition, book references for laypeople should be offered.

In many cases, even when patients do not volunteer concerns with sex in the course of the visits, they will acknowledge concern during a sexual history. Assuming that the workup and management of treatable conditions have been addressed and intercourse will not be possible, the physician should explore with the patient modes of sexual expression that may not involve actual coitus.

Marital discord in elderly couples who have remained together will usually have led to acceptable compromises that may not be wise to disrupt. In such situations, one or both partners may be interested in self-stimulation for sexual release and pleasure and should be reassured if necessary that masturbation is safe at any age. Couples who are interested in intimacy should be advised that sexual satisfaction with or without an orgasmic end point can be achieved in one or both partners without penetration. Such counseling sessions should begin by asking patients what currently happens during sexual encounters, as well as what used to happen before performance became impaired, in order to build from a starting point. This information is best acquired from each partner separately, although considerable tact may be needed when partners ask the physician to keep some points secret about the other partner.

Single and widowed patients may need specific advice to increase social contacts. Occasionally adult children may need counseling when they object to a surviving parent engaging in a new intimate relationship.

Reference

1. U.S. Bureau of the Census: 1986.

Suggested readings

Feldman HA et al: Impotence and its medical and psychological correlates: results of the Massachusetts Male Aging Study, *J Urol* 11:54-61, 1994.

Greselnfeld M, Newman J: *Love, sex, and intimacy after 50,* New York, 1991, Fawcett Combine.

NIH Consensus Conference: Impotence. NIH Consensus Development Panel on Impotence, *JAMA* 270:83-90, 1993.

Shabsign R, Fishman IJ, Scott FB: Evaluation of erectile impotence, *Urology* 32:83-90, 1988.

 PRESSURE ULCERS
Fred F. Ferri, MD

Epidemiology

1. Pressure sores affect up to 3 million persons annually
2. Annual expenditures exceed $5 billion[11]
3. The cost estimate to heal each pressure ulcer ranges from $5000 to $50,000
4. The prevalence of pressure sores varies between 3% and 14% in the community and acute care setting to 15% to 25% in long-term care facilities[8]
5. Less than 20% of pressure sores develop in the nursing home and in the home care setting; over 60% develop in the acute care setting[1]
6. There are over 17,000 litigations annually for the development of pressure sores,[10] with settlements as high as $4 million[3]
7. Sixty thousand people die each year from complications of pressure sores
8. The development of a pressure sore quadruples the risk of death for institutionalized patients
9. Osteomyelitis is present in 26% of nonhealing pressure ulcers
10. Bacteremia occurs in 50% of patients following ulcer debridement

Pathophysiology and risk factors[5-7]

1. Pressure ulcers occur as a result of four major factors
   a. **Excessive and prolonged pressure over a limited surface area**
      (1) Pressure is the most significant risk factor in the development of decubitus ulcers
      (2) Pressure results in decreased transcutaneous oxygen tension, vessel leakage, lack of nutrients, and accumulation of toxic metabolites with subsequent necrosis of muscle, subcutaneous tissue, dermis, and epidermis
      (3) The area of ischemia is cone shaped, with the wide base in the deeper tissues
      (4) Nearly all pressure ulcers develop at five classic sites (sacrum, ischium, greater trochanter, tuberosity of calcaneus, and lateral malleolus)
   b. **Shearing force**
      (1) Term refers to the sliding of adjacent surfaces with distortion of subcutaneous vessels and resulting tissue ischemia and necrosis
      (2) It typically occurs when the head of the bed is raised and the body slides downward, causing a compressive force on the posterior sacral tissues
   c. **Friction**
      (1) It usually occurs when an individual is pulled across the bed linen

    (2) Friction removes the protective stratum corneum and can result
        in development of intraepidermal blisters
  d. **Moisture**
    (1) It macerates tissue and predisposes to skin breakdown
    (2) It is generally secondary to fecal and urinary incontinence and per-
        spiration
2. Contributing factors
  a. Age-related skin changes: these may facilitate skin breakdown and
     may mask signs of ischemia (e.g., erythema and warmth from RBC
     engorgement in the capillaries may not be evident because of reduced
     local blood flow)
    (1) Delayed wound healing caused by slower epithelialization
    (2) Decreased proliferative ability and turnover in the stratum
        corneum results in altered skin barrier
    (3) Diminished pain sensation caused by decreased Pacini's and
        Meissner's corpuscles
    (4) Decreased elasticity favors skin breakdown
    (5) Decreased cell-mediated immunity (decreased density of Langer-
        hans' cells)
  b. Poor nutritional status: may be secondary to immobility, poor finan-
     cial status, isolation, poor dentition, and dementia
  c. CVA, fractures, bed or wheelchair confinement, impaired level of con-
     sciousness, weight loss, and hypotension are all independently asso-
     ciated with pressure sore formation

Prevention

1. Decrease pressure by repositioning (e.g., turning bedridden patient at
   2-hour intervals) and by using pressure-relieving mattresses
2. Minimize shearing force by avoiding prolonged "head elevated" position
   in bed and preventing patients from sliding down in bed with use of a
   footboard
3. Decrease friction by using drawsheets to position patients
4. Minimize moisture by improving bladder continence (see Section 5.2).
   Prompted toileting in nursing homes can reduce incontinent episodes in
   some demented patients to less than one wet episode per 12-hour period.[12] Fecal incontinence collectors, fashioned after an ostomy bag, are
   useful to minimize perineal irritation
5. Assess and improve nutritional status
6. Encourage activity and mobility. Assessment by physical/occupational
   therapist and rehabilitation nurse is useful to develop a mobilization
   plan
7. Institution of preventive measures for high-risk patients has been shown
   to decrease the incidence of pressure sores by more than 50%

Screening for development of pressure sores

Various screening instruments are available (e.g., Braden scale,[2] Norton
scale[9]) to assess risk factors in pressure ulcer development by taking into
account continence, mobility, mental status, general physical condition, and
nutritional status (Tables 5-10 and 5-11).

Treatment*

A pressure ulcer is defined as any lesion caused by unrelieved pressure resulting in damage of underlying tissue. Pressure ulcers are usually located over bony prominences and are graded or staged to classify the degree of tissue damage observed; however, pressure ulcers do not necessarily progress from stage I to stage IV or heal from stage IV to stage I. The staging of pressure ulcers recommended for use here is consistent with the recommendations of the National Pressure Ulcer Advisory Panel[4] Consensus Development Conference:

- *Stage I:* nonblanchable erythema of intact skin, the heralding lesion of skin ulceration. In individuals with darker skin, discoloration of the skin, warmth, edema, induration, or hardness may also be indicators.
- *Stage II:* partial-thickness skin loss involving epidermis, dermis, or both. The ulcer is superficial and presents clinically as an abrasion, blister, or shallow crater.
- *Stage III:* full-thickness skin loss involving damage to or necrosis of subcutaneous tissue that may extend down to, but not through, underlying fascia. The ulcer presents clinically as a deep crater with or without undermining of adjacent tissue.
- *Stage IV:* full-thickness skin loss with extensive destruction, tissue necrosis, or damage to muscle, bone, or supporting structures (e.g., tendon, joint capsule). Undermining and sinus tracts also may be associated with stage IV pressure ulcers.

These staging definitions recognize the following limitations:

- Stage I ulcers may be superficial, or they may be a sign of deeper tissue damage.
- Stage I pressure ulcers are not always reliably assessed, especially in patients with darkly pigmented skin.
- When eschar is present, a pressure ulcer cannot be accurately staged until the eschar is removed.
- It may be difficult to assess pressure ulcers in patients with casts, other orthopedic devices, or support stockings. Extra vigilance is required to assess ulcers under these circumstances.

HIGHLIGHTS OF PATIENT MANAGEMENT

Effective pressure ulcer treatment is best achieved through a team approach involving patients, their families or caregivers, and health care providers. The clinician should

- Discuss pressure ulcer treatment options with patients and their families.
- Encourage patients to be active participants in their care.
- Develop an effective plan of care that is consistent with the patient's goals and wishes.

The recommended treatment program should focus on the following areas

*Modified from Bergstrom N et al: *Pressure ulcer treatment: clinical practice guideline.* Quick reference guide for clinicians, No. 15., AHCPR Pub. No. 95-0653, Rockville, MD, Dec 1994, U.S. Department of Health and Human Services, Public Health Service, Agency for Health Care Policy and Research. Dec. 1994. *Text continued on p. 119.*

Table 5-10   Braden scale for predicting pressure sore risk

Patient's Name		Evaluator's Name
Sensory Perception Ability to respond meaningfully to pressure-related discomfort	1. **Completely limited:** unresponsive (does not moan, flinch, or gasp) to painful stimuli because of diminished level of consciousness or sedation, OR limited ability to feel pain over most of body surface.	2. **Very limited:** responds only to painful stimuli. Cannot communicate discomfort except by moaning or restlessness, OR has a sensory impairment that limits the ability to feel pain or discomfort over half of body.
Moisture Degree to which skin is exposed to moisture	1. **Constantly moist:** skin is kept moist almost constantly by perspiration, urine, etc. Dampness is detected every time patient is moved or turned.	2. **Moist:** skin is often but not always moist. Linen must be changed at least once per shift.
Activity Degree of physical activity	1. **Bedfast:** confined to bed.	2. **Chairfast:** ability to walk severely limited or nonexistent. Cannot bear own weight and/or must be assisted into chair or wheelchair.
Mobility Ability to change and control body position	1. **Completely immobile:** does not make even slight changes in body or extremity position without assistance.	2. **Very limited:** makes occasional slight changes in body or extremity position but unable to make frequent or significant changes independently.

From Braden BJ, Bergstrom N: *Decubitus* 2(3):44-51, 1989.
*TPN Total parenteral nutrition

Date of Assessment				
3. **Slightly limited:** responds to verbal commands but cannot always communicate discomfort or need to be turned, OR has some sensory impairment that limits ability to feel pain or discomfort in one or two extremities.	4. **No impairment:** responds to verbal commands. Has no sensory deficit that would limit ability to feel or voice pain or discomfort.			
3. **Occasionally moist:** skin is occasionally moist, requiring an extra linen change approximately once per day.	4. **Rarely moist:** skin is usually dry; linen requires changing only at routine intervals.			
3. **Walks occasionally:** walks occasionally during day but for very short distances, with or without assistance. Spends majority of each shift in bed or chair.	4. **Walks frequently:** walks outside the room at least twice per day and inside room at least once every 2 hours during waking hours.			
3. **Slightly limited:** makes frequent although slight changes in body or extremity position independently.	4. **No limitations:** makes major and frequent changes in position without assistance.			

Continued

Table 5-10 Braden scale for predicting pressure sore risk—cont'd

Patient's Name		Evaluator's Name
Nutrition Usual food intake pattern	1. **Very poor:** never eats a complete meal. Rarely eats more than one third of any food offered. Eats two servings or less of protein (meat or dairy products) per day. Takes fluids poorly. Does not take a liquid dietary supplement, OR is NPO and/or maintained on clear liquids or IV for more than 5 days.	2. **Probably inadequate:** rarely eats a complete meal and generally eats only about half of any food offered. Protein intake includes only three servings of meat or dairy products per day. Occasionally will take a dietary supplement, OR receives less than optimum amount of liquid diet or tube feeding.
Friction and Shear	1. **Problem:** requires moderate to maximum assistance in moving. Complete lifting without sliding against sheets is impossible. Frequently slides down in bed or chair, requiring frequent repositioning with maximum assistance. Spasticity, contractures, or agitation leads to almost constant friction.	2. **Potential problem:** moves feebly or requires minimum assistance. During a move skin probably slides to some extent against sheets, chair, restraints, or other devices. Maintains relatively good position in chair or bed most of the time but occasionally slides down.

	Date of Assessment				
3. **Adequate:** eats over half of most meals, eats a total of four servings of protein (meat, dairy products) each day. Occasionally will refuse a meal but will usually take a supplement if offered, OR is on a tube feeding or TPN* regimen, which probably meets most of nutritional needs.	4. **Excellent:** eats most of every meal. Never refuses a meal. Usually eats a total of four or more servings of meat and dairy products. Occasionally eats between meals. Does not require supplementation.				
3. **No apparent problem:** moves in bed and in chair independently and has sufficient muscle strength to lift up completely during move. Maintains good position in bed or chair at all times.					
	Total score				

Table 5-11 The Norton scale

Name	Date	Physical Condition		Mental Condition		Activity		Mobility		Incontinent		Total Score
		Good 4 Fair 3 Poor 2 Very bad 1		Alert 4 Apathetic 3 Confused 2 Stupor 1		Ambulant 4 Walk/help 3 Chairbound 2 Bed 1		Full 4 Slightly limited 3 Very limited 2 Immobile 1		Not 4 Occasional 3 Usually/urine 2 Doubly 1		

From Norton D: *Decubitus* 2(3):24-31, 1989.

- Assessment of the patient and the pressure ulcer or ulcers
- Managing tissue loads
- Ulcer care
- Managing bacterial colonization and infection
- Operative repair of the pressure ulcer or ulcers
- Education and quality improvement

Figure 5-3 provides an overview of the activities related to treatment of pressure ulcers. When applied to individual patients, this algorithm should be adapted to accommodate patient preferences and overall patient goals. Additional algorithms are provided throughout this section to summarize approaches to nutritional assessment and support, management of tissue loads, ulcer care, and management of bacterial colonization and infection.

ASSESSMENT

Assessment is the starting point in preparing to treat or manage an individual with a pressure ulcer. Assessment involves the entire person, not just the ulcer, and is the basis for planning treatment and evaluating its effects. Adequate assessment is also essential for communication among caregivers.

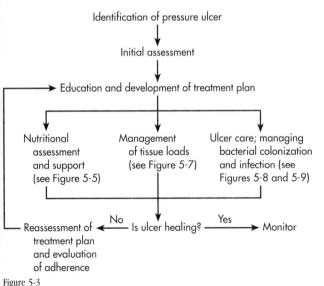

Figure 5-3
An overview of the management of pressure ulcers. (From Bergstrom N et al. *Pressure ulcer treatment: clinical practice guideline.* Quick reference guide for clinicians, No. 15. AHCPR Pub. No. 95-0653, Rockville, Md, Dec 1994, U.S. Department of Health and Human Services, Public Health Service, Agency for Health Care Policy and Research.)

This section discusses recommendations for assessing the pressure ulcer and the individual.

Assessing the pressure ulcer

Initial assessment. Assess the pressure ulcer or ulcers initially for location, stage, size (length, width, and depth), sinus tracts, undermining, tunneling, exudate, necrotic tissue, and the presence or absence of granulation tissue and epithelialization. (See Figure 5-4 for a sample pressure ulcer assessment guide.)

Reassessment. Reassess pressure ulcers at least weekly (as shown in Figure 5-4). If the condition of the patient or wound deteriorates, reevaluate the treatment plan as soon as any evidence of deterioration is noted.

Monitoring progress. A clean pressure ulcer with adequate innervation and blood supply should show evidence of some healing within 2 to 4 weeks. If no progress can be demonstrated, reevaluate the adequacy of the overall treatment plan as well as adherence to this plan, making modifications as necessary.

Assessing the individual

Assessment of the individual should address physical health, complications, nutritional assessment and management, pain assessment and management, and psychosocial assessment and management.

Physical health and complications

History and physical examination. Perform a complete history and physical examination, because a pressure ulcer should be assessed in the context of the patient's overall physical and psychosocial health.

Complications. Clinicians should be alert to the potential complications associated with pressure ulcers, such as amyloidosis, endocarditis, heterotopic bone formation, maggot infestation, meningitis, perineal-urethral fistula, pseudoaneurysm, septic arthritis, sinus tract or abscess, squamous cell carcinoma in the ulcer, and systemic complications of topical treatment (e.g. iodine toxicity and hearing loss after topical neomycin and systemic gentamicin). Three other complications—osteomyelitis, bacteremia, and advancing cellulitis—are discussed later in the recommendations for managing bacterial colonization and infection.

Nutritional assessment and management

Since many studies have linked pressure ulcers with malnutrition, screening for nutritional deficiencies is an important part of the initial assessment. The goal of nutritional assessment and management is to ensure that the diet of

---

Figure 5-4

Sample pressure ulcer assessment guide. (From Bergstrom N et al: *Pressure ulcer treatment: clinical practice guideline.* Quick reference guide for clinicians, No. 15. AHCPR Pub. No. 95-0653, Rockville, Md, Dec 1994, U.S. Department of Health and Human Services, Public Health Service, Agency for Health Care Policy and Research.)

Patient name: _____ Date: _____ Time: _____

Ulcer 1:		Ulcer 2:	
Site _____		Site _____	
Stage*_____		Stage*_____	
Size (cm) _____		Size (cm) _____	
Length _____		Length _____	
Width _____		Width _____	
Depth _____		Depth _____	

	No	Yes		No	Yes
Sinus tract	☐	☐	Sinus tract	☐	☐
Tunneling	☐	☐	Tunneling	☐	☐
Undermining	☐	☐	Undermining	☐	☐
Necrotic tissue	☐	☐	Necrotic tissue	☐	☐
Slough	☐	☐	Slough	☐	☐
Eschar	☐	☐	Eschar	☐	☐
Exudate	☐	☐	Exudate	☐	☐
Serous	☐	☐	Serous	☐	☐
Serosanguineous	☐	☐	Serosanguineous	☐	☐
Purulent	☐	☐	Purulent	☐	☐
Granulation	☐	☐	Granulation	☐	☐
Epithelialization	☐	☐	Epithelialization	☐	☐
Pain	☐	☐	Pain	☐	☐
Surrounding skin	☐	☐	Surrounding skin	☐	☐
Erythema	☐	☐	Erythema	☐	☐
Maceration	☐	☐	Maceration	☐	☐
Induration	☐	☐	Induration	☐	☐

Description of ulcer(s):
_____
_____

Indicate ulcer sites:

Anterior   Posterior
(Attach a color photo of the pressure ulcer(s) (optional))

*Classification of pressure ulcers:
Stage I: Nonblanchable erythema of intact skin, the heralding lesion of skin ulceration. In individuals with darker skin, discoloration of the skin, warmth, edema, induration or hardness may also be indicators.
Stage II: Partial-thickness skin loss involving erpidermis, dermis, or both.
Stage III: Full-thickness skin loss involving damage to or necrosis of subcutaneous tissue that may extend down to, but not through, underlying fascia. The ulcer presents clinically as a deep crater with or without undermining adjacent tissue.
Staage IV: Full-thickness skin loss with extensive destruction, tissue necrosis or damage to muscle, bone, or supporting structures (e.g., tendon or joint capsule).

Figure 5-4
For legend see opposite page.

the individual with a pressure ulcer contains nutrients adequate to support healing. The following recommendations and the algorithm in Figure 5-5 are designed to help the clinician meet this goal.

Adequate dietary intake. Ensure adequate dietary intake to prevent malnutrition to the extent compatible with the individual's wishes.

Nutritional assessment. Perform an abbreviated nutritional assessment, as defined by the Nutrition Screening Initiative, at least every 3 months for individuals at risk for malnutrition. These individuals include patients who are unable to take food by mouth or who experience an involuntary change in weight. (See Figure 5-6 for a sample nutritional assessment guide.)

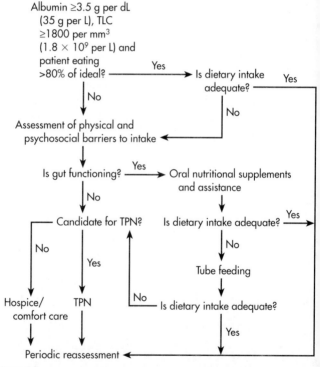

Figure 5-5

Nutritional assessment and support. *TLC,* Total lymphocyte count; *TPN,* total parenteral nutrition. (From Bergstrom N et al: *Pressure ulcer treatment: clinical practice guideline.* Quick reference guide for clinicians, No. 15. AHCPR Pub. No. 95-0653. Rockville, Md, Dec 1994, U.S. Department of Health and Human Services, Public Health Service, Agency for Health Care Policy and Research.)

Nutritional support. Encourage dietary intake or supplementation if an individual with a pressure ulcer is malnourished. If dietary intake continues to be inadequate, impractical, or impossible, nutritional support (usually tube feeding) should be used to place the patient into positive nitrogen balance

---

Patient name: _____ Date: _____ Time: _____

To be filled out for all patients at risk on initial evaluation and every 12 weeks thereafter, as indicated. Trends will document the efficacy of nutritional support therapy.

Protein compartments

Somatic

Current weight (kg) _____

Previous weight (kg) _____ (Date: _____)

Percent change in weight _____

Height (cm) _____

Height/weight _____

Current body mass index (BMI) _____ (wt/[ht]²)

Previous BMI _____ (Date: _____)

Percent change in BMI _____

Visceral

Serum albumin _____

(Normal ≥3.5 g per dL [35 g per L])

Total lymphocyte count _____ (optional)

(White blood cell count × percent lymphocytes/100)

Guide to total lymphocyte count:

• Immune competence ≥1800 per mm³ (1.8 × 10⁹ per L)

• Immunity partly impaired <1800 per mm³ (1.8 × 10⁹ per L) but ≥900 per mm³ (0.9 × 10⁹ per L)

• Anergy <900 per mm³ (0.9 × 10⁹ per L)

State of hydration

24-Hour intake _____ mL   24-Hour output _____ mL

Note: Thirst, tongue dryness in non-mouth-breathers and tenting of cervical skin may indicate dehydration. Jugular vein distension may indicate overhydration.

Estimated nutritional requirement

Estimated nonprotein calories _____ /kg   Estimated protein _____ (g/kg)

Actual nonprotein calories _____ /kg   Actual protein _____ (g/kg)

Recommendations/plan

1. _____

2. _____

3. _____

4. _____

Figure 5-6

Nutritional assessment of patient with pressure ulcers. (From Bergstrom N et al: *Pressure ulcer treatment: clinical practice guideline.* Quick reference guide for clinicians, No. 15. AHCPR Pub. No. 95-0653, Rockville, Md, Dec 1994, U.S. Department of Health and Human Services, Public Health Service, Agency for Health Care Policy and Research.)

(approximately 30 to 35 kcal/kg/day and 1.25 to 1.50 g of protein per kilogram per day) according to the goals of care. As much as 2 g of protein per kilogram per day may be needed.

Vitamin and mineral supplements. Give vitamin and mineral supplements if deficiencies are suspected or confirmed.

Pain assessment and management

The goal of pain management in the patient with pressure ulcers is to eliminate the cause of the pain, to provide analgesia, or both.

Assessment. Assess all patients for pain related to the pressure ulcer or its treatment. Caregivers should not assume that because a patient cannot express or respond to pain it does not exist.

Management. Manage pain by eliminating or controlling the source of pain (e.g., covering wounds, adjusting support surfaces, repositioning). Because pain may be evoked or may be especially acute during dressing changes and debridement, the caregiver should try to prevent such discomfort or take steps to relieve it. Provide analgesia as needed and appropriate.

Psychosocial assessment and management

The goal of a psychosocial assessment is to gather the information necessary to formulate a plan of care consistent with individual and family preferences, goals, and abilities. The goal of psychosocial management is to create an environment conducive to patient adherence to the pressure ulcer treatment plan.

Assessment of the individual. All individuals being treated for pressure ulcers should undergo a psychosocial assessment to determine their ability to comprehend the treatment program and their motivation to adhere to it. The assessment should include but not be limited to mental status, learning ability and signs of depression; social support; polypharmacy (i.e., taking many drugs concurrently) or overmedication; alcohol and/or drug abuse; goals, values, and life-style; sexuality; culture and ethnicity; and stressors. Periodic reassessment is recommended.

Assessment of resources. Assess resources (e.g., availability and skill of caregivers, finances, equipment) of individuals being treated for pressure ulcers in the home.

Goal setting. Set treatment goals consistent with the values and life-style of the individual, family, and caregiver.

Interventions. Arrange interventions (e.g., psychologic counseling, education) to meet identified psychosocial needs and goals. Follow-up care should be planned in cooperation with the individual and the caregiver.

MANAGING TISSUE LOADS

The goal of tissue load management is to create an environment that enhances soft tissue viability and promotes healing of the pressure ulcer. The term *tissue load* refers to the distribution of pressure, friction, and shear on the tissue. The interventions are designed to decrease the magnitude of tissue load and provide levels of moisture and temperature that support tissue health and growth. Tissue load management can be achieved through the vigilant use of proper positioning techniques and support surfaces, whether the individual is in bed or sitting in a chair. The algorithm in Figure 5-7 will guide clinical decisions on the management of tissue loads.

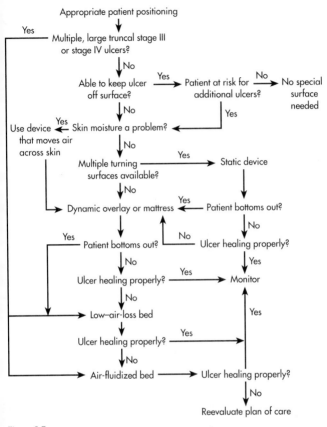

Figure 5-7

Management of tissue loads. (From Bergstrom N et al: *Pressure ulcer treatment: clinical practice guideline.* Quick reference guide for clinicians, No. 15. AHCPR Pub. No. 95-0653, Rockville, Md, Dec 1994, U.S. Department of Health and Human Services, Public Health Service, Agency for Health Care Policy and Research.)

Positioning techniques and support surfaces for patients in bed are important factors in the management of tissue loads.

Positioning techniques while in bed

Staying off the ulcer. Avoid positioning patients on a pressure ulcer.
Positioning devices. Use positioning devices to raise a pressure ulcer off the support surface. If the patient is no longer at risk for developing pressure ulcers, these devices may reduce the need for pressure-reducing over-

lays, mattresses, and beds. Avoid using donut-type devices, which are more likely to cause pressure ulcers than to prevent them.

Written schedules. Establish a written repositioning schedule based on the patient's risk for additional ulcers and on the response of the tissue to pressure. Patients at higher risk of additional ulcers and those with a longer duration of reactive hyperemia should be turned more frequently. Written repositioning schedules should be developed even when patients are using pressure-reducing support surfaces, because these surfaces are only adjuncts to strategies for positioning and careful monitoring of at-risk patients.

Positioning at-risk patients. Assess all patients with existing pressure ulcers to determine their risk for developing additional pressure ulcers.

- Avoid positioning immobile individuals directly on their trochanters, and use devices such as pillows and foam wedges that totally relieve pressure on the heels, most commonly by raising the heels off the bed.
- Use positioning devices such as pillows or foam to prevent direct contact between bony prominences (e.g., knees or ankles).
- Maintain the head of the bed at the lowest degree of elevation consistent with medical conditions and other restrictions. Limit the amount of time the head of the bed is elevated. The shear forces generated when an individual slides down in bed contribute to ischemia and necrosis of sacral tissue and undermining of existing sacral ulcers.

Support surfaces while in bed

When selecting a support surface for a patient, the primary concern should be the therapeutic benefit associated with the product. Various support surfaces have been shown to be useful in the improvement of pressure ulcers, but no compelling evidence shows that one support surface consistently performs better than all others under all circumstances. Therefore the caregiver should consider a variety of factors when selecting a support surface, including the clinical condition of the patient, the characteristics of the care setting, and the characteristics of the support surface.

Table 5-12 categorizes the various classes of support surfaces according to their performance in counteracting the different forces that contribute to the development of pressure ulcers. After determining which of these forces might be increasing an individual's risk for pressure ulcers, the caregiver may find this table useful in selecting a support surface for a particular patient. In addition to considering the features listed in Table 5-12, caregivers also need to consider other performance factors, such as ease of use, requirements for maintenance, cost, and patient preference.

It is important to remember that support surfaces are only one part of a comprehensive treatment plan. If an ulcer does not heal, the entire plan should be reevaluated before the support surface is changed.

The support surface should match the clinical condition and needs of the patient. The following patient characteristics should be considered when selecting a support surface.

Risk for additional ulcers. Assess all patients with existing pressure ulcers to determine their risk for developing additional pressure ulcers. If the patient remains at risk, use a pressure-reducing surface.

Table 5-12   Selected characteristics for classes of support surfaces

Performance Characteristics	Support Devices					
	Air-Fluidized	Low–Air Loss	Alternating-Air	Static Flotation (Air or Water)	Foam	Standard Mattress
Increased support area	Yes	Yes	Yes	Yes	Yes	No
Low moisture retention	Yes	Yes	No	No	No	No
Reduced heat accumulation	Yes	Yes	No	No	No	No
Shear reduction	Yes	?	Yes	Yes	No	No
Pressure reduction	Yes	Yes	Yes	Yes	Yes	No
Dynamic	Yes	Yes	Yes	No	No	No
Cost per day	High	High	Moderate	Low	Low	Low

From Bergstrom N et al: *Pressure ulcer treatment: clinical practice guideline. Quick reference guide for clinicals*, No. 15. AHCPR Pub. No. 95-0653, Rockville, Md. Dec 1994, U.S. Department of Health and Human Services, Public Health Service, Agency for Health Care Policy and Research.

Indications for static support surfaces. Use a static support surface if a patient can assume a variety of positions without bearing weight on a pressure ulcer and without "bottoming out." The caregiver can determine whether the patient has bottomed out by placing an outstretched hand (palm up) under the overlay below the pressure ulcer or below the part of the body at risk for a pressure ulcer. If the caregiver feels less than 1 inch of support material, the patient has bottomed out and the support surface is inadequate.

Indications for dynamic support surfaces. Use a dynamic support surface if (1) the patient cannot assume a variety of positions without bearing weight on a pressure ulcer; (2) the patient fully compresses the static support surface; or (3) the pressure ulcer does not show evidence of healing within 2 to 4 weeks.

Indications for low–air loss and air-fluidized beds. If a patient has large stage III or stage IV pressure ulcers on multiple turning surfaces, a low–air loss bed or an air-fluidized bed may be indicated. A low–air loss bed may also be indicated if the individual bottoms out or fails to heal on a dynamic overlay or mattress.

Need to control moisture. When excess moisture on intact skin is a potential source of maceration and skin breakdown, a support surface that provides airflow (e.g., air-fluidized and low–air loss beds) can be important in drying the skin and preventing additional pressure ulcers. While lying on this type of support surface, patients should not wear incontinence briefs because the briefs obstruct airflow to the skin. Follow manufacturers' instructions for using linen and underpads.

•   •   •

Positioning techniques and support surfaces for patients who are sitting are important factors in the management of tissue loads.

Positioning techniques while sitting

Avoiding pressure on the ulcer. A patient who has a pressure ulcer on a sitting surface should avoid sitting. If pressure on the ulcer can be relieved, limited sitting may be allowed.

Proper positioning. Consider postural alignment, distribution of weight, balance, stability, and pressure relief when positioning sitting individuals.

Frequent repositioning. Reposition the sitting individual so the points under pressure are shifted at least every hour. If this schedule cannot be kept or is inconsistent with overall treatment goals, return the patient to bed. Individuals who are able should be taught to shift their weight every 15 minutes.

Support surfaces while sitting

Cushion selection. Select a cushion based on the specific needs of the individual who requires pressure reduction in a sitting position. Avoid donut-type devices, which are more likely to cause pressure ulcers than to prevent them.

Written plan. Develop a written plan for the use of positioning devices.

ULCER CARE

Initial care of the pressure ulcer involves debridement, wound cleansing, the application of dressings, and possibly adjunctive therapy. In some cases, operative repair will be required. In all cases, specific wound care strategies should be consistent with overall patient goals. Figure 5-8 offers a recommended management approach to ulcer care.

Debridement

Moist, devitalized tissue supports the growth of pathologic organisms. Therefore the removal of such tissue favorably alters the healing environment of

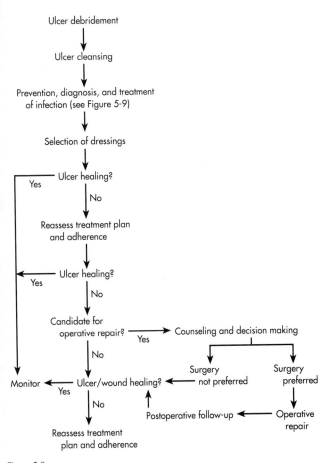

Figure 5-8
Ulcer care. (From Bergstrom N et al: *Pressure ulcer treatment: clinical practice guideline.* Quick reference guide for clinicians, No. 15. AHCPR Pub. No. 95-0653, Rockville, Md, Dec 1994, U.S. Department of Health and Human Services, Public Health Service, Agency for Health Care Policy and Research.)

a wound. Although debridement is a time-honored modality for treating pressure ulcers, it has not been studied in a randomized trial.

Removal of devitalized tissue. Remove devitalized tissue in pressure ulcers when appropriate for the patient's condition and when consistent with patient goals.

Selection of a method. Select the method of debridement most appropriate to the patient's condition and goals.

- Sharp, mechanical, enzymatic, and/or autolytic debridement techniques may be used when there is no urgent clinical need for drainage or removal of devitalized tissue.
- Sharp debridement involves the use of a scalpel, scissor, or other sharp instrument to remove devitalized tissue. This method is the most rapid form of debridement and may be the most appropriate technique for removing areas of thick, adherent eschar and devitalized tissue in extensive ulcers.
- If there is an urgent need for debridement, as with advancing cellulitis or sepsis, sharp debridement should be used.
- Those performing sharp debridement should have demonstrated the necessary clinical skills and should meet licensing requirements.
- Although small wounds can be debrided at the bedside, extensive wounds are usually debrided in the operating room or in a special procedures room. When debriding extensive stage IV ulcers in the operating room, the surgeon should consider performing a bone biopsy to detect osteomyelitis.
- Mechanical debridement techniques include wet-to-dry dressings, hydrotherapy, wound irrigation, and dextranomers.
- Enzymatic debridement is accomplished by applying topical debridement agents to devitalized tissue on the wound surface.
- Autolytic debridement involves the use of synthetic dressings to cover a wound and allow devitalized tissue to self-digest from enzymes normally present in wound fluids. This technique should not be used if the wound is infected.

Dressings during and after debridement. Use clean, dry dressings for 8 to 24 hours after sharp debridement associated with bleeding; then reinstitute moist dressings. Clean dressings may also be used in conjunction with mechanical or enzymatic debridement techniques.

Stable heel ulcers, an exception. Heel ulcers with dry eschar need not be debrided if they do not have edema, erythema, fluctuance, or drainage. Assess these wounds daily to monitor for pressure ulcer complications that would require debridement (e.g., edema, erythema, fluctuance, drainage).

Pain. Prevent or manage pain associated with debridement as needed.

Wound cleansing

Wound healing is optimized and the potential for infection is decreased when all necrotic tissue, exudate, and metabolic wastes are removed from the wound. The process of cleansing a wound involves selecting both a wound-cleansing solution and a mechanical means of delivering that solution to the wound. The benefits of obtaining a clean wound must be weighed against the potential trauma to the wound bed as a result of such cleansing. Routine wound cleansing should be accomplished with a minimum of chemical and mechanical trauma.

Cleansing. Cleanse wounds initially and at each dressing change.

Nontraumatic technique. Use minimal mechanical force when cleansing the ulcer with gauze, cloth, or sponges.

Avoidance of antiseptics. Do not clean ulcer wounds with skin cleansers or antiseptic agents (e.g., povidone-iodine, iodophor, sodium hypochlorite solution [Dakin's solution], hydrogen peroxide, acetic acid), because they are cytotoxic. Table 5-13 delineates a toxicity index by listing the dilutions required for various skin and wound cleansers to maintain the viability and phagocytic function of white blood cells exposed to these agents.

Normal saline. Use normal saline for cleansing most pressure ulcers.

Appropriate irrigation pressures. Use enough irrigation pressure to enhance wound cleansing without causing trauma to the wound bed. Safe and effective ulcer irrigation pressures range from 4 to 15 pounds per square inch (psi). Irrigation pressures below 4 psi may not cleanse the wound adequately, and pressures greater than 15 psi may cause trauma and drive bacteria into the wound tissue. Irrigation devices that deliver 8 psi of pressure are significantly more effective in removing bacteria and preventing infection than is a bulb syringe. Table 5-14 lists the irrigation pressure delivered by various clinical devices.

Whirlpool. Consider whirlpool treatment for cleansing pressure ulcers that contain thick exudate, slough, or necrotic tissue. Note that trauma can result if the wound is positioned too close to the high-pressure water jets. Discontinue whirlpool when the ulcer is clean.

Dressings

Pressure ulcers require dressings to maintain their physiologic integrity. An ideal dressing should protect the wound, be biocompatible, and provide ideal

Table 5-13 Toxicity index for wound and skin cleansers

Test Agent	Toxicity Index*
Shur Clens	1:10
Biolex	1:100
Saf Clens	1:100
Cara Klenz	1:100
Ultra Klenz	1:1000
Clinical Care	1:1000
Uni Wash	1:1000
Ivory Soap (0.5%)	1:1000
Constant Clens	1:10,000
Dermal Wound Cleanser	1:10,000
Puri-Clens	1:10,000
Hibiclens	1:10,000
Betadine Surgical Scrub	1:10,000
Techni-Care Scrub	1:100,000
Bard Skin Cleanser	1:100,000
Hollister	1:100,000

From Foresman PA et al: *Wounds* 5(5):226-231, 1993.
*The dilution required to maintain white blood cell viability and phagocytic efficiency.

Table 5-14   Irrigation pressures delivered by various devices

Device	Irrigation Impact Pressure (PSI)
Spray bottle—Ultra Klenz* (Carrington Laboratories, Inc., Dallas, Tex.)	1.2
Bulb syringe* (Davol Inc., Cranston, R.I.)	2.0
Piston irrigation syringe (60 ml) with catheter tip (Premium Plastics, Inc., Chicago, Ill.)	4.2
Saline squeeze bottle (250 ml) with irrigation cap (Baxter Healthcare Corp., Deerfield, Ill.)	4.5
Water Pik at lowest setting (#1) (Teledyne Water Pik, Fort Collins, Colo.)	6.0
Irrijet DS Syringe with tip (Ackrad Laboratories, Inc., Cranford, N.J.)	7.6
35 ml syringe with 19-gauge needle or angiocatheter	8.0
Water Pik at middle setting (#3)† (Teledyne Water Pik, Fort Collins, Colo.)	42
Water Pik at highest setting (#5)† (Teledyne Water Pik, Fort Collins, Colo.)	>50
Pressurized Cannister-Dey-Wash† (Dey Laboratories, Inc., Napa, Calif.)	>50

From Beltran KA, Thacker JG, Rodeheaver GT: *Impact pressures generated by commercial wound irrigation devices*, unpublished research report, Charlottesville, 1994, University of Virginia Health Science Center.

*These devices may not deliver enough pressure to adequately cleanse wounds.

†These devices may cause trauma and drive bacteria into wounds. They are not recommended for cleansing of soft tissue wounds.

hydration. The condition of the ulcer bed and the desired dressing function determine the type of dressing needed. The cardinal rule is to keep the ulcer tissue moist and the surrounding intact skin dry.

Selection of a dressing.   Use a dressing that will keep the ulcer bed continuously moist. (Wet-to-dry dressings should be used only for debridement and are not the same as continuously moist saline dressings, which keep the ulcer bed moist.) The following criteria should be considered when selecting a dressing:

- Dry surrounding skin. Choose a dressing that keeps the surrounding intact (periulcer) skin dry while keeping the ulcer bed moist.
- Exudate control. Choose a dressing that controls exudate but does not desiccate the ulcer bed. Excessive exudate may delay wound healing and macerate surrounding tissue.
- Caregiver time. Consider caregiver time when selecting a dressing. Film and hydrocolloid dressings require less caregiver time than do continuously moist saline gauze dressings.

  Clinicians should also consider the following:

- Prevention of abscess formation. Eliminate wound dead space by loosely filling all cavities with dressing material. Avoid overpacking the wound. Overpacking may increase pressure and cause additional tissue damage.

- Maintenance of dressings. Monitor dressings applied near the anus, because they are difficult to keep intact. Taping the edges of dressings (picture framing) may reduce this problem.

Adjunctive therapies

The roles of several adjunctive therapies in enhancing pressure ulcer healing have been investigated. The therapies considered by the panel included electrotherapy; hyperbaric oxygen; infrared, ultraviolet, and low-energy laser irradiation; ultrasound; miscellaneous topical agents (e.g., sugar, vitamins, elements, hormones, cytokine growth factors, skin equivalents), and systemic drugs other than antibiotics (e.g., vasodilators, hemorrheologics, serotonin inhibitors, fibrolytic agents).

At this time, electrotherapy is the only adjunctive therapy with sufficient supporting evidence to warrant recommendation by the panel. The panel recommends that clinicians consider a course of treatment with electrical stimulation for stage III and IV pressure ulcers that have proved unresponsive to conventional therapy. Electrical stimulation may also be useful for recalcitrant stage II ulcers.

To date this therapy has been limited to a small number of research centers. Clinicians considering electrical stimulation therapy should ensure that they have proper equipment and trained personnel who are following protocols shown to be effective and safe in appropriately designed and properly conducted clinical trials.

MANAGING BACTERIAL COLONIZATION AND INFECTION

Stage II, III, and IV pressure ulcers are invariably colonized with bacteria. In most cases, adequate cleansing and debridement prevent bacterial colonization from proceeding to the point of clinical infection. Recommendations regarding the management of colonization and infection follow. Figure 5-9 guides the clinician through a preferred pathway for managing ulcer colonization and local and systemic infection.

Pressure ulcer colonization and infection

Cleansing and debridement. Minimize pressure ulcer colonization and enhance wound healing by effective wound cleansing and debridement. If purulence or foul odor is present, more frequent cleansing and possibly debridement are required.

No swab cultures. Do not use swab cultures to diagnose wound infection because all pressure ulcers are colonized. Swab cultures detect only the surface colonization and may not truly reflect the organism or organisms causing the tissue infection.

Trial of topical antibiotic. Consider a 2-week trial of topical antibiotics for clean pressure ulcers that are not healing or are continuing to produce exudate after 2 to 4 weeks of optimal patient care (as defined in this guideline). The antibiotic should be effective against gram-negative, gram-positive, and anaerobic organisms (e.g., silver sulfadiazine, triple antibiotic). Monitor for allergic sensitization and other adverse reactions.

Diagnosis of soft tissue infection and osteomyelitis. Healing may be impaired if bacterial levels exceed 10^5 organisms per gram of tissue or if the patient has osteomyelitis. When the ulcer does not respond to topical anti-

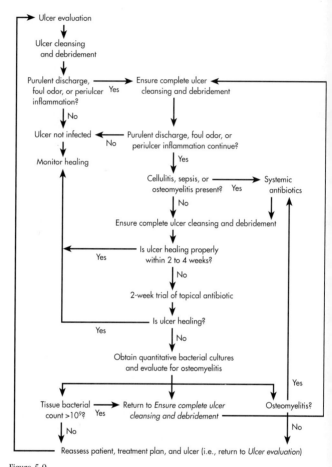

Figure 5-9

Managing bacterial colonization and infection. Suspicion of sepsis requires urgent medical evaluation and treatment. (From Bergstrom N et al: *Pressure ulcer treatment: clinical practice guideline.* Quick reference guide for clinicians, No. 15. AHCPR Pub. No. 95-0653, Rockville, Md, Dec 1994, U.S. Department of Health and Human Services, Public Health Service, Agency for Health Care Policy and Research.)

biotic therapy, the clinician should perform quantitative bacterial cultures of the soft tissue and evaluate the patient for osteomyelitis.

When cultures are required to diagnose a soft tissue infection, the Centers for Disease Control and Prevention recommend obtaining fluid through needle aspiration or tissue through ulcer biopsy.

Examination of a bone biopsy specimen is the gold standard for diagnosing osteomyelitis, but this invasive diagnostic technique is not always appropriate. A combination of three tests (white blood cell count, erythrocyte sedimentation rate, and plain radiography) has a positive predictive value of 69% when all three tests are positive.

No topical antiseptics. Do not use topical antiseptics (e.g., povidone-iodine, iodophor, sodium hypochlorite [Dakin's solution], hydrogen peroxide, acetic acid) to reduce bacteria in wound tissue.

Systemic antibiotics for systemic infections. Institute appropriate systemic antibiotic therapy for patients with bacteremia, sepsis, advancing cellulitis, or osteomyelitis.

Urgent medical attention is required for patients with pressure ulcers who develop clinical signs of sepsis (e.g., unexplained fever, tachycardia, hypotension, deterioration in mental status). It is appropriate to rule out other causes of the symptoms, obtain blood cultures, and treat with antibiotics that will combat these organisms. Systemic antibiotics are not required for pressure ulcers with only clinical signs of local infection.

Prevention of contamination. Protect pressure ulcers from exogenous sources of contamination (e.g., feces).

Infection control

The fear of cross contamination of microorganisms within institutions is realistic. The following recommendations are provided to prevent cross contamination of pathologic organisms.

Body substance isolation. Follow body substance isolation precautions or an equivalent system appropriate for the health care setting and for the patient's condition when treating pressure ulcers.

Clean gloves. Use clean gloves for each patient. When treating multiple ulcers on the same patient, attend to the most contaminated ulcer last (e.g., in the perianal region). Remove gloves and wash hands between patients.

Sterile instruments for debridement. Use sterile (as opposed to clean) instruments to debride pressure ulcers. Following debridement, monitor the patient's temperature and be alert for signs of bacteremia or sepsis (e.g., unexplained fever, tachycardia, hypotension, deterioration in mental status).

Clean dressings. Use clean dressings, rather than sterile ones, to treat pressure ulcers in health care facilities, as long as dressing procedures comply with institutional infection-control guidelines. Clean dressings may also be used in the home setting. Disposal of contaminated dressings should be done in a manner consistent with local regulations.

Keeping dressings clean. Procedures to keep dressings clean and prevent cross-contamination should be established and rigorously followed. These procedures include the following:

- Strict adherence to body substance isolation precautions and good hand-washing between patients.
- Multipatient treatment carts taken to the bedside should not be used to house dressing supplies. Individual patients should have their own dressing supplies that are protected from inadvertent environmental contamination by water damage, dust accumulation, or contact contaminants.
- Clean bundled dressings can be purchased less expensively than can individual dressings; however, measures should be taken to ensure that they remain clean (e.g., keeping dressings in the original package or in other plas-

tic packaging; storing them in a clean, dry place; and discarding the entire package if any of the dressings become wet, contaminated, or dirty).

- Caregivers must wash their hands before contact with the supply of clean dressings or dressing supplies. Before the dressing or treatment, only the number of dressings necessary for each dressing change should be removed from containers. Once the hands of the caregiver are soiled with wound secretions, they should not come in contact with the remaining clean dressings and other supplies until the gloves are removed and hands are washed. Dressings, instruments, and solutions should be obtained from suppliers who can ensure that shipment and handling will not expose the dressings and supplies to damage or contamination.

Disposal. Local regulations vary on the disposal of soiled dressings. The Environmental Protection Agency recommends that soiled dressings be placed in securely fastened plastic bags before being added to other household trash.

OPERATIVE REPAIR OF PRESSURE ULCERS

Operative procedures to repair pressure ulcers include one or more of the following: direct closure, skin grafting, skin flaps, musculocutaneous flaps, and free flaps. Although more research is needed to develop clear criteria for selecting those individuals most likely to benefit from surgical management, the panel has provided some general criteria. Preoperative patient counseling should include information about the operative procedures available and the anticipated benefits and potential risks of each. Factors that might impair healing should be addressed preoperatively. Vigilant postoperative follow-up is essential to healing and prevention of recurrence.

Patient selection

Determine patient need and suitability for operative repair when clean stage III or stage IV pressure ulcers do not respond to optimal patient care (as defined in this section). Potential candidates are medically stable and adequately nourished and can tolerate operative blood loss and postoperative immobility. Quality of life, patient preferences, treatment goals, risk of recurrence, and expected rehabilitative outcome are additional considerations.

Controlling factors that impair healing

Promote successful surgical closure by controlling or correcting factors that may be associated with impaired healing, such as smoking, spasticity, levels of bacterial colonization, incontinence, and urinary tract infection.

Selection of methods

Use the most effective and least traumatic method to repair the ulcer defect. Wounds can be closed by direct closure, skin grafting, skin flaps, musculocutaneous flaps, and free flaps. To minimize recurrence, the choice of operative technique is based on the individual patient's needs and overall goals as well as on the specific site and extent of the ulcer.

Avoid prophylactic ischiectomy

Prophylactic ischiectomy is not recommended since it often results in perineal ulcers and urethral fistulas, which are more threatening problems than ischial ulcers.

Postoperative care

Minimize pressure to the operative site by use of an air-fluidized bed, a low–air loss bed, or a Stryker frame for a minimum of 2 weeks. Assess postoperative viability of the surgical site as clinically indicated. Have the patient slowly increase periods of time sitting or lying on the flap to increase its tolerance to pressure. To determine the degree of tolerance, monitor the flap for pallor, redness, or both that do not resolve after 10 minutes of pressure relief. Ongoing patient education is imperative to reduce the risk of recurrence.

Prevention of recurrence

Assess for recurrence of pressure ulcers as an ongoing component of care. Caregivers should provide education and encourage adherence to measures for pressure reduction, daily skin examination, and intermittent relief techniques.

References

1. Allman RM: Epidemiology of pressure sores in different populations, *Decubitus* 2(3):40-43, 1989.
2. Braden BJ, Bergstrom N: Clinical utility of the Braden scale for predicting pressure sore risk, *Decubitus* 2(3):44-51, 1989.
3. Braun JL, Silvetti AN, Xakellis GC: Decubitus ulcers: what really works? *Patient Care* 22:22-31, 1988.
4. Garrell M: Prevention and treatment of pressure sores, *Hosp Physician,* p 39, 1991.
5. Goode PS, Allman RM: The prevention and management of pressure sores, *Med Clin North Am* 73:1511-1524, 1989.
6. Levine JM, Simpson M, McDonald RJ: Pressure sores: a plan for primary care prevention, *Geriatrics* 44:75-90, 1989.
7. Moss RJ, LaPuma J: The ethics of pressure sore prevention and treatment in the elderly: a practical approach, *J Am Geriatr Soc* 39:905-908, 1991.
8. National Pressure Ulcer Advisory Panel: Consensus development conference statement on pressure ulcers, *Decubitus* 2:24-28, 1989.
9. Norton D: Calculating the risk: reflections on the Norton scale, *Decubitus* 2(3):24-31, 1989.
10. Perdue RW, Wilson JL: Decubitus ulcers, *J Am Board Fam Pract* 2(1):43-48, 1989.
11. Pinchcofsky-Devin GD, Kaminsk MO: Correlation of pressure sores and nutritional status, *J Am Geriatr Soc* 24:435-440, 1986.
12. Schnelle JF: Treatment of urinary incontinence in nursing home patients by prompted voiding, *J Am Geriatr Soc* 38:356-360, 1990.

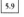

COOPERATION WITH CARE PLAN
Marsha D. Fretwell, MD

Critical to successful care of all patients is a cooperative relationship between the providers and recipients of the care. In the case of older patients, the barriers that may interfere with accomplishing the care plan can be related to the three groups involved in the care

- Clinicians
- The older patient
- Spouses, children, or other caretakers

ROLE OF PHYSICIAN IN SUCCESSFUL CARE PLAN

The physician is responsible for making accurate diagnoses and prognoses, educating the patient and/or family about the appropriate treatments, respecting the personal preferences of the patient about the treatments, and monitoring the outcomes of treatments undertaken.

1. Failure of the physician to listen fully to the patient so that a treatment or care plan can be directed at the issues of most concern is a major barrier to a patient's cooperation with that care plan. An inappropriate care plan will fail
2. Failure to educate the patient about the potential risks and benefits of new medications and other types of treatment often impairs the patient's and the family's ability to cooperate

Role of older patient in successful care plans

Several attributes of an older patient may lead to either active or passive uncooperativeness with a care plan.

1. Personality traits: the characteristic emotional, interpersonal, experiential, and motivational styles that are stable over an individual's life span and form the basic elements of the personality. A cluster of personality traits—or in their extreme, personality disorders—can interfere with cooperation with a successful care plan
   a. Eccentric, or odd, group
      (1) Paranoid type: mistrustful of others
      (2) Schizoid type: indifferent to social relationships
   b. Dramatic, emotional, or erratic group
      (1) Antisocial personality disorder: unable to conform to social norms and rules
      (2) Histrionic personality disorder: emotionally labile and self-centered; has many minor complaints
      (3) Narcissistic personality disorder: has an extreme sense of self-importance with entitlement
   c. Anxious group
      (1) Avoidant personality disorder: extremely shy
      (2) Dependent personality disorder: unable to make decisions or take responsibility for his or her role in the care plan
      (3) Obsessive-compulsive personality disorder: characterized by perfectionism and a focus on details
      (4) Passive-aggressive personality disorder: appears to understand the care plan but then covertly does not follow through with recommendations
2. Change in personality: on the whole, personality traits do not change over one's life span
   a. A review of past emotional, interpersonal, and motivational styles in an older individual can provide valuable prognostic information about response to the stress of the current situation
   b. If an individual experiences a change in personality, think first about the diseases, medications, changes in sites of care, or overwhelming personal losses that may underlie the change

Role of spouses, children, and other family caretakers in successful care plans

When an appropriate care plan is not succeeding, it is important to examine the cognitive and emotional capacities of the spouse (most often the primary caretaker) and the overall functioning of the family support network.

1. Spouses: spouses of older patients are often older themselves and subject to the same diseases, difficulties with hearing and vision, and barriers to communication as are the patients. Brief screening examinations for vision, hearing, cognition, and anxiety/depression are indicated, especially if the patient has a dementia and no progress is being made in the care plan

2. Children and other family caretakers: "What goes around, comes around" is a phase that succinctly captures how children and other family caretakers can become a barrier to a successful care plan. Because they are often the most critical element for a successful care plan, it is important to recognize and address the problem. In some families the critical step of the parent-child relationship—separation and individuation of the child—has not been successfully navigated. Many years later, when the child is called on to take care of the parents, two responses may interfere with a successful care plan

   a. In the overly connected family, the child is often unable to set limits on the parent's behavior that are necessary to appropriate and safe care. This is particularly difficult if the parent has a dementia but may also be true for physically impaired patients who are demanding and abusive to caretakers. It is critical to recognize and obtain counseling and support for these children caretakers. It is also crucial to obtain prior directives from these older patients while they are cognitively intact, since the children may be emotionally unable to function as a proxy for substituted judgment (see Chapter 10)

   b. In the disconnected family, the physician may become the target of unresolved anger at the parent/authority figure or inappropriate expectations of physician responsibility for the well-being of the parent. It then becomes important that the physician set limits, identify responsible family members, and clarify roles and responsibilities early in the course of the care plan. Again, obtaining prior directives from the patient/parent while cognitively intact greatly facilitates implementation of the successful care plan

Suggested readings

Blazer DG: Schizophrenia and schizophreniform disorders. In Abrams WB, Berkow R, editors: *The Merck manual of geriatrics,* Rahway, NJ, 1990, Merck Sharp & Dohme.

Costa PT, McCrae RR: Personality and aging. In Hazzard WR et al, editors: *Principles of geriatric medicine and gerontology,* New York, 1994, McGraw-Hill.

Holroyd S, Rabins PV. Personality disorders. In Hazzard WR et al, editors: *Principles of geriatric medicine and gerontology,* New York, 1994, McGraw-Hill.

Laitman LB, Davis KL: Paraphrenias and other psychosis. In Hazzard WR et al, editors: *Principles of geriatric medicine and gerontology,* New York, 1994, McGraw-Hill.

Selected Organ System Abnormalities

| 6.1 | **NEUROLOGIC DISORDERS**

| 6.1.a. | ***STROKE AND TRANSIENT ISCHEMIC ATTACK***
Fred F. Ferri, MD

Epidemiology

1. Seventy-five percent of strokes occur in patients older than 65
2. Annual incidence of strokes in the elderly is 2%
3. Incidence of all types of strokes has declined over the past 20 years as a result of better management of risk factors; mortality from stroke has also declined dramatically
4. Eighteen percent of strokes result from intracranial hemorrhage
   a. Subarachnoid hemorrhage (74%)
      (1) Berry aneurysm (51%)
      (2) Arteriovenous malformation (AVM) (6%)
      (3) Vasculitis, endocarditis, coagulopathy (21%)
      (4) Unknown (22%)
   b. Intracerebral (26%)
      (1) Usually secondary to hypertension (80%)
      (2) Less common causes are AVMs, tumors, coagulopathy, amyloid angiopathy
5. Eighty-two percent of strokes result from cerebral infarction. These are caused by the following
   a. Large-vessel atheromatous disease (82%)
   b. Lacunar infarcts (25%)
   c. Cardiogenic embolism (15%)

Clinical presentation

1. Transient ischemic attacks (TIAs) precede strokes in 50% to 70% of cases
2. TIA presentation varies with the vessel involved. Major distinguishing characteristics between carotid and vertebrobasilar TIAs are described in the box on p. 141

Differences Between Carotid and Vertebrobasilar Artery Syndrome

Characteristics of Carotid Artery Syndrome

1. Ipsilateral monocular vision loss (amaurosis fugax); patient often feels as if "a shade" has come down over one eye
2. Episodic contralateral arm, leg, and face paresis and paresthesias
3. Slurred speech, transient aphasia
4. Ipsilateral headache of vascular type
5. Carotid bruit may be present over carotid bifurcation
6. Microemboli, hemorrhages, and exudates may be noted in ipsilateral retina

Characteristics of Vertebrobasilar Artery Syndrome

1. Binocular visual disturbances (blurred vision, diplopia, total blindness)
2. Vertigo, nausea, vomiting, tinnitus
3. Sudden loss of postural tone of all four extremities (drop attacks) with no loss of consciousness
4. Slurred speech, ataxia, numbness around lips or face

From Ferri F: *Practical guide to the care of the medical patient*, ed 3, St Louis, 1995, Mosby.

3. Major characteristics of cerebral thrombosis and embolism are described in Table 6-1; however, the clinical distinction between them is often impossible

Management

1. The primary agents used in the prophylaxis of stroke and TIA are aspirin, ticlopidine, heparin, and warfarin. Antithrombotic therapy for ischemic cerebrovascular disease is summarized in Table 6-2
2. Carotid endarterectomy is highly beneficial to patients with recent hemispheric and retinal TIAs or nondisabling strokes with ipsilateral high-grade stenosis (70% to 99%) of the internal carotid artery
3. Rehabilitation (see Chapter 9) should begin immediately in the acute care hospital with a multidisciplinary team and should continue in rehabilitation units, nursing homes, or the outpatient setting until recovery of function is maximized
4. Potential complications such as dysphagia (30% of stroke patients), urinary incontinence, pressure sores, and depression (60% of patients) must be rapidly identified and addressed. Deep vein thrombosis (DVT) prophylaxis is strongly recommended in immobilized patients since DVT complicates over 30% of strokes and results in lethal pulmonary embolism in 3% of stroke patients

Table 6-1 Characteristics of cerebral thrombosis and embolism

	Thrombosis	Embolism
Onset of symptoms	Progression of symptoms over hours to days	Very rapid (seconds)
History of prior TIA	Common	Uncommon
Time of presentation	Often during night hours while patient is sleeping Classically the patient awakens with a slight neurologic deficit that gradually progresses in a stepwise fashion	Patient is usually awake and involved in some type of activity
Predisposing factors	Atherosclerosis, hypertension, diabetes, arteritis, vasculitis, hypotension, trauma to head and neck	Atrial fibrillation, mitral stenosis and regurgitation, endocarditis, mitral valve prolapse

From Ferri F: *Practical guide to the care of the medical patient,* ed 3, St Louis, 1995, Mosby.

Table 6-2 Current range of antithrombotic therapy for ischemic cerebrovascular disease

Clinical Setting	Therapy*
Acute noncardioembolic stroke	Aspirin; subcutaneous heparin; no specific therapy
Acute cardioembolic stroke	Intravenous heparin; subcutaneous heparin; warfarin; aspirin; no specific therapy
Unstable or progressing stroke	Intravenous heparin; aspirin; no specific therapy
Acute transient ischemic attack	Aspirin; ticlopidine; intravenous heparin†; subcutaneous heparin
After transient ischemic attack or minor stroke (noncardioembolic)	Aspirin; ticlopidine
After major stroke (noncardioembolic)	Ticlopidine; aspirin
Atrial fibrillation	
Primary stroke prevention	Aspirin or warfarin‡
Secondary stroke prevention	Warfarin; aspirin
Asymptomatic carotid stenosis	Aspirin; no specific therapy
Asymptomatic adult sample	No specific therapy; aspirin

From Rothrock JF, Hart RG: Antithrombotic therapy in cerebrovascular disease, *Ann Intern Med* 115:892, 1991.

*The first therapy listed for each clinical setting represents the authors' first choice of treatment.

†Intravenous heparin therapy should be considered only in patients with "crescendo" transient ischemic attacks or vertebrobasilar transient ischemic attack.

‡See Section 6.6.e.

Prognosis

1. Varies with the presence of coexisting illness, extent of stroke, nursing and social support systems, and patient's attitude
2. Overall, 40% of survivors will have significant dysfunction, 40% will have mild residua, 10% will recover completely, and 10% will require institutional care

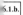

PARKINSONISM
Fred F. Ferri, MD

PARKINSON'S DISEASE

Clinical manifestations (Table 6-3)

1. Classic manifestations
   a. Rigidity
   b. Resting tremor
   c. Akinesia
   d. Gait disturbance
   e. Other: micrographia, orthostatic hypotension, abnormal reflexes
2. Dementia occurs in approximately 50% of patients
3. Depression

Therapeutic approach

1. General principles: physical therapy, encouragement, reassurance, and treatment of possible associated conditions (e.g., depression)
2. Avoidance of drugs that can induce or worsen Parkinson's disease
   a. Neuroleptic agents (especially haloperidol)
   b. Certain antiemetics (e.g., prochlorperazine, trimethobenzamide); these drugs will block dopamine receptors; diphenidol (Vontrol) may be used for nausea
   c. Metoclopramide (Reglan) and cisapride (Propulsid)
   d. Nonselective MAO inhibitors (may induce hypertensive crisis)
   e. Certain antihypertensives (reserpine, methyldopa)
3. Drug therapy should be delayed until symptoms significantly limit patient's daily activities, since tolerance and side effects to antiparkinsonian agents are common. Deprenyl may have some early benefit
4. Treatment (medical and surgical) of Parkinson's disease summarized in Table 6-4

PARKINSONISM-PLUS

Parkinsonism-plus refers to symptoms and signs of parkinsonism occurring in association with other multisystem degenerative diseases (see Table 6-3).

1. **Progressive supranuclear palsy** (Steele-Richardson-Olszweski syndrome)
   a. Usual onset at end of sixth or beginning of seventh decade
   b. Characterized by parkinsonian symptoms plus
      (1) Supranuclear gaze palsies (vertical > horizontal, downward > upward)
      (2) Subcortical dementia, depression

Text continued on p. 150.

Table 6-3 Parkinsonian syndromes

Disorder	Clinical Manifestations	Differential Diagnosis	Tests	Treatment
Parkinson's disease (PD)	Tremor: prerequisite for PD; present at rest; chiefly in fingers and hands at 3–7 Hz. Bradykinesia: paucity of spontaneous movements of face, giving masklike appearance; scarcity of natural limb and trunk movements is less obvious Disturbed body posture and gait; stooped posture; slowed, shuffling gait, sometimes festination and "freezing"; postural instability, causes falls Rigidity: shoulder girdle rigidity pre-	Essential tremor: tremor is only on activity such as holding arms outstretched; voice and head tremor frequent accompaniments; neurologic examination shows no other abnormalities; family history of tremor; tremor dampened by propranolol or small doses of alcohol Symptomatic parkinsonism: structural brain lesions such as frontal lobe meningioma, subdural hematoma, normal-pressure hydrocephalus, Binswanger disease,	Primarily clinical diagnosis Brain CT and MRI: to exclude structural brain lesions but show no abnormalities pathognomonic of PD Serum calcium: for rare cause of hypoparathyroidism Positron emission tomography scan using radioactive fluorodopa shows hypometabolism in basal ganglia but is research tool at present Therapeutic test with L-dopa: dramatic improvement of bradykinesia, rigidity, and sometimes	See text

Continued

shoulder ; neck and trunk rigidity contributes to stooped posture; lower trunk rigidity manifests as low back pain syndrome
Micrographia
Speech: low volume

gnitic infarcts; rarely, infiltrating lesions of midbrain, traumatic (boxer's) encephalopathy
"Metabolic parkinsonism": toxins such as meperidine-related MPTP, carbon monoxide, manganese
Drug induced: phenothiazines, haloperidol, metoclopramide, reserpine
Hypocalcemia of hypoparathyroidism
Degenerative brain disorders (parkinsonism-plus syndrome): Steele-Richardson-Olszewski syndrome, Shy-Drager syndrome, corticobasal ganglionic degeneration

strongly suggests PD; response may take a few weeks; lack of response casts doubt on diagnosis of idiopathic PD

Table 6-3 Parkinsonian syndromes—cont'd

Disorder	Clinical Manifestations	Differential Diagnosis	Tests	Treatment
Steele-Richardson-Olszewski syndrome (progressive supranuclear palsy)	Resembles PD because of rigidity, bradykinesia, gait disorder, and falls; cardinal distinguishing feature: supranuclear gaze palsy with early paresis of downward gaze, which can deteriorate to total gaze paralysis; tremor minimal or absent; dysarthria/dysphagia early; neck held in extension dystonia		Clinical diagnosis	No specific therapy at present, L-dopa is temporarily beneficial in early stages; tricyclic antidepressants ameliorate pseudobulbar emotional lability

Shy-Drager syndrome (multiple-systems atrophy)	Bradykinesia and rigidity mimic PD; distinctive features: progressive autonomic failure with orthostatic hypotension, impotence, anhidrosis, neurogenic bladder, obstipation, dry mouth, impaired pupillary reflexes; vocal cord paralysis and sleep apnea rare	Clinical diagnosis; autonomic function tests clarify clinical dysautonomia	No specific treatment; pharmacologic and physical treatments available for various aspects of dysautonomia
Corticobasal ganglionic degeneration	Increasingly recognized disorder; progressive limb and trunk rigidity, bradykinesia; distinctive features: apraxia, cortical-type sensory loss	Diagnosis clinical and confirmed by brain biopsy	In early stages, slight benefit from L-dopa; no specific treatment

From Noble J et al, editors: *Textbook of primary care medicine*, St Louis, 1996, Mosby.

Table 6-4 Management of Parkinson's disease

Pharmacologic Treatment

Medication	Dosage	Side Effects
Dopaminergic drugs		
Carbidopa/levodopa (L-dopa)	25/100 mg qid; maintenance usually up to 500 mg of L-dopa daily	Orthostatic hypotension; nausea, confusion, especially in elderly; visual hallucinations, nightmares, myoclonus, dyskinesias
Bromocriptine	2.5-mg tablets; start with half tablet, increase gradually; bid or tid dosage; maintenance: 7.5-30 mg	Hypotension, visual hallucinations, confusion, livedo reticularis, cryomelagia of feet
Pergolide	0.05 mg/day; increase up to 1 mg tid or qid	Same as for bromocriptine
Amantadine	100 mg bid	Nausea, confusion, livedo reticularis
Anticholinergic drugs		
Trihexyphenidyl (Artane)	2 mg/day; increase to 2 mg up to tid	Dry mouth, blurred vision; can precipitate narrow-angle glaucoma
Benztropine (Cogentin)	0.5-1.0 mg/day; increase up to 4-6 mg/day	Urinary hesitancy (can precipitate urinary retention), confusion
MAO inhibitor		
Deprenyl	5 mg bid	Nausea, nervousness, insomnia

Surgical Treatment

Procedure	Indication	Comment
Stereotactic thalamotomy	Intractable, unilateral	A few patients with disabling tremor but without severe bradykinesia or rigidity experience marked relief
Fetal adrenal medulla and substantia nigra transplants into caudate nuclei		These treatments remain experimental at present
Stereotactic pallidotomy		

Symptom Management

Symptom	Intervention
Activities of daily living, frozen shoulder prevention, prevention of falls	Physical therapy
Low-volume speech	Speech therapy
Dysarthria	Clonazepam: 0.5-1 mg tid
Spastic bladder	Oxybutynin: 5-10 mg tid
Constipation	High-fiber diet: Metamucil, Colace
Action tremor (frequently coexists with Parkinson's)	Propranolol: 40-80 mg tid
Painful dystonia of limbs	Baclofen: 5-10 mg tid
Paroxysmal drenching sweats	Beta-blockers
Depression	Tricyclic antidepressants, electroconvulsive treatment

From Noble J, editor: *Primary care medicine*, St Louis, 1996, Mosby.

     (3) Pseudobulbar palsy (dysphagia, dysarthria)
     (4) Axial rigidity (increased truncal and neck tone)
   c. Prognosis poor; disease follows a rapid course with significant inca-
      pacity within 2 to 4 years; mean survival: 6 years
2. **Olivopontocerebellar atrophy**
   a. Parkinsonian symptoms
   b. Cerebellar signs (scanning speech, ataxia, tremor of trunk and head)
   c. Mild dementia
3. **Shy-Drager syndrome (multiple systems atrophy)**
   a. Parkinsonian features
   b. Orthostatic hypotension (see Section 6.6.c)
   c. Dizziness, unsteady gait

6.1.c.

TREMORS
Fred F. Ferri, MD

Tremors are characterized by rhythmic oscillations, usually involving distal
parts of the body.
1. Major causes
   a. Metabolic abnormalities: uremia, liver failure
   b. Endocrine disorders: hypoglycemia, pheochromocytoma, thyrotoxico-
      sis
   c. Drugs: theophylline, caffeine, amphetamines, alcohol, lithium, beta-
      agonists, bronchodilators, tricyclics, metoclopramide, valproic acid,
      amiodarone, nifedipine
   d. Anxiety, exercise, fatigue, alcohol withdrawal, benzodiazepine with-
      drawal
   e. Cerebellar disorders
   f. Huntington's disease
   g. Cerebrovascular disease
2. Classification
   a. Behavioral situation
      (1) **Rest tremor:** occurs in absence of voluntary muscle activity (e.g.,
          Parkinson's disease)
      (2) **Movement tremor:** provoked by any movement (e.g., essential
          tremor, brain stem disorders, cerebellar disease)
      (3) **Postural tremor:** occurs with maintenance of posture (e.g., physi-
          ologic tremor, drug-induced, essential tremor, postural tremor of
          parkinsonism)
   b. Disease process: Table 6-5 describes the major distinguishing charac-
      teristics of the various conditions causing tremor

6.1.d.

CHOREIC DISORDERS
Fred F. Ferri, MD

1. **Huntington's disease**
   a. Onset between ages 40 and 55; usually fatal within 15 years of onset
   b. Autosomal dominant; gene localized on chromosome 4
   c. Characterized by choreiform movements, dementia, and emotional
      disturbances

Table 6-5 Characteristics of tremor in selected conditions

Type of Tremor	Frequency (Hz)	Characteristics	Therapy
Parkinsonism	4-7.5	See text	See text
Essential senile tremor	8-12	Commonly affects hands and head Usually begins asymmetrically and tends to remain asymmetric Initially not present at rest Suppressed by alcohol, worsened by fatigue and emotional factors	Propranolol 20 mg tid initially is effective in approximately 50% of patients Primidone 25 mg tid initially may be effective in patients refractory to propranolol
Cerebellar	3-5	Tremor is evident when patient holds arms outstretched Tremor is accentuated by targeting (e.g., finger-to-nose testing) (intention tremor)	No effective therapy
Alcohol withdrawal	Variable	Rapid and coarse Involves entire body Abolished by alcohol intake	Abstinence from alcohol
Hysterical tremor	Variable	Variable frequency from moment to moment Can be rest, movement, or postural tremor Can affect any part of the body Usually diminished when patient is distracted	Psychotherapy

    d. Chorea and psychosis can be initially managed with phenothiazines and haloperidol
2. **Senile chorea**
    a. Spontaneous buccolingual dyskinesias, at times accompanied by involuntary movements of other body regions
    b. Occurs in 10% of nursing home residents and 1% of noninstitutional elderly
    c. Distinguished from Huntington's chorea by absence of autosomal-dominant family history and associated mental disturbance
    d. Symptoms are mild, and course is usually benign
3. **Drug-induced choreas**
    a. Common offending drugs: tricyclic antidepressants, lithium, phenytoin, L-dopa, carbamazepine, isoniazid, antihistamines

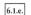

TARDIVE DYSKINESIA
Fred F. Ferri, MD

1. Involuntary movements, usually involving the orofacial structures (e.g., tongue movements, lip smacking, chewing)
2. Different regions of the body can also be affected (e.g., legs, respiratory system, fingers)
3. Usually associated with prolonged exposure to neuroleptics that block and bind dopamine receptors
4. Incidence of neuroleptic-induced tardive dyskinesia exceeds 30% in the elderly after 2 to 3 weeks of cumulative neuroleptic treatment. Psychotic (as opposed to organic) diagnoses and presence of extrapyramidal signs early in treatment are associated with increased tardive dyskinesia vulnerability
5. Prevalence of tardive dyskinesia is increased in the elderly. Age is the most consistently reported risk factor for development
6. Dosage reduction, discontinuation of the offending agent, or intermittent therapy usually does not alleviate the symptoms
7. Reserpine (0.25 mg/day initially, titrated to 5 mg/day over several weeks) may ameliorate orobuccal dyskinesias
8. Table 6-6 compares tardive dyskinesia to other hyperkinetic disorders

HEADACHE
Tom J. Wachtel, MD

Epidemiology

Headache is a very common complaint with more than 90% of all people acknowledging some experience with this complaint. Women are somewhat more likely than men to seek medical care for headache, and when they do, they are more likely to report a longer duration of the problem. Headaches account for 2% to 4% of all primary care office visits, with older patients more likely to visit when they experience headache than their younger counterparts. In addition, many people with headache rely on self-care with over-the-counter medications. When patients consult a physician, many will have some preconceived idea about their headache; in particular, laypeople often misuse the term *migraine* as synonymous with

Text continued on p. 157.

Table 6-6 Hyperkinetic movement disorders

Disorder	Clinical Manifestations	Differential Diagnosis	Tests	Treatment
Chorea, choreoathetosis, tardive dyskinesia	Continuum of abnormal involuntary movements; jerky, nonrhythmic, semipurposive, predominantly in limbs; may affect head, neck, trunk; lips and tongue may participate (buccolingual dyskinesia); often mixed with writhing (choreoathetosis)	Drug induced Phenothiazines L-dopa Phenytoin Cocaine Amiphetamines Tricyclics Oral contraceptives	Urine toxic screen	Withdrawal of toxic drug Symptomatic treatment: clonazepam: 0.5 mg bid up to 4-16 mg/day Haloperidol: 0.5-1.0 mg tid up to 5-15 mg/day
		Liver failure	Liver function tests	Treatment of hepatic encephalopathy
		Wilson's disease: dyskinesia accompanied by dystonia, cerebellar ataxia, dysarthia, proximal limb tremor, emotional lability	Slit-lamp examination for Kayser-Fleischer rings; serum ceruloplasmin, serum copper	Penicillamine
		Thyrotoxicosis	Serum thyroxine, TSH	Antithyroid drugs

Continued

Table 6-6 Hyperkinetic movement disorders—cont'd

Disorder	Clinical Manifestations	Differential Diagnosis	Tests	Treatment
		Polycythemia Systemic lupus erythematosus Sydenham's chorea Huntington's chorea	Hematocrit Antinuclear antibody — Brain CT/MRI, DNA analysis	Phlebotomy Steroids Symptomatic Symptomatic
Hemiballismus	Large, flinging, ballistic limb movements; predominates in arm or leg	Lacunar CVA in vicinity of subthalamic nuclei in basal ganglia; other focal lesions; metastases and toxoplasmosis (in AIDS)	Brain CT/MRI	Therapy of underlying lesion Symptomatic treatment same as for chorea
Focal dystonia	Spasmodic torticollis	Idiopathic	Clinical	Anticholinergics (high dose): trihexyphenidyl (Artane), 2 mg bid up to 10-40 mg/day Benzodiazepines: clonazepam as above; diazepam, 5 mg bid up to 20-60 mg/day Botulin A toxin: focal

Spasmodic dysphonia (laryngeal)	Idiopathic	—	Surgery: peripheral muscle denervation Botulin A toxin: injection into vocal muscles
Essential blepharospasm: dystonia of orbicularis oculi muscle is principal feature; if accompanied by dystonia of facial, tongue, and neck muscles, called Meige syndrome	Idiopathic	—	Clonazepam as above Botulin A toxin: injection into appropriate muscles
Segmental and generalized dystonia May affect different segments of body or be generalized or multifocal	Idiopathic Hereditary Drug induced: Phenothiazines L-dopa Calcium channel blockers	—	Symptomatic treatment: anticholinergics, clonazepam Baclofen: 10 mg bid up to 50-100 mg/day Carbamazepine: 100 mg bid up to 600-1200 mg/day
	Wilson's disease	Same as for chorea	Penicillamine plus symptomatic treatment

Continued

Table 6-6 Hyperkinetic movement disorders—cont'd

Disorder	Clinical Manifestations	Differential Diagnosis	Tests	Treatment
		Diurnal dystonia: childhood onset (Segawa disease type) may have parkinsonian features	Familial	Dramatic response to L-dopa Carbidopa/L-dopa: 25/100 mg bid or tid
Acute dystonic reaction	May be segmental or generalized with oculogyric crisis, torticollis, tongue protrusion, opisthotonos; children more susceptible	Drug induced Prochlorperazine Metoclopramide	—	Benztropine (Cogentin): 1-2 mg IM Diphenhydramine: 50 mg IM
Paroxysmal dystonia	Kinesigenic: brief attacks of dystonia triggered by sudden movements	Idiopathic or familial	—	Carbamazepine: 100-200 mg tid Phenytoin: 100 mg tid
	Nonkinesigenic dystonia: prolonged paroxysm of dystonia unrelated to activity	Idiopathic or familial	—	Carbamazepine, clonazepam Acetazolamide (Diamox): 250 mg tid

From Noble J et al, editors: *Textbook of primary care medicine*, St Louis, 1996, Mosby.

TSH, Thyroid-stimulating hormone; *CT,* computed tomography; *MRI,* magnetic resonance imaging; *DNA,* deoxyribonucleic acid; *CVA,* cerebrovascular accident; *AIDS,* acquired immune deficiency syndrome.

headache, when in reality 80% of all headaches are tension headaches and only 5% are migraine, the second most common cause of a chronic headache condition.

Etiology

1. Tension headaches (muscle contraction headache or stress headache)
2. Vascular headaches
   a. Idiopathic or primary
      (1) Migraine (classic or common)
      (2) Cluster headache
   b. Secondary or associated with vascular disorders
      (1) Temporal arteritis (giant cell arteritis)
      (2) Other vasculitis
      (3) Hypertension
3. Mixed tension/vascular headaches
4. Headaches associated with ophthalmologic, otolaryngologic, facial, or dental diseases
   a. Eye
      (1) Refraction errors
      (2) Acute glaucoma
      (3) Red eye (conjunctivitis, keratitis, iritis, uveitis)
      (4) Miscellaneous painful eye conditions
   b. Nose and sinuses (rhinitis/sinusitis)
      (1) Bacterial infection
      (2) Viral infection
      (3) Allergic rhinitis
      (4) Nasopharyngeal carcinoma
   c. Ear, e.g., otitis media or externa
   d. Oral cavity
      (1) Dental and gingival problems
      (2) Oropharyngeal malignancies
      (3) Oropharyngeal infections (e.g., pharyngitis, tonsillitis, abscess)
   e. Temporomandibular joint (TMJ) disease
   f. Bruxism (teeth grinding)
5. Cranial neuralgias (e.g., trigeminal neuralgia or tic douloureux)
6. Headaches associated with head trauma
7. Cervical spine and neck diseases
   a. Arthritis (degenerative or inflammatory)
   b. Cervical disk disease
   c. Whiplash injuries
   d. Torticollis (stiff neck)
   e. Odynophagia and other referred pain resulting from laryngeal or upper esophageal problems, usually malignancies, or rarely from cervical lymphadenopathy or thyroid enlargement
8. Meningitis or meningoencephalitis (NOTE: pure encephalitis does not cause a headache in the absence of cerebral edema)
9. Headache associated with distant infection or fever (probably a variant of tension headache)
10. Spinal headache (following a lumbar puncture or spinal anesthesia)

11. Medication-induced headache: many prescription and over-the-counter drugs can cause headache as an adverse reaction, some more frequently than others, e.g., nitrates
12. Headache associated with substance abuse or withdrawal
    a. Alcohol
    b. Caffeine
    c. Recreational (illicit) drugs
13. Intracranial mass lesions
    a. Hematoma (epidural, subdural, subarachnoid, intracerebral)
    b. Tumor
       (1) Primary (e.g., astrocytoma, meningioma)
       (2) Metastatic
    c. Abscess
       (1) Protozoan (toxoplasmosis)
       (2) Bacterial
14. Pseudotumor cerebri (benign intracranial hypertension)
15. Malingering
16. Not classifiable

Office evaluation

1. History
   a. Location, especially unilateral vs. bilateral
   b. Temporal features
      (1) Overall duration of the pain (days, months, years)
      (2) Duration of each episode if recurrent
      (3) Circadian rhythm (e.g., does it begin in the morning or the evening?)
   c. Character of the pain (e.g., pounding vs. constant ache)
   d. Severity (e.g., on a scale from 1 to 10)
   e. Precipitating factors
   f. Aggravating factors
   g. Alleviating factors
   h. Associated symptoms (e.g., prodromal or during the headache)
   i. Prior evaluation
   j. Psychosocial background (e.g., family situation, occupational history, drug use)
   k. Functional impact (e.g., disability)
2. Physical examination
   a. A complete physical exam is obviously desirable
   b. Minimum
      (1) Evaluate vital signs
      (2) Do a thorough head, eyes, ears, nose, oral, throat, neck, and neurologic exam, including reflexes; cranial nerves; motor, sensory, and cerebellar functions; and mental status
3. Ancillary tests
   a. Most patients can be managed without any laboratory or imaging studies. The most difficult decision is when to perform a head CT scan or MRI to rule out an intracranial mass lesion
   b. Since the majority of patients will have a tension headache or migraine, it is usually reasonable to initiate treatment based on a clinical

impression and defer a decision regarding further workup based on patient's response during follow-up

c. Similarly, if a high-probability etiologic diagnosis can be made at the first visit (e.g., sinusitis), further diagnostic tests for other causes of headache are not indicated initially. Caution and a low threshold for imaging procedures are advisable when the symptoms are of very recent onset and unusually severe. Imaging is mandatory if the neurologic exam is abnormal

d. Finally, patient failure to improve with a treatment targeted at the most likely etiologic diagnosis will often require cerebral imaging

e. Patients with HIV disease require a high index of suspicion for mass lesions and meningitis

TENSION HEADACHES

Tension headaches can present as mild intermittent headaches or severe continuous daily headaches, the first usually associated with usual life stresses, the latter more likely found in patients with depression or anxiety. In either case the pathophysiology is presumed to be contraction of facial expression muscles, scalp muscles, or neck muscles. See Table 6-7 for the clinical description.

Treatment

1. Nonpharmacologic management
   a. Information and reassurance
   b. Stress reduction and relaxation
   c. Psychotherapy for depression or anxiety if present
   d. Scalp massage or acupressure
   e. Environmental modification, family counseling, vocational counseling
2. Pharmacologic options
   a. Aspirin or acetaminophen
   b. Nonsteroidal antiinflammatory drugs (NSAIDs)
   c. Propoxyphene (Darvon) or aspirin/caffeine/butalbital combinations (Fiorinal) may be used reluctantly for short courses only because of their addictive potential
   d. Narcotic agents should not be used
3. Treatment with antidepressant or anxiolytic drugs may be used when underlying depression or anxiety is present

MIGRAINE

Migraine headache occasionally presents as classic migraine (i.e., preceded by an aura or prodromal symptoms consisting of vague malaise, visual phenomenon [usually scotomas], olfactory or auditory perceptions, or focal neurologic symptoms) or more frequently as common migraine (i.e., without an aura). The pathogenesis is unknown, but the most widely accepted hypothesis (albeit unproven) is an episode of intracranial or extracranial vasoconstriction contemporary of the aura (when present) followed by vasodilation resulting in a unilateral throbbing headache often associated with nausea, vomiting, diarrhea, and photophobia. The onset of migraine is most unusual after age 40, but many patients have a lifelong course of illness requiring knowledge of the condition by geriatricians. See Table 6-7 for a

Table 6-7 Clinical characteristics of selected headaches

Pain	Tension	Migraine	Sinusitis	Mass Lesion
Location	Bilateral (frontal, occipital, bandlike)	Unilateral (but not always on same side)	Bifrontal (may be unilateral)	Unilateral (always on same side) or bilateral
Character	Pressure	Throbbing	Pressure	Pressure
Severity	Mild to moderate	Moderate to severe	Moderate	Progressively worse as mass expands
Time of occurrence	Late in day or any time	Morning or any time	Worse in morning	Constant (may be intermittent early in course)
Frequency	Several times per week	Less than weekly	Daily until resolved	Constant
Aura	No	Sometimes	No	No
Precipitants	Stress	Bright lights, menstruation, alcohol (see text)	None	None but pain aggravated by Valsalva type of provocation (coughing, sneezing, defecation)
Alleviating factors	Relaxation or sleep	Recline in dark room Migraine-specific drugs	Decongestants, antihistamines, antibiotics	None
Associated symptoms	None or stress related	Vomiting, photophobia	Nasal stuffiness or dripping, epistaxis	Projectile vomiting, neurologic symptoms, may have known primary cancer
Age at onset	Any age	10-30 yr	Any age	Any age for primary brain tumor, older for metastatic brain tumor
Gender	Both	Majority female	Both	Both
Family history	Sometimes	Often	No	No
Chronicity	Several months to years	Several months to years	Acute except in allergic rhinitis (may be seasonal)	Progressive

complete clinical description. Note that a migraine headache can lead to a tension headache or a mixed syndrome.

Treatment

1. Acute attack
   a. Mild attacks: same as tension headache (together with lying down in a dark quiet room)
   b. Severe attacks
      (1) Migraine-specific agents
         (a) Ergotamine can be given orally, sublingually, or in suppository. The usual dose is 1 mg to be repeated twice at 30-minute intervals if needed. The dose-limiting factor is nausea and vomiting; however, because of its potent peripheral vasoconstriction effect, most clinicians recommend no more than three doses per attack and ten doses per week. Do not use this drug in anyone with possible or known arteriosclerotic cardiovascular disease
         (b) Alternatively, a single subcutaneous injection of sumatriptan (Imitrex) 6 mg can be administered by the patient at home or by a physician. A second identical dose may be administered after 30 minutes if a partial response is obtained. If no response is achieved after the first dose, a second dose will not be successful. Sumatriptan may also be given orally at a dose of 25 mg followed, if needed, by a second dose of up to 100 mg. The initial dose can be increased up to 100 mg if needed for subsequent attacks. Sumatriptan is contraindicated in patients with known occlusive arterial disease and therefore should be used with caution in anyone over age 40
      (2) If the above migraine-specific treatment is not effective or not tolerated, narcotic analgesic agents should be used. Parenteral drugs are preferred, because patients should not keep oral narcotic agents at home where they may be abused
2. Migraine prophylaxis
   a. Nonpharmacologic
      (1) Avoidance of triggering factors such as drugs (NSAIDs, vasodilators), stress, coffee, identifiable dietary components, bright lights, sleep deprivation, alcohol
   b. Drugs
      (1) Many medications can reduce the frequency and severity of migraine attacks. None are better than 50% effective. Therefore treatment should be reserved for patients with more than six severe attacks per year
      (2) Patients should be instructed to keep a pretreatment and treatment migraine diary to evaluate effectiveness of any prescribed medication
      (3) Beta-blockers (e.g., propranolol 40 to 320 mg/day)
      (4) Calcium channel blockers (e.g., nifedipine 20 to 60 mg/day)
      (5) Amitriptyline 10 to 175 mg/day
      (6) Carbamazepine 400 to 800 mg/day (monitor drug levels)
      (7) Cyproheptadine 12 to 32 mg/day

(8) Ergotamine 2 mg/day (if this drug is used for prophylaxis, it can not be used to treat acute attacks)

(9) Methysergide 2 to 8 mg/day (NOTE: the patient must be taken of this drug for 3 months every year to avoid retroperitoneal fibrosis)

Suggested readings

Kumar KL: Recent advances in the acute management of migraine and cluster headaches, *J Gen Intern Med* 9:339-348, 1994.

Kumar KL, Cooney TG: Vascular headache, *J Gen Intern Med* 8:384-395, 1988.

Linet MS et al: An epidemiologic study of headache among adolescents and young adults, *JAMA* 261:2211, 1989.

Saper JR: Daily chronic headache, *Neurol Clin* 8:891, 1990.

Silberstein SD: Evaluation and emergency treatment of headache, *Headache* 32:396 1992.

Silberstein SD: Treatment of headache in primary care practice, *Am J Med* 77:65, 1984

Smith MJ, Jensen NM: The severity model of chronic headache, *J Gen Intern Med* 8:396-409, 1988.

Weingarten S et al: The effectiveness of cerebral imaging in the diagnosis of chronic headache, *Arch Intern Med* 152:2457, 1992.

 SEIZURES

Tom J. Wachtel, MD

Definition

Seizures are a manifestation of abnormal neural electrical discharge within the brain. The event is typically sudden and unprovoked and can be described as a "spell," sometimes preceded by a premonition or warning symptoms (aura). The seizure can manifest as abnormal motor activity, abnormal sensory phenomena, unusual behavior, and/or impairment of consciousness.

Etiology

1. Idiopathic
2. Perinatal cerebral hypoxia (may also cause cerebral palsy and mental retardation)
3. Intracranial birth injury (may also cause cerebral palsy and mental retardation)
4. Congenital malformations and genetic disorders
5. Metabolic disturbances
   a. Hypoglycemia
   b. Hypocalcemia
   c. Hypomagnesemia
   d. Hypoxia
   e. Hyponatremia
   f. Hepatic or renal failure
   g. Acid-base disturbance
6. Alcohol related
   a. Acute intoxication (rum fit)
   b. Alcohol withdrawal
7. Recreational drug use and withdrawal
8. Benzodiazepine withdrawal

9. Epileptogenic medications (theophylline, lidocaine, penicillins, neuro-leptics)
10. Brain trauma
11. CNS infection
    a. Brain abscess (bacterial, toxoplasmosis)
    b. Encephalitis (viral, e.g., herpes)
    c. Meningoencephalitis (bacterial, tuberculosis)
    d. Cysticercosis
12. Arteriovenous malformations
13. **Brain tumor (primary or metastatic)** ⎫
                                          ⎬ most common etiologies
                                          of new onset seizures in the
14. **Cerebrovascular disease** ⎭ elderly

Clinical classification

1. Generalized
    a. Convulsive
        (1) Tonic-clonic (grand mal)
        (2) Myoclonic
    b. Nonconvulsive
        (1) Typical absence (spike and wave on EEG) (petit mal)
        (2) Atypical absence
        (3) Atonic
2. Focal
    a. Consciousness preserved (simple partial seizure)
        (1) Sensory
        (2) Focal motor
            (a) With marching sequence (jacksonian seizure)
            (b) Without marching
    b. Consciousness impaired (complex partial seizure)
3. Atypical (e.g., unusual or bizarre behavior), often temporal lobe focus

Clinical manifestations

1. History
    a. Loss of consciousness (may be mistaken as syncope)
    b. Description of the spell by witness
    c. History of previous seizure
    d. Drug and alcohol history
    e. Medications
    f. History of head trauma
    g. Signs of infection
    h. History of cancer
    i. History of arteriosclerotic cardiovascular or cerebrovascular disease
2. Physical examination
    a. Signs of trauma (e.g., tongue bite)
    b. Neurologic exam
3. Laboratory
    a. Blood tests: CBC, serum glucose, BUN, creatinine, electrolytes, calcium, magnesium, transaminase, alkaline phosphatase, blood alcohol level, toxicology screen, anticonvulsant drug levels if relevant
    b. Brain imaging (MRI or CT scan)

    b. EEG with activation procedures (hyperventilation, photic stimulation sleep)

Management

1. Recent, new onset convulsive seizure (within 24 hours) requires hospitalization
2. Multiple recent convulsive seizures (several in 24 hours) or status epilepticus requires hospitalization even in known epileptic patients
3. All other situations can be evaluated and treated on ambulatory basis
4. Anticonvulsant medications (whether to treat a single episode of convulsion is controversial and depends on the etiology [e.g., brain tumor and cerebrovascular disease are more likely reasons for immediate anticonvulsant use than alcohol-related seizures])

   a. Generalized tonic-clonic seizures
      (1) Phenytoin (Dilantin) 300 to 400 mg PO qd
         (a) Therapeutic range: 10 to 20 μg/ml
         (b) Main side effects: ataxia, skin rash, gum hyperplasia, lymphadenopathy, hepatotoxicity
      (2) Phenobarbital 30 to 60 mg PO bid
         (a) Therapeutic range: 10 to 50 μg/ml
         (b) Main side effects: sedation, heptatotoxicity
      (3) Carbamazepine (Tegretol) 400 to 600 mg PO bid
         (a) Therapeutic range: 4 to 12 μg/ml
         (b) Main side effects: ataxia, dizziness, bone marrow suppression, hepatoxicity
      (4) Valproic acid (Depakene) 250 to 500 mg bid to tid
         (a) Therapeutic range: 50 to 100 μg/ml
         (b) Main side effects: ataxia, sedation, hepatoxicity

   b. Generalized myoclonic seizures
      (1) Valproic acid
      (2) Clonazepam (Klonopin) 1 to 12 mg PO qd
         (a) Therapeutic range: 5 to 70 mg/ml
         (b) Major side effect: sedation

   c. Simple and complex partial seizures
      (1) Carbamazepine
      (2) Phenytoin

   d. Absence seizures
      (1) Ethosuximide (Zarontin) 250 to 1500 mg PO qd
         (a) Therapeutic range: 40 to 100 μg/ml
         (b) Major side effects: ataxia, sedation, rash, bone marrow suppression
      (2) Valproic acid

   e. Temporal lobe epilepsy
      (1) Carbamazepine
      (2) Phenytoin
      (3) NOTE: phenobarbital is contraindicated

   f. Drug levels are indicated for breakthrough seizures (lack of control) and for suspected toxicity. Some clinicians recommend routine monitoring of drug levels every 3 to 12 months. CBC, transaminase, and alkaline phosphatase should be monitored every 3 to 12 months for patients taking phenytoin, carbamazepine, or valproic acid. Mild he-

patic function abnormalities (less than three times above the normal range) can be accepted if stable and the patient's epilepsy is well controlled. When the first anticonvulsant does not control the seizure, a second should be added. If the patient is still uncontrolled, drug substitution should be tried before adding a third drug

5. The use of newer drugs (e.g., felbamate) or brain surgery should be left to neurologists and neurosurgeons
6. Patient education
   a. Driving forbidden
   b. Occupational and other activities may require modification

Suggested readings

Delgado-Escueta AV, Treiman DM, Walsh GO: The treatable epilepsies, *N Engl J Med* 308:1508, 1576, 1983.

French J: The long-term therapeutic management of epilepsy, *Ann Intern Med* 120:411-422, 1994.

Niedermeyer E: Clinical evaluation and differential diagnosis in epileptic seizure disorders. In *The epilepsies: diagnosis and management,* Baltimore, 1990, Urban and Schwarzenberg.

Niedermeyer E: Epileptic seizure etiologies. In *The epilepsies: diagnosis and management,* Baltimore, 1990, Urban and Schwarzenberg.

Niedermeyer E: Pharmacotherapy: general considerations. In *The epilepsies: diagnosis and management,* Baltimore, 1990, Urban and Schwarzenberg.

Niedermeyer E: Types of epileptic seizures. In *The epilepsies: diagnosis and management,* Baltimore, 1990, Urban and Schwarzenberg.

Shorvon SD: Epidemiology, classification, natural history, and genetics of epilepsy, *Lancet* 336:93-96, 1990.

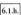 **6.1.h.** ***PERIPHERAL NEUROPATHY***
Tom J. Wachtel, MD

Definitions

Diseases of the peripheral nervous system can be distinguished from central nervous system disorders by the distribution of the neurologic abnormalities. Motor system involvement is characterized by flaccidity and eventually atrophy of involved muscles and areflexia. Peripheral neuropathies can affect all sensory modalities as well.

1. Anatomic classification
   a. Radiculopathies (diseases of the nerve roots)
      (1) Monoradiculopathy: single dermatome
      (2) Polyradiculopathy: multiple dermatomes
   b. Mononeuropathy: single nerve dysfunction
   c. Mononeuropathy multiplex or multifocal mononeuropathies: several nerves are dysfunctional concurrently or sequentially; usually nonsymmetric
   d. Polyneuropathy: symmetric, distal and graded distribution ("stocking and glove")
   e. Autonomic neuropathy: manifests by orthostatic hypotension, gastroparesis, hypoperistalsis, incontinence, impotence; often associated with polyneuropathy
2. Pathophysiologic classification
   a. Axonal neuropathy ("dying-back" neuropathy): usually a toxic poly-

neuropathy most commonly seen in chronic alcohol abuse or diabetes mellitus, and predominantly sensory

b. Demyelinating neuropathy: motor involvement is more likely and may predominate; subjective sensory complaints may be out of proportion to the objective findings such as seen in Guillain-Barré syndrome

c. Mixed axonal/demyelinating is often seen in diabetes

Clinical features

1. Onset: acute vs. chronic
2. Distribution of deficits: dermatome vs. peripheral nerve (Figures 6-1 and 6-2 and Tables 6-8 and 6-9)
3. Past medical history, family history, occupational history, medications and drugs, including alcohol
4. Ancillary tests
   a. Blood work
      (1) In all cases: CBC, sedimentation rate, serum creatinine, urinalysis, fasting blood glucose, transaminase, vitamin B_{12} level, folate level, chest x-ray
      (2) In selected cases: Watson-Schwartz test for acute intermittent porphyria, serum protein electrophoresis for multiple myeloma, heavy metals (lead, mercury, arsenic), B vitamins, human immune virus (HIV) test, antinuclear antibody (ANA), screening for occult cancer
   b. Electromyography looking for evidence of denervation
   c. Nerve conduction studies (mild slowing in axonopathies [40 m/sec], marked slowing in demyelinating neuropathies [10 to 15 m/sec])
   d. Nerve biopsy

Classification

1. Radiculopathies
   a. Acute polyradiculopathy (Guillain-Barré syndrome): patient presents with generalized weakness associated with sensory complaints (subjective and objective) that progress over several days to weeks, following an infectious illness. Weakness begins proximally; cranial nerves and respiratory muscles may be involved. Autonomic neuropathy may also be present (e.g., sphincter dysfunction). CSF characterically shows an elevated protein with few or no cells. Treatment is mainly supportive because the disease is self-limited in most cases (90%). If the disease is severe, plasmapheresis and IV immunoglobulin may be effective
   b. Chronic polyradiculopathy may be idiopathic or associated with malignancies (e.g., multiple myeloma)
   c. Monoradiculopathy
      (1) Cervical disk herniation
      (2) Lumbar disk herniation (sciatica [see Section 6.5])
      (3) Herpes zoster (shingles): acyclovir 800 mg five times daily for 5 days
2. Mononeuropathies (distribution of the deficits is a single nerve)
   a. Chronic compression

Text continued on p. 172.

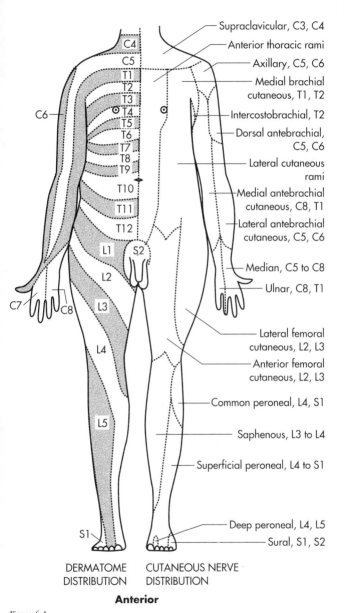

Figure 6-1

Cutaneous sensation on anterior aspect of body. (From DeGowin EL, DeGowin RL: *Bedside diagnostic examination,* ed 4, New York, 1981, Macmillan.)

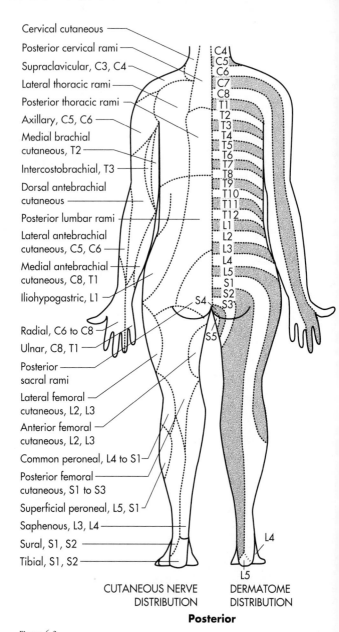

Cervical cutaneous
Posterior cervical rami
Supraclavicular, C3, C4
Lateral thoracic rami
Posterior thoracic rami
Axillary, C5, C6
Medial brachial cutaneous, T2
Intercostobrachial, T3
Dorsal antebrachial cutaneous
Posterior lumbar rami
Lateral antebrachial cutaneous, C5, C6
Medial antebrachial cutaneous, C8, T1
Iliohypogastric, L1
Radial, C6 to C8
Ulnar, C8, T1
Posterior sacral rami
Lateral femoral cutaneous, L2, L3
Anterior femoral cutaneous, L2, L3
Common peroneal, L4 to S1
Posterior femoral cutaneous, S1 to S3
Superficial peroneal, L5, S1
Saphenous, L3, L4
Sural, S1, S2
Tibial, S1, S2

C4 C5 C6 C7 C8 T1 T2 T3 T4 T5 T6 T7 T8 T9 T10 T11 T12 L1 L2 L3 L4 L5 S1 S2 S3 S4 S5 L4 L5

CUTANEOUS NERVE DISTRIBUTION

DERMATOME DISTRIBUTION

Posterior

Figure 6-2

Cutaneous sensation on posterior aspect of body. (From DeGowin EL, DeGowin RL: *Bedside diagnostic examination,* ed 4, New York, 1981, Macmillan.)

Table 6-8   Spinal root signs and symptoms

Spinal Root	Distribution of Pain, Paresthesias, or Sensory Loss	Weak Muscles	Diminished Reflexes
C5	Shoulder, antero-lateral arm and forearm	Deltoids, infraspinatus and supraspinatus, biceps	Pectoralis, biceps
C6	Shoulder, radial forearm, thumb	Biceps and brachioradialis, pronator teres	Biceps, brachioradialis
C7	Pectoral area, axilla, posterolateral forearm, second and third digits	Triceps, wrist extensors	Triceps
C8	Axilla, posteromedial arm, fourth and fifth digits	Hand interossei (ulnar nerve), abductor pollicis brevis (median nerve)	Finger flexors
L4	Hip, anterior thigh, anteromedial leg, great toe	Knee extensors, hip flexors	Knee
L5	Hip, posterolateral thigh, anterolateral leg, middle of foot	Foot extensors, great toe extensors, knee flexors	Medial hamstring
S1	Gluteal area, posterior thigh and leg, lateral foot	Foot flexors	Ankle
S2	Posterior thigh and leg	Toe flexors	—
S3-5	Sacral area	Sphincters	Bulbocavernosus, anal wink

From Stein J, editor: *Internal medicine*, ed 4, St Louis, 1994, Mosby.
C, Cervical; *L*, lumbar; *S*, sacral.

Table 6-9 Common mononeuropathies

Nerve	Clinical Presentation	Causes
Spinal accessory	Shoulder pain, droop and weakness of abduction, trapezius wasting "Winging" of scapula	Nerve trauma
Long thoracic		Backpacking, idiopathic
Axillary	Deltoid weakness, sensory loss over lateral upper arm	Trauma
Radial at spiral groove (Saturday night palsy)	Wrist and finger drop, weakness and areflexia of brachioradialis, sensory loss over dorsum of first web space	Acute compression
Musculocutaneous	Weakness of elbow flexion, sensory loss over radial aspect of forearm	Trauma, elbow hyperextension
Ulnar at elbow	Wasting, weakness of interossei; sensory loss over palmar and dorsal surface of ulnar aspect of hand	Chronic compression
Radial in forearm (posterior interosseous palsy)	Forearm pain, finger drop, radial deviation of extended wrist	Mass lesion, trauma, idiopathic
Median at wrist (carpal tunnel syndrome)	Nocturnal hand "tingling"; weakness, wasting of abductor pollicis brevis; sensory loss over volar aspect of fingers 1-3	Chronic compression

Ulnar at wrist	Weakness, wasting of interossei; variable sensory loss over fourth and fifth fingers	Occupational trauma
Femoral	Hip, groin pain; knee buckling; knee extensor weakness; absent knee jerk; sensory loss over anteromedial thigh and medial calf	Diabetes, retroperitoneal hemorrhage or tumor, postsurgical
Lateral femoral cutaneous at inguinal ligament	Thigh pain; sensory loss over lateral thigh; Tinel's sign in lateral inguinal ligament	Chronic compression
Sciatic	Weakness of dorsiflexion and plantar flexion; foot eversion and inversion; sensory loss over dorsum and sole of foot	Hip surgery, prolonged bed rest
Peroneal at fibular head (peroneal palsy)	Tripping; foot drop; sensory loss over lateral calf and dorsum of foot; normal foot eversion and inversion	Acute compression (i.e., leg crossing)
Posterior tibial at ankle (tarsal tunnel syndrome)	Nocturnal foot pain and tingling; Tinel's sign posterior to medial malleolus	Chronic compression, trauma

From Stein J, editor: *Internal medicine*, ed 4. St Louis, 1994, Mosby.

  (1) Median nerve (carpal tunnel syndrome)
  (2) Ulnar nerve (compression at elbow)
  (3) Lateral femoral cutaneous nerve (tight belt)
  b. Acute compression
  (1) Radial nerve (compression at spiral groove of humerus by some-one's head during sleep)
  (2) Peroneal nerve at fibular head (leg crossing)
  c. Trauma
3. Mononeuropathy multiplex (distribution of deficits is several nerves; eti-ology is a vasculitis)
  a. Polyarteritis nodosa
  b. Vasculitides associated with other collagen vascular diseases
  c. Diabetes
  d. Sarcoidosis
  e. Leprosy
4. Polyneuropathies
  a. Axonal
  (1) Vitamin deficiencies
    (a) B_1 (beriberi)
    (b) B_6
    (c) B_{12}
    (d) Niacin (pellagra)
  (2) Metabolic disease
    (a) Diabetes mellitus
    (b) Uremia
    (c) Thyroid dysfunction
  (3) Infection
    (a) HIV
    (b) Lyme disease
  (4) Paraneoplastic neuropathies
  (5) Neuropathies associated with connective tissue diseases
  (6) Hereditary neuropathies
    (a) Neuropathy associated with Friedreich's ataxia and variants
    (b) Ataxia-telangiectasia
  (7) Neuropathies associated with dysproteinemias and amyloidosis
  (8) Drug-induced neuropathies: nitrofurantoin, isoniazid, hydralazine, vincristine, amiodarone, dapsone, fluoxetine, ddI, phenytoin
  (9) Toxins: acrylamide, arsenic, cyanide, hexacarbons, mercury, meth-ylbromide, organophosphorous esters)
  b. Demyelinating neuropathies
  (1) Lead toxicity
  (2) Dysproteinemias
  (3) Hereditary (Charcot-Marie-Tooth disease)
  (4) NOTE: in clinical practice, demyelinating neuropathies are very dif-ficult to distinguish from polyradiculopathies

Suggested readings

Hallet M, Tandon D, Berardelli A: Treatment of peripheral neuropathies, *J Neurol Neu-rosurg Psychiatry* 48:1193-1207, 1985.

Logigian EL: Disease of peripheral nerve and motor neurons. In Stein JH, editor: *In-ternal medicine*, ed 4, St Louis, 1994, Mosby.

6.2   **ENDOCRINE AND METABOLIC DISORDERS**

6.2.a.   **DIABETES MELLITUS**
Tom J. Wachtel, MD

Criteria for diagnosis of diabetes in nonpregnant adults in a clinical setting*

1. Presence of the classic symptoms of diabetes, such as polyuria, polydipsia, ketonuria, and rapid weight loss, together with gross and unequivocal elevation of plasma glucose, e.g., postprandial or random plasma glucose concentration >200 mg/dl (11.1 mmol/L)

2. Elevated fasting glucose concentration on more than one occasion, venous plasma ≥140 mg/dl (7.8 mmol/L), venous whole blood ≥120 mg/dl (6.7 mmol/L), capillary whole blood ≥120 mg/dl (6.7 mmol/L)

3. Fasting glucose concentration less than that which is diagnostic of diabetes (above) but sustained elevated glucose concentration during an oral glucose tolerance test (OGTT). The NDDG requires that both the 2-hour sample and some other sample taken between administration of the 75-g glucose dose and 2 hours later meet the following criteria; WHO requires only that the 2-hour sample meet these criteria: venous plasma ≥200 mg/dl (11.1 mmol/L); venous whole blood ≥180 mg/dl (10 mmol/L); capillary whole blood ≥200 mg/dl (11.1 mmol/L)

4. In each case, measurement of glucose concentration should be repeated on a second occasion to confirm diagnosis

Etiology

1. Hypoinsulinemic causes
   a. Insulin-dependent diabetes mellitus (type I diabetes, insulin-dependent diabetes, juvenile-onset diabetes, ketosis-prone diabetes, brittle diabetes): rare onset in the elderly; almost all patients are long-term survivors of childhood or young adulthood onset
   b. Pancreatic disease (e.g., pancreatitis, pancreatic cancer, cystic fibrosis, hemochromatosis)
   c. Drugs
      (1) Diuretics (thiazides, diazoxide, furosemide, ethacrynic acid)
      (2) Psychoactive agents (lithium carbonate, neuroleptics, tricyclic antidepressants, marijuana)
      (3) Antineoplastic agents (streptozotocin, cyclophosphamide [Cytoxan])
      (4) Miscellaneous (phenytoin, propranolol [Inderal], isoniazid, nicotinic acid, cimetidine, pentamidine)
   d. Type II diabetes can lead to pancreatic beta–islet cell burnout and become insulin dependent
2. Hyperinsulinemic causes
   a. Non–insulin-dependent diabetes mellitus (type II diabetes, adult-onset diabetes, maturity-onset diabetes, ketosis-resistant diabetes, stable diabetes)
   b. Insulin receptor abnormalities (rare)

*Recommended by the National Diabetes Data Group (NDDG) and the World Health Organization (WHO).

    (1) Hereditary defect in insulin receptor
    (2) Congenital lipodystrophy associated with virilization, acanthosis nigricans
    (3) Antibody to insulin receptor–associated immune disorders
    (4) Ataxia-telangiectasia
    (5) Myotonic dystrophy
  c. Hormonal
    (1) Glucocorticoids (Cushing's syndrome or exogenous)
    (2) Progestins and estrogens
    (3) Growth hormone (acromegaly)
    (4) Glucagon (glucagonoma)
    (5) Epinephrine (pheochromocytoma)

Clinical presentations

1. Symptomless: discovered on routine examination (screening)
2. Acute or subacute onset
   a. Progressive loss of weight despite hyperphagia
   b. Severe polyuria and polydypsia (rare in type II diabetes)
   c. Diabetic ketoacidosis (rare in type II diabetes)
   d. Diabetic hyperosmolar state
   e. Postprandial hypoglycemia
3. Gradual onset
   a. Pruritus, generalized or perigenital
   b. Recurrent infections
   c. Polyuria and polydypsia
   d. Blurring of vision
4. Late manifestations
   a. Neuropathic
     (1) Peripheral polyneuropathy (lower limbs)
     (2) Mononeuropathy
       (a) Vascular (e.g., oculomotor)
       (b) Compression (e.g., carpal tunnel syndrome)
     (3) Autonomic neuropathy
     (4) Amyotrophy
   b. Vascular
     (1) Premature large vessel disease (atherosclerosis)
     (2) Small vessel disease (microangiopathy)
   c. Renal: glomerulosclerosis (nephrotic syndrome and uremia)
   d. Ophthalmic
     (1) Diabetic retinopathy
     (2) Cataract
     (3) Glaucoma
   e. Dermatologic
     (1) Necrobiosis lipoidica
     (2) Foot ulcer

Initial evaluation

1. Medical history
   a. Symptoms and previous laboratory test results related to diagnosis of diabetes

b. Dietary habits, nutritional status, and weight history
c. Details of previous treatment programs, including diabetes education
d. Current treatment of diabetes, including medications, diet, and results of glucose monitoring
e. Exercise history
f. Frequency, severity, and cause of acute complications such as ketoacidosis and hyperosmolar syndrome
g. Prior or current infections, particularly skin, foot, dental, and genitourinary
h. Symptoms and treatment of chronic complications associated with diabetes: eyes, heart, kidney, nerve, sexual function, peripheral vascular, and cerebral vascular
i. Medications that may affect carbohydrate metabolism (see above)
j. Risk factors for atherosclerosis: smoking, hypertension, obesity, hyperlipidemia, and family history
k. Psychosocial and economic factors that might influence management of diabetes
l. Family history
m. Gestation history

Physical examination
a. Height and weight measurement
b. Blood pressure determination (with orthostatic measurements)
c. Ophthalmoscopic examination, if possible with dilation
d. Thyroid palpation
e. Cardiac examination
f. Evaluation of pulses (and arterial auscultation)
g. Foot examination
h. Skin examination (including insulin injection sites)
i. Neurologic examination
j. Dental and periodontal examination

Laboratory evaluation
a. Fasting plasma glucose
b. Glycosylated hemoglobin (Hb A_{1c})
c. Total cholesterol or fasting lipid profile (total cholesterol, HDL cholesterol, and triglycerides)
d. Serum creatinine
e. Urinalysis: ketones, glucose, protein, microscopic if indicated
f. Urine for microalbumin (unless proteinuria on urinalysis)
g. Urine culture: if microscopic is abnormal or if urinary symptoms are present
h. Thyroid function tests (T_4 or TSH)
i. CBC
j. ECG

Management

Diet
a. Calories calculated to achieve ideal body weight (see Section 5.1). Since most adults with diabetes have type II diabetes and are overweight, one usual goal of the diet is weight reduction
b. Carbohydrates should represent 50% to 60% of the diet with

emphasis on complex carbohydrates (starch) and avoidance of simple carbohydrates (sweets). Fruits and vegetables are also encouraged

c. Proteins can represent 15% of the diet as in the general population

d. Fats should comprise 25% to 35% of the diet with emphasis on polyunsaturated fats and avoidance of saturated fats and cholesterol (e.g., animal products except skinned chicken and fish, dairy products, fried foods, tropical oils, and egg yolks)

2. Exercise

a. Aerobic exercises preferred over isometric exercise for cardiovascular protective benefit

b. Exercise should be as consistent as possible from day to day to avoid wide variations in caloric expenditures that impact insulin requirements and glucose metabolism

3. Oral hypoglycemic agents

a. Sulfonylureas

(1) Promote insulin release by pancreatic islet cells; any additional impact on peripheral glucose utilization probably not important clinically

(2) Six agents available currently

(a) First-generation drugs: can be classified as short acting (tolbutamide), intermediate acting (tolazamide and acetohexamide), and long acting (chlorpropamide)

(b) Most clinicians use second-generation sulfonylureas (glyburide and glipizide) because they are more potent and offer dosing flexibility. Glyburide (Micronase, Glynase, Diabeta) is given at doses of 1.25 to 20 mg daily in a single or bid schedule. Glipizide (Glucotrol) is given at doses of 2.5 to 40 mg daily in a single or bid schedule

(3) Major side effects: hypoglycemia and hyponatremia

(4) These drugs are titrated and then monitored, based principally on fasting blood sugar measurements. Good control (i.e., fasting blood sugar <140 mg/dl) can be confirmed with a glycosylated hemoglobin (e.g., Hb A_{1c} <7.5%)

b. Metformin (Glucophage)

(1) Promotes peripheral use of glucose; therefore it can be used alone or in combination with sulfonylureas or insulin

(2) Dose: 500 mg bid to a maximum of 2500 mg/day divided tid

(3) Also reduces LDL cholesterol and does not cause hypoglycemia

(4) Most common side effect: dyspepsia

(5) Most serious adverse reaction: lactic acidosis (very rare)

(6) Contraindicated in patients with renal disease (creatinine >1.5 mg/dl), liver disease, heavy alcohol use, or any metabolic acidosis

4. Insulin

a. Patients with type I diabetes must be treated with insulin; without it, their disease would lead rapidly to ketoacidosis and death. Patients with type II diabetes may benefit from treatment with insulin, but any benefit is difficult to quantitate and probably relates to patient age, level of glycemic control, ease of glycemic control, and other parameters

b. Whereas a strong argument can be made for "tight glycemic control" in patients with type I diabetes, based on the medical literature, a similar claim about type II diabetes can only be made by inference. Major risk of insulin treatment is hypoglycemia. The tighter the control, the higher the risk

c. Based on the desired level of glycemic control, therapy can be divided into

   (1) Minimal therapy, which will provide symptom control and reduce risk of ketoacidosis (type I) or hypersmolar state (type II). Average blood sugar will be 200 to 300 mg/dl and Hb A_{1c} will be 9.5% to 12%. This level of control is probably the best achievable without home glucose monitoring

   (2) Conventional therapy, which in addition to symptom control is intended to postpone onset of long-term degenerative complications of diabetes. Average blood sugar will be 150 to 200 mg/dl and Hb A_{1c} will be 7.5% to 9.5%. This level of control is the best that most patients can hope to achieve and is probably the best that should be offered by most generalists

   (3) Intensive insulin therapy aims at normalizing glycemic control and Hb A_{1c}. This requires multiple-dose insulin programs or continuous insulin infusion pumps

d. Many types and brands of insulin are available in the United States. For practical purposes, only human insulin (genetically engineered) should be used to avoid insulin allergy. Unless intensive therapy is considered, minimal and conventional therapy goals can be achieved with rapid-acting insulin (regular) and intermediate-acting insulin (NPH). Patient should not be admitted to the hospital because caloric intake and expenditure cannot approximate that associated with the patient's usual life-style. Patient should be instructed about home glucose monitoring and insulin self-injection. Injection should be subcutaneous in one part of the body (thigh, arm, or abdominal wall), which should not be rotated because of variable rates of insulin absorption. However, injection sites should be changed within the chosen area. **Goal of insulin treatment is to optimize glycemic control without causing hypoglycemia**

   (1) Insulin pharmacokinetics

	Onset (hr)	Peak (hr)	Duration (hr)
Regular insulin	2	4	6
NPH insulin	3	10	24

Treatment algorithm

   (1) Select a starting dose of NPH insulin (usually 14 units) to be given at 7 AM

   (2) Measure blood sugars at those times in a 24-hour period when

the blood sugar is most likely to be lowest (i.e., 5 PM or before dinner) and fasting the next day (i.e., 7 AM or before breakfast). This can be done on a daily or less frequent basis depending on how quickly one wishes to achieve control

(3) Increase the morning NPH insulin on a daily to weekly basis by 10% to 20% increments until one or both daily blood sugars approach 150 mg/dl

(4) If both 5 PM and 7 AM blood sugars come down together, the patient should check the blood sugar at 11 AM (before lunch) and at 11 PM (bedtime). If either of those are high, they can be treated with regular insulin given 4 hours earlier (begin with 2 units and use 2-unit increments)

(5) If the fasting blood sugar is high when the 5 PM blood sugar approaches 150 mg/dl, the patient should be advised to split the NPH by dividing the current daily dose into two thirds at 7 AM and one third at 7 PM and retitrate from this new starting point with 7 AM and 5 PM blood sugars. Such a patient should also be questioned about night sweats, nightmares, and morning headaches, any of which would suggest a Somogyi phenomenon (nighttime hypoglycemia followed by counterregulatory overcompensation and fasting hyperglycemia); in this case, total insulin should be decreased

(6) Other reasons to split the NPH insulin are a total daily requirement of more than 50 units or a patient with a high 11 PM, who otherwise would inject regular insulin alone at 7 PM as in (4)

(7) If patient's fasting blood sugar approximates 150 mg/dl but the 5 PM blood sugar is still high, one option would be to move some of the daily calories to a snack at bedtime; another option would be to add some regular insulin in the morning because some patients are slow at metabolizing the morning dose of NPH

(8) Again, once the 7 AM and 5 PM are adjusted with the NPH insulin, 11 AM and 11 PM blood sugars should be checked as in (4)

e. It is important to insist that patients check their blood sugar (or have it checked) at the critical times. More useful information is gained from four blood sugars during one typical day in a week than from seven daily fasting blood sugars. Hypoglycemia is much more dangerous in the short term than hyperglycemia; the logic of the algorithm is to prevent it

f. Insulin and oral hypoglycemic agents can be used in combination for patients with type II diabetes, but the indication for this is not clear. Some patients gain weight as a result of pharmacologic treatment of diabetes without dietary compliance. They then become more resistant to insulin and require increasing doses of oral agents or insulin. In such patients the goals of treatment must be reassessed with the therapeutic emphasis placed on diet

5. Current standards for ongoing management of type II diabetes are presented on a chart (Figure 6-3)

NAME: _____

DOB: _____
= = = = = = = = = = = = = = = = = = = =

On insulin   Yes ___   No ___

Year								
Semester	1st	2nd	1st	2nd	1st	2nd	1st	2nd
Not on insulin Number of FBS tests (q3mos)								
On insulin Home glucose monitoring (qid once/week) Y/N								
Hgb A₁C (q6mos)								
U/A (q1year)								
Urine for microalbumin (q1year)								
Creatinine (q1year)								
Cholesterol (q1year)								
TSH (q1year)								
Eye Exam (q1year)								
Foot Exam (q1year)								

Figure 6-3
Diabetes chart.

NONKETOTIC HYPERTONICITY

Definition

Nonketotic hypertonicity (NKH), a complication of type II diabetes, can be defined strictly in patients with severe hyperglycemia (serum glucose >800 mg/dl) and severe hyperosmolarity (serum osmolarity >350 mOsm/L) or more loosely in patients with more modest elevations of serum glucose (600 mg/dl) and osmolarity (320 in Osm/L).

Serum osmolarity can be measured directly in the laboratory but most commonly is calculated from the patient's serum sodium (Na), potassium (K), glucose (glu), and blood urea nitrogen (BUN), which are readily available. The formula used to calculate serum osmolarity is as follows: Osm = 2(Na + K) + glu/18 + BUN/2.8. Some authorities do not include BUN in the calculation of effective serum osmolarity because BUN is freely permeable between extracellular and intracellular spaces.

Epidemiology

The majority of patients with NKH have type II diabetes mellitus and tend to be elderly. The incidence approximates 17.5 cases per 100,000 person years. This figure is very close to the incidence of diabetic ketoacidosis (DKA), which is 14/100,000 person-years. Factors associated with the development of NKH include sociodemographic factors (old age, female sex, nursing home residence); underlying illness (acute infection [especially pneumonia and UTI] pancreatitis, stroke); and medications (thiazide and loop diuretics, phenytoin, beta-blockers, glucocorticoids).

Pathophysiology

The simplest explanation, although unproven, is that hyperosmolarity results from hyperglycemia-induced osmotic diuresis. When a diabetic patient's volume status becomes slightly depleted, one of two events will occur:

1. The sensation of thirst is experienced and the patient drinks high-glucose–containing fluid, thus aggravating the hyperglycemia and diuresis.
2. Thirst is not experienced despite a negative volume status.

In either case the patient enters a vicious circle of worsening hyperosmolarity and osmotic diuresis, which, if untreated, leads to NKH and death. In addition to free water loss and severe dehydration, the patient also loses sodium and potassium. Further, hyperosmolarity and potassium depletion may inhibit insulin secretion, thus perpetuating the cycle.

The mechanism whereby dehydration occurs in DKA is the same. Why some patients become hyperosmolar, yet do not develop ketonemia, is not known. One explanation is that the regulation of lipolysis is so sensitive to insulin that the levels of insulin in many patients with NKH may be sufficient to prevent ketoacidosis but not hyperglycemia. This theory fits neatly with the clinical observation that overlap cases of NKH and DKA are common and dependent on the relative availability of insulin receptors.

Clinical presentation

The most common complaints are weakness or fatigue, followed by polydipsia, polyuria, and nausea. Other symptoms include vomiting, dizziness, seizures, other neurologic complaints with no specific anatomic localization, diaphoresis, and behavior disturbances. A history of diabetes is known in only two thirds of all cases.

The cardinal signs of NKH are alterations of consciousness and hypovolemia. Most patients are at least lethargic and many are confused, stuporous, or unresponsive. The severity of cognitive impairment is directly related to the elevation in osmolarity and to the age of the patient. Hypovolemia manifests itself by sustained or postural hypotension, tachycardia, dry skin and mucous membranes, and cold extremities. Particular care should be taken to rule out an underlying acute infectious process whether or not the patient is febrile; pneumonia or bacterial skin infection may be evident, but the aid of the laboratory is necessary to diagnose a UTI, septicemia, meningitis, or a deep-seated abscess.

Laboratory tests to be obtained immediately include a CBC and differential, blood glucose, BUN, creatinine and electrolytes, urinalysis, ECG, and chest x-ray. If the anion gap is larger than 15 mEq/L, arterial blood gases and serum ketone and lactate levels should be determined. In addition, appropriate cultures should be ordered.

Management

Initial fluid therapy should correct the volume deficit with rapid administration of isotonic saline at the rate of 1 L per 1 or 2 hours until the blood pressure begins to rise or, if the patient is centrally monitored, until the central venous pressure or pulmonary wedge pressure begins to rise. Then a half-normal saline solution should be given at the same rate of infusion until the intravascular volume deficit is replaced. Thereafter, the rate of infusion can be reduced to maintenance at 100 to 200 ml/hr. A rough guideline is to correct one half of the fluid deficit over the first 12 hours and the remainder by 36 hours.

Serum glucose, BUN, and electrolytes should be obtained on an hourly basis until the hyperosmolarity (and acidosis, if present) has been corrected. Potassium deficit may be anticipated during insulin therapy regardless of the presence of acidosis. Although the serum potassium level is often above normal range at the time of presentation, intracellular potassium has been depleted and replacement should begin as soon as the level is in the normal range, by adding potassium chloride to each liter of IV infusion at a concentration of 20 to 40 mEq/L. Insulin treatment in NKH is less important than in DKA, where insulin is the cornerstone of management, but insulin in NKH serves to restore normal glucose homeostasis. Twenty units of regular insulin should be given intravenously at once, followed by infusion at a rate of 5 to 15 U/hr until the patient's blood sugar reaches 250 mg/dl, at which point subcutaneous insulin treatment should replace the IV administration and D5W should be added to the crystalloid in the IV infusion, guided by the patient's blood sugar levels to prevent hypoglycemia. Any underlying infection must be diagnosed and treated with an appropriate antibiotic regimen (and drainage in the case of an abscess).

Prognosis

Mortality from NKH is high, ranging from 14% to 58%. Factors associated with death in NKH include advanced age, nursing home residence, high osmolarity, high BUN, and high sodium.

Prevention

First, since one third of all cases occur in patients who were not previously known to have diabetes, screening the general population for diabetes and educating all diabetic people about the symptoms of hyperglycemia may be useful. In particular, nursing home populations should be screened for diabetes and staffs should be encouraged to monitor each patient's state of hydration regularly.

Second, prompt diagnosis and treatment of pneumonia, UTI, and other infections in diabetic people are likely to prevent a substantial proportion of NKH cases.

Third, drugs known to cause carbohydrate intolerance should be avoided in diabetic patients. Thiazides or beta-blockers, for example, should not be used as agents of choice when hypertension and diabetes coexist; phenytoin should not be used as the first-line anticonvulsant when epilepsy and diabetes coexist; and glucocorticoids should be avoided, if possible, in diabetic persons.

Finally, compliance with diet, oral hypoglycemic agents, or insulin should be promoted.

Suggested readings

The Diabetes Control and Complications Trial Research Group: The effect of intensive treatment of diabetes on the development and progression of long-term complications in insulin-dependent diabetes mellitus, *N Engl J Med* 329: 977-986, 1993.

Hanson RL et al: Comparison of screening tests for non-insulin-dependent diabetes mellitus, *Arch Intern Med* 153:2133-2140, 1993.

Nathan DM: Long-term complications of diabetes mellitus, *N Engl J Med* 328:1676-1685, 1993.

Viberti G et al for the European Microalbuminuria Captopril Study Group: Effect of captopril on progression to clinical proteinuria in patients with insulin-dependent diabetes mellitus and microalbuminuria, *JAMA* 271:275-279, 1994.

Wachtel TJ: The diabetic hyperosmolar state, *Clin Geriatr Med* 6:797-806, 1990.

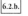

HYPERLIPIDEMIA
Tom J. Wachtel, MD

Who should be tested?

All adults should have their total cholesterol (TC) measured at least every 5 years. Clinicians should measure nonfasting TC and evaluate patients for coronary heart disease (CHD) risk factors during routine office visits.

Alternative screening approaches include measuring nonfasting TC and high-density lipoprotein cholesterol (HDL-C) every 5 years (recommended by the National Cholesterol Education Program [NCEP]) or obtaining a full lipid panel, which requires a 12-hour fasting TC, HDL-C, and triglyceride (TG) level; the low-density lipoprotein cholesterol (LDL-C) can be calculated with the following formula

$$LDL\text{-}C = TC - HDL\text{-}C - TG/5$$

The latter approach is the best strategy for patients who have known arteriosclerotic cardiovascular disease (ASCVD) or who are at high risk of being affected with it.

With the rapid accumulation of evidence proving that lowering cholesterol promotes regression (or at least delays progression) of ASCVD (i.e., effective tertiary prevention), an upper age cutoff for screening and treatment can no longer be justified.

Initial classification based on TC and HDL-C

High blood cholesterol is defined at ≥240 mg/dl for persons with no risk factors or only one risk factor for ASCVD and ≥200 mg/dl for persons with two or more risk factors for ASCVD. An estimated one third of U.S. adults have TC levels above those thresholds. Figure 6-4 outlines the decision pro-

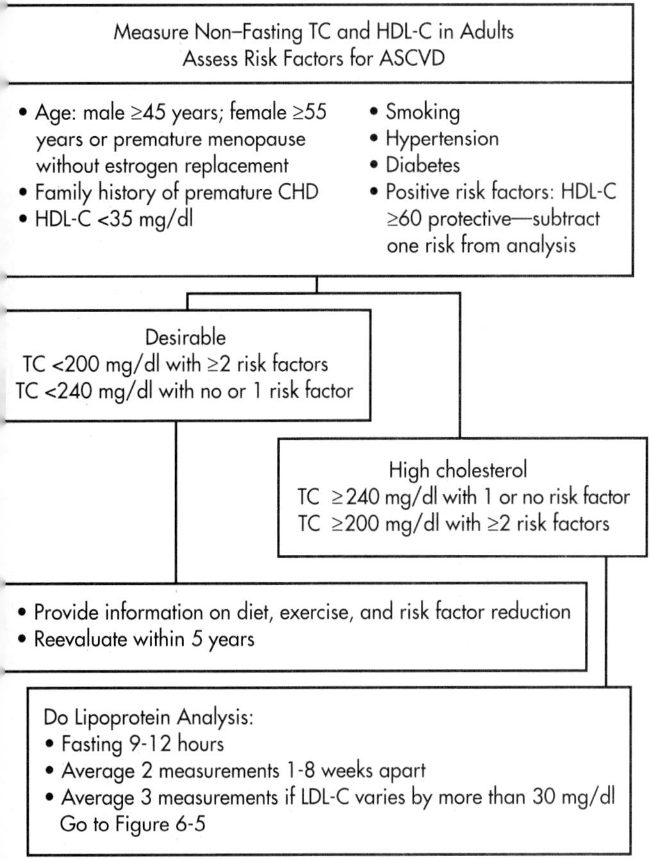

Figure 6-4
Classification based on total cholesterol HDL-C.

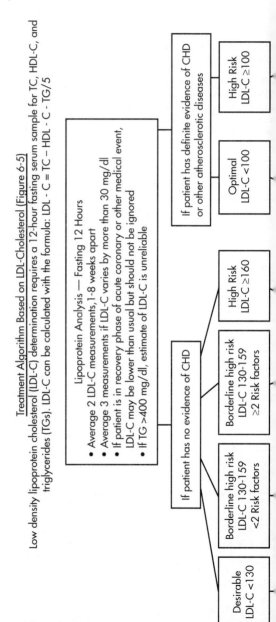

Treatment Algorithm Based on LDL-Cholesterol (Figure 6-5)

Low density lipoprotein cholesterol (LDL-C) determination requires a 12-hour fasting serum sample for TC, HDL-C, and triglycerides (TGs). LDL-C can be calculated with the formula: LDL - C = TC – HDL - C - TG/5

Lipoprotein Analysis — Fasting 12 Hours
• Average 2 LDL-C measurements, 1-8 weeks apart
• Average 3 measurements if LDL-C varies by more than 30 mg/dl
• If patient is in recovery phase of acute coronary or other medical event, LDL-C may be lower than usual but should not be ignored
• If TG >400 mg/dl, estimate of LDL-C is unreliable

If patient has no evidence of CHD

Desirable
LDL-C <130

Borderline high risk
LDL-C 130-159
<2 Risk factors

Borderline high risk
LDL-C 130-159
≥2 Risk factors

High Risk
LDL-C ≥160

If patient has definite evidence of CHD or other atherosclerotic diseases

Optimal
LDL-C <100

High Risk
LDL-C ≥100

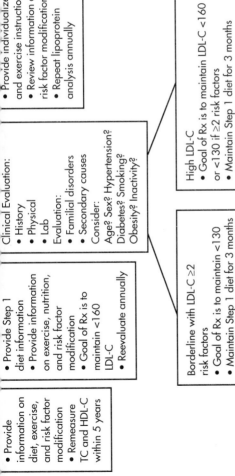

- Provide information on diet, exercise, and risk factor modification
- Remeasure TC and HDL-C within 5 years

- Provide Step 1 diet information
- Provide information on exercise, nutrition, and risk factor modification
- Goal of Rx is to maintain <160 LDL-C
- Reevaluate annually

- Provide individualized diet and exercise instruction
- Review information on risk factor modification
- Repeat lipoprotein analysis annually

Clinical Evaluation:
- History
- Physical
- Lab

Evaluation:
- Familial disorders
- Secondary causes

Consider:
Age? Sex? Hypertension? Diabetes? Smoking? Obesity? Inactivity?

Clinical Evaluation:
- History
- Physical
- Lab

Evaluation:
- Familial disorders
- Secondary causes

Consider:
Age? Sex? Hypertension? Diabetes? Smoking? Obesity? Inactivity?

Begin Diet Step II:
- Begin drug Rx if LDL-C ≥130 after 6-12 weeks
- Goal of Rx is to maintain LDL-C <100
- Provide information on risk factor modification

Borderline with LDL-C ≥2 risk factors
- Goal of Rx is to maintain <130
- Maintain Step 1 diet for 3 months
- Go to Step 2 diet if necessary
- After 6 months, consider drug Rx if LDL-C ≥160

High LDL-C
- Goal of Rx is to maintain LDL-C <160 or <130 if ≥2 risk factors
- Maintain Step 1 diet for 3 months
- Go to Step 2 diet if necessary
- After 6 months, consider drug Rx if LDL-C ≥190 or ≥160 with ≥2 risk factors

Figure 6-5
Treatment algorithm based on LDL-C.

cess for initial determination of risk status in patients without known CHD or other atherosclerotic disease (primary prevention) and is based on the measurement of TC (with or without initial HDL-C determination). Figure 6-5 outlines further management for those who fail the screen and those who require tertiary prevention.

Diet and exercise based on LDL-C

Individualized therapy for high LDL-C is the key to successful intervention and risk reduction. Diet modification and physical activity (exercise) are essential first steps in therapy for all patients, and weight reduction is extremely important in patients who are overweight.

The LDL-C levels at which dietary treatment is initiated depend on whether the clinical objective is primary prevention or tertiary prevention and risk factors for ASCVD (Table 6-10). In primary prevention (patients without CHD or other atherosclerotic disease) most patients who qualify for medical intervention will require dietary therapy and a program of aerobic physical exercise. Begin dietary therapy with the step 1 diet, which calls for a reduction of saturated fat intake to 8% to 10% of total calories and less than 300 mg of cholesterol per day. If the patient is already adhering to the step 1 diet at the evaluation and if this diet proves inadequate to achieve the goal LDL-C level, the patient should proceed to the step 2 diet. This diet calls for further reduction of saturated fat intake to less than 7% of calories and less than 200 mg of cholesterol per day. Dietary therapy should be monitored at 3- and 6-month intervals to determine effectiveness. Diet brochures or books can be given or recommended to patients. Asking patients to keep a food diary for 1 week between visits can help the physician provide individualized advice.

In tertiary prevention (patients with CHD or other atherosclerotic disease) dietary therapy should begin with the step 2 diet and the patient should be watched closely for 1 to 3 months.

The target level of LDL-C lowering depends on the risk status of the patient (Table 6-10).

Drug treatment based on LDL-C

For patients whose diet therapy does not achieve adequate cholesterol lowering, drug therapy is recommended. The LDL-C levels for initiation of drug

Table 6-10 Dietary therapy based on LDL-C level (mg/dl)

Risk Status	Initiation Level	LDL-C Goal
Definite CHD or other atherosclerotic disease	≥100	<100
No CHD, two or more other risk factors	≥130	<130
No CHD, fewer than two other risk factors	≥160	<160

therapy and LDL-C target goals also depend on whether the clinical objective is primary or tertiary prevention (Table 6-11).

1. For patients without heart disease (or other atherosclerotic disease), consider drug therapy in men ≥45 years old and women ≥55 years old when LDL-C is ≥190 mg/dl, with fewer than two ASCVD risk factors and after maximal dietary therapy, or when LDL-C is ≥160 mg/dl, with two or more ASCVD risk factors
2. Drug considerations for patients with CHD (or other atherosclerotic disease)
   a. For CHD patients with LDL-C levels of 100 to 130 mg/dl, clinical judgment of individual patient characteristics will be key in deciding whether to initiate drug treatment
   b. If the LDL-C goal of <100 mg/dl is not attained after 3 months with a single drug, consider adding a second agent. Concomitant use of HMG-CoA reductase inhibitors (statins) and fibrates should generally be avoided. Counsel the patient about benefits and risks (Table 6-11)
3. Available drug therapies
   a. Bile acid sequestrants
      (1) Cholestyramine and colestipol are especially valuable for lowering isolated and moderately elevated LDL-C by 15% to 20%
      (2) Useful in combination with statins in severe forms of hypercholesterolemia
   b. Nicotinic acid
      (1) Lowers LDL-C (10% to 25%) and TG (20% to 50%) and raises HDL-C (15% to 35%)
      (2) Disadvantage: frequency of side effects at high doses (especially flushing, which may be decreased by taking aspirin, 325 mg, 30 minutes before the nicotinic acid)
      (3) Useful in treating high-risk patients with isolated low HDL-C
   c. HMG-CoA reductase inhibitors (statins): fluvastatin, lovastin, pravastatin, simvastatin
      (1) Highly effective in lowering LDL-C (20% to 40%) and TG (10% to 20%) and raising HDL (5% to 15%)
      (2) Easy to administer and generally well tolerated and safe; hepatotoxicity may occur, but the benefit of episodic liver function testing has not been established

Table 6-11   Drug therapy based on LDL-C level (mg/dl)

Risk Status	Initiation Level	LDL-C Goal
If patient has CHD or atherosclerotic disease	Add drug therapy if LDL-C ≥130 after 6 mo of diet therapy	<100
No CHD, two or more other risk factors	≥160 after 6 mo of diet therapy	<130
No CHD, fewer than two other risk factors	≥190 after 6 mo of diet therapy	<160

       (3) Particularly useful in achieving substantial LDL-C reductions in patients with severe hypercholesterolemia, established CHD, and multiple risk factors

       (4) Rapidly replacing bile acid sequestrants as first-line agents

  d. Fibrates: gemfibrozil and clofibrate

       (1) Particularly effective in lowering TG (20% to 50%) and in some patients raising HDL-C (10% to 15%)

       (2) Not listed as major drugs because of their modest effect on lowering LDL-C

       (3) Most useful for treating very high TG, familial dysbetalipoproteinemia, combined hyperlipidemia, and diabetic patients with high TG

  e. Probucol

       (1) Lowers LDL-C only 5% to 15% and is therefore not classified as a major drug

       (2) Also lowers HDL-C in most patients

  f. Estrogen replacement therapy

       (1) Lowers LDL-C and raises HDL-C in postmenopausal women

       (2) In prospective uncontrolled studies, women with and without CHD have a 50% or greater reduction in rates of CHD complications when given estrogen replacement therapy, but no large-scale controlled clinical trials have confirmed this effect

       (3) Epidemiologic evidence for benefit of estrogen therapy is especially strong for tertiary prevention in women with prior CHD

4. Selection of drugs

  a. High LDL-C with TG <200 mg/dl

       (1) Therapeutic goal: to lower LDL-C

       (2) Most effective for lowering LDL-C levels: bile acid sequestrants and statins

       (3) Nicotinic acid is also effective, but daily doses of 3 g are usually required to reduce LDL-C levels by 20% to 25%. If HDL-C is also low, nicotinic acid is the most effective for increasing HDL-C

       (4) Fibrates generally produce only a 10% reduction in LDL-C and thus are not recommended

Single Drug Selection	Combination Therapy
HMG-CoA (statin)	Statin + BAS
Nicotinic acid (NA)	NA + BAS
Bile acid sequestrant (BAS)	Statin + NA

  b. Combined hyperlipidemia (elevated LDL-C with TG 200 to 400 mg/dl)

       (1) Nicotinic acid: drug of first choice. If adequate doses are tolerated, nicotinic acid can favorably modify all of the lipoprotein abnormalities. If LDL-C is substantially elevated, nicotinic acid therapy may not reduce LDL-C to target level. Avoid nicotinic acid or use it with caution in diabetic patients

       (2) Consider statins if nicotinic acid therapy is ineffective

(3) Fibrates effectively lower TG and raise HDL-C but in patients with combined hyperlipidemia they either lower LDL-C to a small extent (only 5% to 10%) or raise the level

Single Drug Selection	Combination Therapy
Nicotinic acid (NA)	NA + Statin
HMG-CoA (statin)	Statin + Gem
Gemfibrozil (Gem)	NA + Gem

c. Patients with low HDL-C
   (1) Low HDL-C, defined as <35 mg/dl, is classified as a major risk factor
   (2) Strong association between low HDL-C and CHD justifies considering HDL-C levels in overall cholesterol management
      (a) Low HDL-C with high LDL-C and without hypertriglyceridemia: nicotinic acid is drug of first choice; if patient cannot successfully take nicotinic acid, a statin is recommended
      (b) Low HDL-C with hypertriglyceridemia; nicotinic acid or fibrates are recommended
      (c) Low HDL-C with "normal" lipids: priority should be given to management of other risk factors (e.g., smoking, hypertension, diabetes); in addition, control patient's weight
d. Patients with isolated hypertriglyceridemia: uncertainty about whether the connection between TG level and CHD is due to the atherogenicity of certain TG-rich lipoproteins (small VLDL and remnants of chylomicrons and VLDL) or to the secondary effects of hypertriglyceridemia (low HDL, small LDL particles, or enhanced thrombogenesis). Not all forms of hypertriglyceridemia impart the same risk for CHD
   (1) Classification by levels of TG (mg/dl)
      (a) Normal TG: <200
      (b) Borderline high TG: 200 to 400
      (c) High TG: 400 to 1000
      (d) Very high TG: >1000
   (2) Management: changes in life-style (low-carbohydrate, low-fat diet, weight reduction, exercise, quit smoking and alcohol) are the principal therapy for dyslipidemias with elevated TG
      (a) Patients with high serum TG who do not respond to diet should probably be treated with TG-lowering drugs because of the potential risk of developing very high TG levels and acute pancreatitis
      (b) Nicotinic acid is the drug choice for patients with high TG level to reduce both VLDL-C and LDL-C while increasing HDL-C
      (c) If nicotinic acid is poorly tolerated, the fibrates provide an alternative therapy
      (d) Statins can be used, although their major effect is to lower LDL-C level; they may moderately reduce TG (and VLDL-C) and mildly increase HDL-C

(e) The presence of a high TG level is a relative contraindication for the use of bile acid sequestrants since they usually raise TG levels

5. Patients with high blood cholesterol and concomitant high blood pressure
   a. Antihypertensive agents can affect serum lipid levels. Thiazides and loop diuretics can cause modest and often transient elevations (5 to 10 mg/dl) in TC, LDL-C, and TG levels with little or no adverse effects on the HDL level
   b. In general, beta-blockers, without intrinsic sympathomimetic activity of alpha-blocking properties, tend to reduce HDL-C, increase TG, and have variable effects on TC; beta-blockers with intrinsic sympathomimetic activity (e.g., acebutolol) and the beta-blocker labetolol (which has alpha$_1$-adrenergic blocking properties) produce no appreciable changes in lipid levels
   c. Alpha$_1$-adrenergic blockers and centrally acting alpha$_2$-receptor agonists have a slight beneficial effect on blood lipid levels by decreasing TC and LDL-C
   d. Calcium channel antagonists, angiotensin-converting enzyme inhibitors, hydralazine, minoxidil, potassium-sparing diuretics, and reserpine have minimal if any effects on serum lipids

Suggested readings

Choice of cholesterol-lowering drugs, *Med Lett Drug Ther* 33(835):1-4, 1991.

Crouse JR III et al: Pravastatin, lipids, and atherosclerosis in the carotid arteries (PLAC-I), *Am J Cardiol* 75:455-459, 1995.

Expert Panel on Detection, Evaluation and Treatment of High Blood Cholesterol in Adults: Summary of the second report of the National Cholesterol Education Program (NCEP) Expert Panel on Detection, Evaluation, and Treatment of High Blood Cholesterol in Adults (adult treatment panel II), *JAMA* 269:3015-3023, 1993.

Furberg CD et al: Effect of lovastatin on early carotid atherosclerosis and cardiovascular events, *Circulation* 90:1679-1687, 1994.

Garber AM et al: Costs and health consequences of cholesterol screening for asymptomatic older Americans, *Arch Intern Med* 151:1089-1095, 1991.

Heudebert GR et al: Combination drug therapy for hypercholesterolemia, *Arch Intern Med* 153:1828-1837, 1993.

Jones PH: A clinical overview of dyslipidemias: treatment strategies, *Am J Med* 93:187-198, 1992.

Jukema JW et al: Effects of lipid lowering by pravastatin on progression and regression of coronary artery disease in symptomatic men with normal to moderately elevated serum cholesterol levels: the Regression Growth Evaluation Statin Study (REGRESS), *Circulation* 91:2528-2540, 1995.

Kronmal RA et al: Total serum cholesterol levels and mortality risk as a function of age, *Arch Intern Med* 153:1065-1073, 1993.

Lewis B, Tikkanen MJ: Low blood total cholesterol and mortality; causality, consequence and confounders, *Am J Cardiol* 73:80-85, 1994.

Lovastatin study groups I through IV: Lovastatin 5 year safety and efficacy study, *Arch Intern Med* 153:1079-1087, 1993.

MAAS investigators: Effect of simvastatin on coronary atheroma: the Multicentre Anti-Atheroma Study (MAAS), *Lancet* 344:633-638, 1994.

The quest for a cholesterol-decreasing diet: should we subtract, substitute or supplement? *Ann Intern Med* 119:627-632, 1993 (editorial).

The Scandinavian Simvastatin Survival Study Group: Randomized trial of cholesterol lowering in 4444 patients with coronary heart disease: the Scandinavian Simvastatin Survival Study (4S), *Lancet* 344:1383-1389, 1994.

Sempos CT et al: Prevalence of high blood cholesterol among US adults, *JAMA* 269:3009-3014, 1993.

Shepherd J et al: Prevention of coronary heart disease with pravastatin in men with hypercholesterolemia, *N Engl J Med* 333:1301-1307, 1995.

Smith GD, Song F, Sheldon TA: Cholesterol lowering and mortality: the importance of considering initial level of risk, *Br Med J* 306:1367-1373, 1993.

Sprecher DL et al: Efficacy of psyllium in reducing serum cholesterol levels in hyper-cholesterolemic patients on high- or low-fat diets, *Ann Intern Med* 119:545-554, 1993.

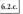

OSTEOPOROSIS
Fred F. Ferri, MD

Definition

Osteoporosis is a disease characterized by low bone mass, microarchitectural deterioration of bone tissue leading to enhanced bone fragility, and a consequent increase in fracture risk. Compression fractures (Figure 6-6) are common with progression of the disease.

Morbidity and financial concerns

1. Osteoporosis affects over 30% of postmenopausal females
2. Over 1 million fractures in the United States each year are attributable to osteoporosis
3. Financial cost of osteoporosis in the United States exceeds $10 billion per year

Risk factors

1. Endocrine
   a. Estrogen deficiency (e.g., early menopause, premenopausal estrogen deficiency)
   b. Prolonged exposure to glucocorticoids
   c. Hyperthyroidism, hyperparathyroidism, Cushing's syndrome, hyperprolactinemia, hypogonadism, diabetes, renal failure
2. Race: Caucasian and Asian females are at greatest risk
3. Body habitus: thin or petite
4. Family history of osteoporosis
5. Life-style: smoking, alcoholism, sedentary life-style
6. Dietary: low dietary intake of calcium, decreased intestinal absorption, vitamin D deficiency, excess caffeine intake, ascorbic acid deficiency, phosphate deficiency
7. Drugs: loop diuretics, phenytoin, aluminum antacids, heparin, warfarin, vitamin A, tetracyclines, excess thyroid hormone, isoniazid, lithium, cyclosporine, methotrexate, medroxyprogesterone
8. Immobilization
9. Multiple myeloma

Diagnosis

Bone mass or bone mineral density accurately reflects fracture risk. It can be measured by several radiologic techniques. Dual-energy x-ray absorptiometry (DEXA) is the most precise method. It also combines low radiation (<3 mrem) and rapid results (takes only 5 to 10 minutes to perform.) Figure 6-7 illustrates DEXA of an osteoporotic spine and femur.

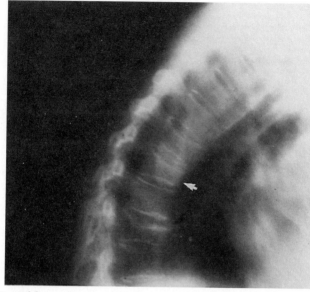

Figure 6-6
Lateral thoracic spine x-ray of woman with osteoporosis. Arrows indicate vertebrae that are compressed centrally and anteriorly. X-ray also shows "codfish" vertebrae, the appearance of oval disk spaces. (From Noble J et al, editors: *Textbook of primary care medicine,* ed 2, St Louis, 1996, Mosby.)

INDICATIONS FOR BONE MASS MEASUREMENT (SHOULD NOT BE PERFORMED INDISCRIMINATELY)

1. Perimenopausal or estrogen-deficient females who are considering long-term therapy
2. Patients with radiologic abnormalities suspicious for osteoporosis (compression fractures, osteopenia) who will consider long-term therapy
3. Monitoring of treatment efficacy in patients with osteoporosis
4. Long-term glucocorticoid therapy
5. Cushing's syndrome, primary hyperparathyroidism, hypogonadism, hyperthyroidism
6. Malabsorption, chronic renal insufficiency

Prevention and treatment

1. Prevention of bone loss should be started earlier in life with modification of risk factors (e.g., regular exercise; avoidance of tobacco, alcohol, and caffeine; elimination of chronic glucocorticoid use); and use of the following agents

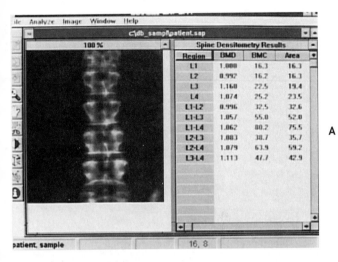

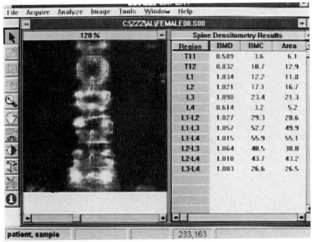

Figure 6-7

Dual-energy x-ray absorption of spine and femur of normal and osteoporotic patient with Lunar Corporation expert system. Views are nearly x-ray quality. **A,** Normal spine. **B,** Osteoporotic spine. **C,** Normal femur. **D,** Osteoporotic femur. (Courtesy Lunar Corp., Madison, Wis.; from Noble J et al, editors: *Textbook of primary care medicine,* ed 2, St Louis, 1996, Mosby.)   *Continued*

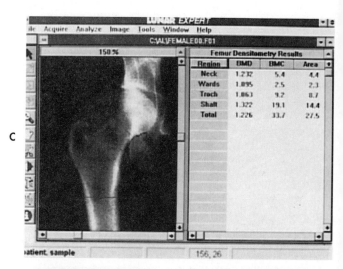

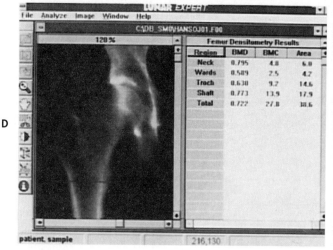

Figure 6-7, cont'd
For legend see p. 193.

a. **Estrogens**

   (1) Estrogen replacement therapy reduces rate of bone loss after menopause by inhibiting bone resorption (e.g., 60% reduction in rate of hip fracture)

   (2) Minimum effective daily oral doses are 0.625 mg of conjugate equine estrogens or 50 to 100 mg of transdermal estradiol

   (3) Estrogen therapy is generally continued for several years

   (4) Additional benefits of estrogen therapy are a reduction of about 40% to 50% in risk of ischemic heart disease and a decrease in mortality from cardiovascular disease

   (5) Potential complications of postmenopausal estrogen replacement therapy

      (a) Increased risk of endometrial cancer: to minimize this risk progestin is added to estrogen. There should also be close monitoring of the patient with annual pelvic exams and Pap smears, looking for RBCs or histiocytes as uterine cancer signals that should be followed up with endometrial biopsy. Addition of a progestinal agent may also result in recurrent episodes of postmenopausal uterine bleeding and may partly reverse some favorable effects of estrogens on serum lipids. Amenorrhea reoccurs in approximately 40% of women within 3 months of initiation of estrogen and progestin therapy. Beneficial effects of estrogen on the skeleton are not affected by the addition of progestins

      (b) Slight increase in incidence of breast cancer (20%). An increase in the risk of breast cancer deaths has not been clearly demonstrated. Addition of progestin to estrogen therapy does not reduce risk of breast cancer in postmenopausal women

      (c) Compliance with estrogen therapy is often a problem

b. **Calcium:** maintenance of an adequate calcium intake (800 to 1500 mg/day) is necessary to prevent osteoporosis; 25% of American females ingest <300 mg/day. Calcium supplementation significantly slows axial and appendicular bone loss in healthy postmenopausal women. If calcium supplementation is necessary, calcium carbonate is preferred because of its low cost. It is also well tolerated and contains more calcium per gram than other forms

c. **Biphosphonates:** these products bind to hydroxyapatite crystals and inhibit ability of osteoclasts to resorb bone. Alendronate (Fosamax) is a newer biphosphonate. Recommended dose is 10 mg daily on an empty stomach. No food should be taken for at least ½ hour after the dose. Etidronate (Didronel) is one of the earlier biphosphonates. It is effective in increasing bone density; however, it can cause mineralization defects when given in large doses or continuously; therefore it is administered cyclically (400 mg/day for 2 weeks followed by 13 weeks without medication)

d. **Vitamin D:** an adequate daily intake of vitamin D (600 to 800 IU) is recommended in the elderly. Calcitriol (1,25-dihydroxyvitamin D_3) can reduce rate of postmenopausal vertebral fractures in women with vitamin D deficiency

e. **Calcitonin:** effective for prevention of bone loss and reduction of vertebral fractures and associated pain. It is available in injectable form (SC) (Calcimar) and as a nasal spray preparation (Miacalcin) administered as one spray in the nostril (200 U) daily

f. **Fluoride:** directly stimulates bone formation and increases bone density; however, it can cause mineralization defects. Use of lower doses and slow-release preparations may prevent mineralization defects

6.2.d.

THYROID DISORDERS IN THE ELDERLY
Fred F. Ferri, MD

Physiologic and anatomic thyroid changes with aging

1. Increased fibrosis, lymphocyte infiltration, and nodularity
2. Decreased T_4 production but normal serum T_4 and free T_4 because of decreased tissue utilization rate for T_4
3. Decreased T_3 and free T_3 because of decreased T_3 production and conversion rate of T_4 to T_3
4. Increased average TSH serum levels, partly caused by increased titers of antithyroid antibodies
5. Despite the above changes, overall thyroid gland function is adequately maintained throughout life

Diagnostic approach to thyroid testing
Refer to Figure 6-8.

HYPOTHYROIDISM

1. The overall incidence of hypothyroidism is 3% to 7% in patients older than 65; incidence is higher in females
2. The diagnosis of hypothyroidism in the elderly can be very difficult on clinical grounds for the following reasons
   a. Fewer than 5% of elderly hypothyroid patients show the classic symptoms of hypothyroidism (fatigue, muscle weakness, cold intolerance, slow speech, and hoarse voice)
   b. Many of the signs of hypothyroidism (e.g., hair loss, slow cerebration with poor memory, leg cramps) are often attributed to old age
   c. Patients may be relatively asymptomatic or may have nonspecific symptomatology
   d. Cognitive impairment, anorexia, decreased mobility, and weight loss are common presentations of hypothyroidism in the elderly
3. Etiology of hypothyroidism in the elderly is primarily autoimmune thyroid disease. Additional causes: previous treatment of hyperthyroidism (radioactive iodine therapy, subtotal thyroidectomy) and radiation therapy to the neck region (usually for malignant disease)
4. Replacement therapy is best given with L-thyroxine. Initial starting dose: 0.025 mg, increased by 0.025 mg every 4 to 6 weeks until TSH level is in the normal range. Rapid replacement should be avoided in the geriatric patient because it may exacerbate underlying cardiac problems. A starting dose of 0.0125 mg of L-thyroxine and smaller incremental doses are recommended in hypothyroid patients with ischemic heart disease

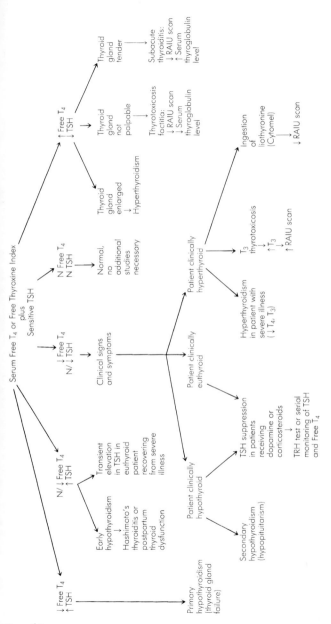

Figure 6-8
Diagnostic approach to thyroid testing. (From Ferri F: *Practical guide to the care of the medical patient,* ed 3, St Louis, 1995, Mosby.)

EUTHYROID SICK SYNDROME

1. Consists of alteration in TSH secretion, thyroid hormone peripheral binding, and metabolism secondary to severe illness or stress
2. More common in the elderly because of the increased frequency of acute and chronic illnesses in the geriatric population
3. Diagnostic laboratory features
   a. Low serum T_3
   b. Increased reverse T_3 (rT_3), decreased T_3 RIA
   c. Blunted TSH response to thyrotropin-releasing hormone (TRH)

HYPERTHYROIDISM

1. Fifteen percent of all clinical hyperthyroidism occurs in patients older than 60 years. Females outnumber males 9:1
2. Clinical presentation
   a. Fewer than 30% of the elderly have the classic complex of symptoms and signs. An enlarged thyroid gland may be absent
   b. Coexisting medical disorders (most commonly cardiac disease) may also mask symptoms. These patients often have unexplained CHF, unstable angina, or new onset atrial fibrillation that is resistant to treatment
   c. In addition to cardiovascular symptoms, other common manifestations are gastrointestinal (weight loss, anorexia), neuropsychiatric (heat intolerance, nervousness), and musculoskeletal (proximal muscle weakness, arthralgia)
   d. *Apathetic hyperthyroidism* refers to an atypical presentation of hyperthyroidism occurring frequently in the elderly and manifesting with lethargy rather than hyperkinetic activity. An enlarged thyroid gland may be absent. Coexisting medical disorders (most commonly cardiac disease) may also mask symptoms. These patients often have unexplained CHF, worsening of angina, or new onset atrial fibrillation resistant to treatment
3. Therapy
   a. Therapy of choice: radioactive iodine after patient is rendered euthyroid with propylthiouracil (PTU) or methimazole
   b. Propranolol: useful to alleviate beta-adrenergic symptoms of hyperthyroidism (unless its use is contraindicated by CHF or bronchospasm)

TOXIC NODULAR GOITER

1. More common than Graves' disease in elderly patients
2. Clinical presentation: onset is usually insidious and clinical phenomena (tachycardia, tremor, heat intolerance) may be masked by manifestations of coexisting diseases
3. Therapy: radioactive iodine after initiation of beta-blockers

THYROID NODULES

1. Prevalence increases from nearly 2% in the population under age 20 to nearly 7% after age 60
2. Four times more common in women than men
3. Cancer: main concern with thyroid nodules. There is increased likelihood that a nodule is malignant if
   a. Nodule increasing in size or larger than 2 cm

b. Regional lymphadenopathy
c. Fixation to adjacent tissues
d. Age less than 40 years; male sex
e. "Cold" on thyroid scan
f. "Solid" on thyroid ultrasound
4. Fine-needle aspiration biopsy is the best initial diagnostic study; accuracy can be over 90% but is directly related to the level of experience of physician and cytopathologist interpreting aspirate

6.3 OTORHINOLARYNGOLOGY

6.3.a. *HEARING LOSS*
Fred F. Ferri, MD

Incidence

1. Hearing loss is the most common sensory impairment in the elderly
2. It affects 28% of elderly and is more prevalent in males

Classification

Hearing loss can be classified according to the component of the auditory system being disrupted

- **Conductive:** disruption of sound transmission from external ear to inner ear (e.g., otitis media, Paget's disease, damage to tympanic membrane)
- **Sensorineural:** caused by dysfunction of hair cells or cochlear nerve (e.g., Meniere's disease, drugs, acoustic neuroma)
- **Central:** secondary to lesions of the auditory centers of the brain (e.g., CVA, neoplasms)

Etiology

1. Frequent causes of hearing loss in the elderly
   a. Cerumen impaction in the external canal: represents a significant reversible factor in 30% of the elderly
   b. Drugs: aminoglycosides, vancomycin, furosemide, ethacrinic acid, cisplatin, nitrogen mustard, NSAIDs, antimalarials
   c. Paget's disease of bone
   d. Meniere's disease
   e. Acoustic neuroma, meningioma
   f. Otosclerosis, otitis media, trauma
2. Most common diagnosis of hearing loss is presbycusis
   a. Characterized by slowly progressive bilateral and symmetric *high-frequency* hearing loss. Patient experiences significant difficulty understanding high-pitched voices (e.g., young children). Background noise (e.g., in restaurants) will also significantly impair speech understanding
   b. Four types of presbycusis, based on the selective atrophy of different morphologic structures in the cochlea (Table 6-12)

Evaluation of hearing loss

1. Initial screening in the office setting can be performed with a tuning fork and a portable audioscope (Sensitivity 90%, specificity 80%)

Table 6-12 Types of presbycusis

Type	Location in Cochlea	Audiometric Profile	
		Pure Tones	Discrimination
Sensory	Basal end	High-tone abrupt slope	Related to frequency range
Neural	All turns	All frequencies	Severe loss
Strial	Apical region	All frequencies	Minimal loss
Cochlear conductive	All turns basal>apical	High-tone gradual slope	Related to steepness of slope

From Goldstein et al: *Geriatric otorhinolaryngology,* Philadelphia, 1989, Decker.

2. Audiologic evaluation with pure-tone threshold audiometry will further define extent of loss and potential for rehabilitation. Figure 6-9 illustrates audiograms of patients with sensory presbycusis (note *abrupt* sloping high-tone hearing loss). Figure 6-10 reveals audiometric profile of patients with cochlear conductive presbycusis (*gradual* sloping high-tone hearing loss)
3. Hearing Handicap In Elderly Screening (HHIE-S): a communication-specific self-assessment scale on social and emotional consequences of hearing loss (Figure 6-11); an accurate screening method to detect hearing loss (specificity is 96% when one obtains a score greater than 24)

Implications of hearing loss in the elderly

1. Hearing loss results in interference with ADLs, reduced socialization, and decreased ability to live independently
2. Misinterpretation of hearing loss as a cognitive, affective, or personality disorder is common
3. Several studies suggest an increased prevalence of hearing impairment among patients with dementia. Seriously hearing-impaired persons have a greater chance of being demented; however, current evidence is inconclusive that poor hearing is associated with cognitive decline in normal elderly persons

Hearing aids

1. Twenty percent of patients older than 80 use hearing aids
2. Five major types of hearing aids
   a. In-the-ear (ITE) aids—most popular type
   b. Behind-the-ear aids—connected to the ear canal by flexible tubing; more durable and easier to adjust
   c. In-the-canal aids—contained entirely within the ear canal
   d. Eyeglass units—popularity of these models has declined significantly
   e. Aids worn on the body—usually reserved for more severe hearing loss
3. Hearing aids can be very expensive (average price is over $500). Their purchase should be conditional to a 30-day trial
   a. Hearing aids dispensed by an audiologist and purchased in a not-for-profit facility can result in significant cost savings to the consumer

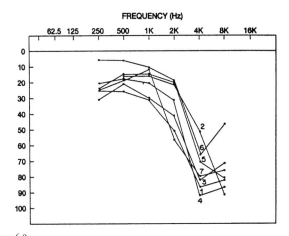

Figure 6-9

Audiogram of seven ears from six subjects showing abrupt sloping high-tone hearing losses. (From Goldstein, Kashima, Koopmann: *Geriatric otorhinolaryngology,* Philadelphia, 1989, BC Decker.)

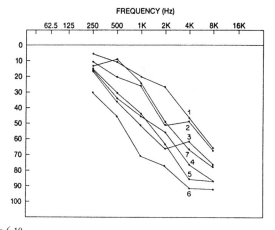

Figure 6-10

Audiogram of seven ears from six subjects showing gradual sloping high-tone hearing losses. (From Goldstein, Kashima, Koopmann: *Geriatric otorhinolaryngology,* Philadelphia, 1989, BC Decker.)

	Yes (4)	**Sometimes** (2)	**No** (0)
1. Does a hearing problem cause you to feel embarrassed when meeting new people?	___	___	___
2. Does a hearing problem cause you to feel frustrated when talking to members of your family?	___	___	___
3. Do you have difficulty hearing when someone speaks in a whisper?	___	___	___
4. Do you feel handicapped by a hearing problem?	___	___	___
5. Does a hearing problem cause you difficulty when visiting friends, relatives, or neighbors?	___	___	___
6. Does a hearing problem cause you to attend religious services less often than you would like?	___	___	___
7. Does a hearing problem cause you to have arguments with family members?	___	___	___
8. Does a hearing problem cause you difficulty when listening to TV or radio?	___	___	___
9. Do you feel that any difficulty with your hearing limits or hampers your personal or social life?	___	___	___
10. Does a hearing problem cause you difficulty when in a restaurant with relatives or friends?	___	___	___

Figure 6-11
Hearing-handicap inventory for the elderly—screening version (HHIE-S). Range of total points: 0 to 40; 0 to 8: no self-perceived handicap; 10 to 22: mild to moderate handicap; 24 to 40: significant handicap. (From Ventry IM, Weinstein BE: *American Speech-Language Hearing Association* 25:37, 1983.)

    b. Diagnostic testing for hearing aids is covered by Medicare, but hearing aid selection, fitting, dispensing, and follow-up are not covered services
4. Patients should be informed of the limitations of hearing aids. Significant hearing improvement can be achieved if hearing loss is 55 to 80 dB, whereas if loss is greater than 80 dB only limited improvement can be expected. Poor discrimination will also limit usefulness of a hearing aid. Successful use of a hearing aid will also depend on
    a. Hearing aid orientation by relistening and auditory-visual communication training

b. Counseling of the hearing impaired and significant others
5. Telephone, TV, radio, and stereo amplifiers are useful to increase loudness of the signal
   a. Telephone amplifiers are usually available from the telephone company. They can be built into the handset of the telephone, or they can be portable
   b. TV, radio, or stereo amplifiers may be connected directly to the audio input. The listener may use standard headphones or pillow speakers. Telephone devices for the deaf (TDD) and telephone caption units are also commonly available

5.3.b.

VERTIGO
Fred F. Ferri, MD

Definitions
1. Dizziness: vague term used by patients to describe various sensations (e.g., vertigo, light-headedness, unsteadiness, near syncope, malaise)
2. Light-headedness: sensation of faintness or giddiness. Patient does not have true vertigo but a perception of difficulty maintaining balance
3. Vertigo: sensation of motion of either the patient with respect to the environment or vice versa; usually accompanied by symptoms of nausea, vomiting, nystagmus, and staggering

Diagnostic approach
1. Vertigo may be multifactorial (e.g., drug toxicity, infection, metabolic abnormalities, nerve conduction abnormalities, hypoxia, mass effect). The history should include the following
   a. Drug and alcohol use
   b. Past and current illnesses (e.g., diabetes, CHF, COPD, CVA)
   c. Duration and lateralization of symptoms, including provoking factors
   d. History of trauma, hearing difficulty, head pain
   e. Intermittent vs. continuous symptoms
2. Physical exam should focus on
   a. Presence/absence of orthostatic blood pressure and pulse changes
   b. Romberg and cerebellar evaluation
   c. Examination for nystagmus, including provocative tests (e.g., Nylen-Barany maneuver) if necessary for diagnosis
      (1) Fast component of nystagmus will be to the "good" ear
      (2) Slow component will be to the affected ear
   d. Hearing testing and tuning fork (including Weber and Rinne tests)
3. Peripheral vertigo can be distinguished from central vertigo by observing nystagmus and which direction the patient tends to fall
   a. Peripheral vertigo: nystagmus is accentuated by looking toward the unaffected ear and is improved by visual fixation. Patient tends to fall away from the fast component of the nystagmus
   b. Central vertigo: nystagmus is accentuated by looking toward the side of the lesion and is not improved by visual fixation. Patient falls toward the fast component of the nystagmus
4. Electronystagmography: can measure nystagmus and distinguish peripheral from central vestibular lesions

Diagnosis and therapy

1. Peripheral vertigo
    a. **Acute labyrinthitis**
        (1) Often follows viral syndrome
        (2) Vertigo is usually associated with tinnitus and can last several days
        (3) Nystagmus is usually more prominent on looking toward the good ear
        (4) Symptoms are exacerbated by positional changes and head movement
        (5) Treatment is symptomatic. Sedatives, antihistamines, decongestants, and antiemetics are commonly used to control symptoms. Caution must be used in the elderly since the risk of potential side effects (urinary retention, delirium, lethargy, falls) is much higher in the geriatric population
    b. **Benign positional vertigo**
        (1) Brief (few seconds) episodes of vertigo occur on assumption of a particular head position
        (2) No hearing loss is found, caloric testing is normal
        (3) Disorder is usually self-limited but can last several months
        (4) Treatment is symptomatic with meclizine prn
    c. **Meniere's disease**
        (1) Classic triad of vertigo, tinnitus, and deafness is seen
        (2) Hearing loss is initially fluctuating
        (3) Vertigo usually lasts 1 or 2 hours
        (4) Treatment includes sedatives, antiemetics, and antihistamines
        (5) Prophylaxis includes diuretics and sodium restriction
        (6) Surgical intervention is controversial
    d. **Vestibular neuronitis**
        (1) Duration of vertigo may be prolonged (several days)
        (2) Deafness or tinnitus is generally not present
        (3) Symptoms are exacerbated by position changes and head movement
        (4) Caloric testing reveals hypofunction of affected side
        (5) Treatment is symptomatic
    e. **Drug toxicity:** elimination of any suspected drugs
2. Central vertigo
    a. **Vertebrobasilar insufficiency**
    b. **Acoustic neuroma**
        (1) Unilateral hearing loss, tinnitus, and dizziness
        (2) Diagnosis
            (a) Brain stem evoked response
            (b) CT scan or MRI directed to cerebellopontine angle and internal auditory canals
        (3) Therapy: surgical excision or palliative subtotal resection depending on size of tumor, severity of symptoms, and overall medical status of patient
    c. **Neoplasms of cerebellopontine angle** (primary or metastatic)
    d. **Cerebellar–brain stem hemorrhage/infarction**
    e. **Basilar migraine:** vertigo associated with occipital headache, tinnitus, and visual disturbances

f. Other common causes of vertigo in the elderly are alcohol and other drug toxicity, electrolyte abnormalities, and hyperventilation

6.4 OPHTHALMOLOGY

6.4.a. *LOSS OF VISION*
Michael D. Stein, MD

Definition

Acute loss of vision is a medical emergency; gradual loss is more frequently encountered in the primary care setting.

History

Ask about
- Onset
- Eye pain
- Unilateral or bilateral symptoms
- Scotomas (blurred or partially blind areas)
- Other medical conditions (diabetes mellitus, multiple sclerosis)
- Trauma
- Headache, jaw claudication, temporal or scalp pain (temporal arteritis)

Examination

1. Inspect eyes, including conjunctiva, cornea, and sclera
2. Check pupillary reflex to determine if there is an afferent defect (no response to direct light), which suggests optic neuritis or acute angle-closure glaucoma
3. Check confrontation visual field for defects
4. Perform funduscopic examination

Differential diagnosis

1. Sudden loss
   a. Vitreous hemorrhage (often caused by diabetes mellitus)
   b. Vascular occlusion of retina
   c. Acute angle-closure glaucoma
   d. Optic neuritis (inflammatory, multiple sclerosis)
   e. Amaurosis fugax (carotid ischemia)
   f. Hysteria
   g. Occipital infarct (may cause bilateral blindness, homonymous hemianopia)
2. Gradual loss
   a. Presbyopia (corrects with refraction)
   b. Chronic or open-angle glaucoma
   c. Cataract
   d. Macular degeneration
   e. Diabetic retinopathy
   f. Corneal degeneration
   g. Corneal opacity

Treatment

1. Dependent on diagnosis
2. Referral to ophthalmologist often recommended

 CATARACTS
Fred F. Ferri, MD

Definition

Cataracts are an opacity in the lens of the eye, usually from denaturation of lens protein caused by aging. The opacity may occur in the cortex, the nucleus of the lens, or the posterior subcapsular region but usually is in a combination of areas. The major age-related changes in the eye are illustrated in Figure 6-12.

Contributing factors

1. Diabetes mellitus
2. Ultraviolet B light (cortical cataract)
3. Systemic corticosteroids (posterior subcapsular cataract)
4. Familial incidence
5. Prolonged glaucoma therapy with topical medications
6. Ocular trauma
7. Intraocular surgery

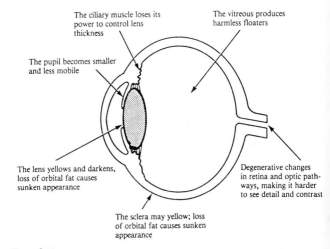

Figure 6-12

Aging changes of the eye. (From Bosker G et al: *Geriatric emergency medicine*, St Louis, 1990, Mosby.)

Prevalence

1. Some stage of cataract development is present in over 50% of persons aged 65 to 74 and 65% to 70% of those over age 75
2. Cataract removal is the most frequent surgical procedure in patients 65 or older (1.3 million operations/yr with an annual cost of approximately $3 billion)

Symptoms and signs

1. The visual abnormalities caused by cataracts vary with the location and stage of the cataract (e.g., distance visual acuity is most significantly impaired by nuclear cataracts)
2. The sclerotic lens results in myopia, which temporarily corrects presbyopia, causing a misconception that eyesight is improving (e.g., patient may be able to read newspaper without glasses): phenomenon called "second sight"

Surgical correction

1. Indicated when corrected visual acuity in the affected eye is greater than 20/50 in absence of other ocular disease; however, surgery may be justified when visual acuity is 20/40 or better in specific situations (e.g., disabling glare, monocular diplopia)
2. In 90% of patients vision improves by two lines or more on a Snellen chart; mental status and timed performance of manual tasks also improve
3. Cataract surgery is generally performed with the patient under local anesthesia on an outpatient basis. It can be accomplished by two methods
   a. Extracapsular extraction (>95% of cataract operations)
      (1) Central portion of anterior capsule is removed and contents of lens are aspirated. Posterior capsule of lens is left behind and an intraocular lens (IOL) is implanted on or within the capsular bag
      (2) Small-incision phacoemulsification is a newer technique that involves fragmenting the lens nucleus with ultrasonic vibrations and subsequent aspiration of lens material
      (3) Most common complication of extracapsular extraction is late opacification of posterior capsule, which occurs in 35% to 50% of patients over a 3-year postoperative period. It manifests by gradual decline in visual acuity, usually 3 to 18 months after surgery. Treatment consists of opening the posterior capsule using a neodymium:YAG laser in outpatient setting
   b. Intracapsular extraction
      (1) Involves removal of entire cataract and surrounding capsule in a single piece
      (2) Since there is no posterior lens capsule to secure an implant, most surgeons use an anterior chamber implant
      (3) Intracapsular extraction is rarely done in the United States and is usually reserved for cases of phacoanaphylaxis and subluxation of lens

6.4.c.   *GLAUCOMA*
Fred F. Ferri, MD

Definition

Glaucoma is a group of disorders characterized by increased intraocular pressure that can lead to cupping and atrophy of the optic nerve head with visual field loss.

Prevalence

1. Glaucoma increases with age and is more common in males than females
2. Can be found in 2% of the population over 40 and 5% to 10% of elderly in the eighth decade of life
3. Ten percent of all blindness in the United States is due to glaucoma
4. It is the second leading cause of blindness in the United States and the leading cause of blindness in African-Americans

Classification

1. Glaucoma can be primary or secondary
2. Primary glaucoma can be subdivided into open-angle (90%) and angle-closure (10%) types
3. Secondary glaucoma is due to processes that anatomically or functionally block the outflow channels (e.g., trauma, diabetes, occlusion of the central retinal vein, uveitis, ocular tumors, cataract extraction)

OPEN-ANGLE GLAUCOMA

Etiology and diagnosis

1. Examination of the affected eyes reveals an increase in intraocular pressure, anatomically normal anterior chamber angle (as determined by gonioscopy), cupping of the optic nerve, and visual field defects
2. The block to the outflow of the aqueous humor in the drainage channels (trabecular meshwork) is poorly understood
3. The visual loss is of insidious onset, slowly progressive, and asymptomatic until very late. Most people are not aware that there is a problem until the disease is far advanced, hence the importance of regular eye care for the elderly
4. The visual loss involves the peripheral field initially, followed by loss of central visual acuity in late stages

Medical therapy

1. **Ophthalmic beta-blockers** (e.g., timolol, levobunolol, betaxolol)
   a. Mechanism of action: suppression of production of aqueous humor in the eye
   b. Systemic side effects: bronchospasm, bradycardia, CHF
2. **Systemic inhibitors of carbonate anhydrase** (e.g., acetazolamide)
   a. Mechanism of action: decreased production of aqueous humor
   b. Systemic side effects: paresthesias, anorexia, nausea and fatigue, metabolic acidosis, renal calculi, bone marrow suppression, cutaneous reactions
3. **Ophthalmic miotics** (e.g., pilocarpine, carbachol)

a. Mechanism of action: pupillary constriction, stimulation of muscle fibers of the ciliary body and improvement of flow through the trabecular meshwork

b. Systemic side effects: headache, nausea, bronchospasm, increased salivation, increased perspiration

4. Ophthalmic adrenergics (e.g., epinephrine)

a. Mechanism of action: decreased production of aqueous humor, increased flow through trabecular meshwork

b. Systemic side effects: hypertension, tachycardia, dysrhythmias, anxiety, headaches

Surgical therapy

1. Argon laser trabeculoplasty

a. Therapeutic step most commonly used after failure of medical therapy

b. Improves drainage of aqueous humor from the eye by using laser burns to create openings on or next to the trabecular meshwork

2. Conventional surgery: a fistula is created between the anterior chamber and the subconjunctival space, allowing passage of the aqueous humor; sometimes augmented by silicone implants

ANGLE-CLOSURE GLAUCOMA

Etiology and diagnosis

1. Results from forward displacement of the iris against the cornea, closing the chamber angle and blocking flow of aqueous humor out of the eye

2. Clinical presentation can be dramatic, with redness and pain in or about the eye associated with abrupt onset of blurred vision

3. Patient may see rainbow-colored haloes around lights, followed by a dramatic loss of vision in involved eye

4. Systemic symptoms of nausea, vomiting, and abdominal pain may accompany acute angle-closure glaucoma

5. Examination of the eye reveals tenderness and firmness of the affected globe, increased intraocular pressure, and fixed, semidilated pupil

Therapy

1. Immediate and frequent instillation of miotics, parenteral or oral administration of acetazolamide or hyperosmotics (glycerol, mannitol)

2. Definitive treatment is laser iridotomy, allowing free flow of aqueous humor

| 6.4.d. | **_MACULAR DEGENERATION_** |

Fred F. Ferri, MD

Etiology

1. Exact etiology unknown

2. The macular area of the retina depends on the choroidal capillaries for nutrition. It is believed that a disruption of the vascular supply to the macula results in changes in the retinal pigmented epithelium (RPE) and separation of the RPE–sensory retina interface with subsequent death of cone photoreceptor cells in the macula and loss of _central_ vision

3. Hyaline deposits (drusen) can accumulate beneath the RPE and are visible as yellow-white pinhead-sized lesions on ophthalmologic exam
4. Leakage or bleeding from retinal neovascularization (choroidal neovascular membranes) can result in further damage to the RPE–sensory retina interface
5. Possible factors may be UV light and retinal adsorption

Prevalence

1. Affects nearly 30% of the geriatric population (females > males)
2. Most common cause of legal blindness (visual acuity 20/200 or less)

Signs and symptoms

1. Painless progressive loss of central vision with complaint of difficulty reading
2. Peripheral vision unaffected; therefore total blindness does not occur

Clinical classification and therapy

1. **Nonexudative** (dry type)
   a. Much more common (90% of cases) but generally less severe (usual visual acuity reduction to 20/50 to 20/100)
   b. Ophthalmoscopic exam may reveal drusen and areas of depigmentation alternating with zones of hyperpigmentation
   c. No specific therapy is available for this type of macular degeneration. Ocuvite with zinc antioxidants may be useful
2. **Exudative** (wet type)
   a. Responsible for 10% of cases of age-related macular degeneration
   b. Results in much more severe loss of visual acuity than the dry type. It causes 90% of cases of legal blindness from macular degeneration
   c. Ophthalmoscopic exam may reveal a detachment of the sensory retina in the macular area
   d. Fluorescein angiography can identify hemorrhagic areas
   e. Therapy with laser photocoagulation may be useful in some patients with focal areas of neovascularization
   f. Monitoring of patients with exudative macular degeneration is done on a regular basis with self-testing using an Amsler grid to detect early distortion in central vision (curvy appearance of the lines or missing squares) indicative of hemorrhage and/or retinal detachment (Figure 6-13)

6.5   RHEUMATOLOGY

6.5.a.   *ARTHRITIS*
Tom J. Wachtel, MD

Musculoskeletal complaints are among the most common reasons for patients to seek medical attention. Laypersons often used the term *arthritis* to describe a wide variety of painful experiences involving the musculoskeletal system. Arthritis specifically refers to an inflammatory or a degenerative process in a joint. It may be mimicked by bursitis, tendinitis,

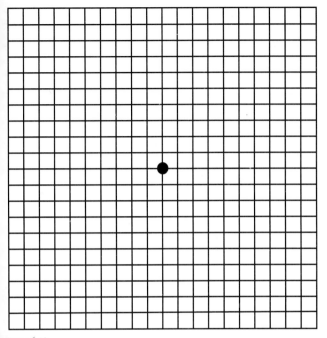

Figure 6-13
Amsler grid. Patient examines Amsler grid with each eye (patients who wear glasses keep their glasses on for this test). Grid is placed on wall or desk at comfortable distance normally used for reading. (From Yoshikawa TT, Cobbs EL, Brummel-Smith K, editors: *Ambulatory geriatric care*, St Louis, 1993, Mosby.)

bone pathologic conditions, cellulitis, phlebitis, myalgia, neuralgia, or ischemia.

Therefore the history and physical exam should always include a complete assessment of any painful limb to ascertain the integrity of the vascular system, nervous system, bones, muscles, and other soft tissue structures of the relevant limb.

Once convinced that the complaint is generated by arthritis, the next step is to differentiate between inflammatory and noninflammatory arthritis. This can be done by looking for the classic signs of inflammation (rubor, calor, tumor, dolor) and asking the patient about the pattern of pain. Inflammatory arthritis is made worse by rest and improved by exercise; degenerative arthritis is worsened by exercise. Although some morning stiffness may be present in either, this lasts only 10 to 15 minutes in degenerative arthritis compared to the 1- to 2-hour loosening-up period in inflammatory arthritis. In addition, often, but not always, inflammatory arthritis tends to be acute or subacute and degenerative arthritis tends to be chronic.

MONOARTICULAR ARTHRITIS

The first step in evaluating monoarticular arthritis is to determine whether signs of acute inflammation (pain, swelling, erythema, heat, and loss of function) are present. Acute monoarticular inflammatory arthritis is a medical emergency because septic arthritis must be treated immediately if present. Further, septic and crystalline arthritides are very painful, and treatment should begin as soon as possible. The key test is arthrocentesis with joint fluid examination for cell count and differential, Gram stain, culture and sensitivity, and a search for crystals (under polarized light).

Noninflammatory monoarticular arthritis can occur as a result of recent trauma; usually the patient will give a history of the traumatic event. Monoarticular osteoarthritis may affect a joint that is subject to repeated microtrauma (occupation or sport), a congenitally abnormal joint, or a joint previously damaged by trauma or infection. Neoplastic disorders (e.g., synovial sarcoma or pigmented villonodular synovitis) may mimic monoarticular arthritis with or without signs of inflammation; a biopsy is required for diagnosis.

Differential diagnosis

1. Infectious arthritis
   a. Bacterial
      (1) Nongonococcal
         (a) *Staphylococcus aureus* (60%)
         (b) Non–group A beta-hemolytic streptococci (15%)
         (c) Gram-negative pathogens (18%)
      (2) Gonococcal
   b. Lyme disease (large joints, intermittent swelling more than pain)
   c. Viral (HIV, hepatitis B)
   d. Mycobacterial (evidence of pulmonary TB present in only 50%)
2. Crystal-induced arthritis
   a. Gout (urate)
   b. Pseudogout (calcium pyrophosphate)
   c. Hydroxyapatite arthropathy
   d. Calcium oxalate arthropathy
3. Trauma
   a. Fracture
   b. Hemarthrosis (acquired or congenital clotting disorders)
4. Osteoarthritis: chronic; made worse after overuse or minor trauma
5. Systemic diseases: rheumatoid arthritis, systemic lupus erythematosus (SLE), inflammatory bowel disease, Reiter's syndrome, psoriasis)

Tests

1. CBC and cultures of blood, skin lesions, cervix, urethra, and urine are important if infectious arthritis is suspected
2. Serum uric acid levels are misleading and may be consistently normal even with gout
3. Arthrocentesis: should be performed in nearly every patient, particularly if infection is suspected; synovial fluid should be examined for
   a. Total leukocyte count and differential
   b. Gram stain and culture

   c. Crystal examination

   d. Interpretation

     (1) Normal synovial fluid contains <180 cells/ml

     (2) Most patients with osteoarthritis have <500 cells/ml

     (3) As leukocyte count increases, so does possibility of infection, especially with >50,000 cells/ml

     (4) More than 90% polymorphonuclear neutrophil leukocytes (PMNs) suggests infection or crystals

     (5) Presence of crystals does not exclude infection

     (6) Cultures are positive in only 25% of patients with gonococcal arthritis

. Radiology: usually not helpful, although fractures, tumors, and chronic osteoarthritis can be discerned; chondrocalcinosis may be seen with pseudogout; MRI can help with sacroiliac involvement, meniscal tears, and ligament damage

Septic arthritis

Septic arthritis is characterized by a cell count greater than 50,000 with more than 90% PMNs. Previously injured joints are more susceptible to infection; therefore a patient with underlying rheumatoid arthritis who presents with fever, chills, and "flare-up" in a single joint should be evaluated in the same manner. The most frequent organism is *Staphylococcus,* but any pathogenic bacterium may be encountered. Disseminated gonococcemia, rare in the elderly, may affect joints and/or the skin. When arthralgia is present, examination of the joint may simply reveal tenosynovitis or an effusion. The latter, if present, should be tapped. Both the Gram stain and culture may be falsely negative in gonococcal arthritis; therefore empiric treatment is indicated if the index of suspicion is high.

TREATMENT

1. Empiric antibiotic therapy is required until cultures are completed if the synovial fluid Gram stain is negative. Normal hosts should be treated for gram-positive organisms (e.g., oxacillin or methicillin)
2. Ceftriaxone should be used to treat gonococcal arthritis
3. Daily closed drainage is mandatory for patients with septic arthritis
4. Joint should be immobilized as long as joint fluid reaccumulates
5. Arthroscopic or open drainage should be considered if response to antibiotics is slow

Crystalline arthritis

Crystalline arthritis is characterized by fewer cells per milliliter (5000 to 20,000) with a predominance of PMNs. The shape and polarizing characteristics of the crystals make the diagnosis of gout or pseudogout. Tapping the first metatarsophalangeal (MTP) joint in podagra may be difficult or refused by the patient. If the diagnosis of gout vs. pseudogout is uncertain, the patient should be treated with indomethacin, an adequate treatment for either condition.

1. Acute gout

   a. Definition: a metabolic disease characterized by hyperuricemia and deposits of monosodium urate crystals in and about joints, with subsequent acute or chronic arthritis

b. Epidemiology: initial acute gouty arthritis occurs primarily in me
over age 30. In women it usually occurs after menopause. Attacks ca
be precipitated by several factors (e.g., trauma, certain foods, ethanc
intake, diuretics, renal failure)

c. Clinical manifestations and diagnosis

(1) Typical presentation is monoarticular and characterized by sud
den severe pain involving the first MTP joint (podagra), althoug
the midtarsal area and ankle are also frequently affected; acut
asymmetric polyarthritis is uncommon

(2) Physical examination reveals a warm, tender, swollen, erythema
tous joint; fever may be present, particularly if several joints ar
involved

(3) Serum uric acid level may be elevated or normal

(4) Aspiration and analysis of synovial fluid from the inflamed join
confirm the diagnosis; examination of the fluid with a polarize
light microscope reveals monosodium urate crystals (needle
shaped, strongly negative, birefringent crystals) with synovia
fluid leukocytes

d. Treatment

(1) NSAIDs: indomethacin, 50 mg q8h for 3 to 4 days, then gradu
ally tapered off over approximately 1 to 2 weeks (depending or
the patient's clinical response); naproxen, sulindac, and othe
NSAIDs are also effective; keterolac may be given IM in NPC
patients

(2) Cochicine can be given PO or IV (0.6 mg q1h until relief i
achieved or side effects [diarrhea, abdominal cramps, nausea
vomiting] require treatment cessation

(3) Glucocorticoids (IV) or ACTH (IM): generally reserved for pa
tients who cannot tolerate PO medication (e.g., postoperatively
and with contraindications to the use of IV colchicine or IM ke
torolac

(4) Intraarticular administration of methylprednisone or betametha
sone is generally reserved for selected patients with monoarticu
lar disease

e. Prevention of recurrences

(1) Workup of hyperuricemia (rarely, gouty arthritis may occur in nor
mouricemic patients) should include a 24-hour determination o
renal urate output: hypoexcretors of uric acid (less than 800 mg/24
hr) may be treated with a uricosuric drug (probenecid or sulfin
pyrazone) or allopurinol; hyperproducers (greater than 800 mg/24
hr) must be treated with allopurinol because uricosuric agents are
contraindicated (increased risk of kidney stones). Because rapid
changes in serum uric acid may precipitate or exacerbate acute
gouty attacks, indomethacin or colchicine should be given for 3
weeks before and at least 3 weeks after the initiation of these
drugs. Allopurinol has many side effects and is usually reserved
for patients with frequent recurrent attacks or gouty nephropathy.
Asymptomatic mild to moderate hyperuricemia need not be treated

(2) Once the acute episode of gout has resolved, avoidance of heavy
alcohol use and foods rich in purines and weight loss can reduce

the likelihood of recurrence. Long-term colchicine therapy (0.6 mg qd or bid) may be necessary in patients with frequent gout attacks despite the use of uric acid–lowering agents

. Joint diseases caused by other chemical species of crystals
  a. Calcium pyrophosphate deposition disease (pseudogout)
    (1) Joints involved: knees, wrists
    (2) Crystal characteristics: rhomboid or polymorphic-shaped, weakly positive, birefringent crystals
    (3) Treatment: NSAIDs, joint immobilization, intraarticular steroids
  b. Hydroxyapatite arthropathy
    (1) Joints involved: knees, hips, shoulders
    (2) Crystal characteristics: crystals form nonbirefringent clumps with synovial fluid when placed on slide; diagnosis often requires electron microscopy because of small size of crystals
    (3) Treatment: NSAIDs, joint immobilization, intraarticular steroids
  c. Calcium oxalate–induced arthritis
    (1) Joints involved: distal interphalangeal (DIP) and proximal interphalangeal (PIP)joints of hands
    (2) Crystal characteristics: bipyramidal-shaped, positive, birefringent crystals
    (3) Treatment: NSAIDs, joint immobilization, intraarticular steroids
  d. Steroids can crystallize following an intraarticular injection and provoke an inflammatory response

POLYARTICULAR ARTHRITIS

Rheumatoid arthritis (RA) and other inflammatory polyarticular arthritides

The evaluation of inflammatory arthritis varies with the acuteness of the disease. The history may provide some clues, but the help of the laboratory may be needed when the symptoms do not resolve rapidly or blossom into a readily recognized clinical entity. Rheumatoid arthritis is the prototype of chronic inflammatory arthritides. The prevalence is 3% in females and 1% in males. The course and prognosis vary in severity; spontaneous long-term remissions may occur, but the disease should be considered incurable.

DIFFERENTIAL DIAGNOSIS

1. Acute arthritis
  a. Rheumatic fever
    (1) Recent strep throat
    (2) Antistreptolysin (ASO) titer greater than 200 Todd units
    (3) Involvement of lower extremity joints
  b. Serum sickness
    (1) Recent administration of a drug
    (2) Rash
  c. Prodrome of hepatitis
    (1) Liver function tests and hepatitis serology
  d. Lyme arthritis
    (1) Recent tick bite
    (2) Characteristic rash

2. Chronic arthritis
   a. Rheumatoid arthritis
   b. Rheumatoid variants
      (1) Still's disease
      (2) Sjögren's syndrome
      (3) Inflammatory bowel disease
      (4) Psoriasis
      (5) Infectious enterocolitis
      (6) Reiter's disease
   c. Connective tissue disease (e.g., lupus)
   d. Sarcoidosis
   e. Amyloidosis
   f. Behçet's syndrome
   g. Whipple's disease

CLINICAL MANIFESTATIONS OF RA

1. Initial manifestations are highly variable. In the majority of patients, the onset is insidious, taking months or years to become clinically evident as a diagnosable entity (Figure 6-14). In other patients, the onset is dramatic, with rapid development of severe manifestations.
2. Disease course is highly variable, characterized by exacerbations and remissions. Approximately 10% of patients will have severe destructive arthritis unresponsive to any therapeutic modalities, whereas 15% of all patients experience a complete remission
3. RA can present with any of the following articular and extraarticular manifestations

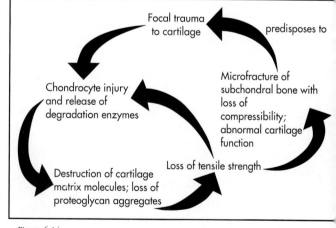

Figure 6-14
Pathogenesis of osteoarthritis. (From Noble J et al, editors: *Textbook of primary care medicine,* ed 2, St Louis, 1996, Mosby.)

a. Articular and periarticular manifestations
   (1) Morning stiffness is often the initial complaint
   (2) Symmetric polyarthritis
     (a) Joint swelling and tenderness to palpation, with significant limitation of motion of involved joints
     (b) Commonly involved joints in RA are metacarpophalangeal (MCP), metatarsophalangeal (MTP), proximal interphalangeal (PIP), wrist, knee, ankle, shoulder, and hip; however, any joint can be affected
     (c) Joint deformities are generally secondary to hyperextension or flexion of joints
       • Hyperextension of PIP joints and flexion of DIP joints (swan-neck deformity)
       • Flexion of PIP joints and extension of DIP joints (boutonniere deformity)
       • Others: ulnar deviation of MCP joints, knee and ankle effusions, hoarseness secondary to cricoarytenoid arthritis, myelopathy secondary to nerve compression
b. Extraarticular manifestations
   (1) Pulmonary involvement consists of one or more of the following
     (a) Pulmonary nodules (usually multiple)
     (b) Pleural effusions (exudative with low glucose concentration)
     (c) Pulmonary vasculitis
     (d) Pleuritis
   (2) Ocular involvement: scleritis, episcleritis, Sjögren's syndrome
   (3) Vasculitis
   (4) Hematologic abnormalities
     (a) Normochromic normocytic/microcytic anemia (multifactorial: chronic disease, blood loss secondary to salicylates and NSAIDs)
     (b) Granulocytopenia (Felty's syndrome)
   (5) Cardiac involvement: pericarditis, conduction defects, myocarditis
   (6) Skin: subcutaneous nodules
   (7) Constitutional symptoms: fever, weight loss, anorexia, malaise
   (8) Others: osteoporosis, myositis, compressive neuropathies, amyloidosis, mesangial glomerulonephritis
c. Laboratory evaluation: no isolated lab test can exclude or prove diagnosis of RA. Any of the following laboratory abnormalities may be present
   (1) Rheumatoid factor (RF): latex positivity may be initially absent, but over the course of the disease approximately 85% of patients become latex positive; RF is not specific for RA and may be found in other conditions (e.g., osteomyelitis, infective endocarditis, liver disease)
   (2) Erythrocyte sedimentation rate (ESR): generally elevated during exacerbations
   (3) ANA: detected in approximately 15% of patients
   (4) Decreased hemoglobin/hematocrit, granulocytopenia
d. Radiographic evaluation

(1) Initially, soft tissue swelling may be the only manifestation
(2) As disease progresses, there is periarticular osteopenia, cortical thinning, and marginal erosion
(3) Subluxation and joint space diminution are late findings

e. Treatment

(1) Improve patient's quality of life with
   (a) Drug therapy to relieve pain and inflammation
   (b) Active rehabilitation with adequate physical therapy program
   (c) Emotional support and social counseling

(2) Arrest or retard disease process with appropriate drug therapy
   (a) Drug therapy generally consists of a stepwise approach based on severity of disease and clinical response. Patients vary markedly in their response to these drugs. Their toxicity results in a high rate of discontinuation. Long-term studies have suggested that the drugs currently used do not prevent disability in many patients with the disease. Use of second-line drugs earlier in the course of RA or their use in combinations may minimize these problems
   (b) Initial treatment generally consists of high doses of salicylates (3 to 6 g/day) or other NSAIDs; frequent side effects: gastric irritation and GI bleeding
   (c) If the above are not effective or not tolerated because of side effects, therapy is generally begun with one of the following agents
   • Hydroxychloroquine: 200 mg PO bid; moderately effective early in RA and has relatively low toxicity compared to other agents; common side effects: nausea, abdominal discomfort, and rash; its use is also associated with retinopathy and requires initial and periodic ophthalmologic examination
   • Methotrexate: 7.5 to 10 mg PO weekly; generally effective and relatively rapid acting; potential toxicity includes bone marrow suppression, interstitial pneumonitis, GI ulceration and bleeding, and liver toxicity
   • Gold preparations: gold injections; 50 mg IM weekly until a total dose of 1 g is reached; then frequency is decreased to biweekly or monthly; complications of therapy: skin rashes, pruritus, stomatitis, leukopenia, thrombocytopenia, and proteinuria
   • Pencillamine: 250 mg PO qd initially, increased in 250-mg monthly increments to a maximum of 750 to 1000 mg/day; can cause proteinuria, bone marrow depression, fever, and rash; nearly 40% of patients discontinue this drug within 1 year because of side effects
   • Azathioprine: 50 to 150 mg/day is effective but can cause bone marrow depression, nausea, vomiting, hepatitis
   (d) Systemic corticosteroids are often used for brief periods in combination with other drugs to minimize symptoms; low-dose prednisone (7.5 mg/day) useful in improving quality of life without significant toxicity when long-term steroid therapy is necessary

(3) Physical and occupational therapy
  (a) Exercise to improve range of motion and strength
  (b) Splinting for synovitis
  (c) Occupational therapy referral for ADLs
(4) Attention to depression, insomnia

Osteoarthritis

Osteoarthritis (degenerative joint disease) is a noninflammatory disorder of moveable joints that is characterized by deterioration and abrasion of articular cartilage and by formation of new bone on the surfaces of the joints.

The diagnosis of degenerative joint disease is generally easy. The disease affects mostly the weight-bearing joints (knees, hips, lumbosacral and cervical spine), DIP joints, and carpometacarpal joints. Symptoms are mostly pain and limitation of function, confirmed on examination by decreased range of motion. Unfortunately, symptoms (occurring in 20% of U.S. adult population) correlate poorly with radiographic evidence of osteoarthritis (present in 80% of patients aged 80 or older).

1. Clinical manifestations
   a. Early osteoarthritis may produce few or no symptoms
   b. Pain: most common symptom; associated with joint activity, particularly after prolonged inactivity and relieved by rest
   c. Mild morning stiffness, lasting less than 30 minutes
2. Specific joint complaints and exams
   a. Hip: patient complains of thigh or groin pain with motion or weight bearing
   b. Knee: significant restriction of movement, bony enlargement, and crepitation (with movement) may be present
   c. Cervical spine: osteophyte formation along margins of vertebral bodies can result in cervical pain, headache, syncope (secondary to vertebral artery and compression), and paresthesias of upper extremities (secondary to nerve compression); areas most commonly involved are C4 to C6
   d. Hands: osteoarthritis generally involves the DIP, PIP, and carpometacarpal joints of the thumb; bony overgrowths (felt as hard, nontender nodules) are known as Heberden's nodes for DIP joints and Bouchard's nodes for PIP joints
   e. Lumbosacral spine: low back pain and stiffness; perispinal muscle spasm may result in translumbar spread of pain and stiffness; facet joint hypertrophy may cause buttock, groin, and iliac crest pain; sciatica may be present if there is accompanying disk prolapse. Spinal stenosis and the clinical syndrome of pseudoclaudication may also complicate spinal osteoarthritis (see Section 6.5.e)
3. Laboratory evaluation: no specific laboratory abnormalities with osteoarthritis
4. Radiographic evaluation
   a. Osteophytes, subchondral sclerosis, cyst formation, and uneven joint space narrowing may be seen (Figure 6-15)
   b. Radiographic progression slow and unpredictable
   c. Symptoms do not parallel radiographic findings

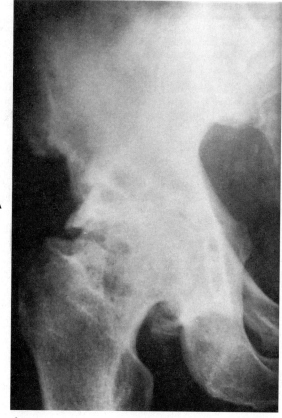

Figure 6-15
Comparison of severe osteoarthritis of the hip **(A)** with a normal hip **(B).** (Courtesy of the American Rheumatism Association; from Noble J et al, editors: *Textbook of primary care medicine,* ed 2, St Louis, 1996, Mosby.)

5. Therapy
   a. Physical measures
      (1) Exercise
         (a) Graded
         (b) Range of motion: active or passive
         (c) Muscle strengthening
      (2) Muscle spasm
         (a) Local heat
         (b) Massage

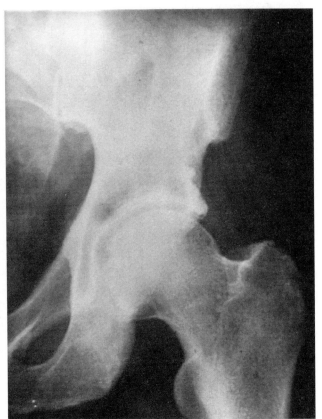

B

Figure 6-15, cont'd
For legend see opposite page.

    (3) Modify activities of daily living (ADLs): posture, sleep position
    (4) Support for joints (e.g., cane, walker, orthoses)
    (5) Weight reduction
    (6) Adapt environment (work, leisure, home)
  b. Medications
    (1) Acetaminophen, propoxyphene, aspirin, or NSAIDs
    (2) Reduction of muscle spasm with muscle relaxants (cyclobenza-
       prine [Flexeril], carisoprodol [Soma], methocarbamol [Robaxin],
       chlorzoxazone [Parafon Forte])

Chapter 6

(3) Corticosteroids
    (a) Systemic therapy not indicated
    (b) Intraarticular injection when inflammation evident (effect lasts about 4 weeks, limit to three injections per year)
  c. Psychologic measures: reassurance, counseling, education about disease
  d. Surgical measures
    (1) Arthroplasty: best results for those <75 years of age and <75 kg
    (2) Osteotomy
    (3) Arthroscopy

Suggested reading

Emmerson BT: The management of gout, *N Engl J Med* 334:445-451, 1996.

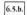

TEMPORAL ARTERITIS
Fred F. Ferri, MD

Definition

Temporal (giant cell) arteritis is a systemic segmental granulomatous inflammation predominantly involving the arteries of the carotid system in patients over 50. However, it can involve any large- or medium-sized arteries.

Demographics

1. Prevalence: 200 cases per 100,000 persons
2. Incidence after age 50: ranges from 17 to 23.3 new cases per 100,000 persons per year

Clinical manifestations

1. Headache, often associated with marked scalp tenderness
2. Tenderness, decreased pulsation, and nodulation of temporal arteries
3. Constitutional symptoms (fever, weight loss, anorexia, fatigue)
4. Polymyalgia syndrome (aching and stiffness of the trunk and proximal muscle groups)
5. Visual disturbances (visual loss, blurred vision, diplopia, amaurosis fugax)
6. Intermittent claudication of jaw and tongue on mastication
7. Cough

Laboratory findings

1. Elevated ESR (usually >50 mm/hr by the Westergren method); however, a normal ESR does not exclude the diagnosis
2. Mild to moderate normochromic normocytic anemia, elevated platelets
3. Liver function test abnormalities (elevation of alkaline phosphatase most common)

Diagnosis

The presence of any three of the following five items allows the diagnosis of temporal arteritis with a sensitivity of 94% and a specificity of 91%:
1. Age of onset ≥50 years
2. New onset or new type of headache

3. Temporal artery tenderness or decreased pulsation on physical exam
4. Westergren ESR $\geq$50 mm/hr
5. Artery biopsy with vasculitis and mononuclear cell infiltrate or granulomatous changes. Because of the presence of "skip lesions" in the artery, the biopsy segment of the temporal artery should be at least 2 cm long

Therapy

1. In stable patients without significant ocular involvement, therapy is usually started with prednisone 40 to 60 mg/day in divided doses, continued for a few weeks until symptoms resolve and ESR returns to normal. If the ESR remains normal, prednisone can be reduced by 5 mg every other week until a dose of 20 mg/day is reached. Subsequent dose reductions should be by 2.5 mg/day every 2 to 4 weeks. When the total dose reaches 5 mg/day, reduction should be by 1 mg every 2 to 4 weeks as tolerated. Usual length of prednisone treatment is 6 months to 2 years
2. In very ill patients and patients with significant ocular involvement (e.g., visual loss in one eye) rapid aggressive treatment with large doses of IV methylprednisolone is indicated to provide optimum protection to the uninvolved eye and offer any chance of visual recovery of the involved eye
3. Temporal arteritis is associated with a markedly increased risk for the development of aortic aneurysm, which is often a late complication and may cause death. Patients with a history of temporal arteritis should have an annual exam, including palpation of the abdominal aorta, and an annual radiograph of the chest, including a lateral view

Suggested reading

Evans JM, O'Fallon WM, Hunder GG: Increased incidence of aortic aneurysm and dissection in giant cell (temporal) arteritis, *Ann Intern Med* 122:502-507, 1995.

6.5.c. | ***POLYMYALGIA RHEUMATICA***
Fred F. Ferri, MD

Definition

Polymyalgia rheumatica is a clinical syndrome predominantly involving individuals over the age of 50 and characterized by pain and stiffness involving mainly the shoulders, pelvic girdle musculature, and torso.

Demographics

1. Prevalence: 600 cases per 100,000 persons
2. Incidence after age 50: 52.5 new cases per 100,000 persons

Clinical manifestations

1. Symmetric polymyalgias and arthralgias involving back, shoulder, neck, and pelvic girdle muscles; duration is generally longer than 1 month
2. Constitutional symptoms (fever, malaise, weight loss)
3. Headache in patients with coexisting temporal arteritis
4. Symptoms worse in the morning (difficulty getting out of bed) and at night

5. Muscle strength usually within normal limits
6. Crescendo of symptoms over several weeks or months

Laboratory findings

Laboratory findings are the same as for temporal arteritis.

Diagnostic criteria

1. Age >50
2. ESR >40 mm in 1 hour
3. At least 1 month of aching and morning stiffness in at least two of the following areas
   a. Neck and torso
   b. Hips and thighs
   c. Shoulders and upper arms
4. Other diseases have been excluded

Treatment

1. Abolish symptoms
   a. Low-dose corticosteroids (e.g., prednisone 10 to 15 mg/day) will generally produce dramatic relief of symptoms within 48 hours and confirm the diagnosis; failure to improve within 1 week suggests other diagnoses (e.g., fibromyalgia, polymyositis, viral myalgias, hypothyroidism, depression, rheumatoid arthritis, occult neoplasm, or infection)
   b. Corticosteroid dosage is then gradually tapered over several months based on repeated clinical observation
   c. In patients with mild symptoms NSAIDs may be used instead of corticosteroids
2. Monitor closely for possible development of temporal arteritis
   a. Instruct patient to immediately report any visual or neurologic symptoms
   b. As many as one third of patients can develop temporal arteritis within 1 year of onset of polymyalgia rheumatica

 BURSITIS, TENDINITIS, AND SELECTED SOFT TISSUE SYNDROMES
Tom J. Wachtel, MD

Definitions

1. Bursa: sac lined with synovial membrane that secretes synovial fluid, which acts as a lubricant between moving structures (e.g., tendons, ligaments, bones)
2. Bursitis: inflammation of a bursa
3. Tendon: noncontractile portion of a muscle; usually inserts on bone
4. Tendinitis: inflammation of a tendon
5. Capsule: fibrous tissue that holds a joint together
6. Ligament: reinforced component of a capsule

BURSITIS AND TENDINITIS

Sometimes specific involvement of a bursa or tendon produces a classic bursitis or tendinitis syndrome (see examples below). More commonly, the distinction between tendinitis and bursitis is tentative at best. The etiology of both conditions is the same, e.g., repetitive microtrauma or mechanical stresses to the structure associated with the patient's occupation or leisure activities. Rarely bursitis or tendinitis is associated with rheumatologic conditions such as rheumatoid arthritis and variants, crystalline arthritis, infection, and osteoarthritis.

The clinical features include pain in the affected area, made worse by any active range of motion that mobilizes the inflamed tendon or bursa. Passive range of motion may be intact or restricted by pain. Palpation of the relevant structure reveals diffuse tenderness and occasionally localized swelling in the case of bursitis. The presence of a well-defined trigger point suggests tendinitis. Diagnostic tests are not required except for a fluctuant inflamed bursa with or without systemic signs of infection; such a bursa should be aspirated and the fluid examined for cell count, Gram stain, cultures, and a search for crystals to rule out septic bursitis and crystalline bursitis.

Treatment

1. Discontinue the causing activity
2. Cold compresses early to provide analgesia and reduce swelling; heat application may be helpful during the recovery phase
3. NSAIDs for 2 weeks
4. Failure to respond to the above is best approached with needle aspiration (in bursitis) and injection of corticosteroid/local anesthetic solutions (e.g., 20 to 40 mg prednisolone with 2 or 3 ml of 1% to 2% xylocaine) inside the bursa (in bursitis) or at the tendon insertion (trigger point) in tendinitis
5. Mobilization should begin as soon as the inflammation (e.g., pain) has subsided, beginning with passive range of motion and progressing to active movements. Heat application should be recommended especially before exercises. Exercise performed alone or in physical therapy is excessive if any induced pain persists for longer than 30 minutes following completion

•   •   •

Common examples of tendinitis, bursitis, and related syndromes are listed in Table 6-13.

OTHER SOFT TISSUE SYNDROMES

1. Stenosing tenosynovitis
   a. Restriction of tendon movement by a fibrotic nodule on the tendon and/or stenosis of a tendon sheath
   b. Examples
      (1) Trigger finger
      (2) De Quervain's disease of the thumb abductor longis and extensor brevis
   c. Treatment: same as tendinitis
2. Nerve entrapment syndromes
   a. Mononeuropathy caused by fibrous tissue compression and resulting nerve degeneration
   b. Example: carpal tunnel syndrome

Table 6-13   Common examples of tendinitis, bursitis, and related syndromes

Bursitis or Tendinitis	Area of Tenderness	Reproducing Syndromes
Shoulder		
Supraspinatus tendinitis	Posterolateral humeral head below acromion	Abduction External rotation
Bicipital tendinitis	Upper medial humerus	Forceful supination with elbow held in flexion
Adhesive capsulitis (frozen shoulder)	Variable	Progressive limitation of all shoulder movements
Elbow		
Tennis elbow	Lateral epicondyle wrist extensor tendon	Forceful extension of wrist and fingers
Olecranon bursitis	Posterior point of elbow	Full elbow flexion
Hip		
Weavers' bursitis	Ischial tuberosities	Sitting on hard surfaces
Trochanteric bursitis	Greater trochanter	External rotation
Knee		
Anserine bursitis	Medial tibia	Ascending and descending stairs
Iliotibial band syndrome	Lateral femur	Repetitive knee flexion and extension (running)
Prepatellar bursitis	Anterior knee	Flexion of knee

    c. Treatment
       (1) Wrist splint
       (2) NSAIDs
       (3) Local steroid injections
       (4) Surgical decompression
3. Reflex sympathetic dystrophy (causalgia)
    a. Unexplained pain and swelling of an extremity sometimes associated with trauma, myocardial infarction, or stroke. Osteoporosis and muscular atrophy of involved extremity may occur
    b. Treatment
       (1) Analgesics, beta-blockers
       (2) Gradual physical therapy
       (3) Nerve block
       (4) Oral corticosteroids

4. Thoracic outlet syndrome
   a. Subclavian artery and/or nerve compression by a cervical rib or by scalene muscles causing symptoms of arterial insufficiency and/or neuropathy
   b. Treatment: surgical decompression if severe symptoms
5. Raynaud's syndrome
   a. Upper extremity vasomotor phenomenon often triggered by cold exposure and resulting in the following clinical temporal sequence
      (1) Hand pallor
      (2) Hand cyanosis
      (3) Erythema and pain caused by hyperemia
   b. Most cases are idiopathic, but syndrome may be associated with a collagen vascular disease (e.g., scleroderma)
   c. Treatment
      (1) Avoid precipitating factors (e.g., cold)
      (2) Calcium channel blockers, except in scleroderma
6. Dupuytren's contracture
   a. Idiopathic hypertrophic fibrosis of the palmar fascia progressing over several years and resulting in a painless flexion contracture of involved hand; often bilateral, may be hereditary, more common in alcoholics
   b. Treatment: surgery

Suggested readings

Bywaters EGL: Tendinitis and bursitis, *Clin Rheum Dis* 5:883, 1979.
Cardelli MD, Kleinsmith DM: Raynaud's phenomenon and disease, *Med Clin North Am* 73:1127, 1989.
Dawson DM: Entrapment neuropathies of the upper extremities, *N Engl J Med* 329:2013-2018, 1993.
Fitzgerald O et al: Prospective study of the evolution of Raynaud's phenomenon, *Am J Med* 84:718, 1988.
Klippel JH: Raynaud's phenomenon: the French tricolor, *Arch Intern Med* 151:2389-2393, 1991.
Kopicky-Burd J: Nonarticular rheumatic disorders. In Barker LR, Burton JR, Zieve PD, editors: *Principles of ambulatory medicine,* ed 3, Baltimore, 1991, Williams & Wilkins.
Spinner RJ, Bachman JW, Amadio PC: The many faces of carpal tunnel syndrome, *Mayo Clin Proc* 64:829-836, 1989.
Stevens JC et al: Conditions associated with carpal tunnel syndrome, *Mayo Clin Proc* 67:541-548, 1992.
Veldman PHJM et al: Signs and symptoms of reflex sympathetic dystrophy: prospective study of 829 patients, *Lancet* 342:1012-1016, 1993.

| 6.5.e. |

LOW BACK PAIN
Tom J. Wachtel, MD

Epidemiology

1. Very common: 75% of all people experience low back pain sometime during their lives; third most frequent office complaint among patients over age 75; 40% of nursing home patients who report pain complain of their backs
2. 20 million new cases per year in the United States and 6.5 million patients bedridden with low back pain every day

Etiology

1. Musculoskeletal causes (Table 6-14)
   a. Acute (lasting up to 6 weeks)
   b. Subacute (lasting 6 to 12 weeks)
   c. Chronic (lasting more than 3 months)
   d. Most common etiologies are age dependent
2. Visceral causes (Table 6-15): any intraabdominal painful process can radiate to the low back or cause pain primarily in the low back

Clinical evaluation and management

1. Acute low back pain
   a. Consider visceral causes first
      (1) Rule out an infectious process by checking for fever and chills, and if they are present, obtain a CBC
      (2) Rule out renal pathology by asking about urinary symptoms and obtaining a urinalysis
      (3) Inquire about female genital symptoms and perform a pelvic exam if there is any question of pelvic pathologic conditions

Table 6-14   Musculoskeletal causes of low back pain

Cause	Duration	Typical Age of Onset
Muscle strain	Acute	Young adult
Disk herniation	Acute to chronic	Young adult
Trauma	Acute	Young adult
Compression fracture		
Secondary to malignancy	Acute to chronic	Elderly
Secondary to osteoporosis	Acute to chronic	Elderly
Osteoarthritis/spinal stenosis	Chronic	Elderly
Paget's disease	Chronic	Elderly
Spondylolisthesis	Acute to chronic	Young adult
Ankylosing spondylitis and variants	Chronic	Young adult
Spinal tumor	Subacute	Any age
Spinal tumor with cord compression	Acute	Any age
Osteomyelitis		
Bacterial	Acute	Any age
Tuberculous	Acute	Any age
Epidural abscess	Acute	Any age
Diskitis	Acute	Any age
Fibromyalgia	Chronic	Any age
Facet joint disease	Acute or chronic	Young adult
Sickle cell crisis	Acute	Young adult
Poor posture	Chronic	Any age
Spine deformities (e.g., scoliosis)	Chronic	Any age
Malingering	Chronic	Any age

b. History
   (1) Onset sudden or insidious?
   (2) Relation to exercise
   (3) Recent trauma (even minor)
   (4) History of fractures

Table 6-15 Visceral causes of low back pain

Cause	Duration	Age
Abdominal aortic aneurysm		
Expanding	Subacute to chronic	Elderly
Ruptured	Acute	Elderly
Dissecting aneurysm	Acute	Elderly
Renal pathology		
Pyelonephritis	Acute	Any age
Renal colic	Acute	Any age
Renal cancer	Subacute	Middle age to elderly
Pancreatic pathology		
Pancreatitis	Acute	Any age
Pancreatic cancer	Subacute	Middle age to elderly
Retroperitoneal mass		
Lymphoma	Subacute to chronic	Any age
Soft tissue sarcomas	Subacute to chronic	Middle age to elderly
Metastatic cancer (uterine, prostate, testicular)	Subacute to chronic	Middle age to elderly
Female pelvic pathology		
Uterine malignancy		
Cervical	Subacute to chronic	Young adult to middle age
Endometrial	Subacute to chronic	Postmenopausal
Uterine leiomyoma	Chronic	Middle age
Ovarian tumor	Subacute to chronic	Middle age to elderly
Pelvic inflammatory disease	Acute	Young adult
Pregnancy	Subacute to "chronic"	Young adult

        (5) Lower extremity symptoms

        (6) History or symptoms of malignancy

  c. Examine spine and lumbar plexus

        (1) Inspect spine for deformities

        (2) Note patient's posture

        (3) Palpate and percuss lumbar spine

        (4) Inquire about symptoms of sciatica (pain, numbness or weakness in buttocks and lower extremities)

        (5) Perform straight leg raising test

        (6) Perform sensory, motor, and reflex examination of lower extremities; any objective neurologic abnormalities require urgent attention and/or neurosurgical referral

  d. Ancillary tests

        (1) Unlike young adults, low threshold for CBC, calcium, ESR, and liver function tests

        (2) Lumbosacral spine x-ray may be useful to rule out osteoporosis, compression fractures, Paget's disease, osteoarthritis, verebral cancer

        (3) Additional tests may be indicated: parathormone level, serum/urine protein/immuneoelectrophoresis, bone scan, MRI of spine

  e. Management

        (1) Majority of patients have a negative or nonspecific exam; should be treated empirically for acute low back syndrome if screening tests are negative (even if sciatica is present)

        (2) Bed rest for 2 days if pain is severe

        (3) Analgesics (aspirin, acetaminophen, NSAIDs, codeine)

        (4) Muscle relaxants (chlorzoxazone [Parafon Forte] cyclobenzaprine [Flexeril] carisoprodol [Soma]). NOTE: avoid benzodiazepines

        (5) Physical therapy, including exercise programs, traction, diathermy, heat or cold application, ultrasound, and transcutaneous electrical nerve stimulation (TENS), not proven effective in management of acute low back syndrome

        (6) Chiropractic or osteopathic manipulative therapy: popular and may be as effective as traditional allopathic management

        (7) Prevention of recurrent episodes

           (a) Exercises to strengthen abdominal and paraspinal musculature

           (b) Pelvic tilt exercises

           (c) Flexion exercises if spinal stenosis is likely

           (d) Improve posture

             • Weight loss if indicated

             • Avoid high heels

             • Avoid standing still; or if not possible, use footstool for one foot when standing (or for both feet when sitting)

           (e) Teach proper lifting techniques (i.e., use thighs, not back)

2. Subacute low back pain

  a. 10% of patients with acute low back syndrome continue to be symptomatic after 6 weeks of conservative treatment. They now have subacute low back pain. At this point, efforts to establish a definitive diagnosis must be made. Often this will be done with imaging using CT or MRI technology that can provide information about the spine, spinal cord, paraspinal soft tissue, retroperitoneal space, and abdominal and pelvic viscera

b. Disk disease (rare onset after age 40)

(1) Pathogenesis: when a person lifts a heavy object using a lumbar extension effort, anterior aspect of vertebral bodies and intravertebral disks become the fulcrum of a lever where considerable force tends to squeeze and express the disk backward. If structural disk injury occurs, process of disk herniation (posterior bulging) will begin

(2) Clinical course

  (a) Stage 1: stretching the sensory receptors in the posterior ligament causes an acute low back syndrome, which should be managed as described in Section 1.e. The pain is aggravated by flexion

  (b) Stage 2: further herniation irritates and then compresses lumbar plexus nerve roots and causes a dermatomal (radicular) neuropathy called sciatica. Lumbar disks most likely to herniate are L4-5 (L5 root) and L5-S1 (S1 root) (98% of all cases)

  (c) Rule out cauda equina syndrome by inquiring about urine and fecal continence and by checking rectal sphincter tone

  (d) Any objective neurologic deficit requires urgent diagnostic evaluation and treatment, albeit not necessarily surgical

  (e) Stage 3: scarring occurs; back pain may decrease or become chronic and neurologic deficits become fixed

(3) Signs of sciatica

  (a) Subjective pain and sensory abnormalities. Subjective symptoms are most likely to be proximal, and objective findings are more likely to be distal (test with light touch or pinprick)

- L5 root: buttock, posterior thigh, lateral leg, dorsum of foot and great toe
- S1 root: buttock, posterior thigh, lateral aspect of ankle and foot, and lateral toes

  (b) Deep tendon reflexes

- L5 root: none
- S1 root: ankle jerk

  (c) Motor function: toe walking and heel walking are adequate tests

- L5 root controls foot dorsiflexion (heel walking and also look for footdrop)
- S1 root controls foot plantar flexion (toe walking)

  (d) Straight leg raising test: dura is stretched around sciatic nerves at angles of 30 to 70 degrees. A positive test is obtained when raising the contralateral leg reproduces sciatica pain on affected side (better than 95% probability of disk disease). Malingering can be detected when distracting the patient produces inconsistent results; or when the leg is lowered to an angle where the sciatic pain disappears, a patient with organic disease should complain on foot dorsiflexion performed at this point

    (4) Management

        (a) Stage 1: managed as a nonspecific acute low back syndrome

        (b) Stage 2: patient may be a candidate for neurosurgery: very successful at relieving the radiculopathy if performed within 12 weeks of onset of neurologic deficit but no more than 50% effective at resolving the back pain

        (c) Stage 3: treatment mainly aimed at pain control, rehabilitative therapy (e.g., exercises), and resolving psychosocial co-morbidities

c. Osteoarthritis

    (1) Many elderly patients with low back pain are found to have radiologic evidence of osteoarthritis; however, poor correlation between symptoms and radiologic findings is the rule rather than the exception in osteoarthritis (see Section 6.5.a)

    (2) Special consideration should be given to the possibility of spinal stenosis, a potentially reversible complication of spinal osteoarthritis. These patients have back pain, bilateral leg pain on standing or walking, resolved by sitting or bending (pseudoclaudication). Lumbosacral spine x-rays are suggestive but CT scan or MRI is diagnostic. Surgical treatment may be required

d. Osteoporosis, compression fractures, and malignant spine lesions

    (1) Osteoporosis per se does not produce symptoms but predisposes patients to acute vertebral compression fractures that can occur spontaneously or during trauma (see Section 6.2.c for diagnosis and management of osteoporosis)

    (2) Sudden onset of low back pain in older women should be presumed to result from a compression fracture, and this can often be confirmed by a simple x-ray of the spine (note that a radiologic diagnosis of a new compression fracture may be difficult in a patient with previous vertebral fracture or severe degenerative changes)

        (a) Pain is variable in severity but may be very severe

        (b) Treatment is symptomatic as in any low back syndrome; however, the first few days following fracture may be complicated by an intestinal ileus often exacerbated by use of narcotic analgesics. Prophylactic stool softeners should be prescribed

        (c) No evidence that back braces or corsets are effective, but many patients report some comfort from their use

    (3) Plain x-ray may also reveal malignant disease involving spine. Primary osteosarcoma is unusual in this location, but multiple myeloma should always be considered as a potential cause of osteoporosis or lytic lesions. Diagnosis can be made by ordering an erythrocytic sedimentation for screening, followed by serum protein electrophoresis, immunoelectrophoresis, and a urine protein electrophoresis

    (4) Metastatic lesions of the spine usually originate from lung (lytic lesions), prostate (blastic lesions), kidney (lytic lesions), breast (blastic or lytic lesions), or thyroid (blastic lesions). Malignant lesions of the spine can cause pain without a compression fracture. This should be suspected when back pain occurs at rest. They also can cause extrinsic cord or root compression, a neurosurgical oncologic emergency

e. Ankylosing spondylarthropathies (onset exceptional after age 40)
   (1) Young men more commonly and severely affected than women. They present with back pain, occasionally with hip, knee, or ankle pain with stiffness, worse in the morning as in any inflammatory arthritis. A positive family history may be elicited
   (2) Findings on examination include reduced chest expansion, increased finger to toe distance, inability to perform the occiput to wall test, and sacroiliac joint tenderness
   (3) Extraarticular manifestations: cardiac complications (A-V block, aortic regurgitation), iritis, pulmonary fibrosis, and amyloidosis; psoriasis or inflammatory bowel disease may coexist
   (4) Diagnosis of ankylosing spondylitis confirmed by an elevated sedimentation rate, evidence of sacroiliitis on pelvic x-ray, evidence of syndesmophytes or common ligament calcification (bamboo spine) on a spine x-ray, and presence of an HLA-B27 antigen
   (5) Symptomatic relief can be achieved with aspirin and NSAIDs. Physical therapy should be performed to preserve mobility or permit ankylosing in the most functional position
   (6) By the time the patient is elderly, the disease usually will have stabilized and the patient will often experience the same problems as those seen in degenerative disease of the spine
f. Osteomyelitis, diskitis, and epidural abscess
   (1) Bacterial infections, or more rarely tuberculosis, can involve the spine and adjacent structures through hematogenous route or from spread of a contiguous focus of infection; infection may be acute (e.g., staphylococcal diskitis) or chronic (e.g., tuberculous osteomyelitis known as Pott's disease)
   (2) Pain characteristically worse at night
   (3) Patient may have particular risk factors (e.g., IV drug abuse) and may have obvious or subtle signs of infection
   (4) Imaging studies needed to establish a definitive diagnosis
g. Posterior facet joint syndrome
   (1) Because posterior articular facets meet each other at an angle, those joints are subjected to a constant shearing force in the erect position; pain is typically of sudden onset (acute lumbago) and rarely lasts more than 1 week
   (2) Posterior facet joint syndrome should be suspected when pain is aggravated by spinal extension; diagnosed more frequently by chiropractors than by allopathic physicians and may be improved by manipulative therapy
h. Fibromyalgia or fibrositis
   (1) Although not restricted to the low back, this controversial condition manifests itself by soft tissue aching and chronic stiffness aggravated by stress
   (2) Young and middle-aged women most commonly affected
   (3) Characterized by the presence of trigger points that, according to some authorities, must be quite specific
   (4) Many patients complain of insomnia and waking up unrefreshed in the morning; substantial proportion of patients also display other depressive symptoms
   (5) Some patients respond to antidepressant drugs, psychotherapy,

NSAIDs, or physical therapy. However, as might be expected in a condition where somatization plays an important part, many patients do not improve and pursue an erratic health care–seeking course

3. Chronic low back pain
   a. Although only 5% of all patients with acute back pain go on to become chronic, the proportion is far greater in the elderly because of high prevalence of osteoarthritis and vertebral collapse fractures; patients often make frequent doctor visits and can cause great bidirectional frustration in the physician-patient relationship. Ideally, workup will have been completed during the subacute phase; if not, it should be done at once
   b. Whether an incurable organic cause is diagnosed (e.g., osteoarthritis, osteoporosis with compression fractures) or patient has unexplained chronic refractory back pain, management should be supportive
      (1) Nonaddictive analgesic agents
      (2) Exercises
      (3) Attention to psychosocial ills, perhaps a trial of antidepressants
      (4) Protection from excessive diagnostic procedures, surgery, and "doctor shopping"
   c. Therapeutic success enhanced by setting realistic symptom and functional expectations with the patient

Suggested readings

Borenstein DG, Burton JR: Lumbar spine disease in the elderly, *J Am Geriatr Soc* 41:167-175, 1993.

Deyo RA: Conservative therapy for low back pain: distinguishing useful from useless therapy, *JAMA* 250:1057-1062, 1983.

Deyo RA: Early diagnostic evaluation of low back pain, *J Gen Intern Med* 1:328-338, 1986.

Deyo RA, Diehl AK, Rosenthal M: How many days of bed rest for acute low back pain? A randomized clinical trial, *N Engl J Med* 315:1064-1070, 1986.

Deyo RA, Loeser JD, Bigos SJ: Herniated lumbar intervertebral disk, *Ann Intern Med* 112:598-603, 1990.

Hall H: Examination of the patient with low back pain, *Bull Rheum Dis* 33:1-8, 1983.

Mooney V: The syndromes of low back disease, *Orthop Clin North Am* 14:505-515, 1983.

Powers R: Fibromyalgia: an age-old malady begging for respect, *J Gen Intern Med* 8:93-105, 1993.

 ### CARDIOVASCULAR DISORDERS

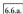 ### *HYPERTENSION*
Fred F. Ferri, MD

Definition

For all adults over age 18, the "Fifth Report of the Joint National Committee on Detection, Evaluation, and Treatment of High Blood Pressure (JNC-V)" defined hypertension as
- Systolic blood pressure (BP) $\geq$140 mm Hg
- Diastolic BP $\geq$90 mm Hg

Isolated systolic hypertension (ISH) is defined as
- Systolic BP $\geq$140 mm Hg
- Diastolic BP <90 mm Hg

Prevalence

1. Arterial hypertension is present in 45% of the elderly and represents the most frequent chronic health problem
2. Isolated systolic hypertension (ISH) is more common in the elderly, occurring in 15% of elderly males and 25% of elderly female

Therapeutic considerations

1. Therapy of hypertension is as beneficial in the elderly as in the younger population
2. ISH is not a normal phenomenon of aging. It increases cardiovascular morbidity and mortality and should be aggressively treated
3. Initial therapy of mild hypertension should be nonpharmacologic
   a. Sodium restriction
   b. Weight loss if the patient is obese
   c. Stress reduction
   d. Regular aerobic exercise
   e. Alcohol restriction
4. If pharmacologic therapy is necessary, the following *age-related cardiovascular and physiologic factors* should be considered
   a. Increased susceptibility to orthostatic hypotension caused by decreased aortic elasticity, myocardial reserve, baroreceptor sensitivity, and plasma renin activity. Medications that can potentiate orthostatic changes (e.g., guanethidine) should be avoided
   b. Decreased regional blood flow can result in impaired perfusion of vital organs if blood pressure is rapidly reduced
   c. Increased total peripheral resistance and decreased cardiac output result in decreased efficacy of agents that reduce sympathetic drive and cardiac output
   d. Decreased renal tubular secretion and concentration may result in impaired drug clearance (e.g., atenolol)
   e. Decreased hepatic function will increase the half-life of lipid-soluble agents
   f. Decreased plasma volume will increase susceptibility to hypotensive effect of diuretics and ACE inhibitors (in hypovolemic patients)
   g. Decreased vascular compliance will impair efficacy of direct-acting vasodilators
5. The increased prevalence of coexisting diseases in the elderly should be considered when choosing a hypertensive agent. The drug's effect on concomitant illnesses must be taken into account
   a. **Diabetes mellitus**—beta-blockers, diuretics, sympathetic inhibitors should be avoided. ACE inhibitors and calcium antagonists are preferred agents
   b. **CHF**—Beta-blockers and calcium antagonists (particularly verapamil) should be avoided. ACE inhibitors and diuretics are preferred agents
   c. **Ischemic heart disease**—diuretics and hydralazine should be avoided. Beta-blockers and calcium antagonists are preferred

6. The risk of drug interactions is much higher in the elderly because of polypharmacy
   a. Nonsteroidal antiinflammatory drugs (NSAIDs): may blunt hypertensive effect of ACE inhibitors
   b. Verapamil and nifedipine: may double digoxin levels
   c. Verapamil: may inhibit hepatic oxidation of theophylline and carbamazepine
   d. Cimetidine: may increase blood levels of metoprolol and propranolol
7. The antihypertensive drug regimen should be simplified. A monotherapeutic regimen with once per day dosage will improve patient compliance
8. Drug therapy should be tailored to the individual patient. It is best to start with a low dose (usually half the standard dose used in younger patients). Dose adjustments should be made in small increments to minimize orthostatic hypotension and potential adverse reactions
9. There is no ideal antihypertensive agent in the elderly. Each drug class has selective advantages and disadvantages
   a. Thiazide diuretics: inexpensive and effective and have been shown to significantly lower the incidence of hip fracture. In the absence of comorbidities, most authors recommend diuretics as first choice in elderly hypertensive patients. Diuretics are, however, associated with potential metabolic side effects; should be only used in low doses (e.g., hydrochlorothiazide 12.5 to 25 mg/day) with close monitoring of electrolytes and renal function
   b. Beta-blockers: effective in controlling hypertension and reducing both cerebrovascular and cardiovascular morbidity and mortality; can, however, cause significant CNS side effects in the elderly; when used, cardioselective beta-blockers are preferred
   c. Calcium inhibitors: generally well tolerated but can result in significant side effects (e.g., constipation with verapamil, pedal edema and impaired learning and memory with nifedipine)
   d. ACE inhibitors: particularly useful in hypertension complicated by CHF; generally well tolerated with minimal side effects (e.g., cough with enalapril, taste disturbances with captopril); can cause significant hypotension in volume-depleted patients
   e. Centrally acting alpha$_2$-agonists, adrenergic antagonists, and direct vasodilators: generally not recommended as initial monotherapy in elderly patients

| 6.6.b. |

CONGESTIVE HEART FAILURE
Fred F. Ferri, MD

Epidemiology

1. Incidence of CHF increases with age. Incidence for age-group 75 to 84 is 13/1000, increasing to over 50/1000 for ages 85 to 94
2. Prevalence of CHF ranges from 3% in individuals aged 45 to 64 to approximately 10% in those aged 75 and above
3. Mortality after the onset of symptoms varies with sex of the patient. It is 20% after 1 year and 62% after 5 years for males; 14% after 1 year and 42% after 5 years for females

Etiology

1. CHF in the elderly: usually secondary to the following conditions
   a. Hypertension (75%)
   b. Arteriosclerotic heart disease
   c. Calcific valvular stenosis
   d. Amyloid infiltration of the ventricles
2. Precipitating factors
   a. Overzealous administration of IV fluids (most common precipitating cause of CHF in hospitalized patients)
   b. Medications (e.g., NSAIDs, prednisone, beta-blockers)
   c. Poor compliance with sodium restriction
   d. Comorbid illness: infection, anemia, hypothyroidism, hypoxia, pulmonary embolus
3. The following age-related changes in the cardiovascular system are not in themselves sufficient to produce CHF but can contribute to it
   a. Myocardial hypertrophy
   b. Impaired myocardial diastolic function
   c. Increased stiffness of the aorta and other major arteries
   d. Impaired response to sympathetic nervous system stimulation

Diagnostic considerations in the elderly

1. The classic clinical history of dyspnea, orthopnea, paroxysmal nocturnal dyspnea, and nocturnal angina may be difficult to elicit, particularly in patients with preexisting dementia and confusional states. The presenting symptom may be fatigue or lethargy secondary to low cardiac output. Poor systemic perfusion may result in delirium and ischemic changes in lower extremities
2. Physical exam may reveal significant loss of lean body mass in addition to the classic findings of S_3 gallop, jugular venous distention (JVD), pulmonary rales, and hepatojugular reflux
3. Radiographic diagnosis may be masked by poor quality of the chest x-ray (portable films, poor inspiratory effort) and by the frequent presence of kyphoscoliosis and associated pulmonary parenchymal disease
4. Table 6-16 summarizes useful tests to evaluate patients with new onset signs or symptoms of heart failure for underlying causes

Therapeutic approach

1. Identify and correct precipitating factors (e.g., anemia, thyrotoxicosis, hypertension, infections, beta-blockers or other cardiac depressants, increased sodium load, medical noncompliance)
2. For therapeutic purposes it is useful to differentiate left ventricular failure (LVF) according to systolic dysfunction (low ejection fraction [EF], e.g., post-MI, cardiomyopathy) and diastolic dysfunction (normal or high EF, "stiff ventricle," e.g., hypertensive cardiovascular disease, valvular heart disease, restrictive cardiomyopathy). A radionuclear ventriculogram or two-dimensional echocardiogram with Doppler is useful to confirm diastolic dysfunction in patients with CHF and normal-sized heart and normal EF on echocardiogram. Table 6-17 compares these two diagnostic modalities

Table 6-16 Recommended tests for patients with signs or symptoms of heart failure

Test Recommendation	Finding	Suspected Diagnosis
Electrocardiogram	Acute ST-segment or T-wave changes	Myocardial ischemia
	Atrial fibrillation or other tachyarrhythmia	Thyroid disease or heart failure caused by rapid ventricular rate
	Bradyarrhythmias	Heart failure caused by low heart rate
	Previous MI (e.g., Q waves)	Heart failure caused by reduced LV performance
	Low voltage	Pericardial effusion
	LV hypertrophy	Diastolic dysfunction
Complete blood count	Anemia	Heart failure caused by or aggravated by decreased oxygen-carrying capacity
Urinalysis	Proteinuria	Nephrotic syndrome
	Red blood cells or cellular casts	Glomerulonephritis
Serum creatinine	Elevated	Volume overload caused by renal failure
Serum albumin	Decreased	Increased extravascular volume caused by hypoalbuminemia
T_4 and TSH (obtain only if atrial fibrillation, evidence of thyroid disease, or patient age >65)	Abnormal T_4 or TSH	Heart failure caused by or aggravated by hypothyroidism or hyperthyroidism
Echocardiogram	Left ventricular function (ejection fraction)	
	Diastolic dysfunction	
	Valvular heart disease	

From *Clinical practice guideline, No. 11* (Pub. No. 94-0612), Rockville, Md, June 1994, AHCPR.
LV, Left ventricular; *MI,* myocardial infarction; *TSH,* thyroid-stimulating hormone.

Table 6-17   Comparison of echocardiography and radionuclide ventriculography in evaluation of LV performance

Test	Advantages	Disadvantages
Echocardiogram	Permits concomitant assessment of valvular disease, LV hypertrophy, and left atrial size Less expensive than radionuclide ventriculography in most areas Able to detect pericardial effusion and ventricular thrombus More generally available	Difficult to perform in patients with lung disease Usually only semi-quantitative estimate of ejection fraction provided Technically inadequate in up to 18% of patients under optimal conditions
Radionuclide ventriculogram	More precise and reliable measurement of ejection fraction Better assessment of right ventricular function	Requires venipuncture and radiation exposure Limited assessment of valvular heart disease and LV hypertrophy

From *Clinical practice guideline, No. 11* (Pub. No. 94-0612), Rockville, Md, June 1994, AHCPR.
LV, Left ventricular.

. Effective drug therapy for systolic heart failure consists of the following agents
   a. **Diuretics**
      (1) Effective and inexpensive; however, associated with frequent metabolic abnormalities (hypokalemia, hypomagnesemia, hyponatremia, hyperuricemia)
      (2) The risk of volume depletion and hypotension can be minimized by using low doses and closely monitoring the patient for early signs of hypovolemia; low-dose hydrochlorothiazide (e.g., 12.5 mg) is nearly as effective as higher doses and causes significantly fewer side effects
      (3) The age-related reduced renal clearance will increase their elimination half-life and the subsequent duration of diuretic-related incontinence in the elderly
      (4) Ototoxicity is also a frequent occurrence because of direct damage to the stria vascularis of the cochlea by loop diuretics
   b. **ACE inhibitors**
      (1) Effective and generally well tolerated
      (2) Duration of action: generally prolonged in the elderly secondary to altered glomerular filtration and CHF

      (3) Hypotension frequent in hyponatremic, volume-depleted patients

      (4) Risk of renal insufficiency secondary to ACE inhibitors: higher in the elderly; reduction of diuretic dose and frequent monitoring of electrolytes and renal function are recommended when adding an ACE inhibitor

  c. **Digoxin**

      (1) Useful in patients with rapid atrial fibrillation, severe CHF, or EF <20%

      (2) One of the most frequently misused drugs; generally not indicated in patients with sinus rhythm and no impairment in ventricular systolic function

      (3) Toxicity occurs in 5% of outpatients and over 10% of hospitalized patients; contributing factors are

          (a) Altered pharmacokinetics in the elderly because of decreased volume of distribution and reduced renal clearance

          (b) Drug interactions (e.g., verapamil, quinidine, procainamide, nifedipine, and amiodarone can significantly increase serum digoxin levels)

          (c) Hypokalemia and hypomagnesemia caused by concomitant use of diuretics

          (d) Excessive dosing in the elderly

          (e) In addition to the classic signs of digoxin toxicity (dysrhythmias, anorexia, nausea, visual disturbances), the elderly can present with atypical manifestations (e.g., fatigue, confusion, irritability). Frequent monitoring of renal function and serum digoxin levels along with heightened awareness of the potential digoxin toxicity will minimize its risk in the elderly

4. Drug therapy for diastolic heart failure differs in the following manner

  a. Diuretics should be used only in small doses since a reduction in preload in patients with a "stiff ventricle" will significantly affect cardiac output. Diuretics are useful in the treatment of CHF caused by diastolic dysfunction from aortic stenosis, hypertension, and mitral stenosis

  b. ACE inhibitors: useful primarily in hypertensive persons with hypertrophy and in diastolic dysfunction from aortic insufficiency and mitral regurgitation

  c. Calcium channel blockers and beta-blockers: useful when hypertrophic cardiomyopathy is present or occasionally for ischemia

6.6.c.   ***ORTHOSTATIC HYPOTENSION***
Fred F. Ferri, MD

Definition

Orthostatic hypotension is a reduction ≥20 mm Hg in systolic blood pressure from lying down to standing upright.

Epidemiology

Orthostatic (postural) hypotension occurs in 20% of elderly. Its incidence increases with age (>30% in population ≥75 years old).

Etiology

The etiology of orthostatic hypotension is usually multifactorial. Contributing factors are

1. Age-associated physiologic changes
   a. Autonomic dysfunction
   b. Decreased venous return
   c. Impaired cerebral autoregulation and volume regulation
   d. Loss of elasticity of arteries
   e. Impaired increase in compensatory heart rate
2. Drugs
   a. Antihypertensives: prazosin, terazosin, methyldopa, clonidine, hydralazine, guanethidine
   b. Antidepressants: imipramine, amitriptyline, monoamine oxidase (MAO) inhibitors
   c. Antipsychotics: chlorpromazine, thioridazine, trifluoperazine
   d. Diuretics
   e. Alcohol
   f. Others: nitrates, narcotics, barbiturates, quinidine, levodopa, anticholinergics, sedatives
3. Organ system abnormalities
   a. Nervous system: parkinsonism, multiple CVAs, peripheral neuropathy, neoplasms, sympathectomy, Shy-Drager syndrome (orthostatic hypotension, parkinsonian features, and other neurologic disturbances involving cerebellar, basal ganglia, pyramidal, and spinal motor neurons)
   b. Cardiovascular: idiopathic hypertrophic subaortic stenosis (IHSS), aortic stenosis, mitral valve prolapse (MVP), CHF, decreased venous return (e.g., large varicose veins)
   c. Endocrine: adrenal insufficiency, hypoaldosteronism, diabetes mellitus (neuropathy), diabetes insipidus (hypovolemia), carcinoid, pheochromocytoma, paraneoplastic syndromes
   d. Anemia
4. Miscellaneous causes: postprandial hypotension, dehydration, malnutrition, electrolyte disturbances, hypovolemia, dysrhythmias, idiopathic orthostatic hypotension, vitamin B_{12} deficiency

Diagnostic approach

1. History
   a. Medications (including over the counter), alcohol use, dietary habits
   b. Previous medical and surgical problems
   c. Autonomic review of systems (e.g., constipation, impotence, neurogenic bladder)
   d. Bleeding
2. Physical examination
   a. Measure blood pressure and pulse rate after the patient has been recumbent for 10 minutes and again at 1 and 5 minutes after the patient has been standing. Absence of pulse increase after standing may indicate autonomic dysfunction
   b. Assess diastolic blood pressure response after isometric handgrip (≥ 10 mm Hg rise indicates adequate sympathetic vasoconstrictor reflexes)

   c. Assess hydration (skin turgor), volume status (jugular venous pres
      sure), presence of heart murmurs (IHSS, MVP), mood (depression)
      presence of tremor and rigidity (parkinsonism), peripheral neuropath
3. Initial laboratory evaluation
   a. CBC, electrolytes, BUN, creatinine, glucose, calcium, albumin, uri
      nalysis
   b. ECG with rhythm strip: useful in patients in regular sinus rhythm t
      evaluate heart rate variability to deep breathing. A variation of 5 to
      beats/min for the longest R-R interval compared with the shortest in
      dicates normal parasympathetic system function

Therapy

1. Eliminate cause (e.g., stop offending medication, correct hypovolemia)
2. Increase sodium intake but monitor closely for onset of CHF
3. Elevate head of bed with 2×6 inch blocks to minimize nocturnal shift
   of interstitial fluid from the legs
4. Minimize daytime bed rest since prolonged bed rest can lead to decon
   ditioning of muscles and reflexes
5. Avoid sudden standing. Patients should rise slowly from supine to sittin
   and wait a few minutes before standing. Dorsiflexion of feet before stand
   ing (to increase venous return) minimizes the risk of postural hypoten
   sion
6. Support stockings may be useful, but they are difficult to get on and un
   comfortable to wear
7. Drug treatment: fludrocortisone acetate (0.1 mg PO initially), sensitize
   blood vessels to the vasoconstrictor effects of catecholamines and pro
   motes fluid retention; potential complications: dependent edema, CHF
   and hypokalemia

  SYNCOPE
Fred F. Ferri, MD

Epidemiology

1. Incidence in elderly noninstitutionalized patients is 6%; recurrence rat
   is nearly 30%
2. Undetermined cause of the syncope in 38% to 47% of patients

Age-related changes predisposing to syncope

1. Altered baroreflex sensitivity
2. Impaired compensatory tachycardic response to stimuli
3. Decreased basal plasma renin and aldosterone concentration result in im
   paired extracellular volume regulation
4. Atherosclerotic loss of blood vessel elasticity

Etiology

1. Syncope can be caused by a variety of diseases. More common causes i
   the elderly are
   a. Vasovagal (vasodepressor)—most common cause of syncope (40% t
      50%)
   b. Orthostatic hypotension

  c. Valvular heart disease
  d. Dysrhythmias
2. The following causes of apparent transient loss of consciousness should be eliminated by careful history and physical exam: seizures, hypoglycemia, alcohol intoxication, CVA, concussion

Diagnostic evaluation

1. History
  a. Review of all medications
  b. Activity at time of syncope
  c. Duration of syncope
  d. Associated and premonitory symptoms
2. Physical exam
  a. Cardiovascular system (e.g., presence of murmurs, orthostatic vital signs)
  b. Neurologic abnormalities (mental status, focal signs)
  c. Carotid sinus pressure can be diagnostic if it reproduces symptoms and other causes are excluded; a pause ≥3 seconds or a systolic blood pressure drop >50 mm Hg without symptoms or a drop <30 mm Hg with symptoms when sinus pressure is applied separately on each side for ≤5 seconds is considered abnormal; this test should be avoided in patients with carotid bruits or cerebrovascular disease; ECG monitoring, IV access, and bedside atropine should be available when carotid sinus pressure is applied
  d. Upright tilt testing and psychiatric exam may be useful in evaluation of recurrent syncope of unknown cause in patients without organic heart disease
3. Initial diagnostic tests: laboratory analysis (CBC, electrolytes, glucose, BUN, creatinine, calcium, magnesium) and 12-lead ECG
4. Additional diagnostic tests (e.g., 24-hour Holter monitor, echocardiogram, drug and alcohol levels, CT scan of head) may be indicated depending on patient's history and physical exam

Prognosis

1. Varies with age of patient and cause of syncope
2. Usually benign in patients ≤70 and having vasovagal/psychogenic syncope or syncope of unknown cause
3. Poor in patients with cardiac syncope (19% chance of dying within 1 year)

6.6.e. **_ATRIAL FIBRILLATION_**
Fred F. Ferri, MD

Definition

Atrial fibrillation (AF) is totally chaotic atrial activity caused by simultaneous discharge of multiple atrial foci.

Demographics

1. Prevalence increases with age and is 5.9% in those older than 65 years
2. Approximately 70% of individuals with AF are between 65 and 85 years

Etiology

1. Coronary artery disease (CAD)
2. Mitral stenosis (MS), mitral regurgitation (MR), aortic stenosis (AS), aortic regurgitation (AR)
3. Thyrotoxicosis
4. Pulmonary embolism, COPD
5. Pericarditis, myocarditis, cardiomyopathy
6. Tachycardia-bradycardia syndrome, Wolff-Parkinson-White syndrome (WPW)
7. MI
8. Alcohol abuse
9. Miscellaneous: left atrial myxoma, atrial septal defect, carbon monoxide poisoning, pheochromocytoma, idiopathic

Diagnostic evaluation

1. ECG: irregular, nonperiodic waveforms and absence of P waves
2. Echocardiogram: useful to evaluate left atrial size and detect valvular disorders
3. Free T_4 level: should be obtained to rule out thyrotoxicosis
4. Serum electrolytes

Therapy of new onset AF

1. Varies with stability of patient
2. Digoxin: initial drug of choice (except in patients with WPW) to control ventricular rate. Conversion to normal sinus rhythm with initial digitalization occurs in 15% to 20% of patients. Quinidine may be added to help convert patient to normal sinus rhythm
3. Cardioversion indicated if ventricular rate >140 beats/min and patient is symptomatic (particularly in acute MI, chest pain, dyspnea, CHF) or when there is no conversion to normal sinus rhythm after 3 days of digoxin and quinidine

Anticoagulation

Recent reports on stroke and nonrheumatic AF recommend

1. Warfarin therapy in all patients older than 75 and patients younger than 75 with any risk factors for stroke (history of prior CVA or TIA, diabetes mellitus, hypertension, CHF, MI, angina)
2. Patients aged 60 to 75 with lone AF may be treated with aspirin, 325 mg/day
3. Anticoagulation not necessary in patients younger than 60 with lone AF
4. Alternatively, warfarin therapy in all patients with AF regardless of etiology or age in absence of contraindication

Suggested reading

Atrial Fibrillation Investigators: Risk factors for stroke and efficacy of antithrombotic therapy in atrial fibrillation: analysis of pooled data from five randomized controlled trials, *Arch Intern Med* 154:1449-1457, 1994.

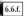
CORONARY ARTERY DISEASE
Jack L. Schwartzwald, MD

Definitions

1. Chronic stable angina: predictable pattern of angina occurring with a characteristic frequency, brought on by a typical level of exertion and relieved by a typical amount of rest or a fixed number of sublingual nitroglycerin tablets or sprays
2. Unstable angina: a changed or unpredictable pattern of angina that includes
   a. Rest angina
   b. Crescendo angina: an increase in frequency, intensity, or duration of anginal episodes or angina precipitated by a lower level of exertion or requiring more rest or nitroglycerin for relief than usual
3. Atypical chest pain: any chest pain that is neither typical angina (retrosternal pressure caused by exercise and relived within 30 minutes by rest or nitroglycerine) nor non–cardiac chest pain (chest pain whose characteristics strongly suggest a non–cardiac cause such as heartburn or pleuritic chest pain)
4. New onset angina: may be difficult to classify as stable or unstable until a pattern is established; clinical judgment assisted by ECG findings will determine urgency of situation
5. Myocardial infarction: implies nonreversible heart muscle injury with diagnosis usually made by electrocardiogram and cardiac isoenzyme (CPK-MB) determination

Epidemiology

Coronary artery disease (CAD) claims the lives of approximately 700,000 people annually in the United States. Increasing age has consistently been shown to be a leading risk for ischemic morbidity and mortality. In 1988 the proportion of the U.S. population over 65 was estimated to be 13%. Nevertheless, this group accounted for 80% of all deaths and 60% of all health care expenditures were attributable to CAD. Risk factors for coronary disease include

1. Reversible factors
   a. Hypertension
   b. Postmenopausal estrogen decline
   c. Tobacco use
   d. Diabetes mellitus
   e. Hypercholesterolemia
2. Irreversible factors
   a. Family history
   b. Increasing age
   c. Male sex

Before menopause, women lag behind men in the development of CAD by approximately 15 years. In postmenopausal women who do not receive estrogen replacement, the disease accelerates and the prevalence between the sexes equalizes by age 75 to 80.

Overview

Coronary disease can produce ischemia (curtailment of myocardial blood flow, and thus oxygen supply, to a level insufficient to meet metabolic demands). The cardinal symptom of ischemia is angina. **Classic anginal chest pain has three features**

1. Substernal or precordial location
2. Exertional precipitant
3. Relief with rest or sublingual nitroglycerin

If only two criteria are met, the pain is said to be atypical. If one or no factors are present, noncardiac etiologies predominate. Ischemic symptoms in the elderly are the same as those in younger patients, but the proportion of atypical presentations increases with age.

1. Silent ischemia is more prevalent in the elderly
   a. Of patients diagnosed with MI after age 65, 25% do not complain of chest pain
   b. In one study 75% of patients with acute MI after age 85 did not complain of chest pain
   c. Chest pain, when present in the elderly, may be of reduced duration and intensity when compared to younger patients with similar ischemic burdens
   d. Even in patients with chest pain, the ratio of silent to symptomatic episodes may be as high as 7:1 as detected by Holter monitoring
   e. Dyspnea may be the lone presenting symptom of angina in the elderly almost as frequently as chest pain (caused by transient LV diastolic dysfunction)

Initial evaluation

1. History
   a. CAD risk factors
   b. Associated symptoms (dyspnea, nausea/vomiting, palpitations, diaphoresis)
   c. Quality, duration, and radiation of pain
      (1) Substernal dull aching, burning, pressure, or squeezing sensation lasting several minutes with or without radiation to jaw or left arm suggests angina
      (2) Sharp, stabbing pains lasting seconds are unlikely to represent angina
      (3) Pleuritic pain is uncommon with angina (consider pneumothorax, pulmonary embolism, pericarditis, bronchitis, or pneumonia in the proper clinical setting)
      (4) Pain reproduced by palpation of the affected area or by changes in body or arm position suggests a musculoskeletal etiology
      (5) Radiation of the pain to the back may suggest pancreatitis or, in the patient with hypertension, aortic dissection
      (6) Pain on lying flat or on bending forward may represent gastroesophageal reflux disease
      (7) Pain associated with peptic ulcer disease may mimic anginal pain but is not exertional and may improve with meals or antacids
   d. Other atherosclerotic disease (carotid, aorta, lower extremities)

e. Previous evaluation (ECG, stress tests, coronary angiogram)

f. Effect on function: New York Heart Association classification (Table 6-18)

2. Physical exam

a. Blood pressure

b. Xanthomas and xanthelasma are associated with familial hypercholesterolemia

c. Arcus cornealis: nonspecific in African-Americans and patients over 50 years but is associated with an increased risk of coronary events in Caucasian patients under 50 years

d. Bruits, diminished peripheral pulses

e. Heart exam may reveal

(1) Normal heart

(2) Diffuse or laterally displaced point of maximal impulse suggesting LV dilation

(3) Double apical impulse suggesting LV aneurysm

(4) S_4: may be a normal variant in elderly patients but suggests atrial contraction against a noncompliant (i.e., ischemic) left ventricle, particularly if associated with a palpable preapical impulse

(5) S_3: hallmark of decompensated LV systolic dysfunction

(6) Mitral regurgitant murmur suggesting ischemic papillary muscle dysfunction or rupture

f. Signs of congestive heart failure (JVD, pulmonary rales, hepatojugular reflux, sacral or pretibial pitting edema)

3. Diagnostic testing in patients with suspected coronary disease

a. Treadmill ECG testing, stress thallium coronary perfusion scan, pharmacologic stress testing (Persantine thallium coronary perfusion scan, dobutamine echocardiography), and cardiac catheterization maintain their sensitivity and specificity in the elderly. Complication rate from cardiac catheterization increases with age of the patient

Table 6-18 New York Heart Association functional classification of angina pectoris

Functional Class	Occurrence of Symptoms	Functional Impairment
I	With unusual activity	Minimal or none
II	With prolonged or slightly more than unusual activity	Mild (can do light and general industrial work)
III	With usual activity of daily living	Moderate (may be able to have desk job)
IV	At rest	Severe (incapacitated)

From Shub C: Angina pectoris and coronary heart disease. In Brandenburg RO et al, editors: *Cardiology: fundamentals and practice*, vol 2, Chicago, 1987, Year Book Medical Publishers.

MANAGEMENT

STABLE ANGINA

1. Since ischemia results when myocardial oxygen demand exceeds supply, ischemic coronary syndromes are treated by bringing these factors back into balance
2. Determinants of myocardial oxygen demand
   a. Heart rate
   b. Ventricular contractility
   c. Systolic ventricular wall tension (function of preload and afterload)
3. Strategies for impacting these determinants
   a. Discontinue tobacco
   b. Diet and exercise (may combine to lower blood pressure in hypertensive patients, improve glycemic control in diabetics, and impact favorably on cholesterol profile)
   c. Medications that slow heart rate decrease cardiac work to decrease oxygen demand and increase time for diastole when coronary perfusion is greatest to increase oxygen supply
   d. Medications that reduce preload and afterload decrease myocardial work and oxygen demand
   e. In general medications should be dosed more judiciously in the elderly because of increased side effects; smaller doses of agents used in combination may avoid major hemodynamic (e.g., hypotension) and other effects seen with higher doses of single agents
4. Medications
   a. Nitrates
      (1) Key actions
         (a) Reduction of LV wall tension through reductions in preload and afterload (preload reduction makes nitrates excellent agents for treatment of ischemic CHF)
         (b) Improved perfusion of ischemic myocardium through preferential dilation of arterioles distal to coronary stenoses
      (2) Side effects: headache, palpitations, dizziness, syncope, reflex tachycardia, hypotension
      (3) A 12-hour nitrate-free period is needed to avoid rapid tachyphylaxis to nitrate actions. Tablets and nitropaste should be given at 10 AM, 2 PM, and 6 PM rather than every 8 hours and transdermal patches should be removed for 12 consecutive hours (usually overnight) to accomplish this
   b. Beta-blockers
      (1) Key actions
         (a) Favorable impact on myocardial oxygen demand
         (b) Proven survival benefit when administered to postinfarction patients who can tolerate them. Agents with intrinsic sympathomimetic (agonist-antagonist) activity (pindolol, acebutolol) may lack this mortality benefit, which is unfortunate because unlike other beta-blockers, they do not elevate serum cholesterol levels
      (2) Side effects: heart block, bradycardia, CHF, fatigue, depression, insomnia, impotence, constipation, exacerbation of bronchospasm

(3) Comorbidity is an important issue in selecting candidates for beta-blockade

    (a) Hypertension, hyperthyroidism, atrial and ventricular ectopy, hypertrophic cardiomyopathy, congestive heart failure caused by LV diastolic dysfunction, migraine or tension headache, and glaucoma may be improved when beta-blockers are used to treat coronary disease

    (b) Bronchospasm, congestive heart failure caused by LV systolic dysfunction, conduction system disease, peripheral vascular disease, Raynaud's phenomenon, depression, and hypercholesterolemia may be exacerbated by use of beta-blockers; in addition, signs and symptoms of hypoglycemia may be masked in diabetics

c. Calcium channel blockers

  (1) Agents of choice for syndrome X (microvascular angina) and Prinzmetal's variant angina (coronary vasospasm); diltiazem may achieve the best mortality benefit in non–Q-wave infarction if LV ejection fraction >40%

  (2) Side effects

    (a) Nifedipine: headache, palpitations, dizziness, peripheral edema, reflex tachycardia (similarity of side effects of nitrates and nifedipine may make them poor choices for combined use)

    (b) Diltiazem: gastrointestinal upset, edema, rash (diltiazem's side effects are typically well tolerated)

    (c) Verapamil: headache, constipation, exacerbation of conduction system disease or CHF (similarity of effects between verapamil and beta-blockers on conduction system disease and CHF may make them a poor choice for combination therapy)

  (3) Calcium blockers are preferred to beta-blockers in the setting of comorbid conditions such as peripheral vascular disease, bronchospasm, diabetes, Raynaud's phenomenon, and hypercholesterolemia

  (4) Calcium blockers may not reduce the heart rate times blood pressure product with exercise in the elderly as well as beta-blockers do. Additionally, constipation and urinary retention from the effect of these agents on smooth muscle become increasingly problematic in the elderly

  (5) Long-acting are safer than short-acting calcium blockers

d. Aspirin 160 to 325 mg qd

e. Cardiac catheterization followed by coronary angioplasty or bypass surgery in selected patients

UNSTABLE ANGINA

1. Admit to hospital to rule out infarction using protocol to include

  a. Bed rest, stool softeners, central telemetry

  b. Aspirin 325 mg po qd

  c. IV heparin plus IV or topical nitroglycerin if suspicion for true unstable angina is high

    d. Obtain CPK and LDH with isoenzymes every 8 hours for three times
    e. Obtain ECG with all episodes of pain and for two consecutive mornings after admission
2. If myocardial infarction is ruled out
    a. Optimize antiischemic therapy and consider cardiac catheterization to rule "active" lesions in moderate- to high-suspicion cases
    b. Consider tapering medications and obtaining a treadmill test in low-suspicion cases to help clarify the diagnosis (true unstable angina is a contraindication to treadmill testing)
3. Add life-style modifications to medical or invasive therapy

MYOCARDIAL INFARCTION

The in-hospital mortality of initial acute MI is approximately sixfold higher in patients over 75 compared to patients under 55. For those who survive hospitalization, 2-year follow-up mortality is fourfold higher in the over-75 group.

1. Acute phase (first week)
    a. Admit to hospital. Confirm diagnosis with serial CPK and LDH determinations with fractionation and follow-up ECGs
    b. Administer thrombolytic therapy for those presenting within 6 hours and perhaps up to 24 hours of the acute event if ECG evidence for infarction is compelling. Streptokinase is less expensive than tPA
      (1) Trials of thrombolytic therapy in acute MI suggest that elderly patients derive equal or greater benefit compared to younger patients. These data are tempered, however, by higher rates of hemorrhage (including fatal intracerebral hemorrhage) in elderly patients
      (2) For patients who do present within 6 hours of onset of symptoms, age should not be used as the criterion for withholding thrombolytic therapy. Certain caveats apply in the elderly population
        (a) Some elderly patients may not be able to perform treadmill tests and should thus be considered for pharmacologic stress testing
        (b) For those elderly patients who can perform treadmill tests, radionuclide imaging is more frequently required as an adjunct than in young patients because of the increased prevalence of baseline ECG abnormalities in the elderly
        (c) Cardiac catheterization carries an increased risk of fatal and nonfatal complications in patients over 65 and should be reserved for high-suspicion cases
    c. Patients with contraindications to thrombolysis (severe hypertension, history of stroke) may be considered for immediate coronary angioplasty
    d. Medical therapy
      (1) Aspirin and beta-blockers have both been shown to reduce mortality in post-MI patient
      (2) Diltiazem may do the same when administered to selected patients with non–Q-wave infarction (see above)
      (3) Nifedipine used alone as an antiischemic in the postinfarction setting may actually *increase* mortality
      (4) Patients with large anterior wall infarctions require anticoagula-

tion with heparin followed by warfarin for 3 to 6 months to avoid LV thrombus formation

   (5) ACE inhibitors may promote healthful remodeling of infarcted left ventricle and may thus reduce mortality by improving LV function

   (6) Antiarrhythmics may be required transiently (24 to 48 hours) for ectopy in the early postinfarction period, but a worse overall prognosis is associated with long-term empiric use of antiarrhythmic therapy after the acute event

e. Invasive therapy

   (1) Patients who experience postinfarct angina or who fail risk stratification (see below) require cardiac catheterization to evaluate the coronary anatomy for possible revascularization by coronary artery bypass grafting (CABG), percutaneous coronary angioplasty (PTCA), or coronary atherectomy

   (2) CABG is a frequent operation in the elderly, but perioperative mortality is up to sixfold higher in patients over 80 compared to patients under 65. Relief of symptoms and 5-year survival approach 80%. PTCA yields similar rates of satisfactory outcome (90%) and restenosis (30%) in elderly and younger populations. The risk of complications from the procedure, however, is increased in the elderly

f. Complications of acute myocardial infarction

   (1) Sinus, atrial, or ventricular arrhythmia

   (2) Conduction system disturbance

   (3) Rupture of ventricular free wall, intraventricular septum, or papillary muscle

   (4) Papillary muscle dysfunction

   (5) Pericarditis

   (6) LV aneurysm

   (7) CHF

   (8) Thromboembolic events

2. Predischarge care: after 5 to 10 days

a. The patient with uncomplicated myocardial infarction who remains pain free should

   (1) Begin cardiac rehabilitation

   (2) Undergo risk stratification

     (a) Assessment of LV function by echocardiogram or radionuclide ventriculography (Muga scan). An EF under 40% connotes an increased risk for ventricular arrhythmia and death. Such patients should be assessed for revascularization by cardiac catheterization

     (b) Low-level or symptom-limited treadmill stress test (ECG or thallium). Low exercise tolerance with inability to achieve predicted heart rate and blood pressure goals, occurrence of ST-segment or T-wave changes, angina, and dyspnea are poor prognostic features as are reperfusing defects on thallium imaging. Patients with these findings should be assessed for revascularization using cardiac catheterization

b. Patients with none of the above findings have a predicted 1-year mortality <2% and can proceed with cardiac rehabilitation. A follow-up full-level treadmill test should be obtained 4 to 6 weeks after infarction (when cardiac remodeling is largely complete) to assess for residual myocardium at risk for injury

3. Postdischarge primary care follow-up
   a. Instructions to patient before first outpatient visit
      (1) Discontinue alcohol and tobacco
      (2) Avoid driving (risk of ischemia or medication-related syncope)
      (3) Avoid heavy exertion and sexual activity but perform light exercise such as walking for 15 to 20 minutes three times per week (increase by 15 to 20 minutes every 1 to 2 weeks)
      (4) Adopt low-fat American Heart Association diet
      (5) Alert physician immediately regarding symptoms of chest pain, dyspnea, syncope, or disturbing medication side effects
   b. First outpatient visit (1 to 2 weeks after infarction)
      (1) Continue to modify risk factors through life-style changes
      (2) Measure and manage cholesterol level (see Section 6.2.b)
      (3) Arrange enrollment in a cardiac rehabilitation program
      (4) Reevaluate regarding anginal symptoms and medication side effects
   c. Second outpatient visit (following full-level treadmill test about 4 to 6 weeks after infarction)
      (1) Patients with inducible ischemia on this test should be evaluated by cardiac catheterization for possible revascularization
      (2) Patients without inducible ischemia have a low probability for coronary events in subsequent 6 months
         (a) Continue risk factor modification
         (b) Advance exercise in a cardiac rehabilitation program
         (c) Promote return to work or leisure activities (delays beyond 6 weeks in the patient with acceptable risk-stratification results may adversely impact employability, insurability, and patient self-image)
         (d) Resume driving and sexual activity
         (e) Reevaluate regarding anginal symptoms and medication side effects
   d. Subsequent visits during first year after infarction
      (1) Have patient return every 3 to 4 months
      (2) Reinforce life-style changes and long-term cardiac rehabilitation
      (3) Consider counseling or antidepressant medications for patients with prolonged depression after infarction (selective serotonin reuptake antagonists are preferred to MAO inhibitors or tricyclics because of safer cardiac side effect profiles)

Suggested readings

All or nothing in MI risk reduction: practical briefings, *Patient Care* 28:20, 1994.
Debrusk RF et al: Post discharge decisions in acute MI, *Patient Care* 27:25-51, 1993.
Debrusk RF et al: Predischarge decisions in acute MI, *Patient Care* 27:69-98, 1993.
Eastaugh JA: The early repolarization syndrome, *J Emerg Med* 7:257-262, 1989.
Edmunds LH et al: Open-heart surgery in octogenarians, *N Engl J Med* 319:131, 1988.
Goldberg RJ et al: The impact of age on the incidence and prognosis of initial acute myocardial infarction: the Worcester Heart Study, *Am Heart J* 117:543-549, 1989.
Grace AA, Shapiro LM: Syndrome X: diagnosis and management, *Practical Cardiol* 15:61-68, 1989.

Gurwitz JH et al: Diagnostic testing in acute MI: does patient age influence utilization patterns? *Am J Epidemiol* 134:948-957, 1991.

Lam JYT, Waters D: Medical management of chronic ischemic heart disease, *Contemp IM* 6:54-69, 1994.

Lazar EJ et al: Angina pectoris and silent ischemia in the elderly: a management update, *Geriatrics* 47:24-36, 1992.

Muller RT et al: Painless myocardial infarction in the elderly, *Am Heart J* 119:202-204, 1990.

Nixon JV: Non-Q-wave myocardial infarction, *Postgrad Med* 95:211-223, 1994.

Shub C: Stable angina pectoris. I. Clinical patterns, *Mayo Clin Proc* 64:1233-1242, 1990.

Shub C: Stable angina pectoris. III. Medical treatment, *Mayo Clin Proc* 65:256-273, 1990.

Singh I: Ischemic heart disease in the elderly, *Int Med World Rep* 10:21, 1995 (excellent review of geriatric considerations in coronary disease).

Subramaniam PN: Complications of acute myocardial infarction, *Postgrad Med* 95:143-148, 1994.

  ### VALVULAR HEART DISEASE
Jennifer Jeremiah, MD

Cardiac murmurs result from vibrations generated by turbulent blood flow. A normal amount of blood passing through an obstruction or an increased amount of blood passing through normal structures may lead to auscultatory changes. The challenge to the primary care physician is to discern those murmurs resulting from physiologic states vs. those caused by pathologic states so that any appropriate diagnostic tests, referrals, and interventions can be pursued.

To make this distinction one must concentrate on the following:

- Identify heart sounds. Are they of normal intensity? Are they single or split? Are there extra sounds or gallops?
- Assess murmur for timing (systole or diastole); shape or configuration; pitch (frequency); location or maximal loudness; radiation; intensity of systolic I-VI and diastolic I-IV; changes with respiration; changes with maneuvers

SYSTOLIC MURMURS

1. **Innocent murmurs**
   a. Ninety-nine percent are systolic, grade I or II, and lack abnormal heart sounds, ejection sounds, radiation. Chest x-ray and ECG within normal limits
   b. Most common murmur in the elderly is murmur of **aortic sclerosis,** caused by roughening and thickening of the valve during aging with the potential to become pathologic. No gradient or obstruction in its benign form

2. **Pathologic murmurs**
   a. **Aortic stenosis (AS)**
      (1) Auscultation: murmur starts after S_1 and ends before S_2. In moderate to severe disease S_2 may be diminished or absent. There may be paradoxic S_2 splitting, an S_4, and an ejection click. It is a rough, medium-pitched, diamond-shaped murmur peaking in midsystole and is heard best in the aortic area and often along the left sternal border with radiation to right midclavicle and carotids

    (2) Etiology: in older persons the newly diagnosed stenotic valve most commonly results from degenerative calcification. Rheumatic fever is a common cause but has generally caused pathologic changes earlier in life

    (3) Symptoms: occur when the valve orifice narrows greater than 30%. Hallmark symptoms of significant AS: angina, exertional dyspnea, and syncope

    (4) Evaluation: echocardiogram and cardiac catheterization when severe AS is suspected

    (5) Management: antibiotic prophylaxis for potential exposure to bacteremia, avoidance of strenuous activity when AS is severe, and cautious diuretic, vasodilator, and inotropic therapy for systolic dysfunction; aortic valve replacement for symptomatic individuals

b. **Hypertrophic cardiomyopathy**

    (1) Auscultation: S_2 usually louder than AS with no ejection sound. Murmur is rough, medium pitched, of long duration, heard loudest along lower left sternal border with radiation to apex; increases with standing and decreases with squatting

    (2) Etiology: abnormal blood flow across LV outflow track below aortic valve. It is important to distinguish from AS since therapies for one may have adverse effects on the other. Approximately 50% of cases are transmitted autosomal dominantly with variable expression

    (3) Symptoms: sudden death during or after physical exertion, dyspnea, angina, fatigue, syncope

    (4) Evaluation: same as for AS

    (5) Management: medical therapy with beta-blockers, calcium channel blockers, and antiarrhythmics. Nitrates, diuretics, and ACE-inhibitors may be helpful but should not be used alone because they can worsen outflow tract obstruction. Antibiotic prophylaxis should be considered for patients with systolic anterior motion of the anterior mitral leaflet, mitral regurgitation, or other valvular abnormalities. Surgical treatment may be considered for those with severe symptoms not controlled by medical therapy

c. **Pulmonic stenosis**

    (1) Auscultation: S_2 may be widely split or single late in the course. Murmur similar to AS in intensity, configuration, and pitch and heard best in the pulmonic area

    (2) Etiology: may be primary (congenital heart disease or rheumatic fever) or secondary to septal defects with left to right shunting (atrial or ventricular septal defect)

    (3) Symptoms: as obstruction progresses there may be fatigue, dyspnea, right ventricular (RV) failure, and syncope

    (4) Evaluation: echocardiography with Doppler ultrasonography can estimate outflow tract pressure gradient

    (5) Management: antibiotic prophylaxis and treatment of right-sided heart failure

d. **Mitral regurgitation**

    (1) Auscultation: murmur is pansystolic, decreases with inspiration, and radiates in a bandlike fashion from left lower sternal border

to apex and midaxillary line; S_3 may be heard in more advanced disease

(2) Etiology: primary mitral regurgitation may result from rheumatic heart disease, MVP, or endocarditis; secondary mitral insufficiency results from papillary muscle dysfunction or cardiomyopathy

(3) Symptoms: CHF

(4) Management: medical treatment for mild chronic mitral regurgitation, severely depressed LV function, and poor surgical candidates includes vasodilator therapy with ACE inhibitors or peripheral vasodilators. Digoxin and diuretics may be added for LV dysfunction. Atrial fibrillation should be treated aggressively including anticoagulation. Surgical repair should be considered to halt progression of LV dysfunction and improve symptoms. Antibiotic prophylaxis recommended

e. **Tricuspid regurgitation**

(1) Auscultation: murmur is high pitched, systolic, and heard at left sternal border in fourth and fifth intercostal spaces and does not radiate to axilla; augmented during inspiration; may be JVD and a pulsating liver

(2) Etiology: may result from rheumatic heart disease, RV failure, or pulmonary emboli

(3) Symptoms: may be well tolerated without therapy for years before development of severe RV failure

(4) Management: treatment of right-sided heart failure and maintenance of high filling pressures. Surgical intervention may be considered for severe disease

DIASTOLIC MURMURS

1. **Mitral stenosis**
   a. Auscultation: murmur is low pitched, rumbling, heard best in apex. Sometimes only heard in a limited location and only with the bell. S_2 may be intensified, and an opening snap may be heard shortly after S_2
   b. Etiology: most cases result from rheumatic fever, but some are congenital; two thirds of patients are women
   c. Symptoms: shortness of breath, pulmonary edema, atrial arrhythmias, and hemoptysis
   d. Evaluation: ECG may reveal evidence of atrial enlargement. The echocardiogram is most sensitive and specific means of diagnosis
   e. Management: prophylaxis against rheumatic fever and infective endocarditis, low-sodium diet, diuretics for symptoms of heart failure, good rate control of atrial fibrillation if present, and consideration of anticoagulation to decrease risk of arterial embolization; surgical treatment for progressive symptoms

2. **Aortic insufficiency**
   a. Auscultation: murmur is high pitched, blowing, heard best with diaphragm of stethoscope in second or third left intercostal space, heard best with patient leaning forward; murmur immediately follows S_2 with rapid diminution
   b. Etiology: rheumatic heart disease, syphilis of aorta, ruptured valve leaflet from endocarditis, Marfan's syndrome, and dissecting aortic aneurysm

c. Symptoms: in chronic aortic insufficiency patients may first complain of palpitations worse on reclining and later develop exertional dyspnea, orthopnea, and chest pain

d. Evaluation: echocardiogram useful for detection, with catheterization and angiography used to guide need for surgical intervention

e. Management: careful serial assessment of LV function is critical to time surgical intervention before irreversible LV damage develops. If surgery cannot be performed, digoxin, diuretics, and afterload-reducing agents may provide symptomatic relief

•   •   •

Once the appropriate classification of the murmur is made, the challenge to the primary care physician is to provide management that will enhance day-to-day function for the patient. The obvious difficulty is to balance the side effects, toxicities, risks, and costs of various cardiac medications and interventions against benefits.

Suggested readings

Gray RJ, Helfant RH: Timing of surgery for valvular heart disease in the elderly. In Breast AN, Frankl WS, editors: *Valvular heart disease: comprehensive evaluation and treatment,* Philadelphia, 1993, FA Davis Co.

Marzo KP, Herling IM: Valvular disease in the elderly. In Breast AN, Frankl WS, editors: *Valvular heart disease: comprehensive evaluation and treatment,* Philadelphia, 1993, FA Davis Co.

6.6.h. ### *PERIPHERAL VASCULAR DISEASE*
Tom J. Wachtel, MD

1. Peripheral arterial occlusive disease (PAD)
   a. Definition: impairment of blood flow to one or more limbs, usually because of atherosclerosis, occasionally because of thromboembolism, and rarely because of arteritis
   b. Epidemiology
      (1) Rare in the third decade (0.5%)
      (2) Uncommon in those aged 30 to 60 (3%)
      (3) Very common above age 75 (20%)
         (a) Symptomatic PAD tends to peak 10 years after CAD onset
         (b) PAD is more common in men than women, whose prevalence rates mirror those of males 10 years later in life
   c. Symptoms
      (1) Intermittent claudication
         (a) Cramping pain caused by ambulation and relieved by rest
         (b) Calf pain associated with superficial femoral or popliteal stenosis
         (c) Buttock, hip, and thigh pain associated with aortoiliac stenosis
         (d) Rest pain indicates more severe disease (narrower stenosis, more extensive stenosis, or fewer collateral arteries as occurs in more rapidly progressive disease)
         (e) see Sections 6.5.a and 6.5.d for differential diagnosis of limb pain
      (2) Arterial leg ulcer
         (a) Painful

      (b) Begins with trauma

      (c) Sites: toes, around first metatarsophalangeal joint, heel, lateral malleolus, distal pretibial region

    (3) Examination

      (a) Abdominal or limb bruits

      (b) Diminished or absent pulses

      (c) Shiny atrophic skin

      (d) Diminished hair growth

      (e) Brittle nails

      (f) Poor capillary filling when skin is blanched

  d. Diagnostic tests

    (1) Noninvasive methods: segmental blood pressure measurement using Doppler technology. Ankle brachial index (ABI) used to stratify severity of PAD (ABI of 1 is normal, <0.4 is severe)

    (2) Invasive procedure: arteriography is the gold standard test to diagnose PAD

  e. Treatment

    (1) Improve cardiovascular risk profile: smoking cessation; treat hypertension, hyperlipidemia, diabetes, and obesity

    (2) Medication

      (a) Aspirin 88 mg to 650 mg daily

      (b) Pentoxifylline (Trental) 400 mg po tid

    (3) Surgery

      (a) Percutaneous angioplasty

      (b) Vascular reconstruction

      (c) Amputation

    (4) Management of arterial ulcer

      (a) Do not elevate limb

      (b) Surgical debridement

      (c) Wet to wet dressings (apply wet, allow it to dry, but wet it again before removing) or wet to dry if continued debridement is desired

2. Peripheral venous disorder

  a. Varicose veins

    (1) Definition and pathophysiology: dilation of superficial veins, resulting from incompetent valves and reversal of blood flow

    (2) Epidemiology prevalence: one third of women and one fifth of men in the United States

    (3) Symptoms

      (a) Dilated, cosmetically displeasing veins

      (b) Calf aching or heaviness; similar symptoms in location of varicose veins

      (c) Acute symptom exacerbation with signs of inflammation and a palpable cord may signify superficial phlebitis

    (4) Treatment

      (a) Avoid a stationary standing position whenever possible

      (b) Leg elevation

      (c) Support stockings

      (d) Weight loss if obese

      (e) Sclerosing therapy (cosmetic indication for small veins)

      (f) Surgery (stripping)

b. Chronic venous insufficiency and venous ulcer
  (1) Definition: chronic venous insufficiency is a sequela of deep vein thrombosis (DVT) during which deep vein valves are permanently disrupted; other causes probably also lead to deep vein valve dysfunction because many patients with chronic venous insufficiency do not have a history of DVT. Stasis dermatitis results from chronic venous hypertension and capillary distention allowing exudation of fibrinogen and red blood cells; hence fibrosis and local hemosiderosis that characterize stasis dermatitis
  (2) Symptoms
    (a) Leg edema often bilateral but asymmetric
    (b) Erythema
    (c) Hyperpigmentation
    (d) Rarely vesicles or bullae may be present
    (e) Dermal fibrosis and loss of skin elasticity (lower leg may look strangulated)
    (f) Ulcer: painless, on medial aspect of leg
  (3) NOTE: Stasis is sometimes mistaken for cellulitis, but cellulitis is typically unilateral and stasis dermatitis is bilateral. However, secondary infection of stasis dermatitis is possible (impetiginization) and should be managed as cellulitis
  (4) Treatment
    (a) Stasis dermatitis
      • Leg elevation as often as practical
      • Weight loss if obese
      • Support stockings
      • Moist compresses (Burow's solution) if skin weeps
      • Corticosteroid cream such as hydrocortisone 1% cream
    (b) Venous ulcer
      • Treat stasis as above
      • Wet to dry dressing if mild debridement is needed
      • Wet to wet dressing if ulcer is free of any necrotic materials
      • Unna boot dressing once epithelialization of ulcer has begun (to be changed weekly); contraindicated if any evidence of infection or arterial insufficiency
      • Occlusive dressing such as foams (Synthraderm), films (Opsite), hydrocolloids (Duoderm), or hydrogels (Vigilon); dressing should be changed when fluid begins to leak

6.7 DERMATOLOGIC DISORDERS

6.7.a. PRURITUS
Fred F. Ferri, MD

Pruritus is the most common dermatologic complaint in the elderly.

Etiology
1. Pruritus in the elderly often due to dry skin (Table 6-19)
2. Other common causes: drug reactions, primary skin disorders, and psychogenic states

Table 6-19   Pruritus in the elderly

Primary skin disorders
    Acute dermatitis (any cause)
    Infestations (scabies, lice)
    Lichen planus
    Lichen simplex chronicus (localized neurodermatitis)
    Infection (varicella, candidiasis)
    Papulosquamous disease (psoriasis)
    Xerosis
    Miliaria (prickly heat)
    Bullous pemphigoid
Drug reactions
    Opiates and derivatives
    Antidepressants
    Aspirin
Psychogenic states
Circulatory
    Stasis dermatitis
Metabolic
    Hepatobiliary disease
    Uremia
    Diabetes mellitus
    Thyroid disease
Hematopoietic
    Iron deficiency anemia
    Polycythemia vera
    Lymphomas, Hodgkin's disease
    Leukemia
Visceral malignancies
    Abdominal cancer
    Central nervous system tumors
Urticaria

From Bosker G et al: *Geriatric emergency medicine,* St Louis, 1990, Mosby, p 511.

Diagnostic approach

1. Pruritus is generally associated with visible skin abnormalities (from the underlying cause or from scratching). Occasionally pruritus may precede skin manifestations. When examining a patient complaining of pruritus, the skin exam should be complete and not limited to selected areas
2. Medical history and laboratory evaluation should focus on potential drug reactions and metabolic disorders
3. Underlying depression and anxiety may cause or exacerbate pruritus
4. Scabies should be suspected when pruritus involves several members of an extended care facility

Treatment

1. Eliminate underlying etiology. Pruritus caused by dry skin may be controlled with use of emollients to lubricate and hydrate the skin, modification of bathing procedures to limit excessive bathing time, and use of mild soaps
2. Topical antipruritic lotions (e.g., pramoxine and hydrocortisone [Pramosone]) may be useful for localized pruritus
3. Topical corticosteroids should be used only in the presence of prominent dermatitis
4. Oral antihistamines (e.g., hydroxyzine) should be reserved for severe cases. Dosage should be decreased in half in the elderly to minimize excessive sedation

 ECZEMA
Fred F. Ferri, MD

Definition

The term *eczema* means bubbling or boiling over and refers to a group of several diseases, including contact dermatitis, stasis dermatitis, atopic dermatitis, nummular dermatitis, and lichen simplex chronicus. The term *dermatitis* is often used to refer to an eczematous eruption.

Clinical manifestations and differential diagnosis

1. The characteristic symptom in patients with eczema is pruritus
2. The differential diagnosis of dermatitis is described in Table 6-20
3. Eczema can also be divided into three evolutionary stages: acute, subacute, and chronic (see Figure 6-16 following p. 272); the clinical appearance of each stage may be modified by scratching and topical treatment

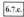 *PSORIASIS*
Fred F. Ferri, MD

Definition

Psoriasis is a chronic skin disorder of unknown origin characterized by excess proliferation of keratinocytes that results in the formation of thickened scaly plaques, itching, and inflammatory changes of the epidermis and dermis. The various forms of psoriasis include guttate, pustular, and arthritic variants.

Demographics

1. Affects 1% to 3% of the world's population
2. Annual cost of outpatient treatment exceeds 2 billion dollars in the United States
3. Peak age of onset is bimodal (adolescence and at 60 years of age)

Clinical manifestations and differential diagnosis

1. Chronic plaque psoriasis generally manifests with symmetric, sharply demarcated, erythematous, silver-scaled patches affecting primarily the intergluteal fold, elbows, scalp, fingernails and toenails, and knees (see Figure 6-17 following p. 272)

Table 6-20 Differential diagnosis of dermatitis

Diagnosis	History	Physical Examination	Laboratory Tests	Management
Atopic dermatitis	Onset by age 5 Family history of atopy Pruritus Exacerbating factors Coexistent hay fever, asthma	Flexural distribution Lichenification Papules, erythema Pustules if secondary *Staphylococcus*	Routine: none Consider culture/pustule; IgE	Topical corticosteroids Control environment Antihistamines Emollients
Contact dermatitis Irritant type	Predisposing history of atopy Frequent water exposure Solvents Job description	Hands commonly Erythema, scales, fissuring	None	Topical steroid ointments Protect from wet exposures Gloves Emollients Wet to dry dressings
Allergic type	Rapid onset Pruritus Exposure to plants or cosmetics	Erythema, vesicles, oozing Location corresponds to exposure	None	Topical or systemic corticosteroids Identify and avoid allergen

Continued

Table 6-20 Differential diagnosis of dermatitis—cont'd

Diagnosis	History	Physical Examination	Laboratory Tests	Management
Stasis dermatitis	Gradual onset Distal legs Previous history Varicosities, leg trauma, etc.	Erythema Pigmentation Edema Fibrosis	None	Acute: steroid ointments Long term: compression, leg elevation, emollient ointments
Xerotic dermatitis	Winter Low humidity Frequent baths Soap use Pretibial common	Patchy, erythema, scales Extensor areas Spares folds	None	Decrease soap and water exposure Liberal use of thick emollients, especially after bath
Dyshidrosis	Pruritic papules and vesicles on hands Recurrent	Papules and small vesicles on hands	None; exclude fungus with KOH and allergen	Steroids short-term prn Systemic or topical steroids Antibiotics
Nummular dermatitis	Gradual onset Pruritic Frequent history Exposure to drying	Round patches Erythema Scaling occasional Oozing occasional	None KOH to exclude fungus	Steroid ointments Tar cream, gel Ultraviolet light

From Noble J, editor: *Primary care medicine*, ed 2, St Louis, 1996, Mosby.

2. Psoriasis can also develop at the site of any physical trauma (sunburn, scratching)
3. Pruritus is variable
4. Beta-blockers, lithium, antimalarials, and systemic steroids may precipitate or exacerbate psoriasis
5. Several skin diseases can easily be confused with psoriasis. Table 6-21 describes the differential diagnosis of psoriasis

Therapy

1. Goal: to decrease epidermal proliferation and dermal inflammation
2. Options vary with degree of psoriasis (Tables 6-22 to 6-24): mild forms treated with topical agents, UV light used in moderate cases, and systemic treatment reserved for severe cases

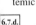

HERPES ZOSTER (SHINGLES)
Fred F. Ferri, MD

Definition

Herpes zoster is a localized infection of peripheral nerves caused by reactivation of varicella-zoster virus that had been dormant in the dorsal root ganglia.

Epidemiology

1. Increased incidence with age (5 cases/1000 between ages 50 and 80, 10 cases/1000 over age 80), possibly secondary to age-related impairment of cell-mediated immunity
2. Incidence also increased in immunocompromised hosts
3. Persons with acute zoster are contagious to persons not immune to chickenpox (varicella)
4. Recurrence of zoster possible but rare

Clinical presentation

1. First symptom is usually dysesthesia or paresthesia of the involved dermatome
2. Sensory changes are usually followed by eruption of grouped vesicles involving one or several dermatomes; in unusual cases, prodromal symptoms are not followed by a rash (zoster sine herpete)
3. Constitutional symptoms (fever, malaise) usually accompany vesicular eruption
4. Vesicles become pustular after 4 or 5 days. They subsequently dry up and crust in 7 to 10 days. Crusts fall off within 3 weeks

Complications

1. Postherpetic neuralgia occurs in over 30% of patients older than 60
2. Extensive dissemination occurs in 2% to 10%; these patients are generally immunocompromised because of immunosuppressive therapy, underlying malignancy, or AIDS
3. Eye involvement (keratoconjunctivitis, iritis) occurs in 40% to 50% of patients with ophthalmic zoster (see Figure 6-18 following p. 272)

Text continued on p. 269.

Table 6-21 Differential diagnosis of psoriasis

Disease	Clinical Features	Cause	Diagnosis
Tinea and onycholysis	Scaling annular to round patches and onycholysis and crumbling nails	Dermatophyte infections	KOH
Seborrheic dermatitis	Diffuse lesions with greasy scales on skin behind ears, nasolabial folds, and presternally	Possibly overgrowth pityrosporum	Skin biopsy may help
Secondary syphilis	Guttate or small scaling plaques over trunk, like pityriasis rosea, but involves palms and soles	Spirochete	Positive test for syphilis RPR
Cutaneous T-cell lymphoma	Flat to thick plaques with variable scaling, which may be identical to psoriasis anywhere on body; may be erythrodermic—Sézary syndrome	T-cell lymphoma	Skin biopsy; Sézary cells in circulation; T-cell gene rearrangement studies

Reiter's syndrome	Identical skin changes as psoriasis with pustular lesions on palms and soles (keratoderma blennorrhagicum); balanitis circinata; arthritis nail involvement; mucous membrane changes not seen in psoriasis	Unknown but triggered by certain infectious agents	Clinical features, arthritis, conjunctivitis, urethritis
Pityriasis rubra pilaris	Diffuse salmon-colored papulosquamous lesion areas, normal skin in midst of involved skin—"island, sparing"; keratoderma palm; keratotic papules on dorsum of fingers	Unknown	Clinical features, skin biopsy
Pityriasis lichenoides et varioliformis acuta	Red, purpuric, vesicular lesions over entire body evolve into scaling macular and papular lesions that scar	Unknown	Clinical features, skin biopsy

From Noble J, editor: *Primary care medicine*, ed 2, St Louis, 1996, Mosby.

Table 6-22   Therapeutic options for persons with psoriasis on less than 20% of the body

Treatment	Advantages	Disadvantages	Comments
Topical steroids	Rapid response; controls inflammation and itching; best for intertriginous areas and face; convenient, not messy	Temporary relief (tolerance occurs); less effective with continued use; atrophy and telangiectasia occur with continued use; brief remissions; very expensive	Best results occur with pulse dosing (e.g., 2 wk of medication and 1 wk of lubrication only); plastic occlusion very effective
Calcipotriol (Dovonex)	Well tolerated; long remissions possible	Burning; skin irritation; expensive	Best for moderate plaque psoriasis
Anthralin	Convenient short contact programs; long remissions; effective for scalp	Purple-brown staining; irritating, careful application (only to plaque) required	Used on chronic (not inflamed) plaques; best results occur when used with UVB light
Tar	New preparations are pleasant	Only moderately effective in a few patients	Most effective when combined with UVB (Goeckerman regimen)
UVB and lubricating agents or tar	Insurance may cover part or all of treatment; effective for 70% of patients; no need for topical steroids	Expensive; office-based therapy	Used only on plaque and guttate psoriasis; travel and time required
Tape or occlusive dressing	Convenient; no mess	Expensive; only for limited disease	May be used to occlude topical steroids
Intralesional steroids	Convenient; rapidly effective; long remissions	Only for limited areas; atrophy and telangiectasia occur at injection site	Ideal for chronic scalp and body plaques when small and few in number

Table 6-23   Therapeutic options for persons with psoriasis on more than 20% of the body

Treatment	Advantages	Disadvantages
UVB and tar administered in physician's office	More effective than UVB alone	More expensive and carcinogenic than UVB alone; requires many office visits
PUVA	Allows patient to be ambulatory; effective	Many treatments needed; many office visits required
Systemic Treatments		
Methotrexate	Gold standard for efficacy; helps arthritis	Hepatotoxicity; liver biopsy periodically required
Hydrea	Effective in the few for whom it works at all	Hematopoietic toxicity; flulike syndrome
Etretinate	Effective for palmar-plantar-pustular, erythrodermic, and pustular types of psoriasis; fast, effective; helps arthritis	Teratogenic; usually ineffective as a single therapy for plaques
Cyclosporine	Fast, effective, helps arthritis	Experimental; hepatotoxic; nephrotoxic; immunosuppressive
Hospitalization or office day treatment for tar, anthralin, and combinations of all therapies above	Most effective for those who are unresponsive to topical agents or for whom systemic agents are inappropriate	Time consuming; expensive

From Habif TP: *Clinical dermatology*, ed 3, St Louis, 1996, Mosby.

Table 6-24 Eczematous inflammation

Stage	Primary and Secondary Lesions	Symptoms	Etiology and Clinical Presentation	Treatment
Acute	Vesicles, blisters, intense red	Intense itch	Contact allergy (poison ivy), severe irritation, id reaction, acute nummular eczema, stasis dermatitis, pompholyx (dyshidrosis), fungal infections	Cold wet compresses, oral or intramuscular steroids, topical steroids, antihistamines, antibiotics
Subacute	Red, scales, fissuring, parched appearance, scalded appearance	Slight to moderate itch, pain, stinging, burning	Contact allergy, irritation, atopic dermatitis, stasis dermatitis, nummular eczema, asteatotic eczema, fingertip eczema, fungal infections	Topical steroids with or without occlusion, lubrication, antihistamines, antibiotics, tar
Chronic	Thickened skin, skin lines accentuated (lichenified skin), excoriations, fissuring	Moderate to intense itch	Atopic dermatitis, habitual scratching, lichen simplex chronicus, chapped fissured feet, nummular eczema, asteatotic eczema, fingertip eczema, hyperkeratotic eczema	Topical steroids (with occlusion for best results), intralesional steroids, antihistamines, antibiotics, lubrication

From Habif TP: *Clinical dermatology*, ed 3, St Louis, 1996, Mosby.

4. Ramsay Hunt syndrome is caused by herpes zoster of the geniculate ganglion. It consists of facial palsy associated with vesicles in the pharynx and external auditory canal. Auditory nerve involvement occurs in 37% of patients, resulting in hearing deficits and vertigo
5. Secondary bacterial infections can occur, particularly in diabetic persons; systemic antibiotics are indicated in suspected infection

Therapy

1. Local care: application of cool compresses for 30 to 60 minutes four times daily. Calamine lotion may be useful for relief of pruritus
2. Analgesics: acetaminophen in high doses is effective for relief of acute pain
3. Antiviral therapy: acyclovir 800 mg PO five times/day for 7 to 10 days will reduce duration of lesions and severity of acute pain. It should be started as early as possible to be effective. Intravenous acyclovir (5 mg/kg q8h) is usually reserved for disseminated zoster or neurologic complications. Valacyclovir (Valtrex, 500-mg caplets) or famciclovir (Famvir, 500-mg tablets) can also be used. Valacyclovir is converted to acyclovir after absorption and is better absorbed. Dosage is 1 g PO tid for 7 days. Famciclovir dosage is 500 mg tid for 7 days
4. Evidence for use of corticosteroids (prednisone 60 mg/day for 10 days, then tapered over 3 weeks) is inconclusive; generally beneficial in patients with Ramsay Hunt syndrome
5. Postherpetic neuralgia may respond to treatment with
   a. Capsaicin (Zostrix) cream (0.025%) applied three to five times/day to the affected skin after the blisters have resolved; works by depleting substance P from cell bodies and nerve terminals
   b. Amitriptyline (10 mg PO at bedtime initially) may decrease pain by blocking reuptake of serotonin and norepinephrine; should be used only in severe cases because of its significant side effects in the elderly
   c. Transcutaneous electrical stimulation (TENS), intracutaneously injected triamcinolone, and neurosurgical intervention may also be effective in postherpetic neuralgia
6. Ophthalmologic consultation mandatory in all cases of ophthalmic herpes zoster

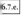 **6.7.e.** ***SCABIES***
Fred F. Ferri, MD

Definition

Scabies is a contagious disease caused by the mite *Sarcoptes scabiei.*

Transmission

1. By direct skin contact with an infested patient
2. Generally associated with poor living conditions and is very common in hospitals and nursing homes
3. Isolation of infested nursing home patients and use of gowns and gloves when entering the infested patient's room are recommended

Signs and Symptoms of Scabies

Nodules on the penis and scrotum
Rash present for 4 to 8 weeks has suddenly become worse
Nocturnal itching
Generalized, severe itching
Pinpoint erosions and crusts on the buttocks
Vesicles in the finger webs
Diffuse eruption sparing the face
Patient becomes better, then worse, after treatment with topical steroids
Rash is present in several members of the same family
Patient develops more extensive rash despite treatment with antibiotics and topical medications

Modified from Habif TP: *Clinical dermatology,* ed 3, St Louis, 1996, Mosby.

4. Linens and recently worn clothing should be washed in hot water, although it is not known whether scabies can be acquired from infested clothing or bed linen
5. Mites can survive out of human skin for approximately 36 hours

Clinical manifestations and diagnosis (see the box above)

1. Primary lesions caused when the female mite burrows within the stratum corneum, laying eggs within the tract she leaves behind; burrow (linear or serpiginous tract) ends with a minute papule or vesicle
2. Primary lesions most commonly found in the web spaces of hands (see Figure 6-19 following p. 272), wrists, buttocks, scrotum, penis, breasts, axillae, and knees (Figure 6-20)
3. Secondary lesions result from scratching or infection
4. Intense pruritus, especially nocturnal, is very common; caused by an acquired sensitivity to the mite or fecal pellets and is usually noted 1 to 4 weeks after the primary infestation

Treatment

1. Following a warm bath or shower, lindane (Kwell, Scabene) lotion should be applied to all skin surfaces below the neck (can be applied to the face if the area is infested); should be washed off 8 to 12 hours after application. Repeat application 1 week later is usually sufficient to eradicate infestation
2. Pruritus generally abates 24 to 48 hours after treatment but can last up to 2 weeks; oral antihistamines are effective in decreasing postscabeic pruritus
3. Topical corticosteroid creams may hasten resolution of secondary eczematous dermatitis
4. Management of scabies epidemic in an extended care facility is described in the box on p. 272

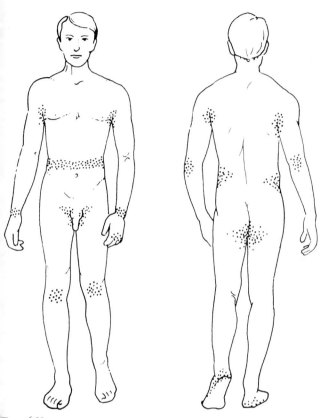

Figure 6-20
Distribution of scabies lesions. (From Habif TP: *Clinical dermatology,* ed 3, St Louis, 1996, Mosby.)

6.8   INFECTIOUS DISEASES

6.8.a.   *INFECTIONS IN THE ELDERLY*
Dennis J. Mikolich, MD

Infections in the geriatric patient may be more problematic because of impairment of cell-mediated and humoral activity, altered physiology secondary to aging, and frequent hospitalizations and institutionalized living, which may lead to altered and often more resistant bacterial flora.

Management of Scabies Epidemic in an Extended Care Facility

1. Educate patients, staff, family, and frequent visitors about scabies and the need for cooperation in treatment.
2. Apply scabicide to all patients, staff, contact staff, and frequent visitors, symptomatic or not. Treat symptomatic family members of staff and visitors.
3. Launder all bedding and clothes worn in the last 48 hours in hot water (or dry clean).
4. Clean beds and floors with routine cleaning agents just before scabicide is removed.
5. Reexamine for treatment failures in 1 week and 4 weeks.

From Habif TP: *Clinical dermatology,* ed 3, St Louis, 1996, Mosby.

URINARY TRACT INFECTIONS

Epidemiology

1. More common in elderly, usually associated with increased pyuria and abnormal genitourinary anatomy
2. Incidence of symptomatic urinary tract infections (UTIs) in the elderly is approximately 10%
3. Asymptomatic bacteriuria, $\geq 10^5$ organisms per millimeter of urine, is as high as 20% in males and 25% in females in nursing homes
4. Asymptomatic bacteriuria does not require antibiotic treatment—has not been shown to have benefit, with often short-lived clearing and common adverse reactions to antibiotic medication
5. Persistent bacteriuria is most commonly caused by *Escherichia coli*
6. Nosocomial UTIs in elderly are most commonly associated with indwelling Foley catheters, with a 15% to 30% case fatality rate if associated with bacteremia; primary cause of bacteremia and sepsis in elderly

Common pathogens

1. *E. coli* and *Proteus:* most common cause of UTIs in the elderly
2. *Pseudomonas klebsiella* and *Enterobacter* species are commonly associated with obstructive processes and neurogenic bladder
3. Nosocomial UTIs are more associated with *Proteus, Klebsiella, Enterobacter, Pseudomonas,* enterococci, whereas *E. coli* is a more common outpatient pathogen

Pathogenesis

1. Obstructive uropathy: calculi; prostatic hypertrophy; cancer of prostate, bladder, or uterus; prostatitis; neurogenic bladder
2. Catheter associated: account for 40% of nosocomial infections in U.S. hospitals, with case fatality rate three times higher than in nonbacteriuric catheterized patients

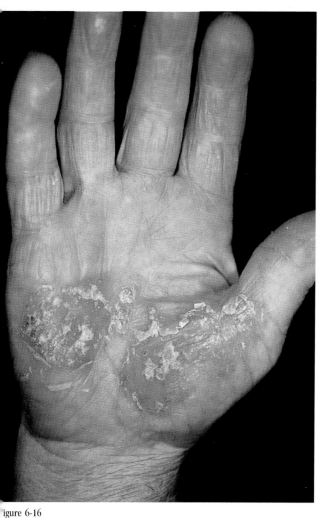

Subacute eczematous inflammation. Acute vesicular eczema has evolved into subacute eczema with redness and scaling. (From Habif TP: *Clinical dermatology*, ed 3,
St Louis, 1996, Mosby.)

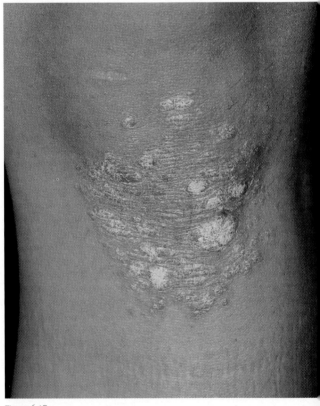

Figure 6-17
Psoriasis. Typical oval plaque with well-defined borders and silvery scale. (From Habif TP: *Clinical dermatology,* ed 3, St Louis, 1996 Mosby.)

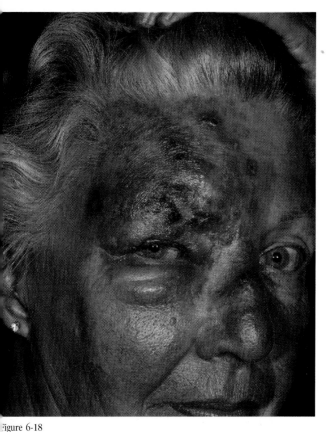

Figure 6-18

Herpes zoster (ophthalmic zoster) involvement of first branch of fifth nerve. (From Habif TP: *Clinical dermatology,* ed 3, St Louis, 1996, Mosby.)

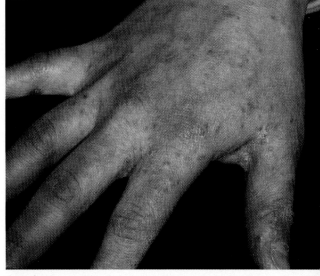

Figure 6-19
Scabies. Tiny vesicles and papules in finger webs and back of hand. (From Habif TP: *Clinical dermatology,* ed 3, St Louis, 1996, Mosby.)

3. Condom catheters: associated with mechanical obstruction (kinking) of urine flow, associated with urinary stasis, bacteriuria, and bladder wall distention
4. Increased uroepithelial adherence of *E. coli* in elderly men
5. Atrophic vaginal mucosa

Diagnosis

1. >5 to 10 WBCs/hpf suggests pyuria
2. White cell counts with infection consistent with pyelonephritis
3. >100,000 bacteria/ml in urine: seen in patients with infection
4. Urine cultures in nursing home setting are necessary for diagnosis; $>10^5$ organisms with associated pyuria and symptoms suggest therapy necessary
5. Not all elderly patients will have classic complaints consistent with UTI, i.e., dysuria, higher frequency and urgency. Upper urinary tract findings of costovertebral angle tenderness (CVAT), fever, flank pain, tenderness may not be present
6. Mental status change, fatigue, loss of appetite may be common complaints in the elderly with UTI. Fever and high white blood cell count may be absent. History often not reliable secondary to dementia or delirium

Treatment

1. Asymptomatic bacteria does not usually require treatment in the elderly. However, treatment is necessary if there is evidence of infection
2. UTI may contribute to mortality in the elderly and should be treated because of associated shock in 26% of cases and bacteremia in 60%
3. Empiric therapy will depend on suspected anatomic involvement and patient presentation. Acute pyelonephritis or suspected bacteremia from obstructive processes can be treated with combination therapy of either extended-spectrum penicillin (piperacillin) or ampicillin, third-generation cephalosporin plus aminoglycoside. This will offer coverage for gram-negative rods and enterococci. Once the organism is identified, removal of aminoglycoside should be entertained to avoid potential nephrotoxicity and ototoxicity
4. Duration of therapy for pyelonephritis: 14 to 21 days. Quinolone therapy, with ciprofloxacin, or ofloxacin may be used if appropriate as a step down from IV
5. Lower UTIs can often be treated empirically with ampicillin, trimethoprim-sulfamethoxazole (Bactrim DS), or quinolone for 7 to 10 days
6. Relapse of infection may require 14 to 21 days of treatment

METHICILLIN-RESISTANT *STAPHYLOCOCCUS AUREUS* (MRSA)

Epidemiology

1. A known pathogen in the United States since 1975
2. Geographically variable prevalence
3. Endemic levels of 30% to 50% of *Staphylococcus aureus* isolates in certain institutions

4. MRSA strains are also resistant to oxacillin, nafcillin, cephalosporin, and carbapenem (imipenem)
5. Acquisition of MRSA colonization associated with prolonged or extended-spectrum antibiotic treatment, exposure to other patients colonized or infected with MRSA, or treatment in an intensive care unit
6. Health-care workers often are colonized with MRSA, both of hands and nasal carriage

Treatment

1. Colonization: treatment with topical mupirocin (Bactroban) to anterior nares qid for approximately 10 days or regimens of oral rifampin/trimethoprim-sulfamethoxazole
2. Infection with MRSA: patients with identified infections, rather than colonization, require systemic IV vancomycin

Criteria for vancomycin use

1. Therapy
   a. Clinical infections when cultures are positive for VRE
   b. Clinical infections caused by ampicillin-resistant enterococcus
   c. Metronidazole-resistant, antibiotic-associated colitis (AAC) (relapse or recurrence 1 to 4 weeks after primary therapy with metronidazole 250 mg qid for 7 to 10 days) OR severe, life-threatening AAC
2. Surgical prophylaxis
   a. GI/GU procedures in high-risk patients (prosthetic heart valves, history of endocarditis or surgically constructed systemic-pulmonary shunts) who are allergic to penicillin
   b. Alternate for dental, oral, or upper respiratory tract procedures in high-risk patients allergic to penicillin (clindamycin is primary choice)
   c. Implantation of prosthetic devices in institutions with high rate of MRSA or methicillin-resistant *Staphylococcus epidermidis*
3. Empiric therapy: suspected nosocomial sepsis in patient with intravascular prosthesis
4. Avoid vancomycin use for
   a. Prophylaxis
      (1) Routine surgery
      (2) Infection or colonization of indwelling intravascular catheters
      (3) Low–birth weight infants
      (4) Continuous ambulatory peritoneal dialysis
   b. Therapy
      (1) Single positive blood culture for coagulase-negative *Staphylococcus*
      (2) Decontamination of the GI tract
      (3) MRSA colonization
   c. Empiric therapy: when cultures are negative for beta-lactamase–resistant organisms

Isolation precautions

1. Patients colonized and/or infected with MRSA in a draining wound or in the sputum should be placed on "contact isolation"

2. Patients with MRSA in their sputum who are actively coughing require a mask on entering. Patients should be placed in private rooms or be cohorted with other patients who are MRSA positive.
3. Gloves must be worn during any direct patient contact
4. A gown is to be worn for close patient contact (i.e., giving a bed bath, assisting patient out of bed, pulling patient up in bed)
5. As with patient examinations on all patients (regardless of MRSA status), hand washing must be performed before and after each patient examination. Hands must be washed following removal of gloves. Following contact with known MRSA-positive patients, bactericidal scrub solution should be used
6. All patients who are MRSA positive should have daily baths with bactericidal soap solution (if tolerated), bacitracin ointment applied to the nares twice daily, and daily change of linen
7. MRSA patients are to have a blood pressure cuff, stethoscopes, Vacutainer sleeve, and tourniquet in the room
8. MRSA status should not restrict the patient's activity. Any wounds should be covered, with drainage contained before patient leaves room. Good personal hygiene should be stressed with the patient. If drainage and secretions cannot be contained, the patient should be restricted to his or her room
9. When the patient is scheduled to go to another department (physical therapy, occupational therapy, radiology), the receiving department should be informed of the patient's MRSA status so appropriate precautions can be observed by the personnel in that department

VANCOMYCIN-RESISTANT ENTEROCOCCI (VRE)

Epidemiology

1. Identified as problem in the United States since 1989
2. Vancomycin resistance as well as to aminoglycosides and ampicillin
3. VRE infection and colonization associated with prior broad-spectrum antibiotic treatment, including PO and IV vancomycin, immunosuppression, intraabdominal surgery
4. Patient to patient transmission, by direct contact or indirect (hands of personnel and patient care equipment, i.e., electronic thermometers, and environmental surfaces)

Isolation precautions

1. Patients colonized and/or infected with VRE are to be placed on gown and glove isolation. The gown and glove isolation sign should be placed in clear view at the entrance to the patient's room. No one should enter the room for any purpose without wearing gowns and gloves. Shoe covers are not required. Masks indicated only if the VRE organism is in the sputum
2. Patients should be placed in private rooms or be cohorted with other patients who are VRE positive. VRE-positive patients must be in a private room if they have fecal incontinence, are unable to contain feces, or have an external foreign body, open wounds, or urinary incontinence with urine colonized and/or infected with VRE

Treatment

1. Evidence for chloramphenicol having activity against this organism
2. Newer agents in the streptogramin family (quinpristin/dalforpristin [Synercid]) have been reported to show some success in clinical trials
3. Teicoplanin: experimental

PNEUMONIA

Epidemiology

1. Most common lethal bacterial infection in elderly
2. Elderly at increased risk related to incidence, morbidity, mortality
   a. Mortality: 40%
   b. Fourth or fifth most common cause of death in elderly
3. Third most common diagnosis for acute care hospitalization

Pathophysiology

Elderly are at increased risk secondary to
- Impaired immunity associated with aging
- Associated multiple chronic medical conditions
- Impairment of clearance of bacteria in oropharynx secondary to decreased cough mechanism and decreased gag reflex
- Aspiration: associated with sedative use, neurodegenerative diseases (dementia)
- Impairment of lung defenses, including cell-mediated and humoral immunity

Etiologic agents

1. *Streptococcus pneumoniae*
   a. Forty to sixty percent of cases
   b. Attack rate >45/1000 persons >65 years old
   c. Most common form of pneumonia in community and in nursing homes
   d. Mortality: 15.20%, 50% if associated with bacteremia
2. *Haemophilus influenzae:* frequently found colonizing oropharynx of elderly patients with COPD, chronic bronchitis
3. Gram-negative bacilli
   a. Lesser role in community-acquired pneumonia in elderly
   b. More commonly associated with patients in nursing homes or chronic care facilities, patients with history of alcoholism, diabetes mellitus, compromised patients on H_2 blockers
   c. *Klebsiella, Pseudomonas aeruginosa, Serratia, Enterobacter*
4. Viral: See section on influenza, also respiratory syncytial virus
5. *Staphylococcus aureus*
   a. Necrotizing pneumonia associated with influenza, 20% of nosocomial pneumonias
   b. MRSA now a concern and more prominent especially in chronic care facilities: requires treatment with vancomycin (see section on MRSA)
6. *Moraxella (Branhamella) catarrhalis:* common cause of bronchitis associated with COPD, usually beta lactamase producing
7. *Legionella pneumophila*
   a. Legionnaires' disease
   b. Often associated with epidemics and contaminated aerosolized water

   c. Approximately 10% community-acquired pneumonia

   d. Increased mortality in elderly: twice that of younger patients

   e. Atypical pneumonic pattern on chest x-ray, associated with bradycardia, diarrhea, abnormal liver chemistries, diagnosis by culture or *Legionella* antigen in urine

Diagnostic dilemmas in elderly

1. Approximately 80% of pneumonia cases in elderly are associated with other underlying or chronic disorders: COPD, diabetes mellitus, dementia

2. Cough and fever commonly absent (25%)

3. Confusion, obtundation commonly seen; elderly are often poor historians secondary to dementia

4. Blood and urine cultures very important. Sputum samples may be difficult to obtain secondary to patient cooperation

5. Chest x-ray: may not initially have findings consistent with infiltrate, should be present within 24 hours

Empiric antibiotic therapy

1. A combination of clinical presentation, sputum Gram stain, and radiographic findings is necessary to choose appropriate antibiotic

2. Demographics of patients important (i.e., community acquired, nursing home, hospitalized) and underlying long-term medical conditions: COPD, diabetes, dementia/CVA

3. If patients residing in institution with known resistant organisms (MRSA, resistant gram-negative rods [GNR]) these should be taken into account

4. If no defined organism, and influenza not suspected, cefuroxime and erythromycin have broad coverage for many pathogens

5. If hospital or immunocompromised acquired and GNR suspected, combination of a third-generation cephalosporin (ceftazidime) or piperacillin plus an aminoglycoside is recommended

6. Dosage based on creatinine clearance with adjustment should be assessed; monitoring of aminoglycoside levels and creatinine should be performed

TUBERCULOSIS

Epidemiology

1. Elderly patients account for approximately 30% of newly diagnosed TB cases yearly

2. Individuals >65 years have a TB case rate higher than any other population, except HIV-positive persons

3. Over 50% of new cases occur in individuals >65 years old

4. Nursing home residents account for 20% of cases in the elderly

5. Ninety percent of TB cases in the geriatric population are due to prior exposure or infection and reactivation

Diagnosis

1. Physical signs and clinical manifestations vary

   a. Asymptomatic or subtle findings including dry nonproductive cough, dyspnea, night sweats, low-grade fever, hemoptysis, anorexia, pleuritic chest pain

b. Atypical chest x-ray presentation, appearing as pneumonia or CHF; high index of suspicion is necessary
2. Physical exam: usually not helpful, rales at apices may not be present
3. Tuberculin skin testing
   a. Five tuberculin units (intermediate strength) of PPD (purified protein derivative) in 0.1 ml of solution is injected intradermally on the forearm
   b. Test should be read at 48 to 72 hours; definition of a positive reaction varies with risk groups (see Section 6.12.d)
   c. In elderly patients, a negative test may require a repeat test 1 week later for booster phenomenon
   d. Factors associated with false-negative tests are given in the box below; 25% of all newly diagnosed cases may have negative PPD secondary to loss of cellular immunity
   e. Patients with a history of prior positive testing should not be tested again
   f. Anergy can be checked by simultaneously applying skin test for other antigens (mumps, *Candida*)

Factors Associated with False-Negative Tuberculin Tests

Technical Errors

Improper administration
Inaccurate reading
Loss of potency of antigen

Patient-Related Factors (Anergy)

Age (elderly)
Nutritional status
Medications—corticosteroids, immunosuppressive agents
Severe tuberculosis
Coexisting diseases
   HIV infection
   Viral illness or vaccination
   Lymphoreticular malignancies
   Sarcoidosis
   Solid tumors
   Lepromatous leprosy
   Sjögren's syndrome
   Ataxia telangiectasia
   Uremia
   Primary biliary cirrhosis
   Systemic lupus erythematosus
   Severe systemic disease of any etiology

From Stein JH, editor: *Internal medicine*, ed 4, St Louis, 1994, Mosby.

4. Acid-fast stain and culture of sputum from three consecutive morning specimens. If TB suspected and patient cannot produce specimen, induction or bronchoscopy may be necessary
5. Chest x-ray study
   a. Reticulonodular infiltration in apical segments
   b. Chest x-ray may be normal
   c. Consolidation caused by tuberculous pneumonia
   d. Nursing home residents with primary infection may have mid and lower lung field involvement
   e. Hilar and paratracheal adenopathy with or without cavitary changes

Treatment

The Centers for Disease Control and Prevention has outlined options for initiation of therapy (Tables 6-25 and 6-26) to prevent emerging resistant organisms.

Prophylaxis

1. Isoniazid (INH) prophylaxis not necessary in elderly patients with known prior positive PPD skin testing
2. Recently converted positive tuberculin tests should be treated with INH 300 mg/day for 6 to 12 months
3. Toxicity: if nausea and vomiting, discontinue INH and have liver function tests obtained. If SGOT >500, discontinue permanently. Lower levels may allow for challenging patients with lower dose
4. Five-percent incidence of nonfatal hepatitis in elderly

Suggested readings

Baldassare JS, Kaye D: Special problems of urinary tract infection in the elderly, *Med Clin North Am* 75:375-390, 1991.

Barker WH: Excess pneumonia and influenza associated hospitalization during influenza epidemics in the United States, *Am J Public Health* 76:761-765, 1986.

Centers for Disease Control and Prevention: Preventing the spread of vancomycin resistance: report from the Hospital Infection Control Practices Advisory Committee, *Fed Regis* 59:25758-25763, 1994.

Centers for Disease Control and Prevention: Recommendations for preventing the spread of vancomycin resistance, *MMWR* 44(RR-12):1-11, 1994.

Crossley KB, Thurn JR: Nursing home-acquired pneumonia, *Semin Respir Infect* 4:64-72, 1989.

Garbaldi RA, Nurse BA: Infections in the elderly, *Am J Med* 81(suppl 1A):53-58, 1986.

Harkness GA, Bentley DW, Roghmann KJ: Risk factors for nosocomial pneumonia in the elderly, *Am J Med* 89:457-463, 1990.

Marrie TJ: Epidemiology of community-acquired pneumonia in the elderly, *Semin Respir Infect* 5:260-261, 1990.

May DS et al: Surveillance of major causes of hospitalization among the elderly, 1988, *MMWR* 40:7-21, 1991.

Strausbaugh LJ et al: Methicillin-resistant *Staphylococcus aureus* in extended-care facilities, *Infect Control Hosp Epidemiol* 12:36-45, 1991.

Wenzel RP et al: Methicillin-resistant *Staphylococcus aureus:* implications for the 1990's and effective control measures, *Am J Med* 91(suppl 3B):2215-2275, 1991.

Table 6-25 Regimen options for the initial treatment of TB among adults

	TB without HIV Infection		TB with HIV Infection
Option 1	Option 2	Option 3	
Administer daily INH, RIF, and PZA for 8 wk, followed by 16 wk of INH and RIF daily or two or three times per week.* In areas where the INH resistance rate is not documented as <4%, EMB or SM should be added to the initial regimen until susceptibility to INH and RIF is demonstrated. Continue treatment for at least 6 r, and 3 mo beyond culture conversion. Consult a TB medical expert if patient is symptomatic or smear or culture is positive after 3 mo.	Administer daily INH, RIF, PZA, and SM or EMB for 2 wk, followed by two times per week* administration of the same drugs for 6 wk (by DOT), and subsequently with two times per week administration of INH and RIF for 16 wk (by DOT). Consult a TB medical expert if the patient is symptomatic or smear or culture is positive after 3 mo.	Treat by DOT, three times per week* with INH, RIF, PZA, and EMB or SM for 6 mo.† Consult a TB medical expert if the patient is symptomatic or smear or culture is positive after 3 mo.	Options 1, 2, or 3 can be used, but treatment regimens should continue for a total of 9 mo and at least 6 mo beyond culture conversion.

From Centers for Disease Control and Prevention: *MMWR* 42 (RR-7), 1993.

DOT, Directly observed therapy; *EMB,* ethambutol; *INH,* isoniazid; *PZA,* pyrazinamide; *RIF,* rifampin; *SM,* streptomycin.

*All regimens administered two times per week or three times per week should be monitored by DOT for the duration of therapy.

†The strongest evidence from clinical trials is the effectiveness of all four drugs administered for the full 6 mo. There is weaker evidence that SM can be discontinued after 4 mo if the isolate is susceptible to all drugs. The evidence for stopping PZA before the end of 6 mo is equivocal for the three times/wk regimen, and there is no evidence on the effectiveness of this regimen with EMB for less than the full 6 mo.

Table 6-26 Dosage recommendation for the initial treatment of TB among adults

	Dosage					
	Daily		Two Times/Wk		Three Times/Wk	
Drugs	Children	Adults	Children	Adults	Children	Adults
Isoniazid	10–20 mg/kg Max, 300 mg	5 mg/kg Max, 300 mg	20–40 µg/kg Max, 900 mg	15 mg/kg Max, 900 mg	20–40 mg/kg Max, 900 mg	15 mg/kg Max, 900 mg
Rifampin	10–20 mg/kg Max, 600 mg	10 mg/kg Max, 600 mg	10–20 mg/kg Max, 600 mg	10 mg/kg Max, 600 mg	10–20 mg/kg Max, 600 mg	10 mg/kg Max, 600 mg
Pyrazinamide	15–30 mg/kg Max, 2 g	15–30 mg/kg Max, 2 g	50–70 mg/kg Max, 4 g	50–70 mg/kg Max, 4 g	50–70 mg/kg Max, 3 g	50–70 mg/kg Max, 3 g
Ethambutol	15–25 mg/kg Max, 2.5 g	5–25 mg/kg Max, 2.5 g	50 mg/kg Max, 2.5 g	50 µg/kg Max, 2.5 g	25–30 mg/kg Max, 2.5 g	25–30 mg/kg Max, 2.5 g
Streptomycin	20–30 mg/kg Max, 1 g	15 mg/kg Max, 1 g	25–30 mg/kg Max, 1.5 g	25–30 mg/kg Max, 1.5 g	25–30 mg/kg Max, 1 g	25–30 mg/kg Max, 1 g

From Centers for Disease Control and Prevention: *MMWR* 42 (RR-7), 1993.

6.8.b.   **SEPSIS AND SEPTIC SHOCK**
Dennis J. Mikolich, MD

Definition

1. Infections occur more frequently in the elderly
2. Forty percent of all sepsis and 60% of all deaths attributed to sepsis occur in patients >60 years
3. Sepsis: presence of an infection with systemic response
   a. Temperature >38° C or <36° C
   b. Tachycardia: pulse >90/min
   c. Respiratory rate >20/min or $Paco_2$ <32
   d. WBC >12,000 cells/mm^3, <5000, or >10% bands
4. Septic shock
   a. Sepsis with hypotension not responsive to fluid resuscitation
   b. Perfusion abnormalities including lactic acidosis, oliguria, mental status changes

Etiology

1. Gram-negative bacteria: *Klebsiella, Escherichia coli, Pseudomonas, Haemophilus influenzae, Salmonella, Neisseria meningitidis*
2. Gram-positive bacteria: *Staphylococcus aureus,* streptococci (including group A strep), *Streptococcus pneumoniae*
3. Fungi: *Candida, Aspergillus, Mucor* spp.
4. Other: *Listeria, Vibrio,* mycobacteria, and viral—herpes simplex virus, cytomegalovirus, varicella, and parasitic

Predisposing factors: sites of infection

1. Genitourinary tract (most common in elderly): associated with UTI, catheters, urinary obstruction, pyelonephritis
2. GI tract: associated with cirrhosis and postoperative surgical patients, cholecystitis, diverticulitis
3. Respiratory tract: second-degree pneumonia
4. Central lines
5. Immunosuppressed patients: steroids, chemotherapy, transplant patients receiving therapy; also seen in patients with cancer, diabetes, and coronary artery disease

Clinical manifestations

1. Elderly patients may have limited focal findings on examination to suggest that they are septic or have an active infection
2. Fever, chills, hypothermia, altered mental status, anorexia, lethargy, tachypnea, and tachycardia; elderly patients may be afebrile
3. Complicated by hypotension, disseminated intravascular coagulation (DIC), leukopenia and organ failure, metabolic acidosis, and oliguria
4. Skin: cellulitis, erythema multiforme, petechial rash associated with meningococcus; ecthyma gangrenosum with *Pseudomonas*
5. Cardiovascular: decreased cardiac output (CO), increased systemic vascular resistance, myocardial dysfunction, tissue hypoperfusion
6. Pulmonary
   a. Increased respiratory rate, respiratory alkalosis
   b. Adult respiratory distress syndrome (ARDS)

7. Hematologic
   a. Leukocytosis early
   b. Neutropenia: overwhelming sepsis
   c. Thrombocytopenia
   d. DIC
8. Renal: acute tubular necrosis associated with volume depletion and hypotension
9. Gastrointestinal: bleeding associated with DIC; elevated transaminases associated with hypotension and/or bacteremia
10. CNS: meningitis—meningeal signs, obtundation, seizures

Diagnosis
See Table 6-27.

Management and therapy

1. Management
   a. Aggressive fluid management with saline intravenously
   b. Swan-Ganz catheter: if needed assess fluid volume status: monitoring pulmonary artery wedge pressure (PAWP), CO, systemic vascular resistance; maintain PAWP between 12 and 15 mm Hg
   c. Vasopressors if blood pressure cannot be maintained $\geq$60 mm Hg
   d. Empiric antibiotic therapy
2. IV antibiotic therapy: early treatment is crucial for patient survival (do not wait until all blood cultures have been obtained); use broad antibiotic coverage with a combination of
   a. Aminoglycoside (amikacin, gentamicin, tobramycin)
   b. Additional agents depending on suspected site of infection; predisposing factors are
      (1) Neutropenic patient: add a beta-lactam (piperacillin or ceftazidime) to provide additional coverage against *Pseudomonas*
      (2) Suspected skin infection: add antistaphylococcal agent (i.e., nafcillin, oxacillin), vancomycin if MRSA suspected
      (3) Suspected intraabdominal focus: add cefotetan, cefoxitin, clindamycin, or metronidazole to cover anaerobic organisms; ampicillin to cover enterococci
      (4) Suspected pulmonary infection: add a cephalosporin (e.g., cefuroxime, ceftriaxone, ceftazidime)
      (5) Suspected UTI: add ampicillin to cover enterococci or vancomycin if ampicillin resistant
   c. Appropriate change of antibiotics pending culture results
3. Monitor with a pulmonary artery catheter and arterial line
4. Low-dose dopamine (1 to 4 μg/kg/min) is useful to maintain perfusion
5. Drain any septic foci; necrotic bowel should be treated surgically
6. Monitor blood gases, electrolytes, and renal function
7. Measure hourly urinary output
8. Measure mixed venous PO_2 to determine tissue oxygenation
9. Correct acid-base and electrolyte disturbances and hypoxia
10. Correct hypocalcemia if present
11. Administer IV hydrocortisone, 100 mg q4h, only if adrenal insufficiency is suspected (elevated K^+ and/or refractory shock)

Table 6-27 Uniform system for defining the spectrum of disorders associated with sepsis

Disorder	Requirements for Clinical Diagnosis
Bacteremia*	Positive blood cultures
Sepsis	Clinical evidence suggests infection *plus* signs of a systemic response to infection (all of the following) Tachypnea (respiration >20 breaths/min [if patient is mechanically ventilated, >10 L/min] Tachycardia (heart rate >90 beats/min) Hyperthermia or hypothermia (core or rectal temperature >38.4° C [101° F] or <35.6° C [96.1° F])
Sepsis syndrome (may also be considered *incipient septic shock* in patients who later become hypotensive)	Clinical diagnosis of sepsis *plus* evidence of altered organ perfusion (one or more of the following) Pao_2/Fio_2 no higher than 280 (in absence of other pulmonary or cardiovascular disease) Lactate level above upper limit of normal Oliguria (documented urine output <0.5 ml/kg body weight for at least 1 hr in patients with catheters in place) Acute alteration in mental status Positive blood cultures not required†
Early septic shock	Clinical diagnosis of sepsis syndrome outlined above, *plus* hypotension (systolic blood pressure below 90 mm Hg or a 40 mm Hg decrease below baseline systolic blood pressure) that lasts for less than 1 hr and is responsive to conventional therapy (IV fluid administration or pharmacologic intervention)
Refractory septic shock	Clinical diagnosis of sepsis syndrome outlined above, *plus* hypotension (systolic blood pressure below 90 mm Hg or a 40 mm Hg decrease below baseline systolic blood pressure) that lasts for more than 1 hr despite adequate volume resuscitation and that requires vasopressors or higher doses of dopamine (>6 µg/kg/hr)

Modified from Bone RC: *Ann Intern Med* 115:457-469, 1991.

*The related term *septicemia* is imprecise and should be abandoned. The sepsis syndrome may result from infection with gram-positive or gram-negative bacteria, pathogenic viruses, fungi, or rickettsia; however, an identical physiologic response may result from such noninfectious processes as severe trauma or pancreatitis. Blood cultures may not be positive.

†Positive blood cultures not required.

12. Use heparin (alone or with fresh frozen plasma [FFP]) in patients with DIC
13. Correct severe thrombocytopenia with platelet concentrates
14. Correct depletion of coagulation factors with FFP

6.8.c.   *INFLUENZA*
Dennis J. Mikolich, MD

Definition

Influenza is an acute viral illness caused by influenza A or B associated with fever, cough, and myalgias in the winter months. It is associated with epidemics and annual changes in antigens and antigenicity. Mortality may be high, especially with pulmonary involvement or pneumonia. Influenza/pneumonia is the fifth leading cause of death in individuals older than 60 years.

Epidemiology

1. Outbreaks occur abruptly, especially influenza A, peaking at 2 to 3 weeks, lasting 1 to 3 months
2. Outbreaks may occur first in a nursing home or in children in the community
3. Epidemics are exclusively in winter months
4. Attack rates can vary between 10% and 50%, often dependent on age

Pathogenesis

1. Transmitted by infected respiratory secretions
2. Small particle–aerosolized virus may be causal in transmission, heightened by talking, coughing, and sneezing
3. Viral replication is approximately 4 to 6 hours, usually adhering to respiratory epithelial cells
4. IgA secretory antibodies and serum antibodies play a role in protection and immunity

Clinical presentation

1. Incubation period: 24 to 48 hours
2. Fever, chills, myalgias, headache, malaise
3. Hypoxia, cyanosis
4. Nonproductive cough
5. Older patients may have mental status changes and confusion accompanying fever, with or without a cough
6. Nasal obstruction frequently observed, with clear nasal discharge
7. Pneumonia
   a. Primary influenza
   b. Secondary bacterial
      (1) *Streptococcus pneumoniae*
      (2) *Staphylococcus aureus*
      (3) *Haemophilus influenzae*
8. Chest x-ray: primary influenza, usually with intestinal-like patterns without consolidation

9. Gram stains in primary influenza pneumonia: without predominant organism, growing normal flora
10. Pneumonia in the elderly from primary influenza may reach 70% of infected individuals

Diagnosis

1. Culture of virus in respiratory secretions: should be used primarily because it allows the quickest diagnosis and treatment intervention
2. Serologic markers by complement fixation and hemagglutination can be used for epidemiologic studies

Treatment

1. Antiviral therapy should be considered for uncomplicated influenza. Amantadine and rimantidine may decrease signs and symptoms by 50% (Table 6-28)
2. Patients with seizure disorders may have increased risk for seizures with amantadine. Other known side effects: anorexia, vomiting, lethargy, agitation, and confusion
3. Bed rest, heightened fluid intake
4. Patients receiving amantadine treatment for Parkinson's disease or multiple sclerosis should not take additional therapy

Vaccination (influenza)

Influenza vaccines usually contain antigens of viral strains that represent influenza viruses presently circulating in the world. The following groups are appropriate for vaccination

1. Individuals at increased risk for influenza-related complications
   a. Adults with chronic disorders of pulmonary or cardiovascular systems
   b. Residents of nursing homes, long-term care facilities, and domiciliary institutions
   c. Persons >65 years
   d. Adults with diabetes mellitus, renal impairment, immunosuppression
2. Groups capable of transmitting influenza to high-risk patients
   a. Nurses, physicians, hospital personnel
   b. Home care providers
   c. Household members of high-risk groups

Table 6-28   Dosage guidelines for amantadine prophylaxis of influenza A among nursing home residents based on serum creatinine

Serum Creatine (mg/dl)	Amantadine Dose
Up to 1.0	100 mg daily
Greater than 1.0 but less than 2.0	100 mg every other day
Greater than 2.0	100 mg twice per week
On dialysis	100 mg once per week

From Gomolin IH et al: *J Am Geriatr Soc* 43:71-74, 1995.

3. Individuals who should not be vaccinated
   a. Known hypersensitivity or anaphylaxis to eggs
   b. Persons with acute febrile illnesses, until symptoms disappear

Side effects and adverse reactions

1. Localized redness at site of vaccine administration (one third of vaccinees)
2. Systemic reactions
   a. Fever, malaise, myalgia
   b. Allergy: hives, angioedema, allergic asthma occur rarely; usually to hypersensitivity of vaccine component
   c. Guillain-Barré syndrome: 1/100,000 or 2/100,000

Isolation recommendations

Recommendations on isolation of nursing home residents with influenza-like illness (ILI) are described in the box below.

Recommendations for Isolation of Nursing Home Residents with ILI

Isolation and cohorting of ill residents are an important component to outbreak control. We recommend the following steps, giving due consideration to quality of life issues:

1. During an influenza outbreak, all residents with ILI should be confined to their rooms for at least 72 hours. For outbreaks of influenza A, this is sufficient time for the prophylactic effects of amantadine to begin among nonill residents.
2. Nonill residents may congregate and eat on the same unit. Travel to other areas of the facility should be discouraged but, if necessary, kept brief. In outbreaks involving high attack rates and/or severe illness, including complications such as pneumonia, consideration should be given to keeping nonill residents in their rooms for the first 72 hours because some may be incubating infection and shedding virus.
3. Centralized activities, such as recreational events, should be decentralized, i.e., unit specific, or postponed for at least 72 hours.

These recommendations apply to the entire facility, including nursing units where no influenza activity has appeared. A possible exception is a facility with separate buildings and for which employees do not share time between buildings. Cohorting of residents and decentralization of activities may be abandoned 72 hours after the onset of the last case of influenza.

---

*From Gomolin IH et al: *J Am Geriatr Soc* 43:71-74, 1995.

6.9   **NEPHROLOGY AND UROLOGY**

6.9.a.   *PROSTATIC HYPERTROPHY*
Fred F. Ferri, MD

Epidemiology

1. Eighty percent of men have evidence of benign prostatic hypertrophy (BPH) by age 80
2. Medical or surgical intervention for problems caused by BPH is required in over 20% of males by age 75
3. Transurethral resection of prostate (TURP) is the tenth most common operative procedure (over 400,000/yr in the United States)

Pathophysiology

1. Multifactorial etiology. Functioning testicle is necessary for its development as evidenced by its absence in males who were castrated before puberty
2. A basic understanding of the pituitary-gonadal axis is crucial to understanding BPH and its therapy. Following is a simplification of this complex endocrine function
   a. Hypothalamus secretes gonadotropic-releasing hormone (GnRH), also known as luteinizing hormone–releasing hormone (LHRH)
   b. LHRH stimulates the pituitary to release luteinizing hormone (LH) and follicle-stimulating hormone (FSH)
   c. LH causes testosterone production by the Leydig cells of the testicles
   d. Testosterone is converted to dihydrotestosterone by the enzyme 5-alpha-reductase
   e. Dihydrotestosterone binds to steroid receptor complexes in the prostate and cell growth occurs

Diagnosis

1. History
   a. Difficulty in initiating urination (hesitancy), decrease in caliber and force of stream
   b. Incomplete emptying of bladder resulting in double voiding (need to urinate again few minutes after voiding), postvoid "dribbling," and nocturia
   c. BPH may be asymptomatic if it does not encroach on the urethral lumen
2. Symptom assessment
   a. Table 6-29 describes the American Urological Association symptom index for benign prostatic hyperplasia. This symptom questionnaire is easy to administer and is useful in treatment planning and periodically in follow-up. In the AUA scoring system, symptoms are classified as mild (0 to 7), moderate (8 to 19), or severe (20 to 35)
   b. Examination: identification of prostatic enlargement on digital rectal exam

Table 6-29 AUA symptom index

Questions To Be Answered	AUA Symptom Score (Circle 1 number on each line)					
	Not At All	Less Than 1 Time in 5	Less Than Half the Time	About Half the Time	More Than Half the Time	Almost Always
1. Over the past month, how often have you had a sensation of not emptying your bladder completely after you finished urinating?	0	1	2	3	4	5
2. Over the past month, how often have you had to urinate again less than 2 hours after you finished urinating?	0	1	2	3	4	5
3. Over the past month, how often have you found you stopped and started again several times when you urinated?	0	1	2	3	4	5

Continued

From Barry M et al: *J Urol* 148:1549-1557, 1992. Used with permission.
Interpretation: mild (0 to 7), moderate (8-19), severe (20 to 25).

Table 6-29 AUA symptom index—cont'd

Questions To Be Answered	Not At All	Less Than 1 Time in 5	Less Than Half the Time	About Half the Time	More than Half the Time	Almost Always
				AUA Symptom Score (Circle 1 number on each line)		
4. Over the past month, how often have you found it difficult to postpone urination?	0	1	2	3	4	5
5. Over the past month, how often have you had a weak urinary stream?	0	1	2	3	4	5
6. Over the past month, how often have you had to push or strain to begin urination?	0	1	2	3	4	5
7. Over the past month, how many times did you most typically get up to urinate from the time you went to bed at night until the time you got up in the morning?	0 (None)	1 (1 time)	2 (2 times)	3 (3 times)	4 (4 times)	5 (5 times or more)

Sum of 7 circled numbers (AUA Symptom Score): _____

  c. Laboratory
    (1) Urinalysis, urine culture, and sensitivity to rule out infection (if suspected)
    (2) BUN and creatinine to rule out postrenal insufficiency
3. Additional diagnostic tests
  a. Uroflowmetry: may be used to determine relative impact of obstruction on urine flow. Urethral pressure profile is useful to predict prostatic hypertrophy within the urethral lumen
  b. Pressure-flow studies, although invasive, are particularly helpful in patients whose history and/or examination suggests primary bladder dysfunction as a cause of symptoms of prostatism. They are also useful in patients for whom a distinction between prostatic obstruction and impaired detrusor contractility might affect the choice of therapy. However, pressure-flow studies may not be useful in the workup of the usual patient with symptoms of prostatism
  c. Postvoid residual urine measurement: has not been proven useful in predicting the need for or response to treatment; may be helpful in monitoring the course of the disease in patients who elect nonsurgical treatment
  d. Urethrocystoscopy: optional during later evaluation if invasive treatment is being planned
  e. Prostate-specific antigen (PSA): protease secreted by epithelial cells of prostate. It is elevated in 30% to 50% of patients with BPH. Testing for PSA increases detection rate for prostate cancer and tends to detect cancer at an earlier stage. However, the PSA test does not discriminate well between patients with symptomatic BPH and those with prostate cancer, particularly if the cancers are pathologically localized and curable. Test may also trigger additional evaluation, including ultrasound and biopsy of the prostate

Treatment*

Asymptomatic patients with prostate enlargement caused by BPH generally do not require treatment. For those patients who have specific complications from BPH, prostate surgery is usually the most appropriate form of treatment. All other patients should, in consultation with their physicians, decide on the treatment after understanding the likely outcomes of each potential treatment.

The depth of information needed will vary from patient to patient. To make a treatment decision, the patient needs to consider how "bothered" he is by his symptoms and his attitude toward the likely benefits and risks of each treatment option. The health-care provider can help guide the patient in making the most appropriate treatment decision.

WATCHFUL WAITING

Watchful waiting is an appropriate treatment strategy for the majority of patients. The probability of disease progression or the development of BPH complications is uncertain. Until research defines these probabilities, patients

*From McConnell JD et al: *Benign prostatic hyperplasia: diagnosis and treatment.* Quick reference guide for clinicians. AHCPR Publication No. 94-0583, Rockville, Md, 1994, Agency for Health Care Policy and Research, Public Health Service, U.S. Department of Health and Human Services.

treated by watchful waiting should be monitored periodically by reassessment of symptom level, physical findings, routine laboratory testing, and optional urologic diagnostic procedures. No studies define the optimal interval for follow-up. Annual follow-up is reasonable but supported only by subjective judgment.

SURGERY

Of all treatment options, prostate surgery offers the best chance for symptom improvement. However, surgery also has the highest rates of significant complications. Transurethral resection of the prostate (TURP) is the most commonly used surgical treatment for BPH. Transurethral incision of the prostate (TUIP), a procedure of almost equivalent efficacy, is limited to prostates whose estimated resected tissue weight (if done by TURP) would be 30 g or less. TUIP can be performed in ambulatory settings or during a 1-day hospitalization. Open prostatectomy is typically performed on patients with very large prostates.

Given proper patient selection, benefits are probably equivalent for each surgical procedure, but complication rates differ among the procedures. Open prostatectomy, for example, has greater incisional morbidity and a longer recovery time than other procedures. TUIP has the lowest morbidity and ejaculatory disturbance rates. Given that prostates of men undergoing surgery average less than 30 g of resected weight, TUIP is an underutilized procedure.

Surgery need not be a treatment of last resort for most patients; that is, patients need not undergo other treatments for BPH before they can have surgery.

However, recommending surgery on the ground that a patient's surgical risk will "only increase with age" is inappropriate. BPH progresses slowly and quite variably among patients.

BALLOON DILATION

Balloon dilation of the prostatic urethra is clearly less effective than surgery for relieving symptoms but is associated with fewer complications. Recent studies suggest that improvement may be temporary, with recurrence of symptoms within 2 years. At present, balloon dilation is a reasonable treatment option for patients with smaller prostates and no middle lobe enlargement. However, TUIP can be performed in the same patients with superior efficacy, with similar morbidity, and in similar outpatient settings.

ALPHA-BLOCKERS

Alpha-$_1$-adrenergic receptor blockers (e.g., doxazosin, prazosin, and terazosin) relax smooth muscle of the bladder neck and prostate. In the average patient, they cause a small increase in peak urinary flow rate (Q_{max}) and a small but perceptible reduction in symptoms. Approved by the U.S. Food and Drug Administration (FDA) for treating hypertension, alpha-blockers are also widely used by physicians for treating BPH.

Titration of dose is necessary. Long-term efficacy has not been determined. Side effects include orthostatic hypotension, dizziness, tiredness, and headache. The nonselective alpha-blocker phenoxybenzamine is not recommended because of a higher incidence of side effects. Also, there is no evilence that alpha-blockers reduce BPH complication rates or the need for future surgery.

FINASTERIDE

The drug finasteride was approved in 1992 by the FDA for treatment of BPH. Finasteride is a 5-alpha reductase inhibitor that blocks conversion of testosterone to dihydrotestosterone, the major intraprostatic androgen in men. The drug is taken orally once daily. It can reduce the size of the prostate. It causes a small average increase in Q_{max} and for some men a small yet perceptible reduction in symptoms. Six months or more are required for maximal effects. Long-term efficacy has not been documented.

Side effects are mainly sexually related and include decreased libido, ejaculatory dysfunction, and impotence. Finasteride also lowers serum PSA approximately 50%. How this affects the utility of PSA as a cancer-detection tool is unknown. As with alpha-blockers, there is currently no evidence that finasteride reduces BPH complication rates or the need for future surgery.

NEW TECHNOLOGIES

Emerging technologies for treating BPH include lasers, coils, stents, thermal therapy, and hyperthermia. The BPH panel reviewed these new therapies but found the data currently insufficient to permit conclusions regarding the safety and efficacy of these modalities in routine practice. Laser prostatectomy appears promising, but its benefits and risks relative to TURP and TUIP are uncertain and long-term effectiveness has not yet been demonstrated.

 ## *KIDNEY STONES*
Tom J. Wachtel, MD

Types of kidney stones and etiology (stones may be mixed)

1. Calcium oxalate (75%)
   a. Radiodense
   b. Size: small (<2 cm)
   c. Color: shades of gray
   d. Etiology
      (1) Hyperparathyroidism
      (2) Idiopathic hypercalciuria
      (3) Hyperoxaluria
      (4) Hyperuricosuria
      (5) Hypocitraturia
2. Calcium phosphate (2%)
   a. Radiodense
   b. Etiology: renal tubular acidosis
3. Uric acid (14%)
   a. Radiolucent
   b. Size: small to staghorn
   c. Color: orange
   d. Etiology: hyperuricosuria

4. Struvite (8%)
    a. Radiodense
    b. Size: small to staghorn
    c. Color: brown
    d. Etiology: urinary infection with urease splitting organism (e.g., *Proteus, Klebsiella, Pseudomonas,* and enterococci)
5. Cystine (1%)
    a. Radiodense
    b. Size: small to staghorn
    c. Onset long before middle age
    d. Color: yellow
    e. Etiology: cystinuria

Presentation

1. Renal colic
    a. Sudden onset of severe costovertebral angle or flank pain that radiates around flank anteriorly toward groin and is associated with the descent of a urinary calculus through a ureter
    b. Nausea, vomiting, urinary frequency, and dysuria may be associated with the pain
    c. Pain persists until stone passes into bladder or is removed
    d. Gross or microscopic hematuria may be present
2. Recurrent UTI
3. Hematuria
4. Obstructive uropathy that may remain silent
5. Incidental radiologic findings
6. Passage of gravel through urethra

Management of renal colic

1. Diagnosis: 90% of all kidney stones are radiopaque and theoretically visible on a plain x-ray. Sonography or IV pyelography may be required
2. Pain control: narcotic analgesics typically required
3. Stone removal
    a. Spontaneous passage can be expected of stones smaller than 0.5 cm and is possible for stones 0.5 to 0.7 cm
    b. Stones that progress, then become lodged in the distal ureter (below the pelvic brim on x-ray) can be moved ureteroscopically with a basket or disrupted by lithotripsy
    c. Stones lodged in the upper ureter can be pushed back into the renal pelvis endoscopically and disrupted later by lithotripsy
        (1) If lithotripsy fails or if the stone is larger than 2 cm, percutaneous nephrolithotomy is performed
        (2) Surgical (i.e., open) ureterolithotomy is indicated only after all else fails

Treatment

1. Treatment at home is reasonable for stones smaller than 0.7 cm for which spontaneous passage is likely
2. Patient should strain all urine to recover the stone, which should then be analyzed for its chemical composition

Diagnostic evaluation of nephrolithiasis

Defining the chemical composition of the stone and the pathophysiology of the stone formation in order to propose a preventive treatment is important because more than half of all patients who pass one stone will pass another.

1. Urinalysis

	Urine pH	Shape of Crystal
Calcium oxalate	Acid to neutral	Envelope shape
Uric acid	Acid	Plates, prisms, clumps, needles, or fan shapes
Struvite	Alkaline	Coffin lid
Cystine	Acid	Hexagonal

2. Stone analysis if stone available
3. Metabolic workup (NOTE: if stone unavailable, it is most likely calcium oxalate)
   a. Calcium oxalate stone
      (1) Serum calcium, phosphorus, and alkaline phosphatase
      (2) Parathormone level if serum calcium is high and phosphorus is low
      (3) Twenty-four–hour urine collection on normal diet for creatinine, calcium (normal urinary calcium <250 mg/24 hr in women and <300 mg/24 hr in men), and oxalate (normal <150 mg/24 hr)
      (4) Effect of a low calcium diet on 24-hour urinary calcium can diagnose idiopathic hypercalciuria that does not respond to diet
      (5) If hypercalcemia is present, consider the various causes, e.g., hyperparathyroidism, malignancy, sarcoidosis, milk-alkali syndrome, Paget's disease, immobilization, hyperthyroidism, vitamin D toxicity
   b. Uric acid stone
      (1) Serum uric acid
      (2) Twenty-four–hour urine collection for creatinine and uric acid (normal urinary uric acid <750 mg/24 hr)
   c. Struvite stone
      (1) No metabolic studies
      (2) Urinalysis and urine culture with sensitivity
   d. Cystine stone
      (1) Urine cystine screen

Preventive treatment

1. General measures
   a. Increase fluid intake (3 L/24 hr)
   b. Avoid dehydration
2. Calcium stone formers
   a. Surgical treatment of primary hyperparathyroidism if present
   b. Treatment of underlying cause of hypercalcemia if relevant
   c. Low calcium diet unless diagnosis is idiopathic hypercalciuria

d. In hyperoxaluria, low oxalate diet (avoid tea, spinach, rhubarb) and treat ilial disease if present; consider pyridoxine deficiency

e. Thiazide diuretics (e.g., hydrochlorothiazide 25 to 50 mg bid): drug of choice to manage hypercalciuria

f. Citrate (e.g., Polycitra) inhibits calcium stone formation and alkalinizes urine

3. Uric acid stones (or calcium or mixed stone former with hyperuricosuria)

a. Avoid purine-rich foods (e.g., liver, kidney, cold cuts)

b. Alkalinize urine (with citrate)

c. Allopurinol (Zyloprim) titrated upward from 200 mg qd to reduce urinary uric acid to below 600 mg/24 hr

d. Avoid uricosuric drugs (e.g., probenecid)

4. Struvite stones: referral to urology for complete stone removal combined with specific antibiotics is treatment of choice

5. Cystine stones

a. Alkalinize urine (with citrate)

b. D-penicillamine (4 g/day until stone is dissolved, then 1 g/day maintenance)

Suggested readings

Coe FL, Parks JH, Asplin JR: The pathogenesis and treatment of kidney stones, *N Engl J Med* 16:1141-1152, 1992.

Consensus Conference: Prevention and treatment of kidney stones, *JAMA* 260:977-981, 1988.

RENAL FAILURE

Tom J. Wachtel, MD, Michael D. Stein, MD, and James Grant, MD

Definition

Renal failure refers to a decrease in renal function that increases the concentration of nitrogenous waste in the blood (e.g., creatinine).

Etiology

The kidneys ultrafilter blood, secrete and absorb the filtrate in the renal tubules, and eliminate urine through the ureters, bladder, and urethra. Acute renal failure results from a problem at any stage of this process. Prerenal azotemia occurs because of a decrease in blood delivered to the kidney, renal azotemia from a malfunction within the renal parenchyma, and postrenal azotemia from an obstruction of urinary flow.

Epidemiology

Because renal failure is associated with a sixfold to eightfold increase in mortality among hospitalized patients, identification of high-risk patients and attention to kidney insults are critical.

Causes

1. Prerenal

a. Fluid volume loss (diarrhea, diuresis)

b. Impaired cardiac output

    c. Renal vasoconstriction (nonsteroidal antiinflammatory medications, ACE inhibitors)

    d. Decreased systemic vascular resistance as seen in sepsis, pancreatitis, cirrhosis, and afterload-reducing drugs

    e. Decreased oncotic vascular volume support: nephrosis, severe catabolic states

    f. Hepatorenal syndrome: labeled "prerenal" because when the involved kidney is transplanted into a normal host, it functions normally

2. Renal

    a. Acute tubular necrosis (ATN)

      (1) Perfusional deficits (prolonged prerenal failure, shock, hypovolemia, sepsis, pancreatitis, low-output states, coronary artery bypass graft [CABG] surgery, aortic aneurysm repair)

      (2) Pigment nephropathy: myoglobinuria (rhabdomyolysis), hemoglobinuria

      (3) Contrast-agent toxicity

      (4) Drug toxicity: aminoglycosides, cisplatinum, pentamidine, lithium, amphotericin

      (5) Crystal-induced ATN: acyclovir, sulfonamides, methotrexate, oxylate from ethylene glycol ingestion or high dose of vitamin C

      (6) Uric acid deposition in the tumor lysis syndrome

    b. Acute and subacute glomerulonephropathies (GNs)

      (1) Poststreptococcal glomerulonephritis (PSGN)

      (2) IgA nephropathy glomerulonephritis (Berger's disease)

      (3) Membranous nephropathy

      (4) Membranoproliferative nephropathy

      (5) Lupus nephritis

      (6) Focal segmental glomerulosclerosis

      (7) Rapidly progressive GN (50% loss of renal function in 3 months)

      (8) Diabetic nephropathy (Kimmelstiel-Wilson syndrome)

    c. Drug-induced interstitial nephritis

      (1) Penicillins, cephalosporins

      (2) Trimethoprim-sulfamethoxazole

      (3) Rifampin

      (4) NSAIDs

      (5) Diuretics

      (6) Cimetidine, allopurinol, amphetamines, sulfinpyrazone

    d. Chronic tubulointerstitial nephritis

      (1) Analgesic nephropathy

      (2) Lead

    e. Acute or chronic renal failure secondary to vascular disorders

      (1) Atheromatous emboli

      (2) Major renal vascular occlusive disease

      (3) Disseminated coagulopathy with acute renal failure

        (a) Hemolytic/uremic syndrome

        (b) Thrombotic thrombocytopenic purpura

        (c) Malignant hypertension

      (4) Nephrosclerosis secondary to chronic essential hypertension: characteristic benign sediment and minimum proteinuria

    f. Myeloma of the kidney; must be differentiated from hypercalcemic nephropathy, ATN, and amyloid disease

    g. Renal tubular acidosis

3. Postrenal
   a. Urethral obstruction (prostatic hypertrophy, urethral stricture)
   b. Bladder calculi or neoplasms
   c. Pelvic or retroperitoneal neoplasms
   d. Bilateral ureteral obstruction (neoplasm, calculi)
   e. Retroperitoneal fibrosis

Diagnosis

The first step is to distinguish among prerenal, intrarenal, and postrenal causes by reviewing recent clinical events and drug therapy. The clinical evaluation should include

- Orthostatic changes
- Daily weights
- Urinary output (in particular, anuria)
- Fluid loss
- Heart failure
- Vascular catheterization within the last month
- Systemic diseases that may cause glomerulonephritis (e.g., lupus) or intestinal disease (e.g., myeloma)
- Past renal disease
- Medications
- Uremic symptoms (confusion, itching, pericarditis, asterixis)

Laboratory tests

1. CBC
2. BUN, creatinine
3. Serum electrolytes
4. Urine creatinine and sodium
5. Urinalysis (Table 6-30)
6. Bladder catheterization if urinary retention is a possibility
7. Renal ultrasound (for kidney size and to rule out obstructive uropathy)
8. Special tests for specific causes of glomerulonephritis
9. Renal biopsy in selected cases of "renal" failure

Effects of uremic toxins

1. General
   a. Anorexia, early satiety
   b. Nausea and vomiting
   c. Pruritus
   d. Fatigue, weakness
2. Cardiovascular
   a. Cardiomyopathy: with chronic fluid overload; concentric hypertrophy is common
   b. Pericarditis
   c. Accelerated atherogenesis: elevated triglycerides, decreased HDL
   d. Hypertension: multifactorial (sodium retention, disturbances of renin/angiotensin axis)

able 6-30   Findings in urine

Diagnosis	Urinary Sediment	Fractional Sodium Excretion $\dfrac{(\text{Urine}_{\text{Na}}/\text{Plasma}_{\text{Na}} \times 100)}{\text{Urine}_{\text{Creat}}/\text{Plasma}_{\text{Creat}}}$
Prerenal	Normal or few hyaline or granular casts	$<1\%$
Postrenal	Normal or hematuria, pyuria, and crystals	Not helpful
Renal		
Vascular	RBCs	Not helpful
Glomerulonephritis	RBCs, RBC casts, proteinuria	Not helpful
Interstitial nephritis	WBCs, WBC casts, eosinophils	Not helpful
Acute tubular necrosis	Pigmented granular casts	$>1\%$

- CNS: abnormalities range from neuromuscular irritability (e.g., "restless legs") to asterixis and coma (metabolic encephalopathy)
- Endocrine
  a. Abnormal glucose metabolism secondary to
    (1) Increased insulin resistance
    (2) Prolonged insulin half-life
    (3) Decreased gluconeogenesis
    (4) Increased renal threshold for glucose
  b. Decreased T_4: secondary to decreased protein binding; normal free T_4
- Hematopoietic
  a. Anemia*: usually normochromic, normocytic; multifactorial
    (1) Chronically depressed erythropoietin levels
    (2) Hemolysis
    (3) Blood loss
    (4) Folate deficiency
  b. Iron overload from transfusions
  c. Coagulopathy: platelet count is normal but with decreased platelet aggregation and adhesiveness
- Gastrointestinal
  a. Increased incidence of duodenitis (increased gastrin levels)
  b. Increased incidence of angiodysplasia of stomach and proximal intestine
  c. Autonomic neuropathy in diabetics
- Divalent ion disturbances
  a. Hyperphosphatemia and hypocalcemia

*Epoetin alfa, a recombinant human erythropoietin, is effective for treating anemia of chronic renal ailure.

    b. Hyperparathyroidism from hypocalcemic stimulus with increase bone resorption

    c. Aluminum retention from dietary phosphate binders (e.g., Amphojel

Management of acute renal failure

1. Prerenal
   a. Correct hypovolemia if present; treat heart failure
   b. Halt medications that could worsen the renal insufficiency (diuretics NSAIDs, ACE inhibitors)
2. Renal
   a. Halt medications that may be nephrotoxic
   b. Treat pyelonephritis if present
   c. If renal vascular disease is possible, consider obtaining a renal scan
   d. With euvolemic patients, fluid intake should equal urinary and othe losses, allowing insensible losses of 300 to 500 ml/day
   e. During recovery, urinary volumes will increase markedly with eac day, so observe for dehydration
3. Postrenal
   a. Bladder catheterization is usually necessary. A residual volume c more than 100 ml suggests obstruction. Ultrasonography can be use to investigate the ureter or renal pelvis for hydronephrosis. Uretera stents, percutaneous nephrostomy following urologic consultation
   b. Partial obstruction may yield variable daily urinary volumes (500 m to 4 L/day); during recovery urinary volumes increase gradually
   c. Polyuria and dehydration may occur after relief of obstruction
4. In general, monitor clinical biochemical status, particularly serum potas sium, and adjust doses of renally excreted medications

Management of chronic renal failure

1. Before dialysis is necessary
   a. Low-protein diet (40 g/day) may prolong remaining renal life
   b. Avoid dehydration (e.g., diuretics)
   c. Strict control of hypertension (emphasis should be on vasoactiv drugs)
   d. Adjust drug doses to correct for prolonged half-lives (particularl digoxin and aminoglycosides)
   e. Start phosphate binder and 1,25-dihydrocholecalciferol (Rocaltro therapy when serum calcium and phosphorus levels become abnorma
   f. Consider starting erythropoietin before dialysis
   g. Consider using ACE inhibitors to reduce glomerular hyperfiltration
2. Initiation of dialysis
   a. Urgent indications: pericarditis, neuropathy, CHF, hyperkalemia, an neuromuscular abnormalities (asterixis, seizures)
   b. Judgmental indications: creatinine clearance below 10 to 15 ml/mir progressive anorexia, weight loss, reversal of sleep pattern, pruritu uncontrolled fluid gains with hypertension and signs of CHF

Considerations in evaluating patient receiving long-term hemodialysis

1. Fluid overload caused by excessive interdialytic weight gain
2. Acute hyperkalemia

3. Pericarditis with tamponade
4. Hypoglycemia
5. Hyperosmolarity and hyperkalemia (frequent in diabetics)
6. Infection and sepsis (vascular access site, infective endocarditis)
7. Subdural hematoma secondary to heparin use during dialysis
8. Seizures secondary to osmotic shifts produced by dialysis
9. Arrhythmias caused by electrolyte shifts
10. GI bleeding secondary to coagulopathy, duodenitis, angiodysplasia
11. Hypercalcemia caused by excessive vitamin D replacement
12. Bone fractures secondary to osteodystrophy
13. Dementia possibly caused by elevated CNS aluminum concentrations
14. Rupture of a berry or aortic aneurysm in patients with polycystic kidneys
15. Higher incidence of pancreatitis, diverticular disease, carpal tunnel syndrome
16. Psychosocial disturbances (depression, loss of independence, denial)
17. Hepatitis and carrier state

Suggested readings

Bennet WM et al: *Drug prescribing in renal failure: dosing guidelines for adults,* ed 3, Philadelphia, 1994, American College of Physicians.

Finn WF: Diagnosis and management of acute tubular necrosis, *Med Clin North Am* 74:873-891, 1990.

Fiscihereder M, Trick W, Nath KA: Therapeutic strategies in the prevention of acute renal failure, *Semin Nephrol* 14:41-52, 1994.

Guidnard JP et al: Acute renal failure, *Crit Care Med* 21:5349-5351, 1993.

Levison SP: Renal disease in the elderly: the role of the renal biopsy, *Am J Kidney Dis* 16:300-306, 1990.

Lindeman RD, Tobin J, Schock NW: Longitudinal studies on the rate of decline in renal function with age, *J Am Geriatr Soc* 33:278-285, 1985.

Montoliu J et al: Acute and rapidly progressive forms of glomerulonephritis in the elderly, *J Am Geriatr Soc* 29:108-116, 1981.

Roy AT et al: Renal failure in older people, *J Am Geriatr Soc* 38:239-253, 1990.

Salvetti A et al: How to treat the hypertensive patient with early renal damage, *Am J Kidney Dis* 21:95-99, 1993.

 6.9.d.   ### HEMATURIA

Tom J. Wachtel, MD, and Jack L. Schwartzwald, MD

Definition

Hematuria is defined as red blood cells (RBCs) in the urine. Hematuria may indicate significant systemic or genitourinary disease. Hematuria is termed *gross* when bleeding discolors the urine and *microscopic* if bleeding is discovered by urinalysis.

In both cases the most common cause is UTI, which can easily be confirmed by urine culture and appropriately treated.

Differential diagnosis

1. Coagulopathy, anticoagulant medication
2. Pseudohematuria
   a. Urinalysis negative for blood and RBCs (beets, food dyes, pyridium, rifampin, porphyria)

     b. Urinalysis positive for blood, negative for RBCs (hemoglobin, myoglobin)

3. Glomerular lesions
   a. Glomerulonephritis
   b. Collagen vascular disease or vasculitis
   c. Benign familial hematuria
4. Nonglomerular lesions
   a. Pyelonephritis or UTI
   b. Polycystic kidney disease
   c. Granulomatous disease (TB)
   d. Interstitial nephritis
   e. Papillary necrosis
   f. Neoplasm (renal cell carcinoma and transitional cell carcinoma)
   g. Nephrolithiasis
   h. Inflammation of ureter, bladder, urethra, epididymis, or prostate
   i. Benign prostatic hyperplasia or prostate cancer
5. Trauma involving urinary tract
   a. History
      (1) Systemic disease
      (2) Prior kidney stone
      (3) Dysuria, frequency, urgency, hesitancy
      (4) Flank pain
      (5) Family history of renal disease (e.g., polycystic kidneys)
      (6) Weight loss, fever
      (7) Bleeding disorders, warfarin use
      (8) Recent urethral catheterization
   b. Physical exam
      (1) Abdomen, including bimanual for renal mass
      (2) Costovertebral angle area for tenderness
      (3) Rectal exam in male for prostate
      (4) Pelvic exam in female to ascertain urinary vs. genital source of bleeding
   c. Laboratory evaluation
      (1) Urinary dipstick (blood) test with urinalysis (for RBCs)
      (2) Urine culture
      (3) Urine for AFB (if tuberculosis suspected)
      (4) Serum creatinine
      (5) Urinary cytology
      (6) Further tests: if cause is unclear after history, examination, and basic laboratory tests, consider the following
         (a) Isolated hematuria on urinalysis or gross hematuria
            • CT scan or ultrasound of kidneys and ureters or IV pyelography to rule out a structural lesion in the upper urinary tract
            • Cytoscopy to evaluate bladder, urethra, and prostate
         (b) Nephritic sediment on urinalysis (proteinuria out of proportion to the RBCs or RBC or granular casts)
            • Tests for secondary glomerular diseases (fasting serum glucose, ANA, ASLO titer, complement levels)
            • Renal biopsy if primary glomerulonephritis suspected

Suggested readings

Abuelo JG: The diagnosis of hematuria, *Arch Intern Med* 143:967-970, 1983.

Abuelo JG: Proteinuria: diagnostic principles and procedures, *Ann Intern Med* 98:186-191, 1983.

Bartlow BG: Microhematuria: picking the fewest tests to make an accurate diagnosis, *Postgrad Med* 88:51-61, 1990.

Froom P, Ribak J, Benbassat J: Significance of microhaematuria in young adults, *Br Med J* 288:20-22, 1984.

Mariani AJ et al: The significance of adult hematuria: 1000 hematuria evaluations including a risk benefit and cost effectiveness analysis, *J Urol* 141:350-355, 1989.

Sutton JM: Evaluation of hematuria in adults, *JAMA* 263:2475-2480, 1990.

Woolhandler S et al: Dipstick urinalysis screening of asymptomatic adults for urinary tract disorders, *JAMA* 262:1215-1219, 1989.

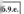 **6.9.e.**

ELECTROLYTES AND ACID-BASE DISORDERS
Tom J. Wachtel, MD

Sodium

1. Hyponatremia (serum Na <135 mEq/L) occurs when total body water is in relative excess to body Na. Total body water may be low, normal, or high
   a. Symptoms: confusion, lethargy, anorexia, cramps. Rapid Na drop can cause seizures
   b. Causes
      (1) Hypovolemia
         (a) Extrarenal sodium loss (urinary Na<10 mmol/L): diaphoresis; vomiting or diarrhea or both; pancreatitis
         (b) Renal loss (urinary Na >20 mmol/L): renal failure, diuretics, Addison's disease, salt-losing nephropathy
      (2) Isovolemia
         (a) Water intoxication (urinary Na <10 mmol/L)
         (b) Water retention (urinary Na >20 mmol/L): syndrome of inappropriate secretion of antidiuretic hormone (SIADH) (urinary osmolarity greater than serum osmolarity)
         (c) Sodium loss greater than water loss (urinary Na >20 mmol/L) with water intake compensation: Addison's disease, salt-losing nephropathy, hypothyroidism
      (3) Hypervolemia or edematous states (urinary Na <10 mmol/L)
         (a) Congestive heart failure
         (b) Cirrhosis
         (c) Nephrotic syndrome
2. Hypernatremia (serum Na >150 mEq/L) occurs in setting of a greater deficit of total body water relative to Na
   a. Symptoms: confusion, muscle twitching, seizures, coma
   b. Causes
      (1) Hypovolemia (water loss greater than sodium loss)
         (a) Extrarenal water loss: diaphoresis; vomiting or diarrhea or both; pancreatitis
         (b) Renal water loss: renal failure, diuretics, osmotic diuresis (e.g., hyperglycemia)
      (2) Isovolemia: diabetes insipidus

(3) Hypervolemia (gain of sodium greater than water)
  (a) Primary hyperaldosteronism
  (b) Cushing's syndrome
  (c) Hypertonic solution administration

Potassium

1. Hypokalemia (serum K <3.5 mEq/L)
   a. Symptoms: muscle weakness, cramps, ileus, ECG changes (U waves, increased Q-T interval, flat T waves); with severe hypokalemia: flaccid paralysis and cardiac arrest
   b. Causes
      (1) GI potassium losses (vomiting, diarrhea, villous adenoma, ureterosigmoidostomy)
      (2) Renal losses
         (a) Metabolic acidosis
         (b) Diuretics (thiazides, loop diuretics)
         (c) Excessive mineralocorticoid effect
            • Primary hyperaldosteronism
            • Secondary hyperaldosteronism
            • Cushing's syndrome and exogenous steroids
            • Licorice ingestion
         (d) Renal tubular acidosis and Liddle's syndrome
         (e) Hypomagnesemia
      (3) Potassium shift into cells
         (a) Insulin effect
         (b) Alkalosis
         (c) Hypokalemic periodic paralysis (may be associated with Graves' disease)
2. Hyperkalemia (serum K >5.5 mEq/L)
   a. Symptoms: ECG changes (peaked T waves→diminished R wave→wide QRS→loss of P wave→sine wave), arrhythmias; all exaggerated by decreased Na and Ca, increased Mg, acidosis, digitalis
   b. Causes
      (1) Inadequate excretion
         (a) Renal disease
         (b) Addison's disease
         (c) Potassium-sparing diuretics, ACE inhibitors
      (2) Potassium shift from intracellular to extracellular space
         (a) Crush injury
         (b) Acidosis
         (c) Hyperkalemic periodic paralysis
      (3) Excessive intake
      (4) Artifactual (in vitro hemolysis and poor venipuncture technique)

Metabolic acidosis (pH <7.35)

1. Low serum bicarbonate caused by addition of acids (increased anion gap acidosis: Na − [Cl + HCO$_3$] > 12 mEq/L) or loss of HCO$_3$ (normal anion gap acidosis)
2. Anion gap acidosis
   a. Diabetic ketoacidosis
   b. Renal failure

   c. Lactic acidosis
   d. Alcoholic ketoacidosis
   e. Starvation ketosis
   f. Salicylate poisoning
   g. Methanol poisoning
   h. Ethylene glycol poisoning
. Non–anion gap acidosis
   a. Diarrhea
   b. Renal tubular acidosis
   c. Enterostomy
   d. Ureterosigmoidostomy
   e. Hyperalimentation
   f. Acetazolamide
   g. Ammonium chloride, lysine HCl, arginine HCl

Metabolic alkalosis (pH >7.45)

. High serum bicarbonate caused by loss of acid (NaCl responsive, low urine chloride <10 mEq/L) or by hyperaldosteronism or hypokalemia (NaCl resistant, high urine chloride >20 mEq/L)
. NaCl responsive
   a. GI losses
      (1) Vomiting
      (2) Nasogastric suction
      (3) Chloride-wasting diarrhea
      (4) Villous adenoma (colon)
   b. Diuretic therapy
   c. Posthypercapnia
   d. Penicillin, carbenicillin
. NaCl resistant
   a. Hyperaldosteronism
   b. Cushing's syndrome
   c. Licorice
   d. Bartter's syndrome
   e. Refeeding alkalosis
   f. Alkali ingestion

Respiratory acidosis

. CO_2 retention caused by ventilating failure
. Symptoms: confusion, lethargy
. Causes
   a. COPD
   b. Sedative overdose
   c. Stroke
   d. Airway obstruction
   e. Neuromuscular diseases

Respiratory alkalosis

. CO_2 loss caused by hyperventilation
. Symptoms: tetany, seizures, syncope, arrhythmias
. Causes
   a. Anxiety, panic disorder

b. Lung diseases (e.g., asthma, pneumonia)
c. Sepsis
d. Salicylate poisoning
e. Hepatic failure
f. Hyperestrogenemic status
g. CNS lesions

6.9.f.   **PROTEINURIA**
Tom J. Wachtel, MD, and Jack L. Schwartzwald, MD

Epidemiology

Routine screening for proteinuria in asymptomatic adults is not currently recommended because fewer than 1.5% of patients with a positive result on qualitative testing will have significant treatable disease. However, proteinuria is frequently encountered when urinalysis is performed for other indications.

Patients with an underlying disease known to cause proteinuria should be offered episodic urine dipsticks for proteinuria (e.g., hypertension, lupus, multiple myeloma, diabetes) or a test for urinary microalbumin that detects 1/10 the concentration of albumin detectable by ordinary dipstick.

Pathophysiology

1. Excess protein can escape into the urine by three mechanisms
   a. Alteration of glomular permeability to protein secondary to pathologic or functional glomerular injury (glomerular proteinuria)
   b. Inadequate tubular reabsorption of normally filtered proteins secondary to tubulointerstitial disease such as a drug-induced or hereditary lesion (tubular proteinuria)
   c. Oversaturation of tubular reabsorptive capacity caused by increased production of low–molecular weight proteins that easily traverse filtration barriers such as occurs with light chains in patients with multiple myeloma (overload proteinuria)
2. Pathologic glomerular injury and overload proteinuria frequently cause >2 g of protein from 24-hour urine collection; functional glomerular injury (i.e., impaired glomerular function in the absence of structural lesions) and tubular injury are generally associated with <2 g/24 hr
3. Clinical manifestations of nephrotic syndrome are the result of specific protein deficiencies. Hypoalbuminemia results in edema, hypovolemia, hyperlipidemia, and toxicity of albumin-bound drugs. Antithrombin III deficiency results in hypercoagulability that can induce renal vein thrombosis and worsen the nephrotic syndrome. Hormone-binding globulin deficiencies result in falsely abnormal laboratory tests (e.g., low total thyroxine level), hypocalcemia, and osteomalacia. All are treated symptomatically

Etiology

1. Vasculitis or connective tissue diseases
2. Diabetes mellitus
3. Amyloidosis
4. Multiple myeloma
5. Endocarditis

6. Pyelonephritis
7. Medications: NSAIDs (e.g., tolmetin), high-dose ACE inhibitors (e.g., captopril), allopurinol, gold, pencillamine, amphotericin B, gentamicin, penicillin analogs
8. Congestive heart failure
9. Hypertension
10. Exposure to extremes of temperature
11. Febrile illness
12. Seizures
13. Strenuous exercise
14. Emotional stress
15. Primary glomerulonephritis or nephrotic syndrome
   a. Idiopathic nephrotic syndrome
      (1) Minimal change glomerulopathy (10% to 15%) responds to steroids and alkylating agents; relapse occurs in 30% of cases
      (2) Focal sclerosing glomerulopathy (10% to 15%) does not respond to steroids; course is relapsing or unremitting with progressive renal failure in 33% of cases; relapse occurs in 67% of grafts
   b. Immune complex disease
      (1) Membranous glomerulopathy (40% to 50%) responds variably to steroids; its course is unremitting in 75% of the cases and leads to progressive renal failure in 25%; recurrence in a graft is rare
      (2) Membranoproliferative glomerulonephritis (5% to 10%) does not respond to steroids; progressive renal failure occurs in 50% of cases and the disease recurs in grafts in 50%
      (3) Mesangial proliferative IgA glomerulonephritis (Berger's disease) (5% to 10%) has a benign course in 90% of cases; steroids may be useful, but 10% develop renal failure; recurrence rate in a graft is unknown
   c. Antiglomerular basement membrane disease (2%)
      (1) Rapidly progressive or crescentic glomerulonephritis (called Goodpasture's syndrome when there is pulmonary involvement) that does not respond to steroids but may respond to plasmapheresis
      (2) Renal failure occurs in 90% of cases and recurrence in grafts occurs in 33%
16. Causes of false-positive results on proteinuria testing
   a. Highly concentrated urine
   b. Gross hematuria
   c. Urinary pH >8.0 (e.g., infection with urea-splitting organisms)
   d. Contamination with the antiseptic used in the collection (chlorhexidine)

Tests

1. Qualitative tests detect presence or absence of proteinuria but can only grossly estimate amount (dipstick)
2. Quantitative tests for proteinuria
   a. Twenty-four–hour urine collection for protein and creatinine: patient discards first urine on the morning of the collection and then collects all samples up to and including the morning urine the next morning; an exact quantitation for protein can be obtained with this method

($>$3.5 g/24 hr represents nephrotic range proteinuria; $>$150 mg/24 hr is abnormal). The acceptability of the sample is confirmed by the quantity of creatinine, which should grossly match the predicted daily creatinine excretion derived from the Cockroft-Gault formulas (as follows)

  (1) Male patients: $(140 - \text{Age})(\text{Weight in kilograms})/5000$
  (2) Female patients: $(140 - \text{Age})(\text{Weight in kilograms})(0.85)/5000$
  b. Alternatively, a protein/creatinine ratio obtained from a single daytime urine sample (other than the first morning sample) correlates well with 24-hour quantitative measurements. A spot urine sample is sent for protein and creatinine determinations. A protein/creatinine ratio $>$3.5 is consistent with nephrotic range proteinuria; a ratio $<$0.2 is within normal limits

Management

1. If urinalysis is performed and proteinuria is present, check
   a. Serum creatinine level
   b. Other abnormalities in urinalysis (in particular hematuria)
   c. Because most of the 2 to 4 g of protein that normally leaks through the glomeruli is reabsorbed, the normal amount of protein excreted over 24 hours is less than 150 mg. This amount can increase with strenuous exercise (up to 300 mg/24 hr). In some patients, upright posture can produce proteinuria up to 1.5 g/24 hr without any underlying renal pathologic condition. Transient proteinuria can accompany a number of acute illnesses such as CHF, seizures, and febrile illnesses (particularly pneumonia). Amount of protein is usually less than 0.5 g/24 hr but can be as high as 2 g/24 hr and does not persist beyond duration of underlying illness
2. If proteinuria is found on qualitative test, repeat testing is indicated for all patients with proteinuria; if any reversible cause (e.g., medications, fever, strenuous exercise) is present, repeat testing should be deferred until the cause has been removed for at least 48 hours
3. If repeat test result is abnormal, proceed to quantitative test; if normal, presume that patient had a false-positive test or transient proteinuria
4. If proteinuria $>$150 mg/24 hr but $<$3.5 g/24 hr, rule out secondary causes (e.g., diabetes, hypertension, lupus and other connective tissue diseases, endocarditis, multiple myeloma); if none is found, refer patient to nephrologist
5. If quantitative test reveals nephrotic range proteinuria, refer patient to nephrologist

Suggested readings

Abuelo JG: Proteinuria: diagnostic principles and procedures, *Ann Intern Med* 98:186-191, 1983.

Ginsberg JM et al: Use of single voided urine samples to estimate quantitative proteinuria, *N Engl J Med* 309:1543-1546, 1983.

Stone RA: Office evaluation of the patient with proteinuria, *Postgrad Med* 86:241-244, 1989.

Woolandler S, Pels RJ, Bor DH: Dipstick urinalysis screening of asymptomatic adults for urinary tract disorders, *JAMA* 262:1214-1219, 1989.

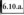 **HEMATOLOGY**

6.10 **HEMATOLOGY**

6.10.a. *ANEMIA*
Bruce Bialor, MD

Definition

Anemia is a reduction in circulating red blood cell (RBC) mass: hemoglobin <12 g/dl (hematocrit <36%) in menstruating women and <14 g/dl (hematocrit <42%) in men and postmenopausal women.

Etiology

1. Decreased RBC production (low reticulocyte index)
   a. Anemias with low mean corpuscular volume (MCV) (microcytic anemias)
      (1) Iron deficiency
      (2) Anemia of chronic inflammation
      (3) Thalassemia
      (4) Sideroblastic anemia
   b. Anemias with high MCV (macrocytic anemias)
      (1) Megaloblastic anemia
         (a) Vitamin B_{12} deficiency
         (b) Folic acid deficiency
         (c) Drugs
      (2) Alcoholism
      (3) Myelodysplastic syndromes
      (4) Hypothyroidism
      (5) Chronic liver disease
   c. Anemias with normal MCV (normocytic anemias)
      (1) Aplastic anemia
      (2) Anemia of chronic inflammation
      (3) Anemia of chronic renal insufficiency
      (4) Anemia associated with endocrine disorders
      (5) Sideroblastic anemia
      (6) Anemia associated with marrow infiltration (myelophthisis)
      (7) Chronic liver disease
2. Increased RBC destruction (appropriate reticulocyte index)
   a. Bleeding
   b. Hemolytic anemias
      (1) Hereditary
         (a) Abnormalities of RBC interior
            • Hemoglobinopathies (e.g., sickle cell, thalassemia, unstable hemoglobin variants)
            • Enzyme deficiencies (e.g., glucose-6-phosphate dehydrogenase [G6PD] deficiency, pyruvate kinase deficiency)
         (b) Membrane abnormalities
            • Hereditary spherocytosis
            • Hereditary elliptocytosis
            • Hereditary stomatocytosis

(2) Acquired
  (a) Splenomegaly
  (b) Immune mediated (immunohemolytic anemias)
   • Warm antibody
   • Idiopathic
   • Lymphomas: chronic lymphocytic leukemia, non-Hodgkin's lymphomas, Hodgkin's disease
   • Systemic lupus erythematosus
   • Drugs: alpha-methyldopa type, penicillin type (hapten), and quinidine type (innocent bystander)
   • Cold antibody
   • Cold agglutinin disease: acute (*Mycoplasma* infection, infectious mononucleosis) or chronic (idiopathic, lymphoma)
   • Paroxysmal cold hemoglobinuria: idiopathic or secondary to acute viral infections (e.g., measles and mumps) or tertiary syphilis
  (c) Trauma in the circulation
   • March hemoglobinuria (secondary to external impact)
   • Cardiac valve prosthesis
   • Microangiopathic hemolytic anemia (secondary to fibrin deposition in microvasculature): malignant hypertension, eclampsia, renal allograft rejection, disseminated cancer, hemangiomas, thrombotic thrombocytopenic purpura (TTP), hemolytic uremic syndrome (HUS), and disseminated intravascular coagulation (DIC)
  (d) Direct toxic effect
   • Infections (e.g., malaria, *Clostridium welchii,* babesiosis)
   • Physical agents (e.g., extensive burns)
   • Chemicals (e.g., copper toxicity in patients with Wilson's disease and in dialysis patients)
  (e) Membrane abnormalities
   • Spur cell anemia (usually seen in adults with advanced cirrhosis)
   • Paroxysmal nocturnal hemoglobinuria (PNH)

Evaluation

1. History
  a. Symptoms: depend on etiology, degree, and rapidity of onset; when onset is gradual, symptoms related to tissue hypoxia (e.g., fatigue, headache, dyspnea, lightheadedness, angina)
  b. Rapidity of onset: sudden onset suggestive of hemolysis or acute hemorrhage; gradual onset suggestive of chronic process (e.g., vitamin B_{12} deficiency, malignancy)
  c. Associated symptoms: e.g., melena, hematochezia, hematuria, menorrhagia (blood loss); jaundice, darkening of urine (hemolysis); paresthesias, confusion, ataxia (vitamin B_{12} deficiency)
  d. Drug and toxin exposures: e.g., alcohol, lead, isoniazid, quinidine, benzene, alkylating agents, methotrexate, sulfa compounds, zidovudine, trimethoprim, colchicine, phenytoin

    e. Family and ethnic history: sickle cell disease, thalassemia, other hereditary hemolytic anemias

    f. Other past medical history: e.g., endocrine disorders, inflammatory disorders, chronic infections; cholelithiasis at an early age (may suggest a hereditary hemolytic anemia); valve replacement

2. Physical exam

    a. General appearance: assess nutritional status

    b. Vital signs: tachycardia, hypotension (the latter in acute blood loss)

    c. Skin: pallor; jaundice (hemolysis); petechiae, purpura (thrombocytopenia); spider angiomas, palmar erythema (liver disease)

    d. Mouth: glossitis (pernicious anemia, Plummer-Vinson syndrome)

    e. Cardiac: prosthetic valve (traumatic hemolysis)

    f. Abdomen: splenomegaly (infiltrative disorders, hemolytic disorders, megaloblastic anemias, liver disease)

    g. Rectal: occult or gross blood in the stool

    h. Lymphadenopathy: infiltrative disease, infections, collagen vascular disease

    i. Neurologic: e.g., impaired vibratory and position sense, impaired cognition suggestive of vitamin B_{12} deficiency; acute mental status changes and/or neurologic deficits seen in TTP

3. Laboratory results

    a. Hemoglobin (Hb) and hematocrit (Hct)

      (1) Estimate of RBC mass

      (2) Does not take into account patient's volume status, so must be interpreted with caution (e.g., Hb normal immediately after acute blood loss, until compensatory mechanisms restore normal plasma volume; Hb low but RBC mass normal in pregnancy because of increased plasma volume)

    b. Reticulocyte count

      (1) Indicator of bone marrow response to anemia

      (2) Reticulocyte index corrects for degree of anemia

$$\text{Reticulocyte index (RI)} = \frac{1}{2}\left(\text{Reticulocyte count} \times \frac{\text{Patient Hct}}{\text{Normal Hct}}\right)$$

      (3) RI >2% to 3% suggests increased RBC destruction

          RI <2% to 3% suggests decreased RBC production

    c. Mean corpuscular volume (MCV)

      (1) Classifies anemia as microcytic, macrocytic, or normocytic

      (2) Should be interpreted in context of an evaluation of peripheral smear, because

         (a) Small and large cells may be present simultaneously, resulting in a normal MCV

         (b) MCV may be spuriously elevated by reticulocytes (which are larger than mature RBCs)

         (c) Abnormal cells may be present in numbers too small to affect the MCV

    d. Red-cell distribution width (RDW)

      (1) A measure of anisocytosis (e.g., multifactorial anemia)

      (2) May be useful in differentiating anemias sharing similar MCV

ranges (e.g., thalassemia and iron deficiency both characterized by low MCV, the former with normal RDW, the latter often with increased RDW)

(3) Elevated before MCV becomes abnormal in early iron, folic acid, and vitamin B_{12} deficiency

e. Peripheral smear: examine for RBC morphology (best done on a portion of the smear where RBCs are just touching one another), white blood cell (WBC) and platelet abnormalities, and other abnormalities

  (1) RBC morphology

    (a) Size: microcytosis, macrocytosis, anisocytosis

    (b) Shape

- Spherocytes (hereditary spherocytosis, immunohemolytic anemia)
- Teardrop cells (myeloproliferative diseases, pernicious anemia, thalassemia)
- Schistocytes (traumatic and microangiopathic hemolysis)
- Sickle cells (sickle cell disease)
- Target cells (liver disease, sickle cell disease, thalassemias, hemoglobin C, hereditary stomatocytosis)
- Burr cells or echinocytes (uremia)
- Acanthocytes or spur cells (spur cell anemia)

    (c) Color: hypochromia (iron deficiency, sideroblastic anemias), hyperchromia (megaloblastic anemia, spherocytosis)

  (2) WBC and platelet abnormalities

    (a) Hypersegmentation: megaloblastic anemias

    (b) Immature WBC forms: marrow infiltrative disorders

    (c) Large or increased numbers of platelets: myeloproliferative disorders

    (d) Bizarre or misshaped platelets: megaloblastic anemias

  (3) Other abnormalities

    (a) Basophilic stippling: lead poisoning, thalassemias, hemolysis, megaloblastic anemias

    (b) Nucleated RBCs: marrow infiltrative disorders, hemolysis, megaloblastic anemias

    (c) Howell-Jolly bodies (nuclear fragments): hemolytic and megaloblastic anemias, functional or anatomic asplenia

    (d) Heinz bodies (precipitated Hb; identification requires supravital stain such as crystal violet): unstable Hb variants, Hb H disease, other hemolytic disorders (e.g., G6PD deficiency)

    (e) Rouleaux formation: multiple myeloma, Waldenstrom's macroglobulinemia

    (f) Cabot ring (nuclear remnants): megaloblastic anemias

    (g) Pappenheimer bodies: hemolytic, sideroblastic, and megaloblastic anemias; postsplenectomy

    (h) Bite cells: anemias associated with Heinz body formation

Further evaluation

1. Microcytic anemia

  a. Serum ferritin

    (1) If <12 µg/dl (normal 12 to 300), indicative of iron deficiency

      (2) Since it is an acute-phase reactant, level may be normal or increased in inflammatory states, liver disease, infection, or malignancy

      (3) If >200 μg/dl, generally indicates adequate iron stores

      (4) Normal or increased in sideroblastic anemia and thalassemias

  b. Serum iron (Fe) and total iron-binding capacity (TIBC) (ratio called transferrin saturation)

      (1) Fe is usually decreased and TIBC is usually elevated in iron-deficiency anemia (rise in TIBC occurs before drop in Fe); however, these changes occur later than does the decline in serum ferritin

      (2) Both Fe and TIBC decreased in anemia of chronic inflammation (transferrin saturation usually $>10\%$)

      (3) Both are normal or increased in sideroblastic anemias and thalassemia

  c. Hemoglobin electrophoresis

      (1) Shows increased Hb A_2 and is the definitive diagnostic test for heterozygous beta-thalassemia

  d. General

      (1) Any adult male or postmenopausal female with iron-deficiency anemia is assumed to have a GI malignancy until proven otherwise

      (2) In iron-deficiency anemia, decline in MCV is usually proportional to degree of anemia. Mild microcytic anemia with MCV decreased out of proportion to degree of anemia (once iron deficiency is ruled out), in which Hb A_2 is normal, is consistent with heterozygous alpha-thalassemia (normal Hb electrophoresis)

      (3) To determine if a patient with a chronic inflammatory disease (e.g., rheumatoid arthritis) has become iron deficient, it may be necessary to either give a trial of iron therapy or check marrow iron stores

      (4) Bone marrow aspiration and biopsy indicated in the evaluation of *any unexplained anemia;* definitive way to diagnose iron deficiency and the only way to diagnose sideroblastic anemia (i.e., by finding ringed sideroblasts)

2. Macrocytic anemias

  a. Thyroid-stimulating hormone level, liver function tests

  b. Reticulocyte count, since reticulocytosis may cause spurious elevation of the MCV (for each increase in the reticulocyte count by 1%, the MCV will increase by 2 fL)

  c. Careful history of drug and toxin exposures (as outlined above)

  d. Serum B_{12} and RBC folate levels

      (1) Serum folate: not a reliable indicator of tissue folate levels, since it may reflect recent changes in dietary intake

      (2) Severe B_{12} deficiency can cause falsely low levels of RBC folate, despite adequate folate intake

      (3) Severe deficiency of either vitamin causes megaloblastic changes in intestinal epithelial cells, which can lead to malabsorption of the other

  e. Schilling test if B_{12} deficient, to investigate cause (e.g., pernicious anemia, bacterial overgrowth, or ileal disease)

f. Bone marrow aspiration and biopsy if macrocytic anemia remains un-explained (to look for a myelodysplastic syndrome), especially if other cell lines also affected

g. Neurologic symptoms of B_{12} deficiency can occur in absence of ane-mia (especially in patients with normal or supranormal levels of fo-late intake) and may not remit completely with treatment

3. Normocytic anemias

a. If no underlying systemic disease (e.g., chronic infection or inflam-mation) is known to exist that would explain anemia, one should search for one of these conditions, as well as renal disease, endocrine disease (e.g., hypothyroidism, hypogonadism, Addison's disease), liver disease, possible occult malignancy

b. If such a condition is found, in addition to treating the underlying dis-order one should look for other factors that may be exacerbating the anemia (e.g., blood loss, nutritional deficiency)

c. If the anemia remains unexplained, bone marrow aspiration and bi-opsy should be considered (looking for aplasia as well as marrow in-filtrative disorders), especially if the WBC and platelet counts are also reduced

4. Hemolytic anemias

a. Coombs' test should be done in all patients with suspected hemolysis

(1) Direct: detects the presence of IgG and C3 on the surface of RBCs

(2) Indirect: detects the presence of anti-RBC antibodies circulating in the patient's serum

b. Other tests

(1) Elevated total bilirubin, elevated lactate dehydrogenase, and decreased or absent haptoglobin can be helpful in establishing the presence of hemolysis but are not helpful in establishing the cause

(2) Other evaluation depends on the results of the initial evaluation

(a) Patients with a Coombs'-positive hemolytic anemia may re-quire ANA, CT scan of chest and abdomen, bone marrow as-piration and biopsy (the latter two to rule out lymphoma), as well as *Mycoplasma* titers

(b) Acid hemolysis or sucrose lysis test to rule out PNH (in the setting of recurrent venous thrombosis and/or mild pancyto-penia)

(c) Osmotic fragility test in a patient with spherocytes on periph-eral smear (to rule out hereditary spherocytosis)

(d) Hb electrophoresis in a patient with target cells on peripheral smear (to look for unstable Hb variants, thalassemia, sickle cell disease)

(e) Liver function tests in a patient with spur cells on peripheral smear (to rule out spur cell anemia)

(f) Platelets, BUN/creatinine, PT/PTT, fibrin degradation prod-ucts, and fibrinogen in a patient with schistocytes on periph-eral smear (to rule out DIC, TTP)

(g) G6PD level in a patient who has had a hemolytic episode (with Heinz bodies on peripheral smear) after certain drug exposures (e.g., sulfonamides, nitrofurantoin, antimalarials)

Treatment

1. Microcytic anemias
   a. Iron deficiency
      (1) Once the cause is determined, iron stores are repleted with either oral $FeSO_4$ (325 mg three times daily) or parenteral iron (i.e., iron dextran for patients with poor absorption, very high iron requirements, or intolerance of oral preparations)
      (2) Therapy usually required for at least 6 months
      (3) Reticulocyte count will peak in 5 to 10 days, Hb will rise over 1 to 2 months
      (4) If response is poor, consider noncompliance, continued blood loss, poor absorption, or a multifactorial anemia
   b. Anemia of chronic inflammation
      (1) Treat underlying condition
      (2) Prevent exacerbating factors, e.g., nutritional deficiencies, marrow-suppressive drugs
      (3) Consider erythropoietin
   c. Thalassemia
      (1) No treatment required for asymptomatic heterozygous forms
      (2) Genetic counseling of couples in which both are heterozygotes (25% chance of a couple, both of whom are heterozygous for beta-thalassemia, having a child who is homozygous for beta-thalassemia)
   d. Sideroblastic anemia
      (1) Eliminate potential precipitants (e.g., isoniazid, alcohol, lead)
      (2) Empiric trial of pyridoxine 50 to 200 mg daily, although response rate is low
      (3) In idiopathic acquired cases (i.e., refractory anemia with ringed sideroblasts, which is one of the myelodysplastic syndromes), therapy is supportive (i.e., transfusions as needed, avoiding marrow-suppressive drugs and nutritional deficiencies)
2. Macrocytic anemias
   a. Megaloblastic anemias
      (1) Eliminate potential precipitants (e.g., drugs such as methotrexate, trimethoprim, phenytoin)
      (2) Folic acid deficiency treated with folic acid 1 mg by mouth daily until deficiency corrected; may be indefinite in patients with high baseline requirements (e.g., patients with chronic hemolytic anemias and patients on hemodialysis)
      (3) Vitamin B_{12} deficiency corrected with cyanocobalamin, typically 1000 μg IM daily for 7 days, then weekly for 1 to 2 months, then every month indefinitely unless reversible cause found. Reticulocyte count usually peaks in 1 week, with Hb rising over 6 to 8 weeks
   b. Myelodysplastic syndromes
      (1) Therapy is supportive, as mentioned above for refractory anemia with ringed sideroblasts
   c. Other causes (i.e., hypothyroidism, liver disease, alcoholism)
      (1) Treat underlying disorder
3. Normocytic anemias
   a. Those associated with systemic disease are best treated by treating underlying condition

b. Treatment of sideroblastic anemia as discussed above
c. Erythropoietin therapy now an important treatment option for patients with anemia of chronic renal insufficiency and for selected patients with anemia associated with HIV infection
d. If aplastic anemia is suspected, urgent referral to a hematologist is recommended. Acutely, therapy is largely supportive. In patients <30 to 35 years, allogeneic bone marrow transplantation is an important consideration

4. Hemolytic anemias: In general, the treatment depends on the cause (see examples below); however, most cases require referral to a hematologist
   a. Sickle cell anemia
      (1) Maintain hydration and oxygenation to minimize frequency of pain crises
      (2) Long-term folic acid supplementation
      (3) Pneumococcal polysaccharide vaccine; aggressive treatment of infections
      (4) During pain crises, adequate analgesia in addition to hydration and oxygenation
      (5) Transfusion only in certain circumstances (e.g., aplastic crisis, severe recurrent pain crises requiring frequent hospitalizations, acute chest syndrome)
   b. G6PD deficiency
      (1) Avoidance of precipitants
      (2) Hydration and supportive therapy during acute hemolytic episodes
   c. Hereditary spherocytosis
      (1) Splenectomy
      (2) Folic acid therapy
   d. Immunohemolytic anemias
      (1) Treatment of underlying cause if discovered
      (2) Discontinuance of potentially offending agents
      (3) Glucocorticoids (prednisone 1.0 to 1.5 mg/kg/day orally until Hct stabilizes, then tapered over several months): initial treatment of choice for clinically significant warm antibody–induced hemolysis; splenectomy: second line of therapy, followed by cytotoxic therapy (specifically azathioprine or cyclophosphamide) in refractory cases

Suggested readings

Gailani D: Anemia and transfusion therapy. In Woodley M, Whelan A, editors: *Manual of medical therapeutics,* ed 27, Boston, 1992, Little, Brown.

Waterbury L: Anemia. In Barker LR, Burton JR, Zieve PD, editors: *Principles of ambulatory medicine,* ed 3, Baltimore, 1991, Williams & Wilkins.

Wilson JD et al, editors: *Harrison's principles of internal medicine,* ed 12, New York, 1991, McGraw-Hill.

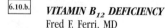

6.10.b.   *VITAMIN B₁₂ DEFICIENCY*
Fred F. Ferri, MD

Prevalence

Vitamin B_{12} (cobalamin) deficiency occurs in 5% to 10% of the elderly.

Etiology

1. Pernicious anemia (antibodies against intrinsic factor and gastric parietal cells)
2. Malabsorption (small bowel disease, pancreatic insufficiency, gastric abnormalities)
3. Inadequate dietary intake
4. Interference with cobalamin absorption (e.g., cholestyramine)
5. Chronic alcoholism (multifactorial)

Clinical presentation

1. Fatigue, anorexia, glossitis, apathy
2. Patients with severe deficiency can present with significant neurologic findings (paresthesia, ataxia, loss of position and vibration senses, memory impairment, depression, dementia)
3. Neuropsychiatric disorders caused by cobalamin deficiency are common and may occur in the absence of anemia or macrocytosis

Diagnosis

1. Diagnosis is crucial because failure to treat may result in irreversible neurologic deficits
2. Low serum cobalamin level is generally sufficient for diagnosis
3. Falsely low levels can be seen in patients with severe folate deficiency, in patients using high doses of ascorbic acid, and when cobalamin levels are measured following nuclear medicine studies (radioactivity interferes with cobalamin RIA measurement)
4. Falsely high or normal levels in patients with cobalamin deficiency can occur in severe liver disease and chronic granulocytic leukemia
5. Absence of anemia or macrocytosis does not exclude the diagnosis of cobalamin deficiency
   a. Anemia is absent in 20% of patients with cobalamin deficiency
   b. Macrocytosis is absent in over 30% of patients at time of diagnosis. It can be blocked by concurrent iron deficiency or anemia of chronic disease and may be masked by thalassemia trait. Red-cell distribution width (RDW) is increased in patients with combined iron and cobalamin deficiency and normal MCV
6. Schilling test: should not be routinely performed in suspected cobalamin deficiency, but is needed to establish its etiology; normal Schilling test is often misleading and may miss cobalamin deficiency in early stages
7. The following tests have been reported as useful in detecting cobalamin deficiency in patients with normal serum B_{12} levels; however, they are expensive and not routinely available in most laboratories
   a. Elevated levels of serum and urine methylmalonic acid
   b. Elevated total homocysteine level
   c. Positive intrinsic factor antibody level

Therapy

1. Traditional therapy of cobalamin deficiency consists of IM injections of 1000 mg weekly for 4 to 6 weeks followed by 1000 mg monthly indefinitely

2. Oral cobalamin (1000 mg PO qd): safe, effective, and inexpensive alternative in patients with inadequate dietary intake, provided normal cobalamin levels are ensured

6.10.c.

HEMATOLOGIC MALIGNANCIES
Tom J. Wachtel, MD

Acute lymphoblastic leukemia

1. Clinical features
   a. Fortyish male
   b. Constitutional symptoms and signs: fatigue, weakness, pallor, weight loss
   c. Easy bruising and bleeding
   d. Infections (pharyngitis, pneumonia, UTI, perirectal abscess)
   e. Lymphadenopathy, hepatosplenomegaly
   f. Meningeal signs
2. Laboratory findings
   a. CBC
      (1) Usually lymphocytosis
      (2) Occasionally lymphopenia
      (3) Peripheral blasts
      (4) Anemia, granulocytopenia, thrombocytopenia
   b. Bone marrow: increased blasts (>30%)
   c. Special studies (cytochemistry and immunologic reactivity studies)
3. Treatment: chemotherapy
4. Prognosis
   a. Complete remission: 90%
   b. Five-year disease-free state: 40%

Hairy cell leukemia

1. Clinical features
   a. Fiftyish male (4:1 male/female ratio)
   b. Constitutional findings: weakness, fatigue
   c. Splenomegaly (90% of cases at presentation)
2. Laboratory findings
   a. CBC
      (1) Single cytopenia
      (2) Pancytopenia
      (3) Peripheral hairy cells
   b. Bone marrow: dry tap
3. Treatment
   a. None if asymptomatic (may remain so for years)
   b. Splenectomy for severe cytopenias
   c. Chemotherapy for severe cytopenias before or after splenectomy
4. Prognosis: long-term survival (median close to 8 years)

Chronic lymphocytic leukemia

1. Clinical features
   a. Disease of the elderly

b. Incidental finding on CBC
c. Constitutional symptoms: weakness, fatigue, weight loss
d. Lymphadenopathy
e. Infections

2. Laboratory
   a. CBC: lymphocytosis ($>$15,000/ml)
   b. Bone marrow examination not needed

3. Treatment: no cure
   a. Palliative chemotherapy indications
      (1) Bone marrow failure (cytopenias)
      (2) Bulky symptomatic disease
      (3) Autoimmune hemolysis
      (4) Extreme lymphocytosis ($>$100,000/ml)
   b. Palliative local radiation

4. Prognosis
   a. Stage 0: lymphocytosis only—$>$10 years
   b. Stage I: lymphocytosis and lymphadenopathy—8 years
   c. Stage II: lymphocytosis and hepatomegaly or splenomegaly—5 years
   d. Stage III: lymphocytosis and anemia—2½ years
   e. Stage IV: lymphocytosis and thrombocytopenia—2½ years

Acute myelogenous leukemia

1. Classification
   a. Myeloblastic (45%)
   b. Promyelocytic (10%)
   c. Myelomonocytic (30%)
   d. Monocytic (10%)
   e. Erythroleukemia (5%)
   f. Megakaryocytic (3%)

2. Clinical features
   a. Signs of anemia (fatigue, pallor, dyspnea)
   b. Signs of thrombocytopenia (bruising, bleeding)
   c. Signs of neutropenia (infections)
   d. Others
      (1) Disseminated intravascular coagulation (promyelocytic)
      (2) Skin or mucosal infiltration (myelomonocytic, monocytic)
      (3) Splenomegaly
      (4) History of myelodysplasia

3. Laboratory findings
   a. CBC
      (1) Peripheral blasts (Auer rods in myeloblastic)
      (2) Pancytopenia
   b. Bone marrow: hypercellular with many blast cells
   c. Special studies (cytochemistry and monoclonal antibodies)

4. Treatment and prognosis
   a. Chemotherapy
   b. Bone marrow transplantation (initial treatment or after first relapse) achieves 50% 5-year survival rate

Chronic myelogenous leukemia

1. Clinical features
   a. Chronic phase
      (1) Asymptomatic (20%)
      (2) Signs of anemia
      (3) Signs of thrombocytopenia
      (4) Splenomegaly
   b. Acute phase (blast crisis) occurs 3 to 4 years after diagnosis
      (1) Fever, weight loss
      (2) Worsening anemia or thrombocytopenia
      (3) Bone pain
      (4) Increasing splenomegaly
      (5) Skin infiltration
2. Laboratory findings
   a. Chronic phase
      (1) CBC
         (a) Granulocytosis (50,000 to 200,000 cells/ml), including a few blasts ($<5\%$)
         (b) Anemia
         (c) Thrombocytosis
      (2) Decreased leukocyte alkaline phosphatase level
      (3) Elevated serum B_{12} level
      (4) Philadelphia chromosome
      (5) Bone marrow hypercellular, but blasts $<5\%$
   b. Acute phase
      (1) CBC
         (a) Increasing granulocytosis with blasts and promyelocytes
         (b) Worsening anemia
         (c) Worsening thrombocytosis or thrombocytopenia
         (d) More basophils
      (2) Bone marrow: increasing fibrosis
3. Treatment and prognosis
   a. Chemotherapy
   b. Bone marrow transplantation achieves 60% 5-year survival rate when done in chronic phase and 40% in acute phase
   c. Without bone marrow transplantation, survival time is 4 months from onset of blast crisis

Essential thrombocytosis

1. Clinical features: bleeding and/or thrombotic events
2. Laboratory findings
   a. CBC: $>1,000,000$ platelets per milliliter
   b. Bone marrow: increased megakaryocytes
3. Treatment: palliative chemotherapy
4. Prognosis: 10 to 15 years median survival time

Polycythemia vera

1. Clinical features
   a. Asymptomatic
   b. Bruising, bleeding

    c. Headaches

    d. Pruritus

    e. Splenomegaly

2. Laboratory findings

    a. CBC

       (1) Hct >55%

       (2) Leukocytosis (not seen in secondary polycythemia)

       (3) Thrombocytosis (not seen in secondary polycythemia)

    b. Bone marrow: trilinear hyperplasia (not seen in secondary polycythemia)

    c. Red cell mass measurement (increased)

3. Differential diagnosis

    a. Relative polycythemia (normal red cell mass)

    b. Secondary polycythemia (elevated red cell mass) seen in

       (1) Chronic hypoxemia

       (2) Elevated carboxyhemoglobin level

       (3) Hemoglobinopathy with high oxygen-affinity Hb

       (4) Renal disease (malignant or benign)

       (5) Hepatic, ovarian, adrenal, cerebellar neoplasms

4. Treatment: palliative reduction of Hct

    a. Phlebotomy

    b. Phosphorus 32 (increases risk of acute leukemia)

    c. Chemotherapy (hydroxyurea)

5. Prognosis: median survival time, 10 to 15 years

Hodgkin's disease

1. Clinical features

    a. Bimodal age distribution: 15 to 40 years or in fifties

    b. Lymphadenopathy

    c. Splenomegaly (40%), hepatomegaly (10%)

    d. Respiratory symptoms (cough, dyspnea)

    e. Pleural effusion

    f. B symptoms: fever, night sweats, weight loss

    g. Pruritus (not a B symptom)

2. Laboratory grade and tests

    a. Lymph node biopsy (frequency of histologic type)

       (1) Lymphocytic predominance (10%): excellent prognosis

       (2) Nodular sclerosis (55%): excellent prognosis

       (3) Mixed cellularity (30%): good prognosis

       (4) Lymphocytic depletion (5%): poor prognosis

         NOTE: (3) and (4) are associated with abundant Reed-Sternberg cells

    b. Staging workup

       (1) Chest x-ray study followed by chest CT scan if chest x-ray film is suspicious

       (2) Abdominal CT scan

       (3) Bone marrow examination

       (4) Lymphangiography

       (5) Staging laparotomy and splenectomy unless obvious advanced disease

        (6) CBC, creatinine, AST, alkaline phosphatase, LDH, uric acid, cal-
cium
  c. Stages
     (1) I: single lymph node region
     (2) II: more than one lymph node region on same side of dia-
phragm
     (3) III: lymph node involvement in both sides of diaphragm
     (4) IV: diffuse extralymphatic involvement
3. Treatment and prognosis
  a. Radiotherapy alone at a specialized center for stages I, II, and III without B symptoms, extranodal spread, extensive splenic involvement,
pelvic nodal involvement, or bulky disease: 75% cure rate
  b. Chemotherapy alone or with radiation therapy for advanced disease:
50% cure rate

Non-Hodgkin's lymphoma

1. Clinical features
  a. Typical age of onset: sixth decade
  b. Lymphadenopathy
  c. Symptoms of anemia
  d. B symptoms
  e. GI symptoms if site involved
  f. Hepatomegaly or splenomegaly
2. Laboratory findings and grade
  a. Lymph node biopsy
     (1) Low grade: favorable prognosis
       (a) Small cell lymphocytic
       (b) Follicular, small cleaved cell
       (c) Follicular, mixed small cleaved cell and large cell
     (2) Intermediate grade: unfavorable prognosis
       (a) Follicular, large cell
       (b) Diffuse, small cleaved cell
       (c) Diffuse, large cell
     (3) High grade: unfavorable prognosis
       (a) Large cell immunoblastic
       (b) Lymphoblastic
       (c) Small noncleaved cell (Burkitt's lymphoma)
  b. Laboratory tests and staging are same as for Hodgkin's disease except that lymphangiography and laparotomy are not necessary
3. Treatment and prognosis
  a. Favorable types are not curable; but median survival time is 6 years,
and 25% of patients live 12 years or longer. Treatment: palliative chemotherapy
  b. Unfavorable types at advanced stages (III and IV) are treated with
combined chemotherapy for potential cure. Complete remission:
achieved in two thirds of cases, half of whom are probably cured (most
relapses occur within 2 years)
  c. Unfavorable types at early stages (I and II): best treated with combined chemotherapy (80% cure rate). Stage I can also be treated with
radiotherapy

Multiple myeloma

1. Clinical features
   a. Typical age of onset: seventh decade (rare before 40 years of age)
   b. More common in African-Americans
   c. Bone pain (two thirds of patients)
   d. Symptoms of anemia
   e. Renal failure
   f. Hypercalcemia
   g. Cord or root compression
   h. Infection (especially pneumococcal pneumonia)
2. Laboratory findings
   a. CBC: anemia
   b. Elevated ESR
   c. Serum protein electrophoresis: monoclonal protein (>3 g/dl) in 90%, hypogammaglobulinemia in 10%
   d. Serum immunoelectrophoresis: monoclonal proteins IgG (50%), IgA (20%), light chain (17%), or IgD (2%)
   e. Urinary electrophoresis shows a globulin peak in 80%
      NOTE: 99% of patients with multiple myeloma have a monoclonal protein in serum or urine
   f. Serum creatinine, calcium, uric acid levels may be elevated
   g. Alkaline phosphatase level may be normal
   h. Bone x-ray films may show osteoporosis, lytic lesion, or fractures (75% have findings at presentation)
   i. Bone scan may be normal
   j. Bone marrow examination reveals at least $>10\%$ plasma cells, often $>20\%$ in sheets
3. Differential diagnosis: mainly that of monoclonal gammopathies
   a. Plasmacytoma
   b. Lymphomas
   c. Waldenstrom's macroglobulinemia
   d. Heavy-chain diseases
   e. Amyloidosis
   f. "Benign" monoclonal gammopathies
   g. Presence of bone pain, anemia, renal failure, bone marrow plasmacytosis ($>10\%$), and a >3 g/dl monoclonal serum protein level indicates multiple myeloma
4. Treatment
   a. Standard chemotherapy (melphalan and prednisone in 6-week cycles)
   b. Combined chemotherapy may be better in more advanced disease
   c. Localized radiation should be avoided because it accelerates bone marrow failure
   d. Biphosphonates (i.e., pamidronate [Aredia])

Suggested readings

Hutton JJ: The leukemias and polycythemia vera. In Stein JH, editor: *Internal medicine*, ed 4, St Louis, 1994, Mosby.

Kyle RA: Multiple myeloma and the dysproteinemias. In Stein JH, editor: *Internal medicine*, ed 4, St Louis, 1994, Mosby.

Miller TP, Grogan TM: Hodgkin's disease and non-Hodgkin's lymphoma. In Stein JH, editor: *Internal medicine*, ed 4, St Louis, 1994, Mosby.

6.11   **ONCOLOGY**

6.11.a.   ***PROSTATE CANCER***
Fred F. Ferri, MD

Epidemiology

1. Prostate cancer has surpassed lung cancer as most common nonskin cancer in men
2. Over 100,000 cases are diagnosed yearly, and nearly 30,000 males die from prostate cancer each year
3. Incidence of prostate cancer increases with age: uncommon before age 50; 80% of new cases are diagnosed in patients 64 or older
4. Average age at time of diagnosis: 73 years
5. African-Americans in the United States have the highest incidence of prostate cancer in the world (one in every nine males)
6. Incidence is low in Asians

Clinical manifestations

1. Generally silent disease until it reaches advanced stages
2. Bone pain and pathologic fractures may be initial symptoms of prostate cancer
3. Local growth can cause symptoms of outflow obstruction

Diagnosis

1. Digital rectal examination may reveal an area of increased firmness. Ten percent of patients will have a negative digital rectal exam
2. Measurement of prostate-specific antigen (PSA) useful in early diagnosis of prostate cancer and also in monitoring efficacy of therapy
3. Transrectal prostatic ultrasonography generally regarded as more sensitive than digital rectal exam and useful to guide the biopsy; however, its use as a primary screening test is limited by cost and availability; most useful to detect an occult lesion in patients with elevated PSA but normal digital exam of prostate

Staging

1. Laboratory: elevation of acid phosphatase usually indicates metastases
2. Bone scan: useful to evaluate bone metastases (present or eventually develop in over 80% of patients with carcinoma of prostate)
3. CT scan and transrectal ultrasonography: may be useful in selected patients to assess extent of prostate cancer
4. Prostate cancer is staged according to criteria shown in Table 6-31
5. Gleason classification is also useful for prognosis (In the Gleason classification, histologic patterns are independently assigned numbers 1 to 5 [best- to least-differentiated]. These numbers are then added to give a total tumor score.)
   a. Prognosis generally good if score <5
   b. Scores 6 to 10 carry an intermediate prognosis
   c. Scores >10 correlate with anaplastic lesions with poor prognosis

Table 6-31 Tumor-Node-Metastasis (TNM) classification of prostate cancer

Primary Tumor

T_x Cannot be assessed
T_0 No evidence
T_1 Clinically unapparent, not palpable or visible by imaging
    T_{1a} Incidental histologic finding in ≤5% of resected tissue
    T_{1b} Incidental histologic finding in >5% of resected tissue
    T_{1c} Identified by needle biopsy (e.g., because of elevated PSA values) but not palpable or visible by imaging
T_2 Confined to prostate
    T_{2a} Involves half of a lobe or less
    T_{2b} Involves more than half of a lobe but not both lobes
    T_{2c} Involves both lobes
T_3 Extends through prostatic capsule
    T_{3a} Extends unilaterally
    T_{3b} Extends bilaterally
    T_{3c} Invades seminal vesicle (or vesicles)
T_4 Fixed or invades adjacent structures other than seminal vesicles
    T_{4a} Invades bladder neck, external sphincter, or rectum
    T_{4b} Invades levator muscles or is fixed to pelvic wall (or both)

Regional Lymph Nodes

N_x Cannot be assessed
N_0 No evidence
N_1 Metastasis in a single regional lymph node (largest dimension, ≤2 cm)
N_2 Metastasis in a single regional lymph node (largest dimension, >2 cm but ≤5 cm) or multiple nodes (largest dimension in all nodes, ≤5 cm)
N_3 Metastasis in a regional lymph node (largest dimension, >5 cm)

Distant Metastases

M_x Cannot be assessed
M_0 None
M_1 Distant metastases
    M_{1a} Nonregional lymph node (or nodes)
    M_{1b} Bone (or bones)
    M_{1c} One or more other sites

From Catalona WJ: Management of cancer of the prostate, *N Engl J Med* 331:997-999, 1994. Reproduced with permission.

Prostate cancer: staging classification

Stage	Sites of Involvement
A	Confined to prostate, no nodule palpable
B	Palpable nodule confined to gland
C	Local extension
D	Regional lymph nodes or distant metastasis

6. The ploidy of the tumor also has prognostic value: prognosis is better with diploid tumor cells, worse with aneuploid tumor cells

Therapy

1. Therapeutic approach varies with the following
   a. Stage of tumor
   b. Patient's life expectancy
   c. General medical condition
   d. Patient's treatment preference (e.g., patient may be opposed to orchiectomy)
2. Table 6-32 describes recommended treatment of prostate cancer according to the stage of the disease and qualifying conditions
3. Table 6-33 describes complications of treatment for prostate cancer

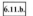 **LUNG CANCER**
Michael D. Stein, MD

Epidemiology

Lung cancer is the leading cause of cancer deaths for both men and women. It is usually discovered by x-ray abnormalities, persistent symptoms, or positive sputum cytology.

Risks

1. Cigarette use
2. Passive smoke inhalation
3. Radon
4. Asbestos
5. Nickel

History

1. Weight loss
2. Chronic cough
3. Hemoptysis (differential diagnosis includes pneumonia, tuberculosis, bronchitis, bronchiectasis, vasculitis, lung abscess, pulmonary embolism, aortic aneurysm, fungal infection, epistaxis)
4. Dyspnea
5. Recurrent or unresolving pneumonia
6. Bone pain
7. Seizure, headache, or other symptom of brain metastasis

Examination findings

1. Distention of neck vein, facial and upper extremity edema (superior vena cava [SVC] syndrome)
2. Pleural effusion
3. Localized wheezing
4. Ptosis, constricted pupil (Horner's syndrome)
5. Myopathy (Eaton-Lambert paraneoplastic syndrome)
6. Neuropathy (paraneoplastic syndromes)
7. Endocrinopathy (paraneoplastic syndromes such as SIADH)

Table 6-32 Recommended treatment of prostate cancer according to the stage of the disease and qualifying conditions

Stage/Qualifying Condition	Recommended Treatment
T_{1a}	
Projected life expectancy <10 yr	Watchful waiting
Projected life expectancy ≥10 yr	Radical prostatectomy, radiation therapy, watchful waiting
T_{1b}, T_{1c}, T_{2a}, T_{2b}, or T_{2c}	
Projected life expectancy <10 yr	Radiation therapy, hormonal therapy
Projected life expectancy ≥10 yr	Radical prostatectomy, radiation therapy, hormonal therapy
Positive surgical margins	
Focal and well or moderately differentiated	Watchful waiting
Diffuse and well or moderately differentiated	Radiation therapy
High-grade, diffuse, and poorly differentiated	Hormonal therapy
Lymph node metastases (with or without prostate removal)	Early or delayed hormonal therapy
Recurrence after surgery	
Without metastases	Radiation therapy
With metastases	Hormonal therapy
Recurrence after radiation	Hormonal therapy
T_3	Radiation therapy
T_4	Hormonal therapy
Persistently elevated serum acid phosphatase	
PSA ≥20 μg/L	Hormonal therapy
PSA <20 μg/L	Lymphadenectomy and radical prostatectomy, radiation therapy with or without lymphadenectomy, hormonal therapy
Disseminated disease	Hormonal therapy
Hormone-refractory disease	Radiation therapy, corticosteroid therapy, supportive therapy, chemotherapy, suramin

From Catalona WJ: Management of cancer of the prostate, *N Engl J Med* 331:997-999, 1994. Reproduced with permission.

Table 6-33 Complications of treatments for prostate cancer

Treatment	Complications (Incidence)	Comment
Radical prostatectomy	Blood loss of 1-2 L	Requires preoperative autologous blood donation with or without erythropoietin administration
	Impotence (30%-60%)	Varies with age and tumor stage; can be restored with vacuum erection device, intracorporeal injection of vasodilators, or implantation of penile prosthesis
	Urinary incontinence (5%-15%)	Can be treated with pelvic-floor muscle exercises, anticholinergic or alpha-adrenergic agonists, periurethral collagen or polytetrafluororethylene injections, antiincontinence clamp, or implantation of inflatable urinary sphincter
	Vesicourethral anastomotic stricture (0.6%-25%)	Corrected by dilation or, in rare cases, transurethral incision
	Rectal injury (0.1%-7%)	Usually repaired at time of primary surgery; occasionally requires temporary diverting colostomy
	Thromboembolism (1%-12%)	
	Myocardial infarction (0.4%)	
	Wound infection (0.4%-16%)	
	Lymphedema (1%-5%)	
	Lymphocele (0.4%-2.3%)	Treated with percutaneous drainage

Obturator nerve palsy (0.1%–0.3%)	Treated with physical therapy
Postoperative bleeding (0.1%)	Treated with surgical reexploration
Ureteral injury (0.1%–0.3%)	Treated with reimplantation
Death (0.1%–2%)	Risk varies with age and general medical condition of patient
External-beam radiation therapy	Acute (30%–50%): proctitis, cystitis, urinary retention, and penoscrotal edema	Treated with anticholinergic drugs or corticosteroid enemas
	Chronic (4%–7%): proctitis (2%), diarrhea (<1%), cystitis (8%), edema (<1%), enteritis (3%), impotence (40%–60%), urethral stricture (4%), incontinence (<1%), and death (<0.1%)	Hospitalization required for 5%–6% of patients, and surgery for 2%
Interstitial radiation therapy (open surgical)		
Intraoperative	Hemorrhage	
Early postoperative	Pelvic abscess, lymphocele, wound infection, hematoma, thrombophlebitis, pulmonary embolism, urinary retention, urinary fistula, and pelvic nerve palsy	
Late postoperative	Voiding symptoms (12%), lower extremity and genital edema (3%), rectal discomfort (3%), impotence (10%), ejaculatory disturbance, and prostatorectal fistula	

Continued

From Catalona WJ: Management of cancer of the prostate, *N Engl J Med* 331:998, 1994. Reproduced with permission.

Table 6-33 Complications of treatments for prostate cancer—cont'd

Treatment	Complications (Incidence)	Comment
Hemibody radiation	Nausea and vomiting, diarrhea, and bone marrow suppression	Treatment of symptoms and supportive measures
Hormonal therapy Orchiectomy	Hot flashes and decreased libido and sexual potency (in most patients), gynecomastia (rare), and wound hematoma or infection (1%-3%)	Hot flashes treated with clonidine (1 mg/day PO) or megestrol acetate (40 mg/day PO)
Diethylstilbestrol (1-3 mg/day PO)	Gynecomastia	Occurs with doses over 1 mg, can be prevented with pretreatment breast irradiation (12-18 Gy)
	Thromboembolism	Treated prophylactically with aspirin
	Fluid retention, GI upset, and decreased libido and sexual potency	
Gonadotropin-releasing hormone agonists		
Leuprolide acetate (depot dose, 7.5 mg/mo IM)	Decreased libido, decreased sexual potency, and hot flashes	Initial disease flare-up (in 5%-10% of patients) can be blocked with antiandrogen agent
Goserelin acetate implant (3.5 mg/mo SC)	Decreased libido, decreased sexual potency, and hot flashes	Initial disease flare-up (in 5%-10% of patients) can be blocked with antiandrogen agent
Flutamide (250 mg tid)	Gynecomastia, nausea, diarrhea, hepatotoxicity, and methemoglobinemia	An antiandrogen agent causing less sexual dysfunction than other hormones but not as effective as more complete androgen-deprivation therapy

Megestrol acetate (40 mg 2 to 4 times daily PO)	Fluid retention, shortness of breath, gynecomastia, and thromboembolism	A progestin with less severe cardiovascular side effects than those associated with estrogen
Ketoconazole (400 mg/8 hr PO)	Nausea and hepatotoxicity	Inhibits adrenal steroidogenesis; therefore hydrocortisone must also be given; used primarily for treatment of spinal cord compression
Chemotherapy		
Estramustine	GI upset and gynecomastia (8%-10%)	Affects mitotic-spindle function
Vinblastine	Neuropathy (12%), leukopenia (8%), and GI upset (20%)	Affects mitotic-spindle function
Suramin		
Earlier regimens (plasma concentration, 350 µg/L)	Malaise, anorexia, fatigue, metallic taste, adrenal necrosis, thrombocytopenia, coagulopathy, hepatitis, renal insufficiency, leukopenia, vortex keratopathy, rash, and polyradiculopathy	Side effects are reversible and are less severe with newer dose schedules; hydrocortisone supplementation is required
Newer regimens (plasma concentration, 150-250 µg/L)		

Evaluation

LABORATORY TESTS

1. CBC, electrolytes, calcium, creatinine, transaminases, PPD, pulmonary function test (if surgery planned)
2. Chest x-ray findings
   a. Often vary by cell type and may be associated with mediastinal adenopathy, pleural effusion, or lobar atelectasis
   b. Adenocarcinoma: peripheral nodule
   c. Squamous cell cancer: peripheral mass
   d. Small cell cancer: perihilar mass
3. Bronchoscopy or needle biopsy
4. Chest CT scan

DIFFERENTIAL DIAGNOSIS OF PULMONARY LESIONS

1. Tuberculosis
2. Sarcoidosis
3. Rheumatoid nodule
4. Fungal disease (histoplasmosis)
5. Septic emboli
6. Pneumonia
7. Aspergillosis
8. Metastatic cancer

STAGING

1. Tumor staging and histopathologic cell type are the two most important prognostic variables for lung cancer. The TNM staging system classifies non–small-cell lung cancer on the basis of primary tumor status *(T)*, regional lymph nodes *(N)*, and metastatic involvement *(M)*.
   a. Present stage

Primary Tumor *(T)*	
T_0	No evidence of primary tumor
T_1	A tumor ≤3 cm in greatest dimension, surrounded by lung or visceral pleura, and without evidence of invasion proximal to a lobar bronchus at bronchoscopy
T_2	A tumor >3 cm in greatest dimension or a tumor of any size that either invades visceral pleura or has associated atelectasis or obstructive pneumonitis that extends to hilar region; at bronchoscopy, proximal extent of demonstrable tumor must be within a lobar bronchus or at least 2 cm distal to carina; any associated atelectasis or obstructive pneumonitis must involve less than an entire lung
T_3	A tumor of any size with direct extension into chest wall (including superior sulcus tumors), diaphragm, or mediastinal pleura or pericardium without involving heart, great vessels, trachea, esophagus, or vertebral bodies or a tumor in main bronchus within 2 cm of carina without involving it

T$_4$ A tumor of any size with invasion of mediastinum or involving heart, great vessels, trachea, esophagus, vertebral bodies, or carina, or with presence of malignant pleural effusion

Nodal Involvement (N)

N$_0$	No demonstrable metastatic involvement of regional lymph nodes
N$_1$	Metastatic involvement of lymph nodes in peribronchial or ipsilateral hilar region, or both, including direct extension
N$_2$	Metastatic involvement of ipsilateral mediastinal lymph nodes and subcarinal lymph nodes
N$_3$	Metastatic involvement of contralateral mediastinal lymph nodes, contralateral hilar lymph nodes, or ipsilateral or contralateral scalene or supraclavicular lymph nodes

Distant Metastatic Involvement (M)

M$_0$	No (known) distant metastatic lesion
M$_1$	Distant metastatic involvement present; specify site(s)

Stage Grouping for Lung Cancer

Occult carcinoma	T$_X$	N$_0$	M$_0$
Stage 0	T$_{is}$	Carcinoma in situ	
Stage I	T$_1$	N$_0$	M$_0$
	T$_2$	N$_0$	M$_0$
Stage II	T$_1$	N$_1$	M$_0$
	T$_2$	N$_1$	M$_0$
Stage IIIa	T$_3$	N$_0$	M$_0$
	T$_3$	N$_1$	M$_0$
	T$_{1-3}$	N$_2$	M$_0$
Stage IIIb	Any T	N$_3$	M$_0$
	T$_4$	Any N	M$_0$
Stage IV	Any T	Any N	M$_1$

b. Tests for staging
   (1) CT scan: usually done of abdomen (liver, adrenals) to detect extrathoracic metastases; other frequent metastatic sites include lymph node, central nervous system, and bone; also used for performing needle biopsies and obtaining tissue specimens
   (2) Bronchoscopy: may be needed for obtaining tissue samples or to evaluate obstructive lesions
c. Prognosis

Stage	5-Year Survival Rate (%)
1	40-75
2	30-50
3	20-25
4	7-10

2. Small-cell cancer accounts for 25% of all pulmonary neoplasms and frequently has early, widespread dissemination; TNM staging does not apply

Treatment

1. Surgical reduction is indicated in patients with limited disease (15% to 30% of new patients) if pulmonary function test results are adequate and patient is otherwise medically stable
2. For unresectable non—small-cell cancers, palliative radiation therapy is used primarily for symptom relief, CNS or skeletal metastases, and SVC syndrome; can be used postoperatively with goal of reducing tumor recurrence in chest
3. Small-cell cancer often responds to chemotherapy or radiation

Suggested readings

Bechtel JJ: Outcome of 51 patients with roentgenographically occult lung cancer detected by sputum cytologic testing: a community hospital program, *Arch Intern Med* 154:975-980, 1994.

Eddy DM: Screening for lung carcinoma, *Arch Intern Med* 112:232-235, 1989.

Johnson BE et al: Ten year survival of patients with small cell lung cancer treated with combination chemotherapy with and without irradiation, *J Clin Oncol* 8:396-403, 1990.

Minna JD, Ihde DC, Glatstein EJ: Lung cancer: scalpels, beams, drugs and probes, *N Engl J Med* 315:1411-1414, 1986.

Mountain CF: A new international staging system for lung cancer, *Chest* 89:225S-233S, 1986.

DISEASES OF THE BREAST
Tom J. Wachtel, MD

Benign tumors

1. Fibroadenoma
   a. Most common cause of unilateral discrete mass in the 15- to 35-year age-group (peak incidence: 20 to 25 years of age)
   b. Multiple lesions in 10% to 15%
   c. Symptoms: painless mass, no discharge
   d. Examination: firm, smooth, nontender, circumscribed tumor
   e. Mammography: usually diagnostic
   f. Treatment: excisional biopsy
   g. Prognosis: not associated with breast cancer risk
2. Intraductal papilloma
   a. Occurs at any age
   b. Symptoms: recurrent serosanguineous nipple discharge

   c. Examination: no palpable lesion, but nipple discharge can be expressed
   d. Mammography: undependable
   e. Treatment: biopsy to exclude intraductal cancer
   f. Prognosis: slightly increased risk of breast cancer

3. Simple cyst
   a. Occurs during menstruating years
   b. Symptoms: painful lump that varies both in size and pain throughout menstrual cycle
   c. Examination: circumscribed, firm, tender lesion that varies in size with serial examinations
   d. Mammography: unreliable, but ultrasonography may be diagnostic
   e. Treatment: observation or biopsy
   f. Prognosis: not associated with breast cancer

4. Other benign lesions
   a. Fat necrosis
   b. Mammary duct ectasia
   c. Hamartomas
   d. Radial scars
   e. Granular cell tumors
   f. Cystosarcoma phyllodes (NOTE: 25% are malignant)

Fibrocystic changes

1. Not a disease: present in varying degrees in 90% of all women
2. Symptoms: dull ache in areas of most nodularity, most severe during premenstrual phase of cycle
3. Examination: lumpy breasts with tender moveable masses that vary over the cycle
4. Mammography: often difficult to interpret
5. Treatment: close observation by patient with self–breast exams and by physician with regular physical exams (at least yearly after age 40) and yearly mammography (beginning at age 35 to 40); danazol and tamoxifen can be used for pain control
6. Prognosis: association with breast cancer depends on other breast cancer risk factors (e.g., family history) and on the degrees of hyperplasia and atypia on biopsy if one is done. The 40% lifetime risk of breast cancer in patients with atypical hyperplasia and a positive family history may justify consideration of prophylactic simple bilateral mastectomy with breast reconstruction

Breast cancer

1. Epidemiology
   a. Lifetime cumulative incidence: one in nine adult women, increasing incidence with age
   b. 180,000 annual new cases per year in the United States and 40,000 annual deaths
   c. Risk factors
     (1) Age >50
     (2) Personal history of prior breast cancer

(3) First-degree relative with breast cancer, especially if bilateral or premenopausal

(4) Upper socioeconomic class

(5) Fibrocystic breast changes with atypical hyperplasia (less with simple hyperplasia)

(6) Personal history of endometrial or ovarian cancer

(7) Role of postmenopausal estrogen replacement not established but probably increases risk by 30%

2. Clinical features

   a. Screening

      (1) Breast self-exam monthly

      (2) Physical exam by physician every 3 years to age 40 and yearly thereafter

      (3) Mammography baseline at age 35, every 2 years from age 40 to 50, and yearly thereafter with no upper limit

   b. Evaluation of a breast mass

      (1) Under age 30, a palpable breast mass is most likely a fibroadenoma; mammography is not needed; elective excision is preferred treatment

      (2) Over age 30, mammography is always the first step in management. Other indications for diagnostic mammography include breast pain, skin thickening, nipple retraction, nipple discharge, nipple eczema, and axillary lymphadenopathy

      (3) For a palpable breast mass, a fine needle aspirate or a core needle biopsy should be done; accuracy is 90%; if aspirate or biopsy is benign, scrupulous follow-up is advised (see screening above)

      (4) For a nonpalpable suspicious lesion found on mammography, a stereotactic-guided fine needle aspirate should be performed. If sterotactic needle aspiration is negative, it should be repeated or patient should undergo open biopsy

      (5) If aspirate or biopsy is positive for breast cancer, patient should undergo surgical staging

3. Pathologic findings

   a. Ductal carcinoma in situ (20% of all cancer, 2% risk per year of developing invasive cancer)

   b. Lobular carcinoma in situ (2% : 1% risk per year of developing invasive cancer)

   c. Infiltrating ductal cancer (most common invasive cancer: 65%)

   d. Infiltrating lobular cancer (5%)

   e. Medullary cancer (5%)

   f. Mucinous cancer (2%)

   g. Tubular cancer (1%)

   h. Others (2%)

4. Staging

   a. In situ cancers: consider four-quadrant random biopsies to confirm in situ stage (controversial)

   b. Invasive cancer: two staging modalities

      (1) Modified radical mastectomy with axillary dissection

      (2) Lumpectomy with axillary node sampling

    c. Estrogen and progesterone receptor status of cancer must be done

    d. Flow cytometry may be useful prognosticator

    e. In addition, a complete physical exam, CBC, AST, alkaline phosphatase, and chest x-rays should be performed routinely. A bone scan is indicated only in patients with relevant symptoms, although some clinicians advise a baseline bone scan in all confirmed invasive cancer patients

4. Stage

    a. Tumor

      (1) T_0: no evidence of primary breast tumor

      (2) T_{is}: carcinoma in situ

      (3) T_1: tumor <2 cm in greatest dimension

        (a) Not fixed to pectoral muscle

        (b) Fixed to pectoral muscle

      (4) T_2: tumor 2 to 5 cm in greatest dimension

        (a) Not fixed to pectoral muscle

        (b) Fixed to pectoral muscle

      (5) T_3: tumor >5 cm in greatest dimension

        (a) Not fixed to pectoral muscle

        (b) Fixed to pectoral muscle

      (6) T_4: tumor fixed to chest wall or involving skin

    b. Lymph nodes

      (1) N_0: no regional lymph nodes

      (2) N_1: palpable, movable, ipsilateral lymph nodes

      (3) N_2: palpable, fixed, ipsilateral lymph nodes

      (4) N_3: ipsilateral, internal mammary lymph nodes

    c. Metastases

      (1) M_0: none

      (2) M_1: distant metastases present

5. Treatment guidelines

    a. Ductal carcinoma in situ

      (1) Diffuse disease confirmed by four-quadrant biopsies

        (a) Rx: simple mastectomy

      (2) Localized disease

        (a) Rx choice: simple mastectomy or breast-conserving surgery excision of lesion with clear microscopic margins followed by radiation

      (3) Consider tamoxifen 20 mg daily for 5 or more years

    b. Lobular carcinoma in situ

      (1) Rx choice: close follow-up or bilateral simple mastectomy (usually with breast reconstruction)

    c. Invasive breast cancer, early disease (stages T_1 and T_2) (currently 80% of all new breast cancers)

      (1) Step 1: definitive local treatment

        (a) Stage T_{1a} or T_{2a}—Rx choice: preferred option (breast-conserving surgery [lumpectomy] with axillary node dissection followed by radiation) or alternate option (modified radical mastectomy)

        (b) Stage T_{1b} or T_{2b}—Rx: modified radical mastectomy

(2) Step 2

    (a) Pathologic staging

    (b) Estrogen receptor (ER) and progesterone receptor (PgR) status

    (c) Flow cytometry

(3) Step 3: adjuvant therapy

    (a) T_{1a} N_0 with tumor <1 cm or too small for ER and PgR assay—Rx: observation or tamoxifen 10 to 20 mg daily for 5 years or longer

    (b) T_{1a} N_0 with ER+ or PgR+—Rx: observation (low-risk tumor by flow cytometry) or combined chemotherapy and/or tamoxifen (high-risk tumor by flow cytometry)

    (c) T_{2a} N_0 with ER+ or PgR+ or T_{1a}/T_{2a} N_0 with ER− and PgR−—Rx: combined chemotherapy and/or tamoxifen

    (d) T_1 or T_2 N_1 with ER+ or PgR+ and premenopausal—Rx: combined chemotherapy ± tamoxifen

    (e) T_1 or T_2 N_1 with ER+ or PgR+ and postmenopausal—Rx: tamoxifen ± combined chemotherapy

    (f) T_1 or T_2 N_1 with ER− and PgR−—Rx: combined chemotherapy

(4) NOTE: treatment in advanced age (e.g., 85+) has not been standardized; lumpectomy followed by tamoxifen is often recommended

d. Invasive advanced breast cancer

    (1) Stage T_3: preoperative debulking systemic chemotherapy followed by simple mastectomy (axillary node sampling is controversial) followed by chemotherapy. If complete tumor resection is not possible, treatment is palliative

    (2) Stage T_4: palliative treatment

7. Prognosis

  a. Favorable prognostic factors

    (1) Older age

    (2) Postmenopausal status

    (3) Small tumor size

    (4) Absent axillary lymph node involvement

    (5) High steroid hormone receptor content

    (6) Good tissue differentiation (by flow cytometry)

    (7) Absent intratumor lymphatic invasion on pathologic examination

    (8) Absent metastases

  b. Survival statistics by lymph node involvement

	5-year survival	10-year survival
Negative lymph node	78%	65%
1-3 positive lymph nodes	62%	37%
>4 positive lymph nodes	32%	13%

Gynecomastia (breast enlargement in men)

1. Causes
   a. Drugs
      (1) Estrogens and gonadotropins
      (2) Testosterone inhibitors (cimetidine, spironolactone, metronidazole, ketoconazole, antitumor agents)
      (3) Digitalis
      (4) Others: INH, methyldopa, narcotics, benzodiazepines, tricyclic antidepressants, penicillamine
   b. Increased estrogen secretion
      (1) Liver disease
      (2) Choriocarcinoma and other hCG-producing tumors
      (3) Adrenal cancer
      (4) Thyrotoxicosis
      (5) Hermaphroditism
   c. Decreased testosterone secretion
      (1) Castration
      (2) Orchitis
      (3) Renal failure
      (4) Various congenital defects (e.g., Klinefelter syndrome, testicular feminization)
   d. Idiopathic

6.11.d.   ***COLON CANCER***
           Tom J. Wachtel, MD

Epidemiology

1. 150,000 new cases per year in the United States
2. Risk factors for adenocarcinoma
   a. Family history (particularly first-degree relatives of persons with adenocarcinoma, including colon cancer, endometrial cancer, and ovarian cancer)
   b. Hereditary colon polyposis syndromes
   c. Diet: high fat, high refined carbohydrate, low fiber (i.e., typical Western diet)
   d. Inflammatory bowel disease (ulcerative colitis more so than Crohn's disease)
   e. Adenomatous polyps, usually villous adenoma, are premalignant lesions with respective <5% and 30% malignant transformation rates; hyperplastic polyps and hamartomas are not
3. Other colon tumors: carcinoid tumors (large ones >2 cm tend to metastasize), leiomyomas (rarely leiomyosarcomas), and lipomas

Pathologic findings

1. Grade
   a. Well differentiated are less aggressive than anaplastic tumors
   b. Mucin-producing tumors are the most malignant

2. Stage
   a. T_{is}:   carcinoma in situ
   b. T_1:   involvement of submucosa

   Duke's stage A if N_0

   c. T_2:   involvement of muscularis
   d. T_3:   involvement of subserosa

   Duke's stage B if N_0

   e. T_4:   involvement of visceral peritoneum
   f. N_0:   no lymph node involvement
   g. N_1:   involvement of <3 lymph nodes

   Duke's stage C if M_0

   h. N_2:   involvement of ≥4 lymph nodes
   i. N_3:   involvement of perivascular trunk
                lymph nodes
   j. M_0:   no distant metastases
   k. M_1:   any distant metastases (Duke's stage D)

Clinical presentation

1. Asymptomatic and discovered by screening (recommendations follow)
   a. Yearly digital rectal examination after age 40
   b. Yearly stool tests for occult blood (three pairs) after age 50 in low-risk persons and after age 40 in high-risk persons
   c. Flexible sigmoidoscopy at ages 50 and 51 and then every 5 years in low-risk persons (controversial)
   d. Colonoscopy or double air-contrast barium enema every 3 years after age 40 to 50 in high-risk persons (less controversial)
2. Occult fecal blood discovered for any reason or gross lower GI hemorrhage (may be melena if source is cecal; otherwise, hematochezia) must lead to appropriate tests to exclude colon cancer (e.g., colonoscopy and/or double air-contrast barium enemas) in all patients over age 40 even if hemorrhoids or other known causes of potential GI bleeding are present NOTE: if the search for a colonic lesion is negative, the upper GI tract should be evaluated (e.g., upper endoscopy)
3. Iron-deficiency anemia in any person above age 40 must be investigated similarly to patient with GI bleeding, regardless of presence or absence of blood in stool; right-sided colon cancers are more likely than left-sided lesions to present this way
4. Right lower quadrant mass (or less commonly elsewhere in the abdomen) may produce discomfort or may be discovered incidentally during a physical examination
5. Lower intestinal obstructive symptoms are more likely associated with a left-sided colon cancer; symptoms include constipation or diarrhea (new onset change in bowel movement is always worrisome in an older person) and abdominal pain; abdominal distention indicates (near) complete obstruction
6. Tenesmus and thin stools: signs of rectal cancer
7. Anorexia and weight loss: tend to be associated with advanced cancer
8. Liver: site of most metastases and rarely a patient will present with signs of hepatic failure or painless jaundice; hepatomegaly is usually found in such cases

Diagnostic tests

1. Double air-contrast barium enema
2. Colonoscopy alone or after barium enema is used to identify or confirm the lesion and obtain biopsy. In addition, it may identify a second cancer (in up to 5%) or polyps (in 50%)
3. CBC
4. Liver function tests (e.g., AST, alkaline phosphatase, and prothrombin time) followed by abdominal CT scan if abnormal
5. Preoperative carcinoembryonic antigen (CEA) that returns to normal after successful (complete) surgical cancer resection

Treatment

1. Right hemicolectomy for right-sided colon cancer
2. Left hemicolectomy for left-sided colon cancer
3. Abdominoperineal resection for rectal cancer within 6 to 8 cm of the rectal verge (sometimes preceded and followed by radiation)
4. Consider adjuvant chemotherapy with 5-fluorouracil and levamisole in advanced resectable cases
5. Palliative chemotherapy and radiation produce marginal benefits
6. Second-look surgical procedure in patient with rising CEA levels and surgical resection of localized liver metastasis may also provide marginal benefits

Prognosis

1. Duke's A: 90% to 95% cure rate
2. Duke's B: 70% to 80% cure rate
3. Duke's C: colon—50% cure rate; rectum—30% cure rate
4. Duke's D: not curable

Suggested readings

Barillari P et al: Relationship of symptom duration and survival in patients with colorectal carcinoma, *Eur J Surg Oncol* 15:441-445, 1989.

Friedman GD, Selby JV: Colorectal cancer: have we identified an effective screening strategy? *J Gen Intern Med* 5(suppl):S23-S27, 1990.

Lieberman DA: Colon cancer screening: the dilemma of positive screening tests, *Arch Intern Med* 150:740-744, 1990.

Ransohoff DF, Lang CA: Screening for colorectal cancer, *N Engl J Med* 325:37-41, 1991.

Stein W et al: Characteristics of colon cancer at time of presentation, *Fam Pract Res J* 13:355-363, 1993.

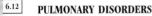

6.12   PULMONARY DISORDERS

6.12.a.   *CHRONIC OBSTRUCTIVE PULMONARY DISEASE*
Michael D. Stein, MD

Definition

Chronic obstructive pulmonary disease (COPD) is a spectrum of chronic respiratory illnesses characterized by dyspnea, cough, sputum production, impaired gas exchange, and airflow limitation.

Epidemiology

COPD affects approximately 15 million Americans and is the fifth leading cause of death in the United States. Because of less lung reserve and life-long exposures to risk factors, persons over 65 are more susceptible. Mortality 10 years after diagnosis is more than 50%.

Diagnosis

Abnormal pulmonary function test results with lower-than-expected ratio of forced expiratory volume in 1 second to the forced vital capacity (FEV_1/FVC) is indicative of airflow obstruction. Differential diagnosis includes

- Congestive heart failure
- Respiratory infections
- Anxiety disorders

Management

1. Reduce airflow obstruction
   a. Reversibility of airflow obstruction is minimal and variable
   b. Performing spirometry before and after using a bronchodilator and showing a 10% to 15% increment in FEV_1 with bronchodilator usage: indication for bronchodilator therapy. A trial of inhaled bronchodilators also can be attempted in other patients. Therapy individualized based on patient factors and contraindications (see the box below)
   c. Little evidence that thinning secretions provides clinical improvement. Acetylcysteine may loosen mucous plugs but does not increase FEV_1 and may induce bronchospasm
2. Correct secondary physiologic abnormalities (supply oxygen)
   a. For hypoxemic patients long-term oxygen therapy for 18 or more hours per day is effective
   b. Goal: to maintain oxygen saturation >90%
   c. Nocturnal administration of oxygen increase sleep quality, reduces nocturnal arrhythmias, and improves daytime activities

---

Indications for Supplemental Oxygen for COPD

Recommended indications
  Pao_2 ≤55 mm Hg or Sao_2 ≤89 at rest
  Pao_2 ≤55 mm Hg or Sao_2 ≤89 with exercise
  Pao_2 ≤55 mm Hg or Sao_2 ≤89 during sleep
Evidence of pulmonary hypertension or cor pulmonale, mental or psychologic impairment, or polycythemia and a Pao_2 of 56 to 59 mm Hg or Sao_2 ≤90% at any time
Medicare criteria for reimbursable oxygen supplementation
  Pao_2 ≤55 mm Hg or Sao_2 ≤89
  Pao_2 ≤56 to 59 mm Hg or Sao_2 ≤89 if evidence of cor pulmonale (P pulmonale, polycythemia, or congestive heart failure)

3. Improve functional status
   a. Exercise conditioning to improve maximal oxygen consumption and reduce ventilation and heart rate is critical for rehabilitation. This should be done in conjunction with an exercise physiologist or physical therapist. Focus on upper extremities may reduce dyspnea. Continuous positive airway pressure during exercise may allow longer periods of exertion
   b. Undernutrition (<90% ideal body weight) is common and is associated with reduced respiratory muscle function and increased mortality; nutritional supplementation may be necessary
4. Education and prevention
   a. Vaccination with pneumococcal vaccine once and influenza vaccine annually
   b. Smoking cessation
   c. Exacerbations with increased or purulent sputum should be treated with antibiotics such as trimethoprim-sulfamethoxazole (Septra) or ampicillin
   d. Education about medications and technique for using inhalers with spacers (see the box below) and suboptimal dosing (too little or too much)
   e. Advise patient to take medications before physical activity
   f. Suggest support groups to help patients overcome anger and depression
   g. Encourage activity as tolerated
   h. Regular spirometry to follow changes in lung function over time

Medications

1. Beta-agonist inhaler
   a. Two puffs qid: usual dose (with spacer)
   b. Side effects: palpitations, hypokalemia
2. Ipratropium (anticholinergic)
   a. Three to six puffs qid (with spacer)
   b. Can be combined with beta-agonist
   c. Slow onset, long duration make it more suitable for regular use rather than as-needed use
3. Theophylline
   a. Start with long-acting agent, 200 to 300 mg q12h
   b. Monitor for serum level of 10 to 20 mg/dl
   c. Controversial role because there is little bronchodilator effect beyond

---

Technique for Using Metered-Dose Inhaler

Point inhaler opening downward and shake.
Exhale normally.
Inhale slowly and spray during deep inhalation.
Hold breath 5 to 10 seconds.
Exhale slowly.
Second puff should be delivered 2 to 5 minutes later in same manner.

inhaled agent and has side effect risks (insomnia, tremor, nausea, seizures) that may limit use
   d. Should avoid caffeine, which may contribute to side effects, during use
4. Inhaled corticosteroids
   a. May have role in both short- and long-term administration
   b. Consider if airflow limitation continues despite therapy with beta-agonist or ipratroprium
   c. Two to four puffs qid
5. Oral steroids: prednisone, 40 mg/day for 14 days, then reduce dose to minimum possible (0 to 10 mg) to maintain FEV_1 and limit dyspnea and nocturnal symptoms

Suggested readings

Ferguson GT, Chermack RM: Management of chronic obstructive pulmonary disease, *N Engl J Med* 328:1017-1022, 1993.

St John RC, Gadek JE, Pacht ER: Chronic obstructive pulmonary disease: less common causes. An algorithm for the primary care physician, *J Gen Intern Med* 8:564-572, 1993.

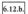 **ASTHMA**
Michael D. Stein, MD

Definition

Asthma is airway hyperresponsiveness to a variety of stimuli in which the underlying process is inflammation, leading to airflow obstruction and intermittent coughing, dyspnea, wheezing, chest tightness, or recurrent episodes of shortness of breath.

Epidemiology

Asthma is estimated to affect approximately 10% of Americans over 65 years old. Mortality has been increasing over the past two decades and is higher than in younger patients with asthma.

Differential diagnosis

1. Viral bronchitis
2. Allergic bronchitis
3. Recurrent pneumonia
4. Foreign body
5. Tracheomalacia
6. COPD
7. Congestive heart failure
8. Gastroesophageal reflux
9. Drug-induced cough (ACE inhibitor)
10. Tumor involving upper or lower respiratory tract

Physical examination

1. Decreased breath sounds
2. Wheezing
3. Expiratory slowing
4. Check for nasal polyps, sinusitis, eczema
5. Exclude congestive heart failure

Laboratory evaluation

1. Spirometric measures to demonstrate airflow obstruction
   a. Increase in forced expiratory volume (FEV_1) of at least 15% in first second after inhaling a bronchodilator
   b. Methacholine or exercise provocation of airway obstruction in patients with mild disease or symptoms only with exertion
   c. Chest x-ray study to evaluate other possible causes
   d. Allergy evaluation when history suggests specific allergens

Therapy

GOALS

1. 24-hour symptom control
2. Normal physical activity
3. Prevention of acute exacerbation

MANAGEMENT

1. Patients should be active in their own asthma care
2. Objective measurements of lung function in day-to-day management are useful because patients and physicians often underestimate extent of impairment. Use of home peak flowmeters daily in morning and evening allows for alterations in medication type or schedule. When morning-to-evening flow difference exceeds 20%, increase in antiinflammatory medication may be indicated
3. Attention to environmental triggers: 75% of patients demonstrate skin testing reactivity. Most common allergen is the house dust mite. If allergen avoidance is not possible and medications do not control symptoms, consider immunotherapy. When successful, immunotherapy should be continued monthly for 3 to 5 years; if there is no improvement during allergen seasons, therapy should be halted
4. Effective use of pharmacologic therapies depends on severity of asthma
5. Written lists of dosing schedules to optimize compliance
6. Attention to anxiety that may exacerbate symptoms

Medications

1. Mild asthma: short duration of symptoms, once or twice per week
   a. Use inhaled beta-agonist when symptoms are present
   b. Increasing doses of inhalers (daily use) suggest patient has moderate asthma
   c. Patients must be taught how to use inhalers properly, with or without a spacer device, and demonstrate their proficiency during physician visits
2. Moderate asthma: frequent symptoms only incompletely controlled by episodic inhaled beta-agonists; peak expiratory flow: 60% to 80% of predicted volume; nocturnal symptoms frequently interrupt sleep
   a. Inhaled beta-agonists should be primary medication for symptom relief
   b. Regular use of antiinflammatory agent (beclomethasone, triamcinolone, flunisolide) also required
   c. Consider using cromolyn (two puffs qid): takes several weeks to provide benefit
   d. Anticholinergics (e.g., ipratroprium)

6.13   **GASTROINTESTINAL DISORDERS**

6.13.a   *GASTROESOPHAGEAL REFLUX DISEASE*
Thomas A. Parrino, MD

Epidemiology

Approximately 4 in 10 adult Americans have heartburn at least monthly. Consequently, this symptom is very commonly presented to the general physician for evaluation and management. In the general medical office, issues arise as to the appropriateness of the initial evaluation, how to treat for resistant disease, when to refer for radiologic and endoscopic evaluation, and treatment for refractory symptoms.

Etiology and pathogenesis

Gastroesophageal reflux symptoms result from the retrograde flow of low-pH gastric contents into the esophagus. Esophageal mucosa lacks the ability to resist the effect of refluxing acid, and typical symptoms occur as a result (see below). Gastroesophageal reflux often occurs as a result of dysfunction of the lower esophageal sphincter (LES), which protects the esophageal mucosa. A number of substances affect esophageal sphincter function and predispose to the regurgitation of acidic gastric contents into the esophagus. These include nicotine, caffeine, and beta-blocking agents. Moreover, anatomic changes that adversely affect esophageal sphincter function, such as obesity, the development of ascites, and local anatomic distortion (by surgery, myotomy, dilation, and chronic esophagitis per se), predispose to the symptoms of gastroesophageal reflux.

History and physical examination

The history of esophageal reflux is typified by burning retrosternal discomfort, often accompanied by excessive salivation, or "water brash." The pain often occurs at night, when the patient is recumbent, and is often relieved by sitting up or walking about. Antacids, food, or water often relieves the symptoms. Associated symptoms may include belching and eructation. Because of the location of the pain, patient and physician may suspect a cardiac etiology, and both may be confused by relief from nitroglycerin. The physical examination is usually unremarkable, but the physician should take note of such factors as obesity and any additional medical problems.

Differential diagnosis

Peptic ulcer disease often presents with similar heartburn symptoms; however, midepigastric pain is a frequent feature of ulcer disease not seen with gastroesophageal reflux disease (GERD). Esophageal spasm (one variant of this is known as nutcracker esophagus) is another cause of severe retrosternal pain of sudden onset, occasionally relieved by nitroglycerin.

Related conditions and complications

Barrett's esophagus is a complication of long-standing esophageal reflux, wherein the appearance of the lining epithelium changes from squamous to columnar. With this histologic reversion, the risk of esophageal cancer begins to increase. Patients identified as having Barrett's esophagus are considered to be at risk for esophageal cancer, and regular surveillance endoscopies are therefore appropriate.

Cancer of the esophagus may be accompanied by reflux symptoms; however, the cardinal symptom is usually dysphagia (difficulty swallowing) or odynophagia (pain on swallowing). With increasing obstruction, the patient may no longer be able to take solids and must adopt a liquid diet.

Patients with local esophageal myopathies and systemic diseases, such as scleroderma and polymyositis, may present with reflux symptoms. The principal symptoms in such cases relate to the location of the physiologic dysfunction. With midesophageal involvement, obstructive symptoms may predominate. When the upper esophagus is involved, reflux symptoms rarely occur; the principal symptoms here relate to regurgitation of esophageal contents, often through the nose, on attempts to swallow.

Esophageal reflux disease is a common cause of *nocturnal asthma* and *night cough*. Here, the mechanism seems to be related to aspiration of acidic esophageal contents. It is important to recognize the contributing role of esophageal reflux in such cases, because the treatment is obviously different from that for primary disease of the airways. The chest pain of GERD may be confused with cardiac pain for several reasons

- It may be very severe, with a heavy quality, mimicking angina pectoris
- It may be relieved by nitroglycerin
- Gastroesophageal reflux can serve as a stimulus for the development of angina pectoris, sometimes through the activation of specific cardioesophageal reflexes, mediated through the vagus nerve

Hence, when symptoms are suggestive, cardiac evaluation should be conducted as part of the evaluation for midline chest pain thought to be caused by gastroesophageal reflux.

Diagnostic evaluation

RADIOLOGIC EVALUATION

Since heartburn is a common problem and many patients will complain of it, questions often arise as to the proper time to institute radiologic studies to rule out alternative possibilities, such as esophageal spasm, and exclude such conditions as esophageal cancer. As a general rule, radiologic evaluation is indicated when symptoms are very severe or if they do not respond to first-line therapy.

RADIOLOGIC FEATURES

On barium swallow, reflux of barium from stomach to esophagus is an important finding. Also important are contributing anatomic factors, such as the presence of strictures, diverticula, and hernias. The demonstration of hiatus hernias and esophageal rings (such as that described by Schatzki), once thought pathognomonic for GERD, are now noted only as associated features.

ENDOSCOPIC EVALUATION

Endoscopy should be carried out when there are concerns about the presence of Barrett's esophagus, esophageal cancer, or associated peptic ulcer disease. Endoscopic features of GERD may include the presence of inflammation in the lower esophagus (a consequence of acid reflux), bleeding points, and the specific features of Barrett's esophagus or esophageal cancer, if present.

ESOPHAGEAL MANOMETRY

Esophageal manometry is occasionally carried out to rule out the contribution of underlying neuromuscular disease.

Treatment

LIFE-STYLE CHANGE

Usually, the most important aspects of treatment revolve around life-style change. Weight reduction is often very helpful for obese patients. To prevent symptoms caused by recumbency, the patient should be counseled to elevate the head of the bed and to take antacids at bedtime. Also, patients should be cautioned against heavy meals, ingestion of aggravating foodstuffs, or use of alcohol late in the evening.

PHARMACOLOGIC APPROACHES

Antacids and coating agents

The mainstay of treatment for GERD has always been antacids, often taken in anticipation of symptoms, e.g., at bedtime. To minimize the production of gastric acid (and hence esophageal reflux of acid), a seven-dose antacid regimen (1 and 3 hours after meals and at bedtime) has proven effective. However, many patients find it inconvenient to adhere to such a regimen and are often inconvenienced by associated diarrhea caused by the antacids themselves. Sucralfate, a gastric coating agent, has been found effective, as well.

Anticholinergic agents

Agents such as atropine have long been used to reduce gastric acid secretion and are still recommended in some situations. However, such agents cause a number of problematic side effects, including urinary retention and exacerbation of glaucoma. Moreover, the effect of such agents on lower esophageal function may actually result in an increase in gastroesophageal acid reflux.

H_2 blockers

The appearance of H_2 blockers, such as cimetidine and ranitidine, has resulted in the relegation of antacids to a secondary role in the management of acid-peptic disease and GERD. H_2 blockers were initially thought ineffective (or marginally effective) for the treatment of GERD. Recently, however, studies showing the value of high-dose regimens (usually given at night) have been published, and H_2 blockers are considered to be among the mainstays of therapy for GERD.

PGE_1 analogs

Prostaglandins, such as misoprostol, reduce gastric acid secretion very effectively and therefore may be of adjunctive value in the management of GERD.

Proton pump inhibitors

The newer proton pump inhibitors, such as omeprazole and lansoperazole, have proven effective in treatment for GERD, but their expense has been a limiting factor. Recently, it has been shown that omeprazole may be the most cost-effective treatment for GERD when there is evidence of erosive esophagitis or after failure of H_2 blockers.

Prokinetic agents

Metaclopramide, the first of the prokinetic agents to become available, has been found effective in relief of reflux symptoms. However, the use of this medication in the elderly has been associated with a high prevalence of parkinsonism, tardive dyskinesia, and akathisia.

Combination therapy

Many clinicians have adopted a step care approach to the management of GERD, wherein pharmacologic agents are substituted for or added to the regimen, one at a time, until symptomatic relief occurs. One possible sequential approach might be as follows: antacid, H_2 blocker, sucralfate, metaclopramide or cisapride, proton pump inhibitor. If the patient remains symptomatic on "ideal" therapy, it may be reasonable to check the pH of the gastric contents to assess effectiveness/compliance with the regimen.

SURGERY

Surgery was at one time an important adjunct in the therapy of refractory GERD. Here, the objective was to fold the gastric fundus about the lower esophagus (fundoplication) to reduce acid reflux. With the advent of new pharmacologic approaches, surgery is performed much less frequently. Nonetheless, there has been extensive experience with surgery as an effective approach in difficult cases of GERD.

Gastroesophageal reflux in the elderly

Since the elderly patient may be subjected to the effects of gastroesophageal reflux over many years, the cumulative effects of the disease may not become readily evident for some time. In elderly patients, heartburn may be absent or mild, presumably because of decreased HCl secretion, and sometimes because of reduced awareness of such symptoms by the patient. Consequently, the disease and its complications may go unrecognized for some time. Elderly patients may also have a higher incidence of atypical complaints, such as night cough and asthma.

Suggested readings

Hillman AL et al: Cost and quality of alternative treatments for persistent GERD, *Arch Intern Med* 152:1467-1492, 1992.

Raiha I: Prevalence and characteristics of symptomatic gastroesophageal reflux disease in the elderly, *J Am Geriatr Soc* 40:1209-1211, 1992.

Richter JE: Surgery for reflux disease: reflections of a gastroenterologist, *N Engl J Med* 376:825-827, 1992.

Sontag SJ: Two doses of omeprazole v. placebo in symptomatic erosive esophagitis: the U.S. Multicenter study, *Gastroenterology* 102:109-118, 1992.

6.13.b.   **DYSPEPSIA**
Peter S. Margolis, MD

The many symptoms that characterize dyspepsia are very common complaints in the elderly. The prevalence of these symptoms may reach as high as 25% of this population. This prevalence is equal among men and women age 65 or older. Interestingly, the majority of elderly persons who experience dyspeptic-like symptoms report the onset within the previous 5 years.

A clear description of the symptoms will help separate these from the also very common reflux-related disease.

Definition

1. Dyspeptic pain
   a. Location: midepigastric; upper abdominal; possible right quadrant
   b. Character: variable
      (1) Sharp
      (2) Dull ache
      (3) Crampy
      (4) Bloating
      (5) Burning (most common)
   c. Timing
      (1) Classically related to meals
         (a) Either 30 to 60 minutes after, or
         (b) Later postprandial awakening at night
      (2) Often weekly to daily
2. Nausea
   a. Very frequent
   b. May occur with or without pain
   c. Postprandial (either immediate or late)
3. Associated symptoms
   a. Belching
   b. Bloating
   c. Flatulence
   d. Change of appetite
   e. Changes of weight

Etiology

1. Cause is often multifactorial but functional/motility disorders occur most frequently. The following are important risk factors
   a. NSAIDs/aspirin products
   b. Other medications
   c. Smoking
   d. *Helicobacter pylori*
   e. Alcohol
   f. Changes in eating arrangements or life-style
   g. Depression
   h. Death of or changes in caregiver
2. Aspirin/NSAIDs
   a. Very important risk factors with approximately 100 million prescribed annually

    b. Represent most frequently prescribed medication for elderly individuals

    c. Most likely medication to cause dyspepsia in this population

3. Medications (excluding NSAIDs)
    a. People 65 years and older represent 10% to 15% of the population yet receive >25% of prescription medication in the United States
    b. Many medications cause reproducible nausea (side effect)
    c. Others cause idiosyncratic response in individual patients

4. *H. pylori*
    a. Cause of peptic ulcer disease
    b. Probable cause of nonulcer dyspepsia
    c. Eradication recommended for documented ulcer disease
    d. Not proven beneficial for nonulcer dyspepsia

Workup

1. History and physical exam
2. Medication review (prescribed and homeopathic)
3. Upper endoscopy (EGD)
4. Upper GI radiology (UGI)
    a. EGD more sensitive and specific, will allow biopsy and therapy if needed
    b. UGI may complement EGD in selected patients; may be more accessible in rural settings

Treatment

1. Generally agreed to initiate therapy and workup together
    a. Discontinue offending agents
    b. Infrequent or mild symptoms: occasional antacid
    c. Frequent or more severe symptoms: histamine-2-reception antagonists (H2RA)
    d. Duration of therapy and dosage depends on endoscopic findings
    e. Proton pump inhibitor if H2RAs fail
2. Prophylaxis if NSAIDs needed
    a. Remains controversial
    b. Ranitidine may prevent duodenal ulcer
    c. Mesoprostil (Cytotech) may prevent both gastric and duodenal ulcers
    d. Must be individualized to patient

Suggested readings

Chandrakumaran K, Vaira D, Hobsley M: Duodenal ulcer, Helicobacter pylori, and gastric secretion, *Gut* 35:1033-1036, 1994.

Hawkey CJ: Gastroduodenal problems associated with non-steroidal, anti-inflammatory drugs (NSAIDs), *Scand J Gastroenterol Suppl* 200:94-95, 1993.

Jones RH, Tait CL: Gastrointestinal side effects of NSAIDs in the community, *Br J Clin Pract* 49:67-70, 1995.

Kay L: Prevalence, incidence and prognosis of gastrointestinal symptoms in a random sample of an elderly population, *Age Ageing* 23:146-149, 1994.

Kay L, Avlund K: Abdominal syndromes and functional ability in the elderly, *Aging* 6:420-426, 1994.

McCarthy C et al: Long-term prospective study of Helicobacter pylori in nonulcer dyspepsia, *Dig Dis Sci* 40:114-119, 1995.

Talley NJ et al: Nonsteroidal anti-inflammatory drugs and dyspepsia in the elderly, *Dig Dis Sci* 40:1345-1350, 1995.

Tham TC et al: Possible role of Helicobacter pylori serology in reducing endoscopy workload, *Postgrad Med J* 70:309-312, 1994.

Zaitoun AM: The prevalence of lymphoid follicles in Helicobacter pylori associated gastritis in patients with ulcers and non-ulcer dyspepsia, *J Clin Pathol* 48:325-329, 1995.

6.13.c. **HEPATOBILIARY DISEASES**
Jack L. Schwartzwald, MD

Age-related anatomic and functional changes in the liver are minimal. Liver chemistry tests in the elderly are expected to remain in normal range in the absence of disease. The ability of the aged liver to metabolize drugs may be mildly compromised because of reduced liver mass and cell number.

JAUNDICE

Jaundice in the elderly is more frequently a manifestation of biliary obstruction than hepatocellular disease. As a result, even in the setting of transaminitis it may be prudent to rule out an obstructing lesion with ultrasound imaging in geriatric patients. Elderly patients with nonobstructive jaundice are more likely to have drug-induced injury than the viral and alcohol-related causes seen most frequently in younger patients.

HEPATOBILIARY DISEASE

1. Although gallstones are more common in elderly than in young patients, a first episode of obstructive jaundice in a geriatric patient is more likely to be caused by malignancy (particularly cancer in the head of the pancreas) than by gallstones
2. Cancers of liver and biliary tree
   a. Hepatocellular carcinoma
      (1) Arises in chronically inflamed livers; alcohol and chronic viral hepatitis are leading risk factors
      (2) Adenocarcinoma is predominant cell type
      (3) Incidence low in the United States but high worldwide
      (4) Tumors are typically unresectable at the time of diagnosis because of advanced stage or underlying liver pathologic findings
      (5) Hepatic transplantation may be curative but is frequently shunned because of high rates of recurrent cancer
   b. Cancers of gallbladder and bile ducts are rare and do not usually present until after age of 50
      (1) Adenocarcinoma is most common cell type
      (2) Surgical resection is optimal therapy
3. Gallstones in the elderly
   a. Incidence increased because of prolonged cholesterol supersaturation of bile
   b. Prophylactic cholecystectomy for asymptomatic gallstones becomes riskier with increasing age; must be weighed against higher complication rate seen with surgery reserved for symptomatic cholelithiasis in the elderly
   c. Oral bile acids (chenodeoxycholic acid, ursodiol) have produced disappointing results in treatment of asymptomatic gallstones

d. Symptomatic (acute) cholecystitis may have an atypical or subtle presentation in the elderly, frequently resulting in delayed diagnosis. Cholecystectomy is the only effective therapy but carries a mortality approaching 10% in some series of elderly patients. Laparoscopic procedures are better tolerated than open procedures but carry a higher risk of common bile duct injury

e. Choledocholithiasis managed by endoscopic sphincterotomy and stone extraction

HEPATOCELLULAR DISEASE

1. Drug-induced injury: primary consideration in elderly patients with hepatocellular disease

   a. Hepatotoxicity from drugs more common and more severe in the elderly and may manifest as either acute or chronic insult

   b. Hundreds of prescription drugs are hepatotoxic. Discontinuation of the medication usually results in normalization of liver function tests; however, stable mild to moderate liver function test abnormalities (up to four times the upper normal limits) can be accepted if the medication is essential (e.g., anticonvulsants)

2. Alcoholic hepatitis less common in geriatric patient with transaminitis than in younger patients. Typical 2:1 ratio of AST/ALT seen with alcoholic hepatitis holds in the elderly population and may aid in diagnosis. Alcoholics at high risk for acetaminophen toxicity even at submaximal doses

3. As in younger patients, viral hepatitis should be ruled out with a hepatitis screen including types A, B and C, in elderly patients with transaminitis

4. Differential diagnosis of chronic hepatitis (transaminitis detected in the patient with stigmas of chronic liver disease or persisting >6 months) includes

   a. Drug induced

   b. Chronic active autoimmune hepatitis (positive antinuclear and anti–smooth muscle antibodies; portal infiltrates of lymphocytes and plasma cells on biopsy)

   c. Chronic hepatitis B or C

CIRRHOSIS

Hepatic cirrhosis implies diffuse hepatic fibrotic scarring with focal areas of nodular regeneration. It is a leading cause of death from the sixth to the eighth decades in the United States.

Definition

Hepatic cirrhosis implies diffuse hepatic fibrotic scarring with focal areas of nodular regeneration.

Etiology

1. Alcohol abuse
2. Postnecrotic

   a. Necrotizing infection (hepatitis B, hepatitis C)

   b. Drugs (isoniazid, amiodarone, methotrexate, metyldopa, acetaminophen [Tylenol])

   c. Toxins (carbon tetrachloride)

   d. Chronic autoimmune hepatitis

3. Metabolic disease
   a. Wilson's disease (rare in the elderly)
   b. Hemachromatosis
   c. Alpha$_1$-antitrypsin deficiency
   d. Glycogen storage disease (rare in elderly)
4. Cardiac cirrhosis (prolonged, recurrent, right-sided heart failure caused by tricuspid regurgitation, cardiomyopathy, or constrictive pericarditis)
5. Primary biliary cirrhosis
6. Impaired venous drainage of liver
   a. Portal vein thrombosis
   b. Inferior vena cava or hepatic vein occlusion (Budd-Chiari syndrome)
7. Chronic biliary tree obstruction
8. Other
   a. Schistosomiasis
   b. Infiltrative disease (amyloidosis)
   c. Sarcoidosis
   d. Cryptogenic

Evaluation

1. History
   a. May reveal clues to the etiology such as alcohol, drug, or toxin ingestion and risk factors for infectious hepatitis
   b. Hemochromatosis typically strikes older patients and features skin hyperpigmentation and hyperglycemia (bronze diabetes) as well as CHF, testicular atrophy, and arthritis
   c. Primary biliary cirrhosis seen most frequently in older women who present with jaundice, pruritus, hypercholesterolemia, and xanthomas
   d. Travel to an endemic area may raise suspicion for schistosomiasis
2. Physical exam
   a. Frequently reveals stigmas of chronic liver disease such as palmar erythema and Dupuytren's hand contracture, spider angiomas, caput medusae, gynecomastia or testicular atrophy in males, ecchymoses, and alopecia
   b. Hepatomegaly or a small nodular liver may be noted; splenomegaly occurs in portal hypertension
   c. Ascites and peripheral edema (anasarca) most likely to occur in setting of combined portal hypertension and hypoalbuminemia
   d. Jaundice accompanies cases with intrahepatic biliary obstruction
   e. Rectal exam may reveal hemorrhoids
   f. Other complications of cirrhosis may also yield physical exam findings, e.g., occult blood–positive stools or melena in patient with esophageal varices; asterixis and altered mental status in patient with hepatic encephalopathy
3. Laboratory evaluation
   a. Common findings: hypoalbuminemia, elevated prothrombin time, low BUN, hyponatremia, hypokalemia, and elevated MCV of red blood cells. Anemia may be seen in patients who experience GI bleeding
4. Liver biopsy indicated in all unexplained cases of cirrhosis
5. Hepatic imaging (CT or MRI) to evaluate sudden worsening where hepatoma may be the culprit

Management

1. General considerations
   a. All patients with cirrhosis should abstain from alcohol and other hepatotoxins
   b. Low-sodium diet and protein restriction (4.5 g/day) should be considered
   c. Monitor for hypokalemia and provide potassium replacement where indicated
   d. Oral or subcutaneous injection of vitamin K (10 mg/day for 3 days) in patients with elevated prothrombin time
   e. Consider multivitamins and folic acid
   f. Consider liver transplantation for otherwise healthy patients with refractory decompensated cirrhosis

2. Complications of cirrhosis
   a. Ascites (most common complication, affecting 50% of cirrhotic patients)
      (1) Sequestration of fluid in peritoneal cavity. Paracentesis with analysis of ascitic fluid can offer clues to etiology. Fluid should be sent for cell count with differential, Gram stain, culture and sensitivity, albumin and total protein levels. Sample of serum for albumin should be obtained on the same day. Infection is suggested by ascitic fluid neutrophil count exceeding 250 cells/ml. The finding of organisms on Gram stain is even more compelling. The gold standard for diagnosis involves culture of the ascitic fluid (85% yield with bedside inoculation of fluid into blood culture bottles as opposed to 50% if fluid is simply forwarded to the microbiology department)
      (2) Portal hypertension is diagnosed or excluded with calculation of the serum to ascites albumin gradient (i.e., serum albumin level minus ascites albumin level). A gradient ≥ 1.1 is diagnostic of portal hypertension. A value <1.1 excludes this diagnosis. Portal hypertension occurs with cirrhosis or impaired hepatic venous drainage (Budd-Chiari syndrome [hepatic vein thrombosis], severe right-sided heart failure, constrictive pericarditis). Ascites in absence of portal hypertension suggests biliary outflow obstruction or extrahepatic etiology (pancreatitis, extrahepatic neoplasm with peritoneal seeding [e.g., ovarian cancer], tuberculous peritoneal seeding). Repeat paracentesis for cytology, AFB smear and culture, amylase and bilirubin levels should be performed in these patients
      (3) Ascitic fluid total protein level may further clarify etiology or provide prognostic information. Ascitic protein >2.5 in patient with portal hypertension is consistent with cardiac cirrhosis. Ascitic protein <1.0 imparts high risk for spontaneous bacterial peritonitis because it indicates fluid depleted of all proteins including complement and opsonins. Polymicrobial infection with an ascitic protein greater than 1.0, however, suggests bowel perforation, requiring surgical intervention. Cefotaxime: agent of choice for empiric therapy of spontaneous bacterial peritonitis. Norfloxacin (400 mg/day) may prevent recurrent episodes

    (4) Therapy for transudative ascites

       (a) Sodium restriction to 88 mmol/day

       (b) Initiation of diuresis with a potassium-sparing and potassium-wasting diuretic combination starting with spironolactone 100 mg and furosemide 40 mg each morning. Dosage may be increased every 2 or 3 days (while keeping this dosage ratio the same to prevent potassium disequilibrium) to a maximum of 400 mg of spironolactone and 160 mg of furosemide daily. Ideally, weight should be monitored daily and daily urinary excretion should be estimated by multiplying a spot urine sodium value by the daily urinary volume. Optimal dosing is achieved when the patient excretes in excess of 88 mmol of sodium per day and is losing 0.5 kg in weight per day. More aggressive diuresis may lead to the hepatorenal syndrome in patients with ascites who do not have peripheral edema

       (c) Patients with tense ascites causing dyspnea or dyspepsia should undergo large-volume (i.e., 5 l) paracentesis

       (d) Patients who are refractory to conservative management may be candidates for surgical or transjugular intrahepatic portosystemic stent shunting, extracorporeal ultrafiltration of ascites fluid, or liver transplantation

  b. Esophageal variceal bleeding (second most common complication of cirrhosis, affecting 30% of patients)

    (1) Therapy of acute bleeding

       (a) Hospitalize

       (b) Temporizing measures before definitive treatment with endoscopic sclerotherapy in patients with active bleeding and hemodynamic compromise include

- IV vasopressin (20-U load over 20 minutes followed by 0.4 U/min drip) **and** IV nitroglycerin (40 μg/min or titrated to a systolic pressure of ~100 mm Hg). Vasopressin achieves splanchnic vasocontriction to reduce portal hypertension while nitroglycerin combats side effects of vasopressin (particularly coronary ischemia). IV fluids may increase variceal engorgement and exacerbate bleeding
- Volume replacement with packed red blood cells
- Treatment failure: consider balloon tamponade of bleeding site with a Sengstaken-Blakemore tube

    (2) Definitive therapy for all variceal bleeds whether active or controlled: endoscopic intravariceal injection of a sclerosing agent (failure to treat with this modality will lead to an expected 12-month recurrence rate of 70%) followed by weekly sclerotherapy for 4 weeks and then biweekly or monthly for up to 3 months or until varices are obliterated; or distal variceal banding (to attain ischemic obliteration of varices)

    (3) Prophylaxis against initial or recurrent variceal bleeding

       (a) Oral beta-blockers (propranolol, nadolol) with dose titrated to a 20% fall in heart rate (but not below 55 beats/min) reduce incidence of initial and recurrent variceal bleeding with a possible mortality benefit

    (b) Calcium channel blockers, nitrates, serotonin antagonists, and alpha$_2$-agonists are being studied as alternatives to beta-blockers

    (c) Invasive therapy
- Shunts (surgical or transjugular [i.e., TIPS: transjugular intrahepatic portosystemic shunt]) attempt to reduce portal vein/hepatic vein pressure gradient to <12 mm Hg (level below which esophageal variceal bleeds become uncommon). Total portal venous shunting may cause ischemic liver failure so some portal flow to liver should be preserved
- Hepatic transplantation should be considered for patients with end-stage hepatic failure

c. Hepatic encephalopathy: implies altered mental status and neurologic function secondary to hepatic failure

  (1) Precipitants: medications (CNS depressants, benzodiazepines), upper GI bleeding, azotemia, infection, high-protein diet, overdiuresis, constipation, and progression of underlying liver disease

  (2) Exact biochemical mediators of hepatic encephalopathy are not known but a CSF glutamine is useful in diagnosis and serum ammonia (NH_3) levels help monitor therapy

  (3) Treatment
    (a) Dietary protein restriction (also substitution of animal proteins by vegetable proteins)
    (b) Promotion of GI ammonia excretion with lactulose 30 ml orally several times per day titrated to a production of two loose stools daily
    (c) Reduction of colonic bacteria that produce ammonia with neomycin (1 g orally every 6 hours) for patients unresponsive to lactulose alone

d. Hepatorenal syndrome: impaired renal function (despite histologically normal kidneys) as a consequence of hepatic disease; syndrome probably occurs as a result of humoral mediators that promote renal vasoconstriction

  (1) Oliguria: a low urine sodium and failure of azotemia to respond to a volume challenge are hallmarks of this condition

  (2) Mortality is 90% during hospitalization in which condition is diagnosed unless patient is a candidate for liver transplantation, which is the only definitive treatment

  (3) Temporizing measures while awaiting liver transplantation may include renally dosed IV dopamine in an effort to improve renal perfusion and combat oliguria

Suggested readings

Badalamenti S et al: Hepatorenal syndrome: new perspectives in pathogenesis and treatment, *Arch Intern Med* 153:1957-1967, 1993.

Brewer TG: Treatment of acute gastroesophageal variceal hemorrhage, *Med Clin North Am* 77:993-1014, 1993.

Conn HO: Transjugular intrahepatic portal-systemic shunts: the state of the art, *Hepatology* 17:148-158, 1993.

Dam JV, Zeldis JB: Hepatic diseases in the elderly, *Gastroenterol Clin North Am* 19:459-472, 1990.

Friedman LS: When patients with liver disease need surgery, *Immunology,* pp 25-34, July 1993.

Hazard WR, Bierman EL, editors: *Principles of geriatric medicine and gerontology,* ed 3, New York, 1994, McGraw-Hill.

Henderson JM et al: Management of variceal bleeding the 1990's, *Cleve Clin J Med* 60:431-438, 1993.

Resnick RH: Management of varices in cirrhosis, *Hosp Pract* 28:123-130, 1993.

Runyon BA: Care of patients with ascites, *N Engl J Med* 330:337-342, 1994.

Optimal
Pharmacotherapy

7

Marsha D. Fretwell, MD

BACKGROUND STATEMENTS

1. Parameters used to determine the best medication
   a. Pharmacodynamic changes related to age
   b. Potential functional impact of a drug
   c. Effect medication may have on patient's quality of life
2. Choosing the correct dose for each medication must incorporate both pharmacokinetic and pharmacodynamic parameters applied to each patient
   a. Larger volume of distribution for fat-soluble medications
   b. Reduced renal excretion of medications: the average 85-year-old has a creatinine clearance of 35 ml/min
   c. Multiple medications competing for the same metabolic site in the liver
   d. Reduced physiologic and functional reserve (i.e., in the brain and bladder, cardiovascular and renal function)
3. Comprehensive functional assessment of acutely ill frail older patients[5]
   a. Decreases inpatient use of medications
   b. Reduces use of medications not linked to identified patient problems
   c. Reduces incidence of inappropriate medication choices
4. Pharmacist can contribute significantly in the process of achieving optimal pharmacotherapy in the older patient

7.2 **DRUG-INDUCED FUNCTIONAL IMPAIRMENTS**

Drug-induced malnutrition

1. Anorexia: loss of appetite can be caused by many drugs (e.g., digoxin, theophylline, hydrochlorothiazide, nonsteroidal antiinflammatory agents, triamterene)
2. Hypogeusia: loss of taste; may be caused by
   a. Allopurinol
   b. Clindamycin
   c. Antihistamines
3. Malabsorption of vitamins and nutrients can be caused by drug use
   a. Vitamin B_6 and niacin: isoniazid\

b. Vitamins A and D: mineral oil
c. Calcium and iron: tetracycline
d. Folate: anticonvulsants, triamterene, trimethoprim
e. Vitamin D: anticonvulsants
f. Vitamin K: mineral oil, salicylates, anticonvulsants
g. Vitamin C: salicylates
h. Zinc deficiency: diuretics

Drug-induced incontinence

1. Usually occurs in patients predisposed to one of three types of incontinence: overflow, stress, and urge (Table 7-1)
2. **Overflow incontinence:** urinary retention may lead to overflow incontinence
   a. Seen with anticholinergics, smooth muscle relaxants, or alpha-agonists
   b. Medications with anticholinergic side effects (rather than pure anticholinergic compounds) (e.g., amitriptyline, imipramine, antihistamines, thioridazine) are often responsible
   c. Smooth muscle relaxant nifedipine may cause overflow incontinence because of its relaxant effect on the detrusor muscle
   d. Alpha-agonists such as phenylpropanolamine may cause incontinence by stimulating the proximal urinary sphincter to contract
3. **Stress incontinence:** alpha-antagonists such as prazosin may cause incontinence by stimulating proximal urinary sphincter to relax
4. **Urge incontinence:** usually associated with drug-induced polyuria caused by diuretics, but a diabetes insipidus–like syndrome can be seen with lithium. Patients prescribed diuretics or other medications causing hyperglycemia or hypercalcemia (e.g., tamoxifen) can also develop polyuria. Older patients who have experienced loss of mobility are at greater risk for urge incontinence caused by drug-induced polyuria

Table 7-1   Drug-induced urinary incontinence[3]

Type of Incontinence	Drugs
Overflow	
Urinary retention	Anticholinergic agents: benztropine
	Agents with anticholinergic effects: amitriptyline, imipramine, thioridazine, antihistamines, disopyramide
	Smooth muscle relaxants: nifedipine
	Alpha-agonists: phenylpropanolamine
Stress	Alpha-antagonists: prazosin
Urge	
Polyuria	Diuretics, lithium
Central inhibition	Neuroleptics
Secondary to oversedation	Benzodiazepines, sedatives, or hypnotics

From Owens NJ, Silliman RA, Fretwell MD: *Ann Pharmacother* 23:847, 1989.

5. **Incontinence secondary to oversedation:** drugs that cause confusional states or delirium in older persons can secondarily cause incontinence. This association warrants special attention because the delirious incontinent patient is at risk for catheter placement and the use of restraints

Drug-induced impairments in cognition

Drug-induced effects on cognitive processes have long been recognized. The subsequent effects of drug-induced cognitive impairment on other functional domains have been described as the cascade effect. A patient who is oversedated with medications will not be able to ambulate, eat, or use the toilet (Table 7-2).

1. Benzodiazepines have been documented in the literature as a cause of memory impairment, specifically anterograde amnesia, and their use should be avoided in older persons whenever possible
2. Long-term phenytoin administration can cause a reversible memory loss
3. Atropine and other anticholinergics have been reported to induce delirium. Patients receiving two drugs with anticholinergic effects (e.g., thioridazine with benztropine to prevent extrapyramidal symptoms) are at greater risk for anticholinergic toxicity
4. H_2-receptor blockers (e.g., cimetidine and ranitidine) are thought to cause confusion or delirium
5. Digoxin toxicity may first manifest as confusion or hallucinations. Nightmares, restlessness or nervousness, hallucinations, and delirium have all been reported as adverse effects of digoxin

Table 7-2   Drug-induced impairments in mental state

Type of Impairment	Drugs
Metabolic alterations	
Hyperglycemia or hypoglycemia	Beta-blockers, corticosteroids, diuretics, sulfonylureas
Electrolyte disturbances	Diuretics
Cognitive impairment	
Dementia, memory loss	Methyldopa, propranolol, hydrochlorothiazide, reserpine, neuroleptics, opiate narcotics, cimetidine, amantadine, benzodiazepines, anticonvulsants
Behavioral toxicity	
Insomnia, nightmares, sedation, agitation, irritability, restlessness leading to delirium, psychosis, hallucinations	Anticholinergics, cimetidine, ranitidine, digoxin, bromocriptine, amantadine, baclofen, levodopa, opiate narcotics, sympathomimetics, corticosteroids
Depression	Reserpine, methyldopa, beta-blockers, corticosteroids

6. Many drugs induce psychoses by their direct effect on dopamine or on the receptors of dopamine and choline (e.g., levodopa, amantadine, baclofen, bromocriptine)
7. Glucocorticosteroids have been reported to induce psychosis at even low doses

Drug-induced depressive disorders

Many agents used to treat hypertension (e.g., reserpine) may cause depression. Methyldopa and beta-blockers (e.g., propranolol) represent well documented causes of depression. It is especially important to avoid drug induced depression in older persons because it may present as cognitive impairment (pseudodementia) rather than classic depression

Drug-induced impairments in mobility

Medications may impair mobility in older persons as a result of a variety of age-related changes (Table 7-3).
1. Depletion of dopamine in the extrapyramidal center of the brain increases the risk for antipsychotic-induced movement disorders (e.g., tremors, rigidity, akathisias, acute dystonic reactions)
2. Hypotension (and therefore the risk of falling) is more likely to occur in older persons because of diminished baroreceptor sensitivity. The following drugs can contribute to postural hypotension
   a. Diuretics—from volume depletion and electrolyte abnormalities
   b. Cardiac medication—from sedation, a decrease in cardiac output, reduced venous return, or decreased peripheral vascular resistance
   c. Sedative-hypnotics—from sedation or autonomic effects

Table 7-3 Drug-induced impairments in mobility

Type of Impairment	Drugs
Supporting structure	
Arthralgias, myopathies	Corticosteroids, lithium
Osteoporosis, osteomalacia	Corticosteroids, phenytoin, heparin
Movement disorders	
Extrapyramidal symptoms, tardive dyskinesia	Neuroleptics, metoclopramide Amoxapine, methyldopa
Balance	
Neuritis, neuropathies	Metronidazole, phenytoin
Tinnitus, vertigo	Aspirin, aminoglycosides, furosemide, ethacrynic acid
Hypotension	Beta-blockers, calcium channel blockers, neuroleptics, antidepressants, diuretics, vasodilators, benzodiazepines, levodopa, metoclopramide
Psychomotor retardation	Neuroleptics, benzodiazepines, antihistamines, antidepressants

3. Some medications may cause mobility problems with both short- and long-term use
   a. Short courses of glucocorticosteroids can cause proximal muscle wasting. Treated patients may find it difficult to get out of bed or rise from a sitting position
   b. When taken for a long period of time, glucocorticosteroids cause osteoporosis by impairing absorption of calcium, enhancing renal excretion of calcium, and decreasing osteoblastic activity in bone
4. Some medications may affect several areas simultaneously (e.g., neuroleptics may cause psychomotor retardation and postural hypotension and at the same time might produce extrapyramidal symptoms such as akathisias, cogwheeling, and muscle rigidity)
5. Risk of falls is increased with long-term neurologic conditions such as Parkinson's disease and any abnormalities in vision, hearing, vestibular function, and proprioception
   a. Drugs that affect the senses must be avoided if possible
   b. Long-acting benzodiazepines, phenothiazines, and tricyclic antidepressants have been shown to increase risk of falls and hip fractures

| 7.3 | **ASSESSMENT FOR OPTIMAL PHARMACOTHERAPY**

1. Collect a comprehensive data base
   a. Interview patient and family; establish influence of family caregiver on patient's medication use
   b. Review old charts, document all adverse drug reactions, calculate creatinine clearance (see Appendix I)
   c. List all medications, including over-the-counter drugs
2. Integrate patient data and organize problem list
   a. Diagnoses: list all diagnoses
   b. Medications
      (1) Link each medication to a documented diagnosis; use this process to identify unnecessary medications or add new diagnoses to problem list
      (2) Evaluate for appropriate medication choice: functional impact of medication, quality of life, and pharmacodynamics
      (3) Evaluate for appropriate medication dosage: pharmacokinetics and pharmacodynamics
   c. Nutrition: evaluate functional impact of each medication (nausea, anorexia, change in bowels) (see Section 5.1)
   d. Continence: evaluate functional impact of each medication (see Section 5.2)
   e. Defecation: evaluate functional impact of each medication (constipation, diarrhea, bloating) (see Section 5.3)
   f. Cognition: evaluate whether patient is cognitively able to manage own medications; if impaired, evaluate functional impact of each medication, paying particular attention to any new medications (see Chapter 4)
   g. Emotion: evaluate functional impact of each medication (see Section 5.5)
   h. Mobility: evaluate functional impact of each medication (see Section 5.6)

    i. Cooperation with care plan: evaluate for cognitive and emotional impairments; evaluate functional impact of each medication

7.4 PRINCIPLES OF CLINICAL MANAGEMENT FOR OPTIMAL PHARMACOTHERAPY

1. Think of medications as external or environmental agents that can have either a positive or negative impact on patient's health and function
2. Initiate all medication trials within the framework of preserving cognitive function and patient's quality of life
3. Use patient functional outcomes as the measure of drug efficacy
4. Monitor drug levels; especially important in
   a. Patients with impaired renal function
   b. Patient taking more than two drugs metabolized by the liver
5. Review all medications regularly
   a. At every office or nursing home visit
   b. Every day in the hospital
6. If patient is having a *new* problem: "Think first what you did to the patient. . . ."

7.5 RECOMMENDATIONS FOR IMPROVING COMPLIANCE IN OLDER PATIENTS[4]

1. Understand patient's values and beliefs regarding health and medical treatment
2. Educate patients about their diseases and repercussions of treatment or no treatment
3. Keep medication regimens as simple as possible
4. Set priorities for which medications are critical to each patient's health
5. Assure patients that there will be careful monitoring for unexpected and expected adverse reactions. Explain adverse effects in terms of their impact on patient function
6. Educate patients and family or caregiver as to name, dose, and indication for every medication. Reinforce this at every encounter
7. Ask patients what techniques they have organized to remind themselves to take their medications
8. Provide printed educational materials for reinforcement of patient knowledge
9. Give patient and family the opportunity to ask questions
10. Ask patient to repeat medication names and instructions for use to allow reiteration of newly acquired medication knowledge

7.6 POLYPHARMACY

1. Very common in the elderly because of the likely presence of multiple disease states
2. Forty-five percent of the elderly take several prescribed drugs with an annual cost of over $10 billion
3. Two thirds of all physician visits lead to a drug prescription; forty percent of office visits involve therapy with two or more drugs

4. Antibiotics are the most commonly misused medications: it has been estimated that over 60% of antibiotic use in hospitalized patients is either unnecessary or inappropriately dosed
5. Highest use of medications is in the institutionalized elderly; average nursing home patient receives eight different drugs per day
6. Average ambulatory elderly person uses seven different drugs (four prescription and three over-the-counter drugs)
7. Ten to seventeen percent of hospital admissions in the elderly are due to inappropriate medication use
8. Risk factors for polypharmacy
   a. Multiple illnesses or multiple physicians
   b. Hospitalization or nursing home placement
   c. Advanced age or severe illness

7.7   **ADVERSE DRUG REACTIONS[1]**

1. The higher frequency of adverse drug reactions in the elderly is attributable to the facts that they consume more medications and are more likely to have baseline illness than younger patients, rather than to the patient's chronologic age[2]
2. Drug reactions can be subdivided into four groups
   a. Primary—a single medication with a narrow toxic/therapeutic ratio is responsible for patient's symptoms (e.g., digoxin, theophylline, lidocaine)
   b. Secondary—result from interaction between two medications (Table 7-4)
   c. Drug withdrawal syndromes—result from sudden cessation of a drug (e.g., angina from beta-blocker withdrawal)
   d. Extrapharmacologic effects (e.g., increased risk of fractured hip with benzodiazepine use)
3. Common types of adverse drug reactions in the elderly
   a. Primary drug reactions (one drug with one side effect)
      (1) Cimetidine psychosis
      (2) Narcotic-induced respiratory depression
      (3) Lidocaine psychosis
      (4) Theophylline seizures
      (5) Insulin reaction
      (6) Chronic salicylism
   b. Secondary drug interactions (requires at least two drugs to cause interaction)
      (1) Sulfonylurea/sulfonamide
      (2) Cimetidine/lidocaine
      (3) Erythromycin/theophylline
      (4) Indomethacin/propranolol
      (5) Tricyclic antidepressant/alpha-sympatholytic
   c. Drug withdrawal syndromes (addictive and nonaddictive withdrawal)
      (1) Beta-blocker withdrawal (angina)
      (2) Calcium channel–blocker withdrawal (angina, hypertension)
      (3) "Addictive drug" withdrawal syndromes (benzodiazepines, narcotics, etc.)

Table 7-4 Drug interactions involving prescription drugs

Drugs	Onset	Severity	Effect	Mechanism	Management
Antacids; iron salts	Delayed	Minor	↓ Hematologic response to Fe	↓ Absorption of Fe because of high gastric pH	Give Fe several hours before antacids, liquid preferred
Benzodiazepines; ethanol	Rapid	Minor	↑ Effects of both; ↑ psychomotor dysfunction and sedation	Synergistic effects and ↓ VD; ↓ elimination of benzodiazepines	Avoid ETOH
Beta-blockers; prazosin	Rapid	Moderate	↑ Severity and duration; hypotension associated with first dose of prazosin	Blocked cardiovascular reflex because of orthostatic hypotension	First prazosin dose at qhs; monitor orthostatic BP
Beta-blockers; indomethacin	Delayed	Moderate	↓ Antihypertensive effect of beta-blockers; BP + 5-10 mm Hg	Inhibition of prostaglandin synthesis	Check BP after 7-10 days
Captopril; indomethacin	Rapid	Moderate	↓ Effect of captopril	Inhibition of prostaglandin synthesis	Check BP day 1 of indomethacin Rx; discontinue if BP too high
Cimetidine; procainamide	Rapid	Moderate	↑ Effect of procainamide, including GI toxicity, weakness, hypotension; ↓ CO, arrhythmias	↓ Renal clearance of procainamide	Decrease procainamide 25%-35% before starting cimetidine; check procainamide and NAPA levels 24 hr after cimetidine

Drugs	Onset	Severity	Effect	Mechanism	Management
Clonidine; tricyclic antidepressants	Rapid	Moderate	↓ Antihypertensive effect of clonidine; hypertensive crisis possible	Unknown	Avoid concomitant use, or increase clonidine dose; beware of risks of high-dose clonidine
Digoxin; quinidine	Delayed	Major	↑ Toxic effects of digoxin	↓ VD; ↓ renal and nonrenal elimination of digoxin	Check ECG, digoxin level, and effect 27-72 hr after starting combination; again 3-5 days; adjust if needed
Digoxin; tetracycline	Delayed	Major	↑ Digoxin toxicity seen in <10% of patients	↑ Bioavailability of digoxin, second-degree change in GI flora	Check digoxin level 5-7 days after starting antibiotic and again in 3-4 mo; adjust dose accordingly
Digoxin; anticholinergics	Delayed	Major	↑ Digoxin toxicity	↑ Bioavailability of slow dissolving digoxin preparation	Use liquid or rapidly dissolving digoxin preparations
Digoxin; thiazide + loop	Delayed	Major	↑ Digoxin toxicity, especially arrhythmias	Diuretic-induced hypokalemia potentiates arrhythmias	Maintain potassium of 4-4.5 with potassium supplementation
Lithium; thiazide	Delayed	Major	↑ Levels and toxicity of lithium; polyuria, weakness, lethargy, ECG changes	↓ Renal excretion of lithium	Use loop diuretics or more carefully monitor lithium levels and reduce dose accordingly

Continued

From Lavizzo-Mourey SC et al: *Practicing prevention for the elderly*, Philadelphia, 1989, Hanley & Belfus.
CO, Cardiac output; *NAPA*, N-acetyl procainamide; *VD*, volume of distribution.

Table 7-4 Drug interactions involving prescription drugs—cont'd

Drugs	Onset	Severity	Effect	Mechanism	Management
Quinidine; rifampin	Delayed	Moderate	↓ Effect of quinidine	↑ Metabolism of quinidine	Monitor quinidine levels 1 wk after starting rifampin; review 3-5 days after discontinuing rifampin
Salicylates; warfarin	Delayed	Major	↑ Anticoagulant effect	Synergistic effect	Avoid combination
Salicylates; antacids	Delayed	Minor	↓ Effect of salicylate	↑ Renal excretion of salicylate	↑ Dose of salicylate; check levels
Sulfonylureas; thiazide diuretics	Delayed	Minor	↓ Hypoglycemic effect	Thiazide-induced glucose intolerance	Monitor glucose, one dose of sulfonylureas
Theophyllines; erythromycin	Delayed	Moderate	↓ Effect of erythromycin; ↑ effect of theophylline	Hepatic metabolism of theophyllines inhibited	↓ Dose or ↑ dosing interval of theophyllines by 60%; monitor levels
Theophyllines; beta-blockers	Delayed	Moderate	↓ Effect of theophylline	↓ Bronchial resistance caused by beta-blockers	Avoid beta-blockers in patients with reactive airway diseases
Warfarin; thyroid hormone	Delayed	Major	↑ Hypothrombinemic effect; bleeding	Unknown	Adjust dose according to patient results
Warfarin; quinidine	Delayed	Major	↑ Hypothrombinemic effect	↓ Vitamin K–dependent factor synthesis	↓ Anticoagulant dose; check patient 5-7 days after starting combination

    d. Tertiary extrapharmacologic effects (measurable only by epidemiologic studies)
       (1) Falls caused by tricyclics, anxiolytics, and antipsychotics (short half-life vs. long half-life agents)
       (2) Traumatic injuries caused by drug-induced orthostatic hypotension

4. Physician factors implicated in adverse drug reactions
    a. Physician prescribes a high-risk drug to vulnerable host (i.e., ASA for patient with peptic ulcer disease)
    b. Physician prescribes highly interactive drug to pharmacologically vulnerable patient (i.e., captopril to patient on potassium-sparing agent, diphenhydramine to patient on anticholinergics)
    c. Physician prescribes inappropriate compensatory drug for unrecognized drug effect (i.e., tricyclic antidepressant to treat beta-blocker depression, major tranquilizer to treat benzodiazepine agitation)
    d. Automatic drug prescribing (i.e., standard orders for ICU, CCU, or chronic care facilities)
    e. Lack of follow-up on drug effects or poor longitudinal monitoring of drug interactions

5. Various suggestions for preventing drug toxicity are outlined in the box below

---

Suggestions for Preventing Drug Toxicity in the Elderly

- Strive for a diagnosis before treating
- Take a careful drug history
- Know the pharmacokinetics of the drug or drugs
- Adjust the dose
- Use smaller doses in the elderly
- Work to simplify the regimen
- Regularly review the regimen
- Avoid polypharmacy at all costs
- Use medication cards
- Keep a record of the Rx on the problem list
- Use medication diary (or containers, such as egg cartons, for daily doses)
- Have patient bring in all medicine bottles
- Check the labels
- Instruct family
- Destroy old medicines
- Use the services of visiting nurses
- Check serum drug levels when appropriate
- Support community education
- Consider overdose risk in elderly patients with clinically evident psychiatric conditions
- Be sure patients are aware that medicines can cause, as well as cure, illness

---

From Bosker G et al, editors: *Geriatric emergency medicine*, St Louis, 1990, Mosby, p 60.

References

1. Albrich JM, Bosker LG: Drug therapy. In Bosker G et al, editors: *Geriatric emergency medicine,* St Louis, 1990, Mosby.
2. Gurwitz JH, Avorn J: The ambiguous relation between aging and adverse drug reactions, *Ann Intern Med* 114:956-966, 1991.
3. Morley JE: Nutrition and aging. In Hazzard WR et al, editors: *Principles of geriatric medicine and gerontology,* ed 2, New York, 1990, McGraw-Hill.
4. Owens NJ, Larrat EP, Fretwell MD: Improving compliance in the older patient. In Cramer JA, Spilker B, editors: *Patient compliance in medical practice and clinical trials,* New York, 1991, Raven Press.
5. Owens NJ, Silliman RA, Fretwell MD: The relationship between comprehensive functional assessment and optimal pharmacotherapy in the older patient, *Ann Pharmacother* 23:847, 1989.

Long-Term Care

HOUSE CALLS
Tom J. Wachtel, MD

Strictly speaking, no one is homebound. There is always a way to bring a homebound person to the hospital or to a physician's office. However, except in the case of a medical emergency, transportation by ambulance is not covered by most health insurance plans; and ambulance trips cost several hundred dollars. For practical purposes a homebound person can be defined as someone who cannot leave the home, transiently (e.g., after surgery) or permanently, using personal or other resources readily available in the community (e.g., friends, relatives, taxi service, senior citizens' transportation, or public transportation). Such a person should receive health services at home.

The house call

Most first visits at home are scheduled well in advance. Therefore it is almost always possible for the informal caregiver (most frequently the patient's daughter) to be present during the visit. Even when a family provides care in shifts, arrangement can be made for a key member of the informal care-giving team to be present. When the patient's condition requires substantial nursing services (e.g., a patient with an active decubitus ulcer), every effort should be made for the visiting nurse to be present during the visit; this will enable the whole team to discuss the plan of care. Unfortunately, Medicare will only reimburse one of the health professionals for a house call on the same day.

Taking a history in the patient's home is no different in its content than a history taken in the office; but because it is done on the patient's turf, often over coffee and muffins, the interaction tends to be less formal. Permission should be requested to inspect the living quarters. What does the home look like? Is it clean? Is it orderly? Can the patient get around, go to the kitchen, go to the bathroom? Is the environment safe? Are there loose rugs, night-lights, rails in the bathroom? An office visit, no matter how comprehensive, cannot provide a complete understanding of the patient's daily routine. The cabinet or drawer that contains the medications should be inspected. Outdated and discontinued medications should be discarded immediately. The refrigerator and food cupboards should also be checked, especially when the homebound patient depends on others for his or her food supply. Aside from appearance, what does the home smell like? Incontinence may be immediately detected. Many elderly patients are reluctant to report incontinence in the office. It is more difficult to hide during a house call.

Observing the interaction between caregivers and patients is also a precious source of information. In the office, patients and families are generally on their best behavior and outbursts are unlikely to occur. In the home setting, people are less inhibited, even in the presence of the physician. Therefore they are more likely to display their usual pattern of interaction. Moreover, the request for a house call is often placed at a time of crisis. Most often, the crisis is not a new medical problem, but rather an exhausted caregiver who needs support or respite.

Although the goal of a house call will certainly vary, like any physician-patient interaction, the content of a home visit should include a number of staple items (see the box on p. 373). Because most candidates for home care are frail or disabled, a functional assessment should always be performed. This includes gathering information on *physical function,* such as activities of daily life (ADLs), instrumental activities of daily life (IADLs), mobility, and continence; *social and role function,* such as visits by friends and relatives, and interest in sexual activity; and *mental function,* such as cognition and affect. Unlike the office setting, where such assessment must be done formally by asking specific questions, much of the above information can be collected by simple observation during a home visit.

Zebley[1] states: "The three minutes it takes you to walk in the door, look around and sit down with the patient may teach you more than all your previous encounters with the patient in the hospital or office setting." A more complete checklist describing the relation between the patient and the home environment is presented in Figure 8-1.

Asking homebound elderly patients to discuss ethical issues such as care intensity should be a routine practice. In the hospital a common and important question is whether to resuscitate. At home the equivalent issue is whether to hospitalize. Whatever decision is made, it is entered into the patient's record. Equally important is the question of surrogate decision makers. Competent patients are routinely requested to think about designating someone who will have durable power of attorney for medical decisions. This is also entered into the medical record.

Homebound patients and their informal caregivers should be given a list of community resources (Figure 8-2).

The physical exam is often less complete at home than in the office or at the hospital. Although technically feasible, a pelvic exam for cancer screening may not be indicated in an elderly patient with Alzheimer's dementia. Although a bimanual exam is possible, expecting to visualize a cervix with an elderly patient lying in a regular bed is unreasonable. Most patients who receive care at home do not expect the same comprehensive services routinely provided to ambulatory patients; nonetheless, it is best to be

Problems to Address During a Geriatric Home Visit

Safety

Household risks (e.g., loose rugs, night-lights, bathroom rails)
Security
Appliances, fire alarm
Dirt, dust, humidity
Access to telephone or other means of calling for help

Psychosocial Situation

Mental status
Affect (rule out depression)
Support (family, friends, rule out loneliness)
Financial resources

Ethical Issues

Intensity of care (especially terminal care)
Decision to (not to) hospitalize
Surrogate decision maker (durable power of attorney) and/or living
    will

Functional Status

Activities of daily life (ADLs)
Instrumental activities of daily life (IADLs)
Mobility
Vision and hearing assessment

Continence

Urine and stool

Nutrition

Availability of food
Ability to prepare and eat meals
Alcoholism

Medical Problems

Tertiary prevention (diagnose, treat, and monitor chronic diseases)
Primary prevention (vaccination, hygiene)
Diagnose and treat acute illnesses
Prognosis
Skin care, foot care

Primary Care

Access and availability of care
Coordination of team of health care professionals
Continuity of care

1. Type of dwelling   ( ) House   ( ) Apartment

2. Previous living situation   ( ) House   ( ) Apartment

3. Who lives at the residence: Name(s), Relation(s) _____
   _____

   ( ) Completely alone   ( ) Alone part of the day   ( ) Rarely/never alone

4. Stairs

   ( ) None (or ramp)   ( ) Stairs to main floor   ( ) Stairs to upstairs

5. Mobility

   ( ) Ambulatory without care ( ) Ambulatory with care   ( ) Ambulatory with walker

   ( ) Chair bound   ( ) Bed bound

6. ADL

7. IADL

8. Function in the home (*I*, independent; *A*, assistance required; *D*, dependent; *NA*, not applicable

A. General Obstacle Negotiation	I	A	D	NA	
Elevator					
Stairs					

Figure 8-1
Checklist for the traditional home evaluation.

explicit and explain to patients the medical goals. Blood and urine tests and an occasional ECG can be obtained as readily in the home as in the office (or community-based laboratories). Portable x-rays can be obtained at great expense and poor quality. Typically, a situation that calls for x-rays or other diagnostic procedures requires evaluation in a hospital.

Logistics and time management

The logistics of house calls may explain why many physicians, busy with their office and hospital work, find house calls an inefficient use of their time. There is obviously some validity to this argument. However, steps can be taken to reduce travel time. The physician with a substantial number of

	I	A	D	NA	
Ramp					
Uneven terrain					
Thresholds					
Through doorways					
Can patient escape safely (e.g., fire)					

NOTE: Stair covering and railing, smoke alarms, emergency exits, extension cords

B. Entrance	I	A	D	NA	
Driveway					
Walkway					
Landing					
Unlock door					
Open door					
Access mail					

NOTE: Lighting, obstacles

C. Living/Family Room	I	A	D	NA	
Ability to maneuver through room					
Ability to transfer on/off chairs					
Ability to manage TV					
Ability to reach and use phone					

NOTE: Lighting, floors, emergency numbers by phone

Figure 8-1, cont'd
For legend see opposite page.

Continued

D. Kitchen	I	A	D	NA	
Ability to maneuver through room					
Ability to use table and chair					
Ability to reach shelves/cabinet					
Ability to use appliances (refrigerator, stove, sink)					
Ability to prepare meals					

NOTE: Lighting, floors, reachability of utensils/dishes/food; the quantity and quality of the food

E. Bathroom	I	A	D	NA	
Ability to maneuver to and through room					
Ability to transfer on/off toilet					
Ability to transfer in/out of tub or shower					
Ability to reach sink, faucet, grooming supplies					

NOTE: Lighting (also between bedroom and bathroom); obstacles; nonskid surface (tub

and shower); tub and shower bench; tub, shower, or toilet rails; hot water temperature

F. Bedroom	I	A	D	NA	
Ability to maneuver to and through room					
Ability to transfer in/out of bed					
Ability to reach phone					

Figure 8-1, cont'd
Checklist for the traditional home evaluation.

Ability to reach light switch					
Ability to use closets and drawers					

NOTE: Lighting, obstacles

G. Medications	I	A	D	NA	
Ability to identify medication					
Ability to follow instructions					
Ability to open containers					

NOTE: What medications are found; outdated, no longer prescribed?

Figure 8-1, cont'd
For legend see opposite page.

homebound patients can arrange to make routine visits to a cluster of patients who live in the same neighborhood. The fact that older members of our society tend to congregate in elderly housing makes clustering easy to accomplish. Except for first encounters, two house calls can be scheduled per hour when several visits are arranged in the same apartment building or neighborhood. In addition, routine house calls can be made to replace idle time caused by cancellations in the office. This can actually improve the efficiency of a geriatric practice (e.g., in the winter).

House calls for urgent problems (e.g., a fever) obviously are impossible to plan in a physician's schedule. Urgent visits can be made at the end of the day on the way home from work. However, it should be made clear to homebound patients that emergencies cannot always be dealt with in the home. The willingness to make housecalls should not eliminate use of traditional emergency services when necessary.

Reference
1. Zebley JW: Geriatric follow-up: what only a home visit can tell you, *Geriatrics* 41:100-104, 1986.

Suggested readings
Ramsdell JW et al: The yield of a home visit in the assessment of geriatric patients, *J Am Geriatr Soc* 37:17-24, 1989.

Community Resources	Telephone #
Council on Aging/Dept. of Elderly Affairs	
Senior Center/Social Day Care	
Home Care Services	
Homemaker	
Home health aide	
V.N.A.	
O.T.	
P.T.	
Adult Day Care	
Housing	
Legal Assistance	
Nutrition/meal sites	
Transportation	
Fuel Assistance	
Life-Line	
Mental Health	
Support Group	
Nursing Home Assistance	

Figure 8-2

List of community resources for the homebound elderly.

Rich MW et al: A multidisciplinary intervention to prevent the readmission of elderly patients with congestive heart failure, *N Engl J Med* 333:1190-1195, 1995.

Rossman I: The geriatrician and the homebound patient, *J Am Geriatr Soc* 36:348-354, 1988.

Stollerman GH: Decisions to leave home, *J Am Geriatr Soc* 36:375-376, 1988.

Stuck AE et al: A trial of annual in-home comprehensive geriatric assessments for elderly people living in the community, *N Engl J Med* 333:1184-1189, 1995.

 RESPITE CARE
Fred F. Ferri, MD

Definition

Respite care is a program designed to provide temporary relief to family caregivers.

Facts about caregivers

1. The vast majority of home care is provided by relatives of the ill or disabled person
2. Caregivers are usually female (wives, mothers, daughters, daughters-in-law) and middle aged or elderly. Average age of a wife who cares for a husband is 65 years; 30% are over 74 years
3. Many caregivers (44%) are in fair or poor health themselves. A recent study revealed that spouse caregivers were more depressed, were more likely to use psychotropic drugs, had more symptoms of psychologic distress, and expressed higher levels of negative affect than the general population[2]
4. Financially 37% of caregivers fall within poverty standards[1]

Respite care programs

1. Most respite care programs involve services in the patient's home
2. The time period varies from several hours on a regular basis (e.g., afternoons or evenings to allow caregivers to run errands) to several days or weeks (e.g., to allow the caregiver a prolonged vacation)
3. Respite care can also be arranged in nursing homes or other institutional settings (e.g., day-care programs can provide a variety of health, social, and related services in a protective setting during daytime hours)

Medicare coverage

1. Inpatient respite care (no more than 5 consecutive days) is partially covered by Medicare Part A
2. Eighty hours of in-home care for chronically dependent patients is covered by Medicare Part B after a deductible has been met

References

1. Older Women's League: *Facts about caregivers,* Washington DC, 1988, The League.
2. Pruchno RA, Potashnik SL: Caregiving spouses: physical and mental health in perspective, *J Am Geriatr Soc* 37:697-705, 1989.

8.3 **NURSING HOME CARE**
Fred F. Ferri, MD

Demographics

1. There are 19,000 nursing homes in the United States, constituting nearly 1.8 million nursing home beds (nursing home beds outnumber hospital beds); average occupancy rate: 92%

2. Approximately 5% of the elderly reside in a nursing home; average age of nursing home residents: 78 years
3. Percentage of elderly residing in nursing homes varies with the age of the patient (2% of those aged 65 to 74, 22% of those older than 85). Risk factors for institutionalization are described in the box below
4. It is estimated that 25% to 50% of Americans 65 or older can expect to enter a nursing home during their lifetime
5. Women comprise the overwhelming majority of nursing home residents
6. Mean length of stay in a nursing home: 19 months
7. Fifty percent of patients admitted to a nursing home die there; annual percentage of nursing home deaths: 21.5%
8. During the first year of nursing home care 20% of patients require hospitalization
9. Forty percent of nursing home patients are discharged to a hospital, and 25% are discharged home

Work force in nursing homes

1. Fewer than 50% of practicing physicians ever visit a nursing home
2. In the majority of nursing homes medical care is provided by fewer than nine physicians
3. The average ratio of registered nurses to patients is 1:50, compared to a ratio of 1:5 in acute care hospitals
4. Nurses' aides constitute greater than 50% of the work force in nursing homes

Financial considerations

1. Seventy-five percent of nursing homes are proprietary and average less than 100 beds; approximately half of U.S. nursing homes are owned by chains
2. Yearly expenditures for nursing home care exceed $30 billion
3. Most patients who require long-term care must exhaust their resources before becoming eligible for government assistance (Medicaid). Medicaid eligibility requirements vary by state. Generally any assets transferred from the patient to others within 30 months of nursing home admission will be considered when determining Medicaid eligibility

Risk Factors for Institutionalization

Over 70 years old	Multiple medical problems
Living alone	Female
Demented	Depressed
Recently bereaved	Socially isolated
Recently discharged from hospital	Incontinent
Immobilized	No supportive relatives nearby

From Ham RJ: *Primary care geriatrics*, Boston, 1983, John Wright.

Clinical care of the nursing home patient[11]

1. Main goal of nursing home care: to maximize quality of life in a safe and supportive environment
2. Subgroups of nursing home patients
   a. Short-stay patients (>50%)
      (1) Terminally ill (life expectancy <6 months)
      (2) Short-term rehabilitation (e.g., following fractured hip)
      (3) Subacute illness (e.g., elderly patient with osteomyelitis)
   b. Long-stay patients
      (1) Significant physical impairment (e.g., end-stage CHF)
      (2) Significant cognitive impairment (e.g., ambulatory patient with dementia)
      (3) Combined physical and cognitive impairment (e.g., patient with CVA and dementia)
3. Goal and approach to each subgroup vary
   a. Provide comfort and dignity for terminally ill patient and family
   b. Restore highest possible level of functional independence in short-term rehabilitation patients
   c. Prevent acute illness and provide a safe and supportive environment for cognitively impaired patient

Common problems encountered in nursing home care

1. Patient usually cannot give a precise history; thus it is difficult to obtain a comprehensive medical data base (unless the physician cared for the patient before nursing home admission); medical histories are especially limited for patients admitted from home or transferred from another nursing home
2. There is often poor recognition of acute illness by the nursing home staff because of limited skills and shortage of staff (particularly on nights, weekends, and holidays); use of nursing pool personnel who are not familiar with the patients exacerbates this problem; increasing use of nurse practitioners and physician assistants to complement physician activities may improve quality of care in nursing homes
3. Many diagnostic procedures (e.g., arterial blood gases [ABGs] in a dyspneic patient) are unavailable or difficult to obtain, necessitating transport of the patient to the local hospital emergency room
4. Restrictive Medicare/Medicaid policies limit physician incentive to provide optimal care (e.g., general policies discourage more than one visit per month)
5. Unreasonable family expectations about nursing home care and guilt about nursing home placement of a loved one can result in conflict among various family members; physician-family conflicts can be lessened by designating only one family member to be the spokesperson for cognitively impaired patients
6. State and federal regulations often limit the availability of several types of drugs and medical equipment

Role of the nursing home medical director[8]

1. The Health Care Financing Administration (HCFA) requires that each long-term facility designate a physician, registered nurse, or other medical staff member to serve as medical director
2. Medical director's responsibilities
   a. Implementation of resident care policies
   b. Development and coordination of resident's treatment plan
   c. Quality of care delivered to each patient
   d. Development of written bylaws and rules delineating responsibilities of attending physicians
   e. Surveillance of employee health
3. Traditionally the medical director served in an advisory role, helping the facility maintain compliance with state and federal regulations (e.g., completion of forms and signing orders for attending physicians who failed to do so). This role has been expanded to include active participation in administrative decision making, quality assurance, and educational programs in addition to the organizing and planning of medical services required by law and regulations

Medicare guidelines for physician reimbursement in nursing home care[9]

1. Maximum number of routine visits allowable for reimbursement: one per month. If the patient develops complications and requires additional visits, the nature of each acute illness must be clearly documented in the patient's chart and additional documentation submitted to Medicare to be considered for reimbursement
2. At each visit the physician must examine the patient and personally
   a. Review the resident's total plan of care, including medications and treatments
   b. Write or dictate a progress note and sign it
   c. Sign and date all orders
3. After the initial visit, and at the option of the physician, a state-licensed clinical nurse specialist may alternate visits with the physician in a skilled nursing facility. At the state's option, any required physician's task may be performed by a nurse practitioner, clinical nurse specialist, or physician assistant who works in collaboration with a physician and who is *not* a facility employee

Medicare coverage of nursing home care

1. Skilled nursing facility services are covered by Medicare Part A benefits for up to 150 days/calendar year
2. Patient is responsible for a copayment (20%) for the initial 8 days/calendar year
3. Prior hospitalization is no longer a requirement for Medicare benefits in admission to a skilled nursing facility
4. Medicare Part A will not cover if
   a. Skilled care is required occasionally (e.g., three times weekly rather than five times weekly or daily)
   b. Services can be provided outside the skilled nursing facility

c. Patient has reached maximum potential and will no longer benefit from skilled care

Cardiopulmonary resuscitation in nursing homes

1. Nursing home residence and age over 65 are associated with poor outcome after CPR attempts. In a recent study only 1.7% of nursing home residents who required CPR survived to hospital discharge. Mean hospital stay of survivors: 45 days.[1] Overall survival from CPR of elderly (both nursing home residents and outpatients): approximately 8%. Half of these survivors are then discharged to a long-term care facility
2. The issue of CPR should be introduced by the physician early in the relationship with the patient, before hospitalization or diminished competency[12]
3. All health care facilities receiving Medicaid or Medicare funds must tell patients on admission of their right to reject or receive life-sustaining treatment

Inappropriate use of medications in nursing homes[3]

Inappropriate drug use in nursing homes is common. Inappropriate prescribing is most common in large nursing homes.

1. The following drugs should be avoided in nursing home residents
   a. Long-acting benzodiazepines
   b. Meprobamate
   c. Combination antidepressant-antipsychotic agents
   d. Certain antihypertensives (methyldopa, reserpine)
   e. Certain nonsteroidal antiinflammatory drugs (NSAIDs) (indomethacin, phenylbutazone) and cyclobenzaprine
   f. Chlorpropamide
   g. Propoxyphene and pentazocine
   h. Dipyridamole
   i. GI antispasmodics
2. Drugs requiring dose modification or limited therapy
   a. Oxazepam, short-acting benzodiazepines, triazolam
   b. Haloperidol, thioridazine
   c. Hydrochlorothiazide
   d. H_2 blockers
   e. Oral antibiotics
   f. Decongestants
   g. Iron supplements

Although these recommendations are mainly for nursing home residents, it is prudent to follow these guidelines for all elderly patients regardless of their residence. To minimize inappropriate prescribing, the following questions should be asked when evaluating medication use in a nursing home resident[2]

- What is the target problem being treated?
- Is the drug necessary?
- Are nonpharmacologic therapies available?
- Is this the lowest practical dose?

- Could discontinuing therapy with a medicine help reduce symptoms?
- Does this drug have adverse effects that are more likely to occur in an older patient?
- Is this the most cost-effective choice?
- By what criteria, and at what time, will the effects of therapy be assessed?

Government regulation of nursing home care[14]

In response to concern over the quality of care in nursing homes, Congress directed the HCFA to study ways to improve nursing home care and regulations. Based on an Institute of Medicine study published in 1986 and a consensus of professional opinion, Congress enacted legislation to improve the quality of care in nursing homes as part of the 1987 Omnibus Budget Reconciliation Act (OBRA). These regulations, known as OBRA 87, mandate patient assessment, limit psychiatric drug use, and ensure residents' rights.

1. **Patient care**
   a. Nursing home residents must be assessed initially and periodically in several areas. This *Minimum Data Set (MDS)* contains 16 sections (Figures 8-3 to 8-18) and must be completed by a registered nurse within 14 days of admission, after major changes in patient status, and annually. The initial section (Figure 8-3) deals with identification and background information. Other categories included in the MDS are
      (1) Cognitive patterns (Figure 8-4)
      (2) Communication/hearing patterns (Figure 8-5)
      (3) Vision patterns (Figure 8-6)
      (4) Physical functioning and structural problems (Figure 8-7)
      (5) Continence in last 14 days (Figure 8-8)
      (6) Psychosocial well-being (Figure 8-9)
      (7) Mood and behavior patterns (Figure 8-10)
      (8) Activity pursuit patterns (Figure 8-11)
      (9) Disease diagnoses (Figure 8-12)
      (10) Health conditions (Figure 8-13)
      (11) Oral/nutritional status (Figure 8-14)
      (12) Oral/dental status (Figure 8-15)
      (13) Skin conditions (Figure 8-16)
      (14) Medication use (Figure 8-17)
      (15) Special treatment and procedures (Figure 8-18)
   b. Problems identified on the MDS are further evaluated using the *Resident Assessment Protocol (RAP)*. These protocols address the following 18 common problem areas encountered in nursing home residents
      (1) Delirium
      (2) Cognitive loss/dementia
      (3) Visual function
      (4) Communication
      (5) ADL functional/rehabilitation potential
      (6) Urinary incontinence and indwelling catheter
      (7) Psychosocial well-being
      (8) Mood state

SECTION A. IDENTIFICATION AND BACKGROUND INFORMATION	
1. **ASSESSMENT DATE**	☐☐ — ☐☐ — ☐☐☐☐ Month　　　Day　　　　　Year
2. **RESIDENT NAME & I.D.#**	(First)　　　(Middle Initial)　　　(Last) ID#_____
3. **SOCIAL SECURITY NO.**	☐☐☐ — ☐☐ — ☐☐☐☐
4. **MEDICAID NO. (If applicable)**	☐☐☐☐☐☐☐☐☐☐
5. **MEDICAL RECORD NO.**	☐☐☐☐☐☐☐☐☐☐
6. **REASON FOR ASSESSMENT**	1. Initial admission assess.　4. Annual assessment 2. Hosp/Medicare reassess.　5. Significant change in status 3. Readmission assessment　6. Other (e.g., UR)
7. **CURRENT PAYMENT SOURCE(S) FOR N.H. STAY**	*(Billing Office to indicate; check all that apply)* a. Medicaid ⬚a.　d. VA ⬚d. b. Medicare ⬚b.　e. Self pay/Private insurance ⬚e. c. CHAMPUS ⬚c.　f. Other ⬚f.
8. **RESPONSIBILITY/ LEGAL GUARDIAN**	*(Check all that apply)* a. Legal guardian ⬚a.　d. Family member responsible ⬚d. b. Other legal oversight ⬚b.　e. Resident responsible ⬚e. c. Durable power attrny./ health care proxy ⬚c.　f. *NONE OF ABOVE* ⬚f.
9. **ADVANCED DIRECTIVES**	*(For those items with supporting documentation in the medical record, check all that apply)* a. Living will ⬚a.　f. Feeding restrictions ⬚f. b. Do not resuscitate ⬚b.　g. Medication restrictions ⬚g. c. Do not hospitalize ⬚c.　h. Other treatment restrictions ⬚h. d. Organ donation ⬚d.　i. *NONE OF ABOVE* ⬚i. e. Autopsy request ⬚e.
10. **DISCHARGE PLANNED WITHIN 3 MOS.**	*(Does not include discharge due to death)* 0. No　1. Yes　2. Unknown/uncertain
11. **PARTICIPATE IN ASSESSMENT**	a. Resident　b. Family ⬚a. 　0. No　　0. No 　1. Yes　　1. Yes ⬚b. 　　　　　2. No family
12. **SIGNATURES**	Signature & Date of RN Assessment Coordinator _____ Signatures & Dates of Others Who Completed Part of the Assessment _____ _____

Figure 8-3
Identification and background information. (Reproduced with permission from Briggs Corp, Des Moines.)

SECTION B. COGNITIVE PATTERNS		
1.	COMATOSE	*(Persistent vegetative state/no discernible consciousness)* *0. No* *1. Yes (Skip to SECTION E)*	

2.	MEMORY	*(Recall of what was learned or known)*
		a. Short-term memory OK—seems/appears to recall after 5 minutes
		   0. Memory OK 1. Memory problem ▲²
		b. Long-term memory OK—seems/appears to recall long past
		   0. Memory OK 1. Memory problem ▲²
			a.
			
			b.

3.	MEMORY/ RECALL ABILITY	*(Check all that resident normally able to recall during last 7 days)* Fewer than 3 ✓ = ▲² a. Current season [a.] b. Location of own room [b.] c. Staff names/faces [c.] d. That he/she is in a nursing home e. *NONE OF ABOVE* are recalled	d. e.
4.	COGNITIVE SKILLS FOR DAILY DECISION- MAKING	*(Made decisions regarding tasks of daily life)* 0. Independent—decisions consistent/reasonable ▲⁴ 1. Modified independence—some difficulty in new situations only ▲⁴ ▲² 2. Moderately impaired—decisions poor; cues/ supervision required ▲⁴ ▲² 3. Severely impaired—never/rarely made decisions ▲²	
5.	INDICATORS OF DELIRIUM —PERIODIC DISORDERED THINKING/ AWARENESS	*(Check if condition over last 7 days appears different from usual functioning)* a. Less alert, easily distracted ●¹ b. Changing awareness of environment ●¹ c. Episodes of incoherent speech ●¹ d. Periods of motor restlessness or lethargy ●¹ e. Cognitive ability varies over course of day ●¹ f. *NONE OF ABOVE*	a. b. c. d. e. f.
6.	CHANGE IN COGNITIVE STATUS	Change in resident's cognitive status, skills, or abilities in last 90 days 0. No change 1. Improved 2. Deteriorated ●¹ ▲¹⁴	

● = **Automatic Trigger**

1 - Delirium	5 - ADL Functional/Rehabilitation Potential
2 - Cognitive Loss/Dementia	6 - Urinary Incontinence and Indwelling Catheter
3 - Visual Function	7 - Psychosocial Well-Being
4 - Communication	8 - Mood State

▲ = **Potential Trigger**

9 - Behavior Problems	13 - Feeding Tubes	
10 - Activities	14 - Dehydration/Fluid Maintenance	17 - Psychotropic Drug Use
11 - Falls	15 - Dental Care	18 - Physical Restraints
12 - Nutritional Status	16 - Pressure Ulcers	

Figure 8-4

Cognitive patterns. (Reproduced with permission from Briggs Corp, Des Moines.)

		SECTION C. COMMUNICATION/HEARING PATTERNS	
1.	HEARING	*(With hearing appliance, if used)* 0. **Hears adequately**—normal talk, TV, phone 1. **Minimal difficulty** when not in quiet setting 2. **Hears in special situation only**—speaker has to adjust tonal quality and speak distinctly 3. **Highly impaired**/absence of useful hearing	
2.	COMMUNI-CATION DEVICES/ TECHNIQUES	*(Check all that apply during last 7 days)* a. Hearing aid, present and used	a.
		b. Hearing aid, present and not used	b.
		c. Other receptive comm. technique used (e.g., lip read)	c.
		d. *NONE OF ABOVE*	d.
3.	MODES OF EXPRESSION	*(Check all used by resident to make needs known)* a. Speech [a.] c. Signs/gestures/sounds	c.
		b. Writing messages to express or clarify needs [b.] d. Communication board	d.
		e. Other	e.
		f. *NONE OF ABOVE*	f.
4.	MAKING SELF UN-DERSTOOD	*(Express information content—however able)* 0. Understood 1. Usually Understood-difficulty finding words or finishing thoughts 2. Sometimes Understood-ability is limited to making concrete requests ▲4 3. Rarely/Never Understood ▲4	
5.	ABILITY TO UNDER-STAND OTHERS	*(Understanding verbal information content-however able)* 0. Understands 1. Usually Understands-may miss some part/intent of message ▲2 2. Sometimes Understands-responds adequately to simple, direct communication ▲2 ▲4 ▲5 3. Rarely/Never Understands ▲2 ▲4 ▲5	
6.	CHANGE IN COMMUNI-CATION/ HEARING	Resident's ability to express, understand or hear information has changed over last 90 days 0. No change 1. Improved 2. Deteriorated ●1	

● = Automatic Trigger

1 - Delirium
2 - Cognitive Loss/Dementia
3 - Visual Function
4 - Communication

5 - ADL Functional/Rehabilitation Potential
6 - Urinary Incontinence and Indwelling Catheter
7 - Psychosocial Well-Being
8 - Mood State

▲ = Potential Trigger

9 - Behavior Problems
10 - Activities
11 - Falls
12 - Nutritional Status

13 - Feeding Tubes
14 - Dehydration/Fluid Maintenance
15 - Dental Care
16 - Pressure Ulcers

17 - Psychotropic Drug Use
18 - Physical Restraints

Figure 8-5
Communication/hearing patterns. (Reproduced with permission from Briggs Corp, Des Moines.)

SECTION D. VISION PATTERNS			
1.	VISION	*(Ability to see in adequate light and with glasses if used)* 0. Adequate—sees fine detail, including regular print in newspapers/books 1. Impaired—sees large print, but not regular print in newspapers/books ●[3] 2. Highly Impaired—limited vision, not able to see newspaper headlines, appears to follow objects with eyes ●[3] 3. Severely Impaired—no vision or appears to see only light, colors, or shapes ●[3]	

2.	VISUAL LIMITATIONS/ DIFFICULTIES	a. Side vision problems—decreased peripheral vision; (e.g., leaves food on one side of tray, difficulty traveling, bumps into people and objects, misjudges placement of chair when seating self) ●[3]	a.
		b. Experiences any of the following: sees halos or rings around lights, sees flashes of light; sees "curtains" over eyes	b.
		c. *NONE OF ABOVE*	c.
3.	VISUAL APPLIANCES	Glasses; contact lenses; lens implant; magnifying glass 0. No 1. Yes	

● = Automatic Trigger

1 - Delirium
2 - Cognitive Loss/Dementia
3 - Visual Function
4 - Communication

5 - ADL Functional/Rehabilitation Potential
6 - Urinary Incontinence and Indwelling Catheter
7 - Psychosocial Well-Being
8 - Mood State

▲ = Potential Trigger

9 - Behavior Problems
10 - Activities
11 - Falls
12 - Nutritional Status

13 - Feeding Tubes
14 - Dehydration/Fluid Maintenance
15 - Dental Care
16 - Pressure Ulcers

17 - Psychotropic Drug Us
18 - Physical Restraints

Figure 8-6

Vision patterns. (Reproduced with permission from Briggs Corp, Des Moines.)

   (9) Behavior problems
  (10) Activities
  (11) Falls
  (12) Nutritional status
  (13) Feeding tubes
  (14) Dehydration/fluid maintenance
  (15) Dental care
  (16) Pressure ulcers
  (17) Psychotropic drug use
  (18) Physical restraints

c. The comprehensive and standardized assessment of the patient's needs is known as the *Resident Assessment Instrument (RAI)* and includes MDS and RAP

d. The RAI is not meant to replace the initial examination and orders provided by the physician but only to serve as a supplement; the physician should be informed if any of the 18 problem areas have been identified (e.g., falls, delirium, incontinence) and address these problems in the plan of care

SECTION E. PHYSICAL FUNCTIONING AND STRUCTURAL PROBLEMS				

1.	ADL SELF-PERFORMANCE *(Code for resident's PERFORMANCE OVER ALL SHIFTS during last 7 days—Not including setup)*
	
	0. *INDEPENDENT*—No help or oversight—OR—Help/oversight provided only 1 or 2 times during last 7 days.
	1. *SUPERVISION*—Oversight encouragement or cueing provided 3+ times during last 7 days—OR—Supervision plus physical assistance provided only 1 or 2 times during last 7 days.
	2. *LIMITED ASSISTANCE*—Resident highly involved in activity, received physical help in guided maneuvering of limbs, or other nonweight bearing assistance 3+ times—OR—More help provided only 1 or 2 times during last 7 days.
	3. *EXTENSIVE ASSISTANCE*—While resident performed part of activity, over last 7-day period, help of following type(s) provided 3 or more times:
	  — Weight-bearing support
	  — Full staff performance during part (but not all) of last 7 days.
	4. *TOTAL DEPENDENCE*—Full staff performance of activity during entire 7 days.				

2.	ADL SUPPORT PROVIDED—*(Code for MOST SUPPORT PROVIDED OVER ALL SHIFTS during last 7 days; code regardless of resident's self-performance classification)* 0. No setup or physical help from staff 2. One-person physical assist 1. Setup help only 3. Two+ persons physical assist	1 SELF-PERFORMANCE	2 SUPPORT
a.	BED MOBILITY	How resident moves to and from lying position, turns side to side, and positions body while in bed 3 or 4 for self-perf = ▲⁵		
b.	TRANSFER	How resident moves between surfaces—to/from: bed, chair, wheelchair, standing position (EXCLUDE to/from bath/toilet) 3 or 4 for self-perf = ▲⁵		
c.	LOCO-MOTION	How resident moves between locations in his/her room and adjacent corridor on same floor. If in wheelchair, self-sufficiency once in chair 3 or 4 for self-perf = ▲⁵		
d.	DRESSING	How resident puts on, fastens, and takes off all items of street clothing, including donning/removing prosthesis 3 or 4 for self-perf = ▲⁵		
e.	EATING	How resident eats and drinks (regardless of skill) 3 or 4 for self-perf = ▲⁵		
f.	TOILET USE	How resident uses the toilet room (or commode, bed-pan, urinal); transfers on/off toilet, cleanses, changes pad, manages ostomy or catheter, adjusts clothes 3 or 4 for self-perf = ▲⁵		
g.	PERSONAL HYGIENE	How resident maintains personal hygiene, including combing hair, brushing teeth, shaving, applying makeup, washing/drying face, hands, and perineum (EXCLUDE baths and showers)		
3.	BATHING	How resident takes full-body bath, sponge bath, and transfers in/out of tub/shower (EXCLUDE washing of back and hair. Code for most dependent in self-performance and support. Bathing Self-Performance codes appear below.) 3 or 4 for (a) = ▲⁵ 0. Independent—No help provided 1. Supervision—Oversight help only 2. Physical help limited to transfer only 3. Physical help in part of bathing activity 4. Total dependence	a.	b.

Figure 8-7

Physical functioning and structural problems. (Reproduced with permission from Briggs Corp, Des Moines.) *Continued*

4.	BODY CONTROL PROBLEMS	*(Check all that apply during last 7 days)*		
		a. Balance—partial or total loss of ability to balance self while standing ▲11	a.	g. Hand—lack of dexterity (e.g., problem using toothbrush or adjusting hearing aid)	g.
		b. Bedfast all or most of the time ▲11	b.	h. Leg—partial or total loss of voluntary movement ▲11	h.
		c. Contracture to arms, legs, shoulders, or hands	c.	i. Leg—unsteady gait	i.
		d. Hemiplegia/ hemiparesis ▲11	d.	j. Trunk—partial or total loss of ability to position, balance, or turn body ▲11	j.
		e. Quadriplegia ▲11	e.	k. Amputation	k.
		f. Arm—partial or total loss of voluntary movement	f.	l. NONE OF ABOVE	l.
5.	MOBILITY APPLIANCES/ DEVICES	*(Check all that apply during last 7 days)*		
		a. Cane/walker	a.	d. Other person wheeled	d.
		b. Brace/prosthesis	b.	e. Lifted (manually/ mechanically)	e.
		c. Wheeled self	c.	f. NONE OF ABOVE	f.
6.	TASK SEG-MENTATION	Resident requires that some or all of ADL activities be broken into a series of subtasks so that resident can perform them. 0. No 1. Yes		
7.	ADL FUNC-TIONAL REHAB. POTENTIAL	a. Resident believes he/she capable of increased independence in at least some ADLs ▲5		a.
		b. Direct care staff believe resident capable of increased independence in at least some ADLs ▲5		b.
		c. Resident able to perform tasks/activity but is very slow		c.
		d. Major difference in ADL Self-Performance or ADL Support in mornings and evenings (at least a one category change in Self-Performance or Support in any ADL)		d.
		e. NONE OF ABOVE		e.
8.	CHANGE IN ADL FUNCTION	Change in ADL self-performance in last 90 days 0. No change 1. Improved 2. Deteriorated ▲14		

● = Automatic Trigger

1 - Delirium	5 - ADL Functional/Rehabilitation Potential
2 - Cognitive Loss/Dementia	6 - Urinary Incontinence and Indwelling Catheter
3 - Visual Function	7 - Psychosocial Well-Being
4 - Communication	8 - Mood State

▲ = Potential Trigger

9 - Behavior Problems	13 - Feeding Tubes	17 - Psychotropic Drug Use
10 - Activities	14 - Dehydration/Fluid Maintenance	18 - Physical Restraints
11 - Falls	15 - Dental Care	
12 - Nutritional Status	16 - Pressure Ulcers	

Figure 8-7, cont'd

Physical functioning and structural problems. (Reproduced with permission from Briggs Corp, Des Moines.)

	SECTION F. CONTINENCE IN LAST 14 DAYS	
1.	**CONTINENCE SELF-CONTROL CATEGORIES** *(Code for resident performance over all shifts.)* **0. CONTINENT**—Complete control **1. USUALLY CONTINENT**—BLADDER, incontinent episodes once a week or less; BOWEL, less than weekly **2. OCCASIONALLY INCONTINENT**—BLADDER, 2+ times a week but not daily; BOWEL, once a week **3. FREQUENTLY INCONTINENT**—BLADDER, tended to be incontinent daily, but some control present (e.g., on day shift); BOWEL, 2-3 times a week **4. INCONTINENT**—Had inadequate control. BLADDER, multiple daily episodes; BOWEL, all (or almost all) of the time.	
a.	**BOWEL CONTINENCE**	Control of bowel movement, with appliance or bowel continence programs if employed
b.	**BLADDER CONTINENCE**	Control of urinary bladder function (if dribbles, volume insufficient to soak through underpants), with appliances (e.g., foley) or continence programs, if employed 2, 3 or 4 = ▲[6]

2.	**INCONTINENCE RELATED TESTING**	*(Skip if resident's bladder continence code equals 0 or 1 AND no catheter is used)* a. Resident has been tested for a urinary tract infection b. Resident has been checked for presence of a fecal impaction, or there is adequate bowel elimination c. *NONE OF ABOVE*	a. b. c.

3.	**APPLIANCES AND PROGRAMS**	a. Any scheduled toileting plan	a.	e. Did not use toilet room/commode/urinal	e.
		b. External (condom) catheter ▲[6]	b.	f. Pads/briefs used ▲[6]	f.
		c. Indwelling catheter ▲[6]	c.	g. Enemas/irrigation	g.
		d. Intermittent catheter ▲[6]	d.	h. Ostomy	h.
				i. *NONE OF ABOVE*	i.

4.	**CHANGE IN URINARY CONTINENCE**	Change in urinary continence/appliances and programs in **last 90 days** 0. No change 1. Improved 2. Deteriorated

● = Automatic Trigger

1 - Delirium	5 - ADL Functional/Rehabilitation Potential
2 - Cognitive Loss/Dementia	6 - Urinary Incontinence and Indwelling Catheter
3 - Visual Function	7 - Psychosocial Well-Being
4 - Communication	8 - Mood State

▲ = Potential Trigger

9 - Behavior Problems	13 - Feeding Tubes	17 - Psychotropic Drug Use
0 - Activities	14 - Dehydration/Fluid Maintenance	18 - Physical Restraints
1 - Falls	15 - Dental Care	
2 - Nutritional Status	16 - Pressure Ulcers	

Figure 8-8

Continence in the last 14 days. (Reproduced with permission from Briggs Corp, Des Moines.)

2. Use of psychotropic drugs[5]

   a. It is estimated that 75% to 94% of nursing home residents have some form of mental disorder.[4] Agitated behavior accompanying mental dysfunction in the elderly is often controlled with pharmacologic therapy

   b. OBRA regulations clearly state that antipsychotic drugs should be used

	SECTION G. PSYCHOSOCIAL WELL-BEING	
1.	**SENSE OF INITIATIVE/ INVOLVE-MENT**	a. At ease interacting with others	a.
		b. At ease doing planned or structural activities	b.
		c. At ease doing self-initiated activities	c.
		d. Establishes own goals	d.
		e. Pursues involvement in life of facility (i.e., makes/keeps friends; involved in group activities; responds positively to new activities; assists at religious services)	e.
		f. Accepts invitations into most group activities	f.
		g. *NONE OF ABOVE*	g.
2.	**UNSETTLED RELATION-SHIPS**	a. Covert/open conflict with and/or repeated criticism of staff ●⁷	a.
		b. Unhappy with roommate ●⁷	b.
		c. Unhappy with residents other than roommate ●⁷	c.
		d. Openly expresses conflict/anger with family or friends ●⁷	d.
		e. Absence of personal contact with family/friends	e.
		f. Recent loss of close family member/friend	f.
		g. *NONE OF ABOVE*	g.

3.	**PAST ROLES**	a. Strong identification with past roles and life status	a.
		b. Expresses sadness/anger/empty feeling over lost roles/status ●⁷	b.
		c. *NONE OF ABOVE*	c.

● = Automatic Trigger

1 - Delirium
2 - Cognitive Loss/Dementia
3 - Visual Function
4 - Communication

5 - ADL Functional/Rehabilitation Potential
6 - Urinary Incontinence and Indwelling Catheter
7 - Psychosocial Well-Being
8 - Mood State

▲ = Potential Trigger

9 - Behavior Problems
10 - Activities
11 - Falls
12 - Nutritional Status

13 - Feeding Tubes
14 - Dehydration/Fluid Maintenance
15 - Dental Care
16 - Pressure Ulcers

17 - Psychotropic Drug U
18 - Physical Restraints

Figure 8-9
Psychosocial well-being. (Reproduced with permission from Briggs Corp, Des Moines.)

only with explicit documentation in the medical chart and only when a specific diagnosis warrants their use (see the box on p. 398). The patient's behavior must be documented quantitatively and objectively by caregivers. Neuroleptics can be used to treat organic mental syndromes (including dementia) with associated psychotic and/or agitated features as defined by

(1) Specific behaviors (e.g., biting, kicking, scratching) that are quantitatively (i.e., periods of time) documented by the facility and that cause the resident to present a danger to self and others (including staff) and actually interfere with the staff's ability to provide care

		SECTION H. MOOD AND BEHAVIOR PATTERNS	
1.	SAD OR ANXIOUS MOOD	*(Check all that apply during last 30 days)*	
		a. **VERBAL EXPRESSIONS of DISTRESS** by resident (sadness, sense that nothing matters, hopelessness, worthlessness, unrealistic fears, vocal expressions of anxiety or grief) ●⁸	a.
		DEMONSTRATED (OBSERVABLE) SIGNS of mental DISTRESS	
		b. Tearfulness, emotional groaning, sighing, breathlessness ●⁸	b.
		c. Motor agitation such as pacing, handwringing or picking ●⁸	c.
		d. Failure to eat or take medications, withdrawal from self-care or leisure activities ●⁸ ▲¹⁴	d.
		e. Pervasive concern with health ●⁸	e.
		f. Recurrent thoughts of death—e.g., believes he/she is about to die, have a heart attack ●⁸	f.
		g. Suicidal thoughts/actions ●⁸	g.
		h. *NONE OF ABOVE*	h.
2.	MOOD PERSISTENCE	**Sad or anxious** mood intrudes on daily life over last 7 days—not easily altered, doesn't "cheer up"	
		0. No 1. Yes ●⁸	
3.	PROBLEM BEHAVIOR	*(Code for behavior in last 7 days)*	
		0. Behavior **not exhibited** in last 7 days 1. Behavior of this type occurred **less than daily** 2. Behavior of this type occurred **daily or more frequently**	
		a. **WANDERING** (moved with no rational purpose; seemingly oblivious to needs or safety) 1 or 2 = ●⁹	a.
		b. **VERBALLY ABUSIVE** (others were threatened, screamed at, cursed at) 1 or 2 = ●⁹	b.
		c. **PHYSICALLY ABUSIVE** (others were hit, shoved, scratched, sexually abused) 1 or 2 = ●⁹	c.
		d. **SOCIALLY INAPPROPRIATE/DISRUPTIVE BEHAVIOR** (made disrupting sounds, noisy, screams, self-abusive acts, sexual behavior or disrobing in public, smeared/threw food/feces, hoarding, rummaged through others' belongings) 1 or 2 = ●⁹	d.
4.	RESIDENT RESISTS CARE	*(Check all types of resistance that occurred in the last 7 days)*	
		a. Resisted taking medications/injection	a.
		b. Resisted ADL assistance	b.
		c. *NONE OF ABOVE*	c.
5.	BEHAVIOR MANAGEMENT PROGRAM	Behavior problem has been addressed by clinically developed behavior management program. (Note: Do not include programs that involve only physical restraints or psychotropic medications in this category.)	
		0. No behavior problem 1. Yes, addressed 2. No, not addressed	
6.	CHANGE IN MOOD	Change in mood in last 90 days	
		0. No change 1. Improved 2. Deteriorated ▲¹	
7.	CHANGE IN PROBLEM BEHAVIOR	Change in problem behavioral signs in last 90 days	
		0. No change 1. Improved 2. Deteriorated ●¹	

Figure 8-10

Mood and behavior patterns. (Reproduced with permission from Briggs Corp, Des Moines.)

SECTION I. ACTIVITY PURSUIT PATTERNS				
1.	TIME AWAKE	*(Check appropriate time periods—last 7 days)* Resident awake all or most of time (i.e., naps no more than one hour per time period) in the:		
		a. Morning	a.	c. Evening	c.
		b. Afternoon	b.	d. *NONE OF ABOVE*	d.
2.	AVERAGE TIME INVOLVED IN ACTIVITIES	**0.** Most—(more than 2/3 of time) ▲10 **2.** Little—(less than 1/3 of time) ▲10 **1.** Some—(1/3 to 2/3 time) **3.** None ▲10		
3.	PREFERRED ACTIVITY SETTINGS	*(Check all settings in which activities are preferred)*		
		a. Own room	a.	d. Outside facility	d.
		b. Day/activity room	b.	e. *NONE OF ABOVE*	e.
		c. Inside NH/off unit	c.		

4.	GENERAL ACTIVITIES PREFER-ENCES (adapted to resident's current abilities)	*(Check all specific preferences whether or not activity is currently available to resident)*			
		a. Cards/other games	a.	f. Spiritual/religious activ.	f.
		b. Crafts/arts	b.	g. Trips/shopping	g.
		c. Exercise/sports	c.	h. Walking/wheeling outdoors	h.
		d. Music	d.	i. Watch TV	i.
		e. Read/write	e.	j. *NONE OF ABOVE*	j.
5.	PREFERS MORE OR DIFFERENT ACTIVITIES	Resident expresses/indicates preference for other activities/choices. **0.** No **1.** Yes ●10			

● = Automatic Trigger

1 - Delirium	5 - ADL Functional/Rehabilitation Potential
2 - Cognitive Loss/Dementia	6 - Urinary Incontinence and Indwelling Catheter
3 - Visual Function	7 - Psychosocial Well-Being
4 - Communication	8 - Mood State

▲ = Potential Trigger

9 - Behavior Problems	13 - Feeding Tubes	17 - Psychotropic Drug U
10 - Activities	14 - Dehydration/Fluid Maintenance	18 - Physical Restraints
11 - Falls	15 - Dental Care	
12 - Nutritional Status	16 - Pressure Ulcers	

Figure 8-11
Activity pursuit patterns. (Reproduced with permission from Briggs Corp, Des Moines.)

      (2) Continuous crying out, screaming, yelling, or pacing, if these behaviors cause an impairment in functional capacity and if they are quantitatively (i.e., periods of time) documented by the facility's staff

      (3) Psychotic symptoms (hallucinations, paranoia, delusions) not exhibited as specific behaviors listed above if these behaviors cause an impairment in functional capacity

SECTION J. DISEASE DIAGNOSES

Check only those diseases present that have a relationship to current ADL status, cognitive status, behavior status, medical treatments, or risk of death. (Do not list old/inactive diagnoses.) (If none apply, check the NONE OF ABOVE box)

1.	DISEASES	HEART/CIRCULATION			
		a. Arteriosclerotic heart disease (ASHD)	a.	r. Manic depressive (bipolar disease)	r.
		b. Cardiac dysrhythmias	b.	**SENSORY**	
		c. Congestive heart failure	c.	s. Cataracts	s.
		d. Hypertension	d.	t. Glaucoma	t.
		e. Hypotension	e.	**OTHER**	
		f. Peripheral vascular disease	f.	u. Allergies	u.
		g. Other cardiovascular disease	g.	v. Anemia	v.
		NEUROLOGICAL		w. Arthritis	w.
		h. Alzheimer's	h.	x. Cancer	x.
		i. Dementia other than Alzheimer's	i.	y. Diabetes mellitus	y.
		j. Aphasia	j.	z. Explicit terminal prognosis	z.
		k. Cerebrovascular accident (stroke)	k.	aa. Hypothyroidism	aa.
		l. Multiple sclerosis	l.	bb. Osteoporosis	bb.
		m. Parkinson's disease	m.	cc. Seizure disorder	cc.
		PULMONARY		dd. Septicemia	dd.
		n. Emphysema/asthma/ COPD	n.	ee. Urinary tract infection- in last 30 days ▲14	ee.
		o. Pneumonia	o.	ff. *NONE OF ABOVE*	ff.
		PSYCHIATRIC/MOOD			
		p. Anxiety disorder	p.		
		q. Depression	q.		
2.	OTHER CURRENT DIAGNOSES AND ICD-9 CODES	260–263.9=●12 276.5=▲14 291.0–293.1=●1			
		a.			
		b.			
		c.			
		d.			
		e.			
		f.			

● = Automatic Trigger

1 - Delirium
2 - Cognitive Loss/Dementia
3 - Visual Function
4 - Communication

5 - ADL Functional/Rehabilitation Potential
6 - Urinary Incontinence and Indwelling Catheter
7 - Psychosocial Well-Being
8 - Mood State

▲ = Potential Trigger

9 - Behavior Problems
10 - Activities
11 - Falls
12 - Nutritional Status

13 - Feeding Tubes
14 - Dehydration/Fluid Maintenance
15 - Dental Care
16 - Pressure Ulcers

17 - Psychotropic Drug Use
18 - Physical Restraints

Figure 8-12

Disease diagnoses. (Reproduced with permission from Briggs Corp, Des Moines.)

SECTION K. HEALTH CONDITIONS				
1.	PROBLEM CONDITIONS	*(Check all problems that are present in last 7 days unless other time frame indicated)*		
		a. Constipation	a.	j. Pain—resident complains or shows evidence of pain daily or almost daily
		b. Diarrhea ▲14	b.	
		c. Dizziness/vertigo ▲14	c.	
		d. Edema	d.	j.
		e. Fecal impaction	e.	k. Recurrent lung aspirations in last 90 days
		f. Fever ▲14	f.	
		g. Hallucinations/ delusions	g.	k.
				l. Shortness of breath l.
		h. Internal bleeding ▲14	h.	m. Syncope (fainting) m.
		i. Joint pain	i.	n. Vomiting ▲14 n.
				o. *NONE OF ABOVE* o.
2.	ACCIDENTS	a. Fell—past 30 days ●11	a.	c. Hip fracture in last 180 days c.
		b. Fell—past 31-180 days ●11	b.	d. *NONE OF ABOVE* d.

3.	STABILITY OF CONDITIONS	a. Conditions/diseases make resident's cognitive, ADL, or behavior status unstable—fluctuating, precarious, or deteriorating.	a.
		b. Resident experiencing an acute episode or a flare-up of a recurrent/chronic problem.	b.
		c. *NONE OF THE ABOVE*	c.

● = Automatic Trigger

1 - Delirium	5 - ADL Functional/Rehabilitation Potential
2 - Cognitive Loss/Dementia	6 - Urinary Incontinence and Indwelling Catheter
3 - Visual Function	7 - Psychosocial Well-Being
4 - Communication	8 - Mood State

▲ = Potential Trigger

9 - Behavior Problems	13 - Feeding Tubes	17 - Psychotropic Drug U
10 - Activities	14 - Dehydration/Fluid Maintenance	18 - Physical Restraints
11 - Falls	15 - Dental Care	
12 - Nutritional Status	16 - Pressure Ulcers	

Figure 8-13

Health conditions. (Reproduced with permission from Briggs Corp, Des Moines.)

    c. A thorough search for a cause of the patient's behavior change should be undertaken before resorting to antipsychotic drug therapy; potentially correctable causes should be eliminated, for example

        (1) *Iatrogenic:* digoxin toxicity, H_2-blocker use

        (2) *Environmental:* activity near the patient's room that may disturb the patient

        (3) *Physiologic:* urinary retention, sepsis

    d. Reductions of medication dosage should be attempted whenever possible

    e. Common behavior problems such as noisiness or uncooperative be-

SECTION L. ORAL/NUTRITIONAL STATUS				
1.	ORAL PROBLEMS	a. Chewing problem		c. Mouth pain ●15
		b. Swallowing problem		d. *NONE OF ABOVE*
2.	HEIGHT AND WEIGHT	*Record height (a) in inches and weight (b) in pounds.* *Weight based on most recent status in* **last 30 days;** *measure weight consistently* ***in accord with standard facility*** *practice— e.g., in a.m. after voiding, before meal, with shoes off, and in nightclothes.* HT (in.) WT (lb.)		
		c. **Weight loss (i.e., 5% + in last 30 days; or 10% in last 180 days)**		
		0. No 1. Yes ●12 ▲14		
3.	NUTRITIONAL PROBLEMS	a. Complains about the taste of many foods ●12		d. Regular complaint of hunger ●12
		b. Insufficient fluid; dehydrated ●14		e. Leaves 25%+ food uneaten at most meals ●12 ▲14
		c. Did **NOT** consume all/almost all liquids provided **during last 3 days** ▲14		f. *NONE OF ABOVE*
4.	NUTRITIONAL APPROACHES	a. Parenteral/IV ▲14 ●12		e. Therapeutic diet ●12
		b. Feeding tube ▲14 ●13		f. Dietary supplement between meals
		c. Mechanically altered diet ●12		g. Plate guard, stabilized built-up utensil, etc.
		d. Syringe (oral feeding) ●12		h. *NONE OF ABOVE*

● = Automatic Trigger

1 - Delirium	5 - ADL Functional/Rehabilitation Potential
2 - Cognitive Loss/Dementia	6 - Urinary Incontinence and Indwelling Catheter
3 - Visual Function	7 - Psychosocial Well-Being
4 - Communication	8 - Mood State

▲ = Potential Trigger

- Behavior Problems	13 - Feeding Tubes	17 - Psychotropic Drug Use
- Activities	14 - Dehydration/Fluid Maintenance	18 - Physical Restraints
- Falls	15 - Dental Care	
- Nutritional Status	16 - Pressure Ulcers	

Figure 8-14

Oral/nutritional status. (Reproduced with permission from Briggs Corp, Des Moines.)

havior alone are not considered adequate justification for use of anti-psychotics (see the box on p. 402)

f. Antipsychotic drugs can be used on a prn basis only in the following situations

   (1) To gradually change the dose for a specific symptom or behavior

   (2) To control episodic symptoms in conjunction with another antipsychotic agent

SECTION M. ORAL/DENTAL STATUS				
1.	ORAL STATUS AND DISEASE PREVENTION	a. Debris (soft, easily movable substances) present in mouth prior to going to bed at night ●¹⁵		a.
		b. Has dentures and/or removable bridge		b.
		c. Some/all natural teeth lost—does not have or does not use dentures (or partial plates) ●¹⁵		c.
		d. Broken, loose, or carious teeth ●¹⁵		d.
		e. Inflamed gums (gingiva), oral abscesses, swollen or bleeding gums, ulcers, or rashes ●¹⁵		e.
		f. Daily cleaning of teeth/dentures	If not checked = ●¹⁵	f.
		g. NONE OF ABOVE		g.

● = Automatic Trigger

1 - Delirium
2 - Cognitive Loss/Dementia
3 - Visual Function
4 - Communication

5 - ADL Functional/Rehabilitation Potential
6 - Urinary Incontinence and Indwelling Catheter
7 - Psychosocial Well-Being
8 - Mood State

▲ = Potential Trigger

9 - Behavior Problems
10 - Activities
11 - Falls
12 - Nutritional Status

13 - Feeding Tubes
14 - Dehydration/Fluid Maintenance
15 - Dental Care
16 - Pressure Ulcers

17 - Psychotropic Drug
18 - Physical Restraints

Figure 8-15

Oral/dental status. (Reproduced with permission from Briggs Corp, Des Moines.)

Indications for which Antipsychotic Medications Should Not Be Used in the Absence of Other Justifying Criteria According to the Interpretive Guidelines of OBRA

1. Wandering
2. Poor self-care
3. Restlessness
4. Impaired memory
5. Anxiety
6. Depression
7. Insomnia
8. Unsociability
9. Indifference to surroundings
10. Fidgeting
11. Nervousness
12. Uncooperativeness
13. Unspecified agitation
14. Prn antipsychotic drug orders should not be used more than five times in any 7-day period without a review of the resident's condition by a physician

SECTION N. SKIN CONDITION			
1.	STASIS ULCER	(i.e., open lesion caused by poor venous circulation to lower extremities) 0. No 1. Yes	
2.	PRESSURE ULCERS	*(Code for highest stage of pressure ulcer)* 0. No pressure ulcers 1. Stage 1 A persistent area of skin redness (without a break in the skin) that does not disappear when pressure is relieved ●12 ●16 2. Stage 2 A partial thickness loss of skin layers that presents clinically as an abrasion, blister, or shallow crater ●12 ●16 3. Stage 3 A full thickness of skin is lost, exposing the subcutaneous tissues—presents as a deep crater with or without undermining adjacent tissue ●12 ●16 4. Stage 4 A full thickness of skin and subcutaneous tissue is lost, exposing muscle and/or bone ●12 ●16	
3.	HISTORY OF RESOLVED/ CURED PRESSURE ULCERS	Resident has had a pressure ulcer that was resolved/cured in **last 90 days** 0. No 1. Yes	

4.	SKIN PROBLEMS/ CARE	a. Open lesions other than stasis or pressure ulcers (e.g., cuts)	a.
		b. Skin desensitized to pain/pressure/discomfort	b.
		c. Protective/preventive skin care	c.
	Nothing Checked From C Thru G = ▲16	d. Turning/repositioning program	d.
		e. Pressure-relieving beds, bed/chair pads (e.g., egg crate pads)	e.
		f. Wound care/treatment (e.g., pressure ulcer care, surgical wound)	f.
		g. Other skin care/treatment	g.
		h. *NONE OF ABOVE*	h.

● = Automatic Trigger

1 - Delirium	5 - ADL Functional/Rehabilitation Potential	
2 - Cognitive Loss/Dementia	6 - Urinary Incontinence and Indwelling Catheter	
3 - Visual Function	7 - Psychosocial Well-Being	
4 - Communication	8 - Mood State	

▲ = Potential Trigger

- Behavior Problems	13 - Feeding Tubes	17 - Psychotropic Drug Use
- Activities	14 - Dehydration/Fluid Maintenance	18 - Physical Restraints
- Falls	15 - Dental Care	
- Nutritional Status	16 - Pressure Ulcers	

Figure 8-16

skin conditions. (Reproduced with permission from Briggs Corp, Des Moines.)

		SECTION O. MEDICATION USE	
1.	NUMBER OF MEDI-CATIONS	*(Record the number of different medications used in the last 7 days; enter "0" if none used.)*	
2.	NEW MEDI-CATIONS	Resident has received new medications during the **last 90 days** 0. No 1. Yes	
3.	INJECTIONS	*(Record the number of days injections of any type received during the last 7 days.)*	
4.	DAYS RECEIVED THE FOLLOWING MEDICATION	(Record the number of days during last 7 days; *Enter "0" if not used; enter "1" if long-acting meds. used less than weekly)*	
		a. Antipsychotics 1-7 = ▲⁹ ▲¹¹ ▲¹⁷	a.
		b. Antianxiety/hypnotics 1-7 = ▲⁹ ▲¹¹ ▲¹⁷	b.
		c. Antidepressants 1-7 = ▲⁹ ▲¹¹ ▲¹⁷	c.
5.	PREVIOUS MEDICATION RESULTS	*(**SKIP this question** if resident currently receiving antipsychotics, antidepressants, or antianxiety/hypnotics— otherwise **code correct response for last 90 days**)*	
		Resident has previously received psychoactive medications for a mood or behavior problem, and these medications were effective (without undue adverse consequences).	
		0. No, drugs not used 1. Drugs were effective 2. Drugs were not effective 3. Drug effectiveness unknown	

● = Automatic Trigger

1 - Delirium
2 - Cognitive Loss/Dementia
3 - Visual Function
4 - Communication

5 - ADL Functional/Rehabilitation Potential
6 - Urinary Incontinence and Indwelling Catheter
7 - Psychosocial Well-Being
8 - Mood State

▲ = Potential Trigger

9 - Behavior Problems
10 - Activities
11 - Falls
12 - Nutritional Status

13 - Feeding Tubes
14 - Dehydration/Fluid Maintenance
15 - Dental Care
16 - Pressure Ulcers

17 - Psychotropic Drug U
18 - Physical Restraints

Figure 8-17

Medication use. (Reproduced with permission from Briggs Corp, Des Moines.)

    g. If an antipsychotic agent is used more than five times in any 7-day period, the resident's plan of care should be reviewed

3. **Use of restraints**

    a. Restraints are a violation of human dignity and should not be used for discipline or convenience

    b. Physical restraints should be used only if the patient is at significan risk of self-injury or injury to others and no safer alternative or setting can be found; in every instance of restraint use, the intervention must be considered temporary and short term

    c. A comprehensive assessment and investigation of the patient's problematic behavior should be undertaken before use of restraints

    d. The order for use of a restraining device must be explained to the

SECTION P. SPECIAL TREATMENTS AND PROCEDURES				
1.	SPECIAL TREAT-MENTS AND PROCE-DURES	**SPECIAL CARE—*Check treatments received during the last 14 days.***		
		a. Chemotherapy	a.	
		b. Radiation	b.	
		c. Dialysis	c.	
		d. Suctioning	d.	
		e. Trach. care	e.	
		f. IV meds		f.
		g. Transfusions		g.
		h. O$_2$		h.
		i. Other _____		i.
		j. *NONE OF ABOVE*		j.
		THERAPIES—Record the number of days *each of the following therapies was administered (for at least 10 minutes during a day) in the last 7 days:*		
		k. Speech—language pathology and audiology services		k.
		l. Occupational therapy		l.
		m. Physical therapy		m.
		n. Psychological therapy (any licensed professional)		n.
		o. Respiratory Therapy		o.
2.	ABNORMAL LAB VALUES	Has the resident had any **abnormal lab values during** the last 90-day period? 0. No 1. Yes 2. No tests performed		
3.	DEVICES AND RESTRAINTS	*Use the following code for last 7 days:* 0 Not used 1 Used less than daily 2 Used daily		
		a. Bed rails		a.
		b. Trunk restraint 1 or 2 = ▲9 ●18		b.
		c. Limb restraint 1 or 2 = ▲9 ●18		c.
		d. Chair prevents rising 1 or 2 = ▲9 ●18		d.

● = **Automatic Trigger**

1 - Delirium
2 - Cognitive Loss/Dementia
3 - Visual Function
4 - Communication

5 - ADL Functional/Rehabilitation Potential
6 - Urinary Incontinence and Indwelling Catheter
7 - Psychosocial Well-Being
8 - Mood State

▲ = **Potential Trigger**

9 - Behavior Problems
10 - Activities
11 - Falls
12 - Nutritional Status

13 - Feeding Tubes
14 - Dehydration/Fluid Maintenance
15 - Dental Care
16 - Pressure Ulcers

17 - Psychotropic Drug Use
18 - Physical Restraints

Figure 8-18

Special treatments and procedures. (Reproduced with permission from Briggs Corp, Des Moines.)

patient or responsible party, use must be valid only for a specific period of time, and its need must be continuously reassessed

e. The medical literature reveals that physical restraints in agitated nursing home patients do not control the symptoms but actually result in increased screaming and agitation[13]

Specific Conditions that Justify the Use of Antipsychotic
Medications in Nursing Home Residents According to the
Interpretive Guidelines of OBRA

1. Schizophrenia
2. Schizoaffective disorder
3. Delusional disorder
4. Psychotic mood disorder (including mania and depression
   with psychotic features)
5. Acute psychotic episodes
6. Brief reactive psychosis
7. Schizophreniform disorder
8. Atypical psychosis
9. Tourette's disorder
10. Huntington's disease
11. Organic mental syndromes (including delirium and dementia)
    with associated psychotic and/or agitated features defined by
    a. Specific behaviors as quantitatively (number of episodes)
       and objectively (e.g., biting, kicking, and scratching) docu-
       mented by the facility, which cause the resident to
       (1) Present a danger to himself or herself
       (2) Present a danger to others (including staff)
       (3) Actually interfere with the staff's ability to provide
           care, or
    b. Continuous crying out, screaming, yelling or pacing if
       these specific behaviors cause an impairment in functional
       capacity and if they are quantitatively (e.g., periods of
       time) documented by the facility, or
    c. Psychotic symptoms (hallucinations, paranoia, delusions)
       not exhibited as specific behaviors listed in a. or b. above
       if these behaviors cause impairment in functional capacity.
12. Short-term (7 days) symptomatic treatment of hiccoughs, nau-
    sea, vomiting, or pruritus

4. **Additional patients' rights**
   a. Patients should be able to choose their own physician
   b. Medical records should be kept confidential
   c. Patients should have a right to make telephone calls, to have visitors,
      and to participate in nursing home activities

Epidemiologic considerations in nursing home care

1. **Tuberculosis testing**[7]
   a. TB occurs with disproportionate frequency among the elderly, particu-
      larly in the nursing home setting (20% of TB cases in the elderly oc-
      cur in nursing home patients)

b. The American Geriatric Society recommends a two-step PPD test for nursing home patients on admission

c. If the initial PPD test is negative, the test is repeated 1 week later; repeat PPD is useful to stimulate a booster phenomenon in patients whose initial infection occurred many years in the past

d. A decision to treat should be based on chest x-ray findings, sputum stain and cultures, and clinical picture in addition to a positive PPD (see Section 6.8.a)

2. **Influenza prevention and treatment** (see Section 6.8.c)

a. Ninety percent of influenza-related deaths occur in those 65 years or older, yet each year only 45% of the elderly receive influenza vaccine

b. Influenza immunization significantly reduces the incidence of hospitalization and death. It should be given to all persons 65 years and older, especially residents of a nursing home. Egg protein allergy is a contraindication to vaccination

c. Amantadine 100 mg/day is effective in preventing or lessening the signs and symptoms of influenza caused by strain A. Dosage should be decreased in patients with renal insufficiency. In a recent study, 22% of amantadine recipients experienced adverse effects (fatigue, nausea, delirium, falls). Frequent monitoring of renal function and dose reduction based on estimated creatinine clearance are recommended to minimize potential toxicity.[6] Amantadine may also lower the seizure threshold in patients with seizure disorders

3. **Pneumococcal vaccination**

a. Pneumococcal vaccine contains antigens to 23 serotypes of pneumococci and can reduce episodes of pneumococcal bacteremia by 70% in older patients with underlying illness (e.g., cirrhosis, renal failure)

b. Vaccination is recommended for anyone 65 years or older. Revaccination may be necessary in persons vaccinated over 10 years ago. The Immunization Practices Advisory Committee of the Public Health Service recommends revaccination for splenectomized patients and those with conditions associated with a rapid decline in pneumococcal antibody levels

c. Egg protein allergy: contraindication to vaccination

d. Most frequent adverse reactions: local erythema and pain at injection site; fewer than 1% of vaccinated patients develop fever or myalgia

e. Simultaneous pneumococcal and influenza vaccinations can be given if injections are given at different sites

Factors contributing to hospitalization of nursing home patients

1. Annual hospitalization rates per nursing home bed range from 0.21 to 0.55. Major reasons for hospitalization are

a. Lack of available IV therapy at the nursing home (70%)

b. Transfer because of poor physician-nurse communication or for the convenience of the physician (e.g., lack of diagnostic services at the nursing home [15%])

c. Pressure from family or nursing home staff (15%)

2. Infection: most common acute medical problem that results in hospitalization

Periodic monitoring of nursing home residents[10]

1. Physicians are generally required by federal and state law to reevaluate nursing home residents every 30 to 60 days
2. Progress notes should follow a standardized format (e.g., SOAP notes)
3. During the periodic evaluation, all reports from nursing staff, other interdisciplinary team members, and consultants should be reviewed
4. All medications should be periodically reviewed and appropriate laboratory monitoring ordered
   a. Patients on diuretics should have BUN/creatinine and electrolytes ordered every 2 to 3 months
   b. Stool for occult blood, Hb/Hct, BUN/creatinine should be evaluated every 1 to 2 months in patients receiving NSAIDs
   c. Monitoring of blood levels for toxicity of specific drugs should be performed every 3 to 6 months (e.g., digoxin, phenytoin [Dilantin], quinidine, theophylline)
   d. ALT/AST and BUN/creatinine should be performed periodically in all patients receiving hepatotoxic and nephrotoxic drugs
   e. Figure 8-19 shows a typical nursing home monitoring flowchart.

NAME:
DOB:

NURSING HOME FLOWCHART

Quarter or month	1st Q			2nd Q			3rd Q			4th Q		
	1/97	2/97	3/97	4/97	5/97	6/97	7/97	8/97	9/97	10/97	11/97	12/97
Weight (q mo)												
BP (q mo)												
Albumin (q yr)												
CBC (q yr)												
FBS (q yr)												
Creat (q yr)												
Cholesterol (q yr)												
Mini Mental Score (q quart)												
Ambulate (Ind/Asst/No) (q mo)												
Continence (U) (Y/N) (q mo)												
Continence (S) (Y/N) (q mo)												
Pressure ulcer (Y/N) (q mo)												
Prescription Meds (#) (q mo)												
OTC Meds (#) (q mo)												
PRN Meds (#) (q mo)												
Falls (Y/N) (q quart)												
Group Activities (Y/N) (q quart)												
Restraints (G/SR/LB/V/M/N)*												
Infections (P/U/O/N)**												

*G, Geri chair; SR, Side rail; LB, Lap belt; V, Vest; M, Mitts; N, None.
**P, Pneumonia; U, UTI; O, Other; N, None.

Figure 8-19
Nursing home flowchart.

References

1. Applebaum GE, King JE, Finucane TE: The outcome of CPR initiated in nursing homes, *J Am Geriatr Soc* 38:197-200, 1990.
2. Avorn J, Gurwitz JH: Drugs in the nursing home, *Ann Intern Med* 123:195-204, 1995.
3. Beers MH et al: Explicit outcome for determining inappropriate medication use in nursing home residents, *Arch Intern Med* 15:1825-1832, 1991.
4. Billig N et al: Pharmacologic treatment of agitation in a nursing home, *J Am Geriatr Soc* 39:1002-1005, 1991.
5. Burke WJ: Neuroleptic drug use in the nursing home, the impact of OBRA, *Am Fam Physician* 43(6):2125-2130, 1991.
6. Degelau J et al: Occurrence of adverse effects and high amantadine concentrations with influenza prophylaxis in the nursing home, *J Am Geriatr Soc* 38:428-432, 1990.
7. Finucane TE et al: The American Geriatric Society Statement on two-step PPD testing for nursing home patients on admission, *J Am Geriatr Soc* 36:77-78, 1988.
8. Levenson S: *Medical direction in long term care: a clinical and administrative guide,* Baltimore, 1988, National Health Publishing.
9. Meiches R: Medicare guidelines for physician reimbursement of nursing home patients, *Am Geriatr Soc Newsletter* 20:1, 1991.
10. Ouslander JG, Osterweil D: Physician evaluation and management of nursing home residents, *Ann Intern Med* 121:584-592, 1994.
11. Ouslander JG, Martin SE: Assessment in the nursing home, *Clin Geriatr Med* 3:155-174, 1987.
12. Stolman CJ et al: Evaluation of patient, physician, nurse, and family attitudes toward do not resuscitate orders, *Arch Intern Med* 150:653-658, 1990.
13. Werner P et al: Physical restraints and agitation in nursing home residents, *J Am Geriatr Soc* 37:1122-1126, 1989.
14. Winograd CH, Pawlson LG: OBRA-87: a commentary, *J Am Geriatr Soc* 39:724-726, 1991.

8.4 HOSPICE CARE AND PAIN MANAGEMENT
Fred F. Ferri, MD, and Tom J. Wachtel, MD

1. Hospice care is reserved for terminally ill patients. The physician must certify that patient's life expectancy is less than 6 months
2. A dignified, comforting, and humane approach along with adequate pain control are important goals of hospice care
3. Hospice services are provided by an interdisciplinary team including physicians, social workers, skilled nurses, counselors, and various allied health professionals
4. Hospice care involves both inpatient and outpatient care; however, Medicare certification requires hospice programs to provide over 80% of its patient days outside institutions
5. Hospice care replaces Part A of Medicare, so to participate in hospice care the patient must waive Medicare benefits for curative services. Medicare covers 210 hospice days. Extended coverage is also available
6. Following entry into the hospice program, a physician can choose to continue to manage the patient's care or relinquish the primary medical responsibility to the hospice program physician
7. Pain is the most feared symptom of terminal illness, so pain control is essential

Pain management*

Figure 8-20 shows the sequence of activities related to pain assessment and management. The flowchart emphasizes the use of multiple modalities concurrently, beginning with the least invasive modalities and advancing treatment to meet the patient's need for pain relief.

1. *Treating cancer pain in the elderly:* like other adults, elderly patients require comprehensive assessment and aggressive management of cancer pain. However, older patients are at risk for undertreatment of pain because of underestimation of their sensitivity to pain, the expectation that they tolerate pain well, and misconceptions about their ability to benefit from opioids. Issues in assessing and treating cancer pain in older patients include

   a. *Multiple chronic diseases and sources of pain:* complex medication regimens place elderly patients at increased risk for drug-drug and drug-disease interactions

   b. *Visual, hearing, motor, and cognitive impairments:* use of simple descriptive, numeric, and visual analog pain assessment instruments may be impeded; cognitively impaired patients may require simpler scales and more frequent pain assessment

   c. *NSAID side effects:* although effective alone or as adjuncts to opioids, NSAIDs are more likely to cause gastric and renal toxicity and other drug reactions such as cognitive impairment, constipation, and headaches in older patients; alternative NSAIDs (e.g., choline magnesium trisalicylate) or coadministration of misoprostol should be considered to reduce gastric toxicity

   d. *Opioid effectiveness:* older persons tend to be more sensitive to the analgesic effects of opioids; peak opioid effect is higher and duration of pain relief is longer

   e. *Patient-controlled analgesia:* slower drug clearance and increased sensitivity to undesirable drug effects (e.g., cognitive impairment) indicate the need for cautious initial dosing and subsequent titration and monitoring

   f. *Alternative routes of administration:* although useful for patients who have nausea or vomiting, the rectal route may be inappropriate for elderly or infirm patients who are physically unable to place the suppository in the rectum

   g. *Postoperative pain control:* Following surgery, surgeons and other health care team members should maintain frequent direct contact with the elderly patient to reassess the quality of pain management

   h. *Change of setting:* reassessment of pain management and appropriate changes should be made whenever the elderly patient moves (e.g., from hospital to home or nursing home)

2. *Pain assessment:* failure to assess pain is a critical factor leading to undertreatment. Assessment involves both the clinician and the patient. It should occur at regular intervals after initiation of treatment, at each new report of pain, and at a suitable interval after pharmacologic or nonpharmacologic intervention, e.g., 15 to 30 minutes after parenteral drug

*Modified from Jacox A et al: *Management of cancer pain: adults quick reference guide No. 9.* AHCPR Pub. No. 94-0593, Rockville, Md, 1994, Agency for Health Care Policy and Research, U.S. Department of Health and Human Services, Public Health Service.

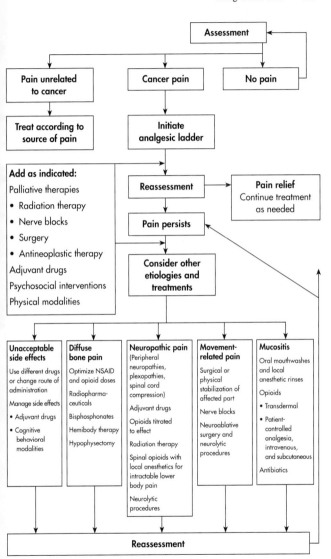

Figure 8-20

Continuing pain management. (Redrawn from Jacox A et al: *Management of cancer pain: adults quick reference guide No. 9.* AHCPR Pub No. 94-0593, Rockville, Md, 1994, Agency for Health Care Policy and Research, US Department of Health and Human Services, Public Health Services.)

therapy and 1 hour after oral administration. Identifying the etiology of
pain is essential to its management. Clinicians treating patients with cancer should recognize the common cancer pain syndromes caused by peripheral neuropathy; prompt diagnosis and treatment of these syndromes
can reduce morbidity associated with unrelieved pain

a. *Initial assessment:* the goal of the initial assessment of pain is to characterize the pain by location, intensity, and etiology. Essential to initial assessment are
   (1) Detailed history
   (2) Physical examination
   (3) Psychosocial assessment
   (4) Diagnostic evaluation
b. *Patient self-report* (Figure 8-21): mainstay of pain assessment; to enhance pain management across all settings, clinicians should teach
   families to use pain assessment tools in their homes. The clinician
   should help the patient to describe
   (1) *Pain:* listen to the patient's descriptive words about the quality of
       the pain; these provide valuable clues to its etiology. Examples of
       simple self-report pain intensity scales include the simple descrip-
       tive, numeric, and visual analog scales shown below

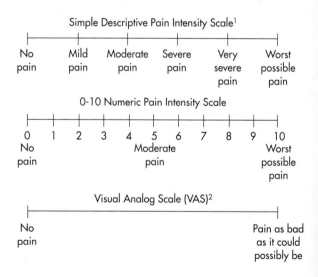

[1]If used as a graphic rating scale, a 10-cm baseline is recommended.
[2]A 10-cm baseline is recommended for VAS scales.

Figure 8-21
Pain intensity scales.

      (2) *Location:* ask the patient to indicate the exact location of the pain on his or her body or on a body diagram and whether it radiates

      (3) *Intensity or severity:* encourage the patient to keep a log of pain intensity scores to report during follow-up visits or by telephone

      (4) *Aggravating and relieving factors:* ask when the patient experiences the most pain and the least pain; document responses in patient's chart

      (5) *Cognitive response to pain:* note behavior suggesting pain in patients who are cognitively impaired or who have communication problems relating to education, language, ethnicity, or culture. Use appropriate (e.g., simpler or translated) pain assessment tools

      (6) *Goals for pain control:* document patient's preferred pain assessment tool and goals for pain control (as scores on a pain scale) in patient's pain history

3. Pharmacologic treatment

  a. NSAIDs: effective for relief of mild pain and have an opioid dose-sparing effect that helps reduce side effects when given with opioids for moderate to severe pain. Acetaminophen is included with NSAIDs because it has similar analgesic potency although it lacks peripheral antiinflammatory activity. Side effects can occur at any time; elderly patients who take acetaminophen or NSAIDs should be observed carefully. Table 8-1 describes dosing data for acetaminophen and NSAIDs in adults. Dose reduction may be necessary in elderly patients

  b. Opioids: can be added for mild to moderate pain. Tables 8-2 and 8-3 describe dose equivalents for opioid analgesics. The predictable consequences of long-term opioid administration—tolerance and physical dependence—are often confused with psychologic dependence (addiction), that manifests as drug abuse; can lead to ineffective prescribing, administering, or dispensing of opioids for cancer pain, with resultant undertreatment. Clinicians may be reluctant to give high doses of opioids to patients with advanced disease because of a fear of serious side effects. The clinician's ethical duty—to benefit the patient by relieving pain—supports increasing doses, even at the risk of side effects. Because many patients with cancer pain become opioid tolerant during long-term opioid therapy, the clinician's fear of shortening life by increasing opioid doses is usually unfounded. Opioids are classified as full morphinelike agonists, partial agonists, or mixed agonist-antagonists, depending on the specific receptors to which they bind and their activity at these receptors. Benefits and risks of using opioids vary among individuals

      (1) *Full agonists,* including morphine, hydromorphone, codeine, oxycodone, hydrocodone, methadone, levorphanol, and fentanyl, are classified as such because their effectiveness with increasing doses is not limited; will not reverse or antagonize effects of other full agonists given simultaneously

        (a) *Morphine:* most commonly used opioid; readily available in several forms, including sustained-acting (8 to 12 hours) tablets of morphine and long-acting (2 to 3 days) transdermal fentanyl patches

        (b) *Other agonists:* for the patient who experiences dose-limiting

Text continued on p. 416.

Table 8-1 Dosing data for acetaminophen and NSAIDs

Drug	Usual Dose for Adults ≥50-kg Body Weight	Usual Dose for Adults[a] <50-kg Body Weight
Acetaminophen and Over-the-Counter NSAIDs		
Acetaminophen[b]	650 mg q4h	10-15 mg/kg q4h
	975 mg q6h	15-20 mg/kg q4h (rectal)
Aspirin[c]	650 mg q4h	10-15 mg/kg q4h
	975 mg q6h	15-20 mg/kg q4h (rectal)
Ibuprofen (Motrin, others)	400-600 mg q6h	10 mg/kg q6-8h
Prescription NSAIDs		
Carprofen (Rimadyl)	100 mg tid	
Choline magnesium trisalicylate[d] (Trilisate)	1000-1500 mg tid	25 mg/kg tid
Choline salicylate (Arthropan)[d]	870 mg q3-4h	
Diflunisal (Dolobid)[e]	500 mg q12h	
Etodolac (Lodine)	200-400 mg q6-8h	
Fenoprofen calcium (Nalfon)	300-600 mg q6h	
Ketoprofen (Orudis)	25-60 mg q6-8h	
Ketorolac tromethamine[f] (Toradol)	10 mg q4-6h to a maximum of 40 mg/day	
Magnesium salicylate (Doan's, Magan, Mobidin, others)	650 mg q4h	
Meclofenamate sodium (Meclomen)[g]	50-100 mg q6h	

Mefenamic acid (Ponstel)	250 mg q6h	
Naproxen (Naprosyn)	250–275 mg q6-8h	
Naproxen sodium (Anaprox)	275 mg q6-8h	5 mg/kg q8h
Sodium salicylate (generic)	325–650 mg q3-4h	
Parenteral NSAID		
Ketorolac tromethamine[f,h] (Toradol)	60 mg initially, then 30 mg q6h Intramuscular dose not to exceed 5 days	

From Jacox A et al: *Management of cancer pain: adults quick reference guide No. 9.* AHCPR Pub. No. 94-0593, Rockville, Md, 1994, Agency for Health Care Policy and Research, U.S. Department of Health and Human Services, Public Health Services.

NOTE: Only the above NSAIDs have FDA approval for use as simple analgesics, but clinical experience has been gained with other drugs as well.

[a]Acetaminophen and NSAID dosages for adults weighing less than 50 kg should be adjusted for weight.

[b]Acetaminophen lacks the peripheral antiinflammatory and antiplatelet activities of the other NSAIDs.

[c]The standard against which other NSAIDs are compared. May inhibit platelet aggregation for ≥1 week and may cause bleeding.

[d]May have minimal antiplatelet activity.

[e]Administration with antacids may decrease absorption.

[f]For short-term use only.

[g]Coombs-positive autoimmune hemolytic anemia has been associated with prolonged use.

[h]Has the same GI toxicities as oral NSAIDs.

Table 8-2 Dose equivalents for opioid analgesics in opioid-naive adults ≥ 50 kg[a]

Drug	Approximate Equianalgesic Dose		Usual Starting Dose for Moderate to Severe Pain	
	Oral	Parenteral	Oral	Parenteral
Opioid Agonist[b]				
Morphine	30 mg q3-4h (repeat around-the-clock dosing) 60 mg q3-4h (single dose or intermittent dosing)	10 mg q3-4h	30 mg q3-4h	10 mg q3-4h
Morphine, controlled-release (MS Contin, Oramorph)	90-120 mg q-12h	N/A	90-120 mg q12h	N/A
Hydromorphone (Dilaudid)	7.5 mg q3-4h	1.5 mg q3-4h	6 mg q3-4h	1.5 mg q3-4h
Levorphanol (Levo-Dromoran)	4 mg q6-8h	2 mg q6-8h	4 mg q6-8h	2 mg q6-8h
Meperidine (Demerol)	300 mg q2-3h	100 mg q3h	N/R	100 mg q3h
Methadone (Dolophine, other)	20 mg q6-8h	10 mg q6-8h	20 mg q6-8h	10 mg q6-8h
Oxymorphone (Numorphan)	N/A	1 mg q3-4h	N/A	1 mg q3-4h
Combination Opioid/NSAID Preparations[f]				
Codeine (with aspirin or acetaminophen)	180-200 mg q3-4h	130 mg q3-4h	60 mg q3-4h	60 mg q2h (IM/SC)

Hydrocodone (in Lorcet, Lortab, Vicodin, others)	30 mg q3-4h	N/A	10 mg q3-4h	N/A
Oxycodone (Roxicodone, also in Percocet, Percodan, Tylox, others)	30 mg q3-4h	N/A	10 mg q3-4h	N/A

(From Jacox A et al: *Management of cancer pain: adults quick reference guide No. 9.* AHCPR Pub. No. 94-0593, Rockville, Md, 1994, Agency for Health Care Policy and Research, U.S. Department of Health and Human Services, Public Health Services.

q, Every. *N/A,* not available; *N/R,* not recommended; *IM,* intramuscular; *SC,* subcutaneous.

NOTE: Published tables vary in the suggested doses that are equianalgesic to morphine. Clinical response is the criterion that must be applied for each patient; titration to clinical responses is necessary. Because there is not complete cross tolerance among these drugs, it is usually necessary to use a lower than equianalgesic dose when changing drugs and to retitrate to response.

[a]CAUTION: Recommended doses do not apply for adult patients with body weight less than 50 kg. For recommended starting doses for adults <50-kg body weight, see Table 8-3.

[b]CAUTION: Recommended doses do not apply to patients with renal or hepatic insufficiency or other conditions affecting drug metabolism and kinetics.

[c]CAUTION: For morphine, hydromorphone, and oxymorphone, rectal administration is an alternate route for patients unable to take oral medications. Equianalgesic doses may differ from oral and parenteral doses because of pharmacokinetic differences. NOTE: A short-acting opioid should normally be used for initial therapy of moderate to severe pain.

[d]Transdermal fentanyl (Duragesic) is an alternative option. Transdermal fentanyl dosage is not calculated as equianalgesic to a single morphine dosage. See the package insert for dosing calculations. Doses above 25 µg/hr should not be used in opioid-naive patients.

[e]Not recommended. Doses listed are for brief therapy. Switch to another opioid for long-term therapy.

[f]CAUTION: Doses of aspirin and acetaminophen in combination opioid/NSAID preparations must also be adjusted to the patient's body weight.

[g]CAUTION: Codeine doses above 65 mg often are not appropriate because of diminishing incremental analgesia with increasing doses but continually increasing nausea, constipation, and other side effects.

Table 8-3 Dose equivalents for opioid analgesics in opioid-naive adults <50 kg

Drug	Approximate Equianalgesic Dose		Usual Starting Dose for Moderate to Severe Pain	
	Oral	Parenteral	Oral	Parenteral
Opioid Agonist[a]				
Morphine	30 mg q3-4h (repeat around-the-clock dosing) 60 mg q3-4h (single dose or intermittent dosing)	10 mg q3-4h	0.3 mg/kg q3-4h	0.1 mg/kg q3-4h
Morphine controlled-release[b,c] (MS Contin, Oramorph)	90-120 mg q12h	N/A	N/A	N/A
Hydromorphone (Dilaudid)	7.5 mg q3-4h	1.5 mg q3-4h	0.06 mg/kg q3-4h	0.015 mg/kg q3-4h
Levorphanol (Levo-Dromoran)	4 mg q6-8h	2 mg q6-8h	0.04 mg/kg q6-8h	0.02 mg/kg q6-8h
Meperidine[d] (Demerol)	300 mg q2-3h	100 mg q3h	N/R	0.75 mg/kg q2-3h
Methadone (Dolophine, others)	20 mg q6-8h	10 mg q6-8h	0.2 mg/kg q6-8h	0.1 mg/kg q3-4h
Combination Opioid/NSAID Preparations[e]				
Codeine[f] (with aspirin or acet-aminophen)	80-200 mg q3-4h	130 mg q3-4h	0.5-1 mg/kg q3-4h	N/R

Hydrocodone (in Lorcet, Lortab, Vicodin, others)	30 mg q3-4h	N/A	0.2 mg/kg q3-4h	N/A
Oxycodone (Roxicodone, also in Percocet, Percodan, Tylox, others)	30 mg q3-4h	N/A	0.2 mg/kg q3-4h	N/A

(From Jacox A et al: *Management of cancer pain: adults quick reference guide No. 9.* AHCPR Pub. No. 94-0593, Rockville, Md, 1994, Agency for Health Care Policy and Research, U.S. Department of Health and Human Services, Public Health Services.

q, Every; *N/A,* not available; *N/R,* not recommended.

NOTE: Published tables vary in the suggested doses that are equianalgesic to morphine. Clinical response is the criterion that must be applied for each patient; titration to clinical responses is necessary. Because there is not complete cross tolerance among these drugs, it is usually necessary to use a lower than equianalgesic dose when changing drugs and to retitrate to response.

aCAUTION: Recommended doses do not apply to patients with renal or hepatic insufficiency or other conditions affecting drug metabolism and kinetics.

bCAUTION: For morphine, hydromorphone, and oxymorphone, rectal administration is an alternate route for patients unable to take oral medications. Equianalgesic doses may differ from oral and parenteral doses because of pharmacokinetic differences. NOTE: A short-acting opioid should normally be used for initial therapy of moderate to severe pain.

cTransdermal fentanyl (Duragesic) is an alternative option. Transdermal fentanyl dosage is not calculated as equianalgesic to a single morphine dosage. See the package insert for dosing calculations. Doses above 25 μg/h should not be used in opioid-naive patients.

dNot recommended. Doses listed are for brief therapy. Switch to another opioid for long-term therapy.

eCAUTION: Doses of aspirin and acetaminophen in combination opioid/NSAID preparations must also be adjusted to the patient's body weight.

fCAUTION: Some clinicians recommend not exceeding 1.5 mg/kg of codeine because of an increased incidence of side effects with higher doses.

side effects with one oral opioid (e.g., hallucinations, nightmares, dysphoria, nausea, or mental clouding), other oral opioids should be tried before abandoning one route in favor of another. Patients receiving opioid analgesics "by the clock" should be provided oral or parenteral rapid-onset short-duration opioid agonists for breakthrough pain

  (c) *Meperidine (Demerol):* useful for brief courses (few days) to treat acute pain; generally should be avoided in treating cancer pain because of its short duration of action (2.5 to 3.5 hours) and its toxic metabolite, normeperidine, accumulation of this metabolite, particularly when renal function is impaired, causes CNS stimulation that may lead to seizures

(2) *Partial agonists,* such as buprenorphine, have less effect than full agonists at the opioid receptor; subject to a ceiling effect and thus are less effective analgesics

(3) *Mixed agonist-antagonists* block or are neutral at one type of opioid receptor while activating a different opioid receptor; contraindicated for use in the patient receiving an opioid agonist because they may precipitate a withdrawal syndrome and increase pain; include pentazocine (Talwin), butorphanol tartrate (Stadol), denocine (Dalgan), and nalbuphine hydrochloride (Nubain); analgesic effectiveness is limited by a dose-related ceiling effect

(4) *Dosage: the appropriate dose is the amount of opioid that controls pain with the fewest side effects.* The need for increased doses of opioid often reflects progression of the disease. As patients develop opioid tolerance, they require more frequent dosing. Tables 8-2 and 8-3 list equianalgesic initial doses of commonly used opioids for adults weighing over and under 50 kg (110 pounds), respectively. Points to keep in mind include

  (a) *Titration:* increase or decrease the next dose by one quarter to one half of previous dose

  (b) *Route conversion:* when changing from the oral to the rectal route, begin with the oral dose, then titrate upward frequently and carefully; lower doses required for parenteral routes but are similar for subcutaneous, intramuscular, and intravenous routes

  (c) *Schedule:* prevent recurring pain rather than having to subdue it; give analgesics on a regular schedule to prevent a loss of effectiveness between doses

  (d) *Tolerance:* assume that patients actively abusing heroin or prescription opioids (including methadone) have some pharmacologic tolerance that will require higher starting doses and shorter dosing intervals

  (e) *Cessation of opioids:* When a patient becomes pain free as a result of cancer treatment or palliation (e.g., nerve destruction), gradually decrease the opioid to avoid withdrawal

c. *Route of administration:* oral administration preferred because it is convenient and usually cost-effective. When patients cannot take oral medications, other less invasive (e.g., rectal or transdermal) routes should be offered. Parenteral methods should be used only when simpler, less demanding, less costly methods are inappropriate or ineffective. Assessing the patient's response to several different oral opioids is usually advisable before abandoning the oral route in favor of anesthetic, neurosurgical, or other invasive approaches

(1) *Rectal:* safe, inexpensive, effective route for delivery of opioids as well as nonopioids when patients have nausea or vomiting; inappropriate for the patient who has diarrhea, anal/rectal lesions, or mucositis; who is thrombocytopenic or neutropenic; who is physically unable to place the suppository in the rectum; or who prefers other routes

(2) *Transdermal (fentanyl):* not suitable for rapid dose titration; hence, use this route for relatively stable pain when rapid increases or decreases in intensity are not likely

(3) *Injection or infusion:* intravenous and subcutaneous routes provide effective opioid delivery. *Avoid the intramuscular route because of unreliable absorption, pain, and inconvenience.* Intravenous administration provides most rapid onset of analgesia, but duration of analgesia after a bolus dose is shorter than with other routes. In patients requiring continuous intravenous access for other purposes, this route of opioid infusion is cost effective and provides a consistent level of analgesia. When intravenous access is not feasible, subcutaneous opioid infusion is practical in the hospital or home

(4) *Patient-controlled analgesia (PCA):* helps patient maintain independence and control by matching drug delivery to need for analgesia; opioid may be administered orally or via a dedicated portable pump to deliver the drug intravenously, subcutaneously, or epidurally (intraspinally)

(5) *Intraspinal:* consider this invasive route for patients who develop intractable pain or intolerable side effects with other routes; requires skill and expertise that may not be available in all settings. Table 8-4 presents advantages and disadvantages. Main indication for long-term administration of intraspinal opioids is intractable pain in the lower part of the body, particularly bilateral or midline pain. Profound analgesia is possible without motor, sensory, or sympathetic blockade

d. *Drugs and routes not recommended:* Table 8-5 presents data on drugs and routes of administration not recommended for management of cancer pain

e. *Side effects:* clinicians who observe patients during long-term opioid treatment should watch for potential side effects and use adjuvant agents to counteract them

(1) *Constipation:* inevitable side effect; treat prophylactically with dietary fiber or regularly scheduled doses of mild laxative; severe constipation may require treatment with a stimulating cathartic (e.g., bisadocyl, standardized senna concentrate, or hyperosmotic agents, orally or via suppository)

(2) *Nausea and vomiting:* treat with antiemetics such as phenothiazines or metoclopramide; depending on antiemetic chosen, monitor patient for increased sedation

Table 8-4 Advantages and disadvantages of intraspinal drug administration

System	Advantages	Disadvantages
Percutaneous temporary catheter	Used extensively both intraoperatively and postoperatively; useful when prognosis is limited (<1 mo)	Mechanical problems: catheter dislodgment; kinking, or migration
Permanent silicone-rubber epidural	Catheter implantation is a minor procedure; dislodgment and infection less common than with temporary catheters; can deliver bolus injections, continuous infusions, or PCA (with or without continuous delivery)	
Subcutaneous implanted injection port	Increased stability, less risk of dislodgment; can deliver bolus injections or continuous infusions (with or without PCA)	Implantation more invasive than external catheters; approved only for epidural catheter in United States; potential for infection increases with frequent injections
Subcutaneous reservoir	Potentially reduced infection in comparison to external system	Difficult to access, and fibrosis may occur after repeated injection
Implanted pumps (continuous and programmable)	Potentially decreased risk of infection	Need for more extensive operative procedure and specialized, costly equipment with programmable systems

(From Jacox A et al: *Management of cancer pain: adults quick reference guide No. 9.* AHCPR Pub. No. 94-0593, Rockville, Md, 1994, Agency for Health Care Policy and Research, U.S. Department of Health and Human Services, Public Health Services.

Table 8-5 Drugs and routes of administration not recommended for treatment of cancer pain

Class	Drug	Rationale for Not Recommending
Opioids	Meperidine	Short (2-3 hr) duration; repeated administration may lead to CNS toxicity (tremor, confusion, or seizures); high oral doses required to relieve severe pain, and these increase risk of CNS toxicity
Miscellaneous	Cannabinoids	Side effects of dysphoria, drowsiness, hypotension, and bradycardia preclude its routine use as an analgesic
	Cocaine	Has demonstrated no efficacy as an analgesic or coanalgesic in combination with opioids
Opioid agonist-antagonists	Pentazocine Butorphanol Nalbuphine	Risk of precipitating withdrawal in opioid-dependent patients; analgesic ceiling; possible production of unpleasant psychomimetic effects (e.g., dysphoria, hallucinations)
Partial agonist	Buprenorphine	Analgesic ceiling; can precipitate withdrawal
Antagonist	Naloxone Naltrexone	May precipitate withdrawal; limit use to treatment of life-threatening respiratory depression
Combination preparations	Brompton's cocktail	No evidence of analgesic benefit to using Brompton's cocktail over single opioid analgesics
	DPT (meperidine, promethazine, and chlorpromazine)	Efficacy poor compared with other analgesics; high incidence of adverse effects

Continued

From Jacox A et al: *Management of cancer pain: adults quick reference guide No. 9.* AHCPR Pub. No. 94-0593, Rockville, Md. 1994, Agency for Health Care Policy and Research, U.S. Department of Health and Human Services, Public Health Services.

Table 8-5 Drugs and routes of administration not recommended for treatment of cancer pain—cont'd

Class	Drug	Rationale for Not Recommending
Anxiolytics alone	Benzodiazepine (e.g., alprazolam)	Analgesic properties not demonstrated except for some instances of neuropathic pain; added sedation from anxiolytics may limit opioid dosing
Sedative/hypnotic drugs alone	Benzodiazepine	Analgesic properties not demonstrated; added sedation from sedative/hypnotic drugs limits opioid dosing

Routes of Administration	Rationale for Not Recommending
Intramuscular (IM)	Painful; absorption unreliable; should not be used for children or patients prone to develop dependent edema or in patients with thrombocytopenia
Transnasal	Only drug approved by FDA for transnasal administration at this time is butorphanol, an agonist-antagonist drug, which generally is not recommended (See opioid agonist-antagonists above.)

(3) *Sedation and mental clouding:* when possible, treat persistent drug-induced sedation by reducing dose and increasing frequency of opioid administration. CNS stimulants such as caffeine, dextroamphetamine, pemoline, and methylphenidate also help decrease opioid sedative effects

(4) *Respiratory depression:* patients receiving long-term opioid therapy generally develop tolerance to the respiratory depressant effects of these agents. When indicated for reversal of opioid-induced respiratory depression, administer naloxone, titrated in small increments to improve respiratory function without reversing analgesia; monitor patient carefully until the episode of respiratory depression resolves

(5) *Subacute overdose:* far more common than acute respiratory depression, subacute overdose manifests as slowly progressive (hours to days) somnolence and respiratory depression; withhold one or two doses until symptoms have resolved, then reduce standing dose by 25%

(6) *Other opioid side effects:* dry mouth, urinary retention, pruritus, myoclonus, altered cognitive function, dysphoria, euphoria, sleep disturbances, sexual dysfunction, physiologic dependence, tolerance, and inappropriate secretion of antidiuretic hormone

f. *Adjuvant drugs:* valuable during all phases of pain management to enhance analgesic efficacy, treat concurrent symptoms, and provide independent analgesia for specific types of pain

(1) *Corticosteroids:* provide a range of effects including mood elevation, antiinflammatory activity, antiemetic activity, and appetite stimulation and may be beneficial in management of cachexia and anorexia; also reduce cerebral and spinal cord edema and are essential in emergency management of elevated intracranial pressure and epidural spinal cord compression

(2) *Anticonvulsants:* used to manage neuropathic pain, especially lancinating or burning pain; use with caution in cancer patients undergoing marrow-suppressant therapies, such as chemotherapy and radiation therapy

(3) *Antidepressants:* useful in pharmacologic management of neuropathic pain; have innate analgesic properties and may potentiate analgesic effects of opioids. Most widely reported experience has been with amitriptyline; therefore, it should be viewed as the tricyclic agent of choice

(4) *Neuroleptics,* particularly methotrimeprazine: have been used to treat chronic pain syndromes. Methotrimeprazine lacks opioid inhibiting effects on gut motility and may be useful for treating opioid-induced intractable constipation or other dose-limiting side effects; also has antiemetic and anxiolytic effects

(5) *Local anesthetics:* used to treat neuropathic pain; side effects may be greater than with other drugs used to treat neuropathic pain

(6) *Hydroxyzine:* mild anxiolytic agent with sedating and analgesic properties that is useful in treating anxious patient with pain; an antihistamine with antiemetic properties

(7) *Psychostimulants:* may be useful in reducing opioid-induced se-

dation when opioid dose adjustment (i.e., reduced dose and increased dose frequency) is not effective

(8) *Placebos should not be used in management of cancer pain*

4. *Physical and psychosocial interventions:* patients should be encouraged to remain active and participate in self-care when possible. Noninvasive physical and psychosocial modalities can be used concurrently with drugs and other interventions to manage pain during all phases of treatment. Effectiveness of these modalities depends on the patient's participation and communication of which methods best alleviate pain

a. *Physical modalities:* generalized weakness, deconditioning, and aches and pains associated with cancer diagnosis and therapy may be treated by

   (1) *Cutaneous stimulation:* noninvasive techniques that can be taught to the patient or family caregiver include

      (a) *Heat:* avoid burns by wrapping heat source (e.g., hot pack or heating pad) in a towel; use of heat on irradiated tissue is contraindicated, and diathermy and ultrasound are not recommended for use over tumor sites

      (b) *Cold:* apply flexible ice packs that conform to body contours for periods not to exceed 15 minutes; provides longer-lasting relief than heat but should not be used in patients with peripheral vascular disease or on tissue damaged by radiation therapy

      (c) *Massage, pressure, and vibration:* help the patient through distraction or relaxation but sometimes increase pain before relief occurs; massage should not be substituted for exercise in ambulatory patients

   (2) *Exercise:* useful in treating subacute and chronic pain; strengthens weak muscles, mobilizes stiff joints, helps restore coordination and balance, enhances patient comfort, and provides cardiovascular conditioning. Therapists and trained family members or other caregivers can assist the functionally limited patient with range-of-motion exercises to help preserve strength and joint function. During acute pain, exercise should be limited to self-administered range-of-motion. Weight-bearing exercise should be avoided when bone fracture is likely

   (3) *Repositioning:* reposition the immobilized patient frequently to maintain correct body alignment and prevent or alleviate pain and, possibly, pressure ulcers

   (4) *Immobilization:* use restriction of movement to manage acute pain or to stabilize fractures or otherwise compromised limbs or joints. Use adjustable elastic or thermoplastic braces to help maintain correct body alignment. Keep joints in positions of maximal function rather than maximal range. Avoid prolonged immobilization

   (5) *Counterstimulation*

      (a) *Transcutaneous electrical nerve stimulation (TENS):* controlled, low-voltage electrical stimulation applied to large myelinated peripheral nerve fibers via cutaneous electrodes to inhibit pain transmission. Although part of the efficacy of TENS can be attributed to a placebo effect, patients with mild pain may benefit from a trial of TENS to see if it is effective in reducing pain

   (b) *Acupuncture:* pain treated by inserting small, solid needles into the skin. Because pain can signal disease progression, infection, or treatment complication, patients who choose acupuncture should be encouraged to report new pain problems to their health care team before using this means of pain relief

b. *Cognitive-behavioral interventions:* an important part of a multimodal approach to pain management; help to give the patient a sense of control and to develop coping skills to deal with pain. Interventions introduced early in the course of illness are more likely to succeed because they can be learned and practiced by patients while they have sufficient strength and energy. Patients and their families should be given information about and encouraged to try several strategies and to select one or more of these cognitive-behavioral techniques to use regularly

   (1) *Relaxation and imagery:* simple relaxation techniques should be used for episodes of brief pain (e.g., during procedures). Brief, simple techniques should be used when the patient's ability to concentrate is compromised by severe pain, a high level of anxiety, or fatigue

   (2) *Cognitive distraction and reframing:* focusing attention on stimuli other than pain or negative emotions accompanying pain may involve distractions that are internal (e.g., counting, praying, or making self-statements such as "I can cope"), external (e.g., music, television, talking, listening to someone read), or exercises (e.g., rhythmic massage or use of a visual focal point.) In the related technique, cognitive reappraisal, patients learn to monitor and evaluate negative thoughts and replace them with more positive thoughts and images

   (3) *Patient education:* both oral and written information and instructions should be provided about pain, pain assessment, and the use of drugs and other methods of pain relief; patient education should emphasize that almost all pain can be effectively managed

   (4) *Psychotherapy and structured support:* some patients benefit from short-term psychotherapy provided by professionals with training in psychotherapy; patients whose pain is particularly difficult to manage (e.g., substance abusers) and those who develop symptoms of clinical depression or another adjustment disorder should be referred to professionals. Relationship among poorly controlled pain, depression, and thoughts of suicide should not be ignored

   (5) *Support groups and pastoral counseling:* because many patients benefit from peer support groups, clinicians should be aware of locally active groups and offer this information to patients and families. Pastoral counseling members of the health care team should participate in meetings to discuss patients' needs and treatment and should be a source of information on community resources for spiritual care and support of patients and families

5. *Invasive interventions: with rare exception, less invasive analgesic approaches should precede invasive palliative approaches.* However, for a minority of patients in whom behavioral, physical, and drug therapy do not alleviate pain, invasive therapies are useful
   a. *Radiation therapy*
      (1) Local or whole-body radiation enhances effectiveness of analgesic drug and other noninvasive therapy by directly affecting the cause of pain (i.e., reducing primary and metastatic tumor bulk); dosage chosen to achieve a balance between amount of radiation required to kill tumor cells and that which would adversely affect normal cells or allow repair of damaged tissue
      (2) A single IV injection of beta particle-emitting agents such as iodine-131, phosphorus-32-orthophosphate, and strontium-89, as well as the investigational new drugs rhenium-186 and samarium-153, can relieve pain of widespread bony metastases; half the patients so treated respond to a second treatment if pain recurs
   b. *Surgery*
      (1) Curative excision or palliative debulking of a tumor has potential to reduce pain directly, relieve symptoms of obstruction or compression, and improve prognosis, even increasing long-term survival
      (2) Oncologic surgeons and other health care providers should be familiar with interactions of chemotherapy, radiation therapy, and surgical interventions to avoid or anticipate iatrogenic complications; should also recognize characteristic pain syndromes that follow specific surgical procedures
   c. *Nerve blocks*
      (1) Control of otherwise intractable pain can be achieved by relatively brief application of a local anesthetic or neurolytic agent
      (2) Reasons for nerve blocks in cancer pain management
         (a) *Diagnostic:* to determine source of pain (e.g., somatic vs. sympathetic pathways)
         (b) *Therapeutic:* to treat painful conditions that respond to nerve blocks (e.g., celiac block for pain of pancreatic cancer)
         (c) *Prognostic:* to predict outcome of long-lasting interventions (e.g., infusions, neurolysis, rhizotomy)
         (d) *Preemptive:* to prevent painful sequelae of procedures that may cause phantom limb, causalgia, or reflex sympathetic dystrophy
      (3) A single injection of a nondestructive agent such as lidocaine or bupivacaine, alone or in combination with an antiinflammatory corticosteroid for a longer-lasting effect, can provide local relief from nerve or root compression. Placement of an infusion catheter at a sympathetic ganglion extends the sympathetic blockade from hours to days or weeks. Destructive agents such as ethanol or phenol can be used to effect peripheral neurolysis at sites identified by local anesthesia as appropriate for permanent pain relief
   d. *Neurosurgery*
      (1) Ablation of pain pathways should, like neurolytic blockade, be re-

served for situations in which other therapies are ineffective or poorly tolerated

(2) Can be performed to implant devices to deliver drugs or to electrically stimulate neural structures

(3) In general, the choice of neurosurgical procedure is based on location and type of pain (somatic, visceral, deafferentation), patient's general condition and life expectancy, and expertise and follow-up available

e. *Management of procedural pain*

(1) Treat anticipated procedure-related pain prophylactically and integrate pharmacologic and nonpharmacologic interventions

(2) Use local anesthetics and short-acting opioids, allowing adequate time for the drug to achieve full therapeutic effect. Anxiolytics and sedatives may be used to reduce anxiety or to produce sedation

(3) Cognitive-behavioral interventions, e.g., imagery or relaxation: useful in managing procedure-related pain and anxiety. Massage, pressure, or vibration may also aid relaxation

Nausea and vomiting

1. Causes of nausea and vomiting can be divided into GI and CNS sources.

a. GI sources include gastric irritation by iron, alcohol, steroids, NSAIDS, antibiotics, blood, constipation, or candidiasis and distal bowel obstruction and gastric outlet obstruction from an enlarging tumor.

b. CNS causes include narcotics, digoxin, antibiotics, estrogens, uremia, hypercalcemia, chemotherapy, mechanical causes such as increased intracranial pressure and vestibular stimulation, emotional causes, and advancing tumor.

2. Treatment begins with eradicating the source of the problem whenever possible and limiting any unnecessary drugs that may complicate the clinical picture.

a. Patterns of symptoms may help determine the cause; thereafter, treatment focuses on medications.

b. Although suppositories and injections may be needed initially to get nausea and vomiting under control, oral therapy is best for long-term prophylaxis.

3. Drugs include

a. Phenothiazines: prochloperazine, 10 mg PO or IM or 25 mg PR q4-6h; chlorpromazine (Thorazine), 10 to 25 mg PO or 25 to 50 mg IM q4-6h; promethazine (Phenergan), 25 to 50 mg PO, IM, or PR q4-6h; haloperidol (Haldol), 0.5 to 2 mg PO or SQ q6-8h

b. Others: metoclopramide (Reglan), 10 to 20 mg PO or IM q6-8h; Dexamethasone (Decadron), 4 to 8 mg PO q8-12h; Meclizine (Antivert), 12.5 to 25 mg PO q6-8h; Transderm scopolamine patch q3d; ondansetron (Zofran), 32 mg IV q4h × 3 for chemotherapy-induced vomiting, or 8 mg PO tid for chemotherapy-induced vomiting

The last three are particularly helpful in treating patients with nausea associated with movement. Dexamethasone and other steroids can be particularly useful in treating patients with increased intracranial pressure, hypercalcemia, or malignant pyloric stenosis and for treating severe nausea resistant to other antiemetic therapy.

Constipation

Constipation is a source of abdominal distention, pain, anorexia, nausea and vomiting, obstruction, and in some cases confusion.
1. Causes
   a. Decreased fluid intake and activity
   b. Narcotics, antidepressants
   c. Low-residue diets
   d. Metabolic abnormalities, including hypercalcemia and hypokalemia
   e. Mechanical obstruction
   f. Sympathetic and parasympathetic imbalances, resulting in reduced peristalsis
   g. Weakness, immobility, and confusion
2. Management
   a. As with pain, the key to the appropriate management of constipation is prevention, along with constant vigilance. A bowel regimen should be in place at or before the point at which opioid narcotics are initiated.
   b. Evacuation should occur at least every 3 days because GI secretions, desquamation, and bacterial matter must be moved despite poor feeding. Constipation can be seen as watery, oozing "diarrhea" around a fixed impaction.
   c. Bowel regimens should begin with stool softeners (e.g., docusate [Colace], 100 mg qd to bid) and gentle stimulation. If bulk agents are used (e.g., psyllium), large amounts of water must be given, or these agents will harden in the GI tract and become a new source of constipation. Lactulose, 1 tablespoon qd, titrated up until the desired number of stools are produced, stimulates the large bowel, and magnesium salts such as magnesium sulfate, 5 to 10 ml with water, stimulate small-bowel peristalsis.

Diarrhea

1. Etiology
   a. Radiation malabsorption
   b. Anxiety
   c. Tumor infiltration
   d. Carcinoid tumor
   e. Bacterial and viral infections
   f. Laxative imbalance
   g. Leakage past an impaction
2. Management: frequent gentle cleansing of the perianal area is important to avoid skin breakdown, particularly if there is incontinence. Antidiarrheal agents include the following:
   a. Attapulgite (Kaopectate), 30 ml after each loose bowel movement, up to 30 to 60 ml PO q4h
   b. Codeine, 15 to 60 mg PO q4h
   c. Diphenoxylate (Lomotil), 2 tabs q4-6h
   d. Loperamide (Imodium), 2 to 4 mg PO q4-6h

Dyspnea

Subjective feelings of dyspnea can be particularly distressing for the terminal patient and frightening for the family.

1. Common causes
   a. Anemia
   b. Congestive heart failure
   c. COPD
   d. Cardiac arrhythmia
   e. Myocardial infarction
   f. Pleural effusion
   g. Bronchospasm and mucus plugging
   h. Pulmonary infection
   i. Enlarging or spreading malignancy in chest
   j. Lung damage from chemotherapy or radiation
   k. Pulmonary embolus
   l. Anxiety
2. Management
   a. Suctioning and positioning
   b. Relaxation and breathing exercises
   c. Medications directed at identifiable causes (e.g., diuretics, antiarrhythmics, bronchodilators, anticoagulants, antibiotics, steroids) and when appropriate, thoracentesis and sclerotherapy
   d. Oxygen
   e. Medications to suppress air hunger: morphine, 5 to 15 mg PO q4h, or SR morphine, 15 to 30 mg q12h; hydromorphone, 1 to 4 mg q4h; diazepam, 5 to 10 mg q6-8h; and chlorpromazine, 10 to 25 mg PO q4-6h
   f. Scopolamine, 0.4 to 0.6 mg SQ q4h prn, to dry pulmonary secretions and relax tracheobronchial smooth muscle
   g. Synthetic cannabis derivative as a bronchodilator and for sedation

Dehydration and anorexia

Dehydration and anorexia are often of greater concern to those around the patient than to the patient. Aside from dry mouth, patients rarely complain of subjective feelings of thirst.

1. Etiology: nausea and vomiting, depression, mouth soreness and infection, pain, dysphagia, constipation, chemotherapy and radiation, increased tumor bulk, hyponatremia, hypercalcemia, uremia, hepatic failure, and many drugs.
2. In most cases IV fluids and feedings are not appropriate. In some instances there are advantages to decreased oral intake in terms of patient comfort from decreased pulmonary secretions, decreased likelihood of vomiting, decreased urinary output, and possible incontinence. Dehydration and anorexia should be corrected when they are distressing to the patient, not just to the provider.
3. Treatment: altering causes whenever possible, relining dentures, providing frequent small meals, providing supplements with or in place of usual meals, serving wine before meals, prescribing metoclopramide, corticosteroids, or anabolic steroids, and allowing the patient to eat or drink whenever he or she desires instead of on a fixed schedule.

Depression (see Section 5.5)

Depression, anticipatory grief, and loss are not uncommon for the terminal patient and his or her significant others. Aggressive symptom management can do much to alleviate depression.

For those patients in whom the depression persists despite appropriate symptom management, antidepressants should be prescribed. Usually it is wise to "start low and go slow."

Confusion or delirium

Misperceptions, disorientation, confusion, and decreasing level of consciousness associated with drug therapy or enlarging tumor are common in the terminal patient.
1. Etiology
   a. Metabolic derangement (uremia, hypoglycemia, hpyercalcemia, hyponatremia, hypomagnesemia, hypoxia, hypercapnia)
   b. Infections
   c. Sepsis
   d. Postictal states
   e. Intracranial malignancy
   f. Altered environment
   g. Underlying dementia
   h. Pain
   i. Fecal impaction
   j. Congestive heart failure
   k. Drug or alcohol withdrawal
2. Management: haloperidol, 0.5 to 1 mg q am and 1 to 2 mg q hs, is the least sedating medication but carries a significant risk of causing pseudoparkinsonism. Prescribing antidepressants and resetting day and night cycles using artificial light often can lessen confusion.

Mouth care

Dry or sore mouth can be a significant source of irritation and pain, resulting in decreased oral intake.
1. Etiology: thrush, dryness, ill-fitting dentures secondary to weight loss, local radiation, mouth breathing, drugs (especially anticholinergics), and vitamin deficiencies
2. Management: relining dentures when possible, ice chips, frequent small sips of fluid, hard candies, vitamins, artificial saliva, and topical anesthetics such as lidocaine (Xylocaine) as part of q2h mouth care

CONCLUSION

Patients (and their families) must be assured that, even though their condition is no longer curable, consistent efforts will be made to ensure symptom palliation up to and including the time of death. The goal of symptom palliation, however, is not simply a "good death" but to improve the quality of life substantially by helping patients to "live until they die."

9.1 GENERAL PRINCIPLES

. Major goal of rehabilitation: restoration of function and improved quality of life (i.e., add "life to years" in addition to adding "years to life")

. Evaluation of the patient should be undertaken by a geriatric rehabilitation team, which should include a geriatrician, physical/occupational therapists, social workers, speech therapist, physiatrist, nutritionist, psychologist, and nursing personnel

. Rehabilitation is a learning process. The patient should be able to understand and retain new information and adapt to any new disability. Any existing musculoskeletal and cognitive impairments will adversely affect the rehabilitation process; therefore realistic individualized goals should be set for each patient

. Age-related factors influencing geriatric rehabilitation[5]

   a. Frequent absence of social and financial support (e.g., diseased spouse, inadequate income from pension)

   b. Presence of significant concurrent illness (e.g., dementia, depression, CHF, COPD)

   c. Impaired mobility (e.g., parkinsonism, degenerative joint disease [DJD])

   d. Impaired homeostatic mechanisms (e.g., propensity for dehydration secondary to impaired thirst mechanism)

   e. Altered pain perception (e.g., occult fracture mistaken for DJD, increased incidence of referred pain)

   f. Increased frequency of adverse reactions to drugs (see Chapter 7)

   g. Impaired equilibrium, resulting in frequent falls (see Section 5.5)

. Rehabilitation is generally initiated during hospitalization for the acute event and continued in one of the following settings[7]

   a. *Inpatient rehabilitation unit:* care is provided by an interdisciplinary team. To qualify for this intensive level of care the patient must require multiple rehabilitative services and must have sufficient cognitive ability to learn on a daily basis and enough stamina to sustain 3 hr/day of therapy

b. *Skilled nursing facility:* indicated for patients who require daily skille[]
   therapy and services 24 hr/day
c. *Home therapy:* indicated for fairly independent patients who have
   supportive family and a suitable home environment
d. *Comprehensive outpatient rehabilitation facility (CORF):* care pr[]
   vided by an interdisciplinary team similar to the inpatient rehabilit[]
   tion unit; indicated for the medically complicated patient who require[]
   multiple services but has adequate community support to live at hom[]

9.2   FINANCIAL CONCERNS IN REHABILITATION[8]

1. Conditions for Medicare reimbursement
   a. Freestanding rehabilitation hospital or hospital-based diagnostic re[]
      lated group (DRG)–exempt rehabilitation unit
      (1) Patient must be able to tolerate up to 3 hr/day of rehabilitatio[]
          therapy
      (2) Documentable progress must be made toward the goal of reha[]
          bilitation; if inadequate progress is made, Medicare coverage wi[]
          no longer be allowed
      (3) Patient's medical status requires daily supervision or availabilit[]
          of a physician
   b. Skilled nursing facility
      (1) Daily therapy, usually for 1 hr/day
      (2) No required minimum daily number of hours of therapy
2. Outpatient rehabilitation reimbursed under Medicare Part B
3. Eighty percent of the cost of adaptive equipment and assistive devices i[]
   generally covered by Medicare if adequate documentation is provided b[]
   the physician
4. Private insurance reimbursement varies with policy and company
5. Medicaid benefits vary with individual states

9.3   ORTHOTIC AND PROSTHETIC DEVICES[1]

1. The nomenclature of orthotic devices is derived from the anatomic nam[]
   of the joints crossed by the device, ending with the letter "O" (e.g., th[]
   Milwaukee brace is known as a cervico-thoraco-lumbo-sacral orthosi[]
   [CTLSO])
2. Common types of orthotic devices
   a. **Ankle-foot orthosis (AFO):** short leg brace, useful for ankle disabil[]
      ity and limb weakness (Figure 9-1)
   b. **Knee-foot orthosis (KAFO):** useful to provide stability during weigh[]
      bearing (e.g., extensor weakness with inability to lock the knee); mos[]
      patients rarely require this and advance to an AFO
   c. **Spinal orthotics:** useful for minimizing pain and allowing early mo[]
      bilization (e.g., cervical collars provide support and protection in pa[]
      tients with cervical disk disease and rheumatoid arthritis)
   d. **Upper extremity orthotics:** useful for nerve entrapment (e.g., cock-u[]
      splint in carpal tunnel syndrome), strokes, and lower motor neuro[]
      lesions; can be static (useful in hemiplegic hands to prevent contrac[]
      ture) or dynamic (allow movement of wrist and fingers)

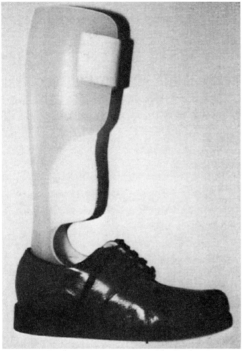

Figure 9-1

Orthosis fabricated for a 64-year-old patient to replace a conventional KAFO with a dorsiflexion assist and a valgus corrective strap that the client was fitted with after a CVA. Three years following the insult she had equinovarus during swing phase, extreme valgus during weight bearing, and genu recurvatum. After the client was fitted with a rigid ankle set in slight dorsiflexion and a valgus corrective flare, her mobility skills improved significantly. (From Umphred DA: *Neurological rehabilitation,* ed 2, St Louis, 1990, Mosby.)

e. **Lower extremity prostheses**[2]: used in amputees; major components are
    (1) **Socket:** a patellar tendon–bearing socket with weight bearing on the patellar tendon and the medial tibial flare is generally used in below-knee amputees. Any fragile pressure points (e.g., surgical scars) should be eliminated. Shrinking of the stump can be accomplished with thigh elastic bandages. A temporary prosthesis can generally be measured 6 to 8 weeks after surgery and a permanent one 12 to 24 weeks after surgery. Suction sockets require significant energy expenditure and coordination, limiting their use in geriatric amputees

(2) **Suspension:** length of the stump and physical condition of the amputee are significant factors in determining suspension for the socket. A prosthesis with greater proximal suspension decreases the sensation of heaviness in the distal prosthesis and is preferred in the elderly amputee

(3) **Shank:** structure that connects the end of the prosthetic foot with the socket

(4) **Foot**

(a) Solid ankle cushion heel (SACH) foot: most often prescribed foot in the elderly amputee because of its low cost and durability; major disadvantage: gradual loss of elasticity

(b) More advanced models such as the Seattle foot allow a more natural gait by releasing energy stored as the patient applies and removes his or her weight on the prosthesis; cost of an energy-storing foot is significantly more

3. **Canes**

   a. Useful in patients with unilateral deficits

   b. Held on the unaffected side in hemiplegic patients; can be held in the hand of preference in patients with foot, ankle, or knee injuries

   c. For proper strength, the elbow should be slightly flexed upward (30 degrees) when the hand is resting on the handle and the tip of the cane is on the ground

   d. Canes with three or four points on the base (tripod or quadripod) provide greater support than single-pronged canes and are preferable in the elderly. If a single-pronged cane is used, an elastic band wrapped around the cane prevents it from falling when placed against a surface

   e. Pistol-shaped grip provides better handling than an evenly rounded handle

4. **Walkers**

   a. Can be pickup, two-wheeled, or four-wheeled

   b. Front-wheeled walkers require less upper extremity strength and standing balance than pickup walkers and are particularly useful in patients with parkinsonism

5. **Wheelchairs**

   a. Two basic types

      (1) Indoor: large wheels are in rear of wheelchair

      (2) Outdoor: large wheels are located in the front

   b. Patients should be fitted and measured for their wheelchair. The width of the wheelchair should enable the patient to clear doorways with at least 2 inches on each side. Proper arm height and positioning of foot rests are necessary for balance and prevention of pressure ulcers

   c. One arm–drive wheelchairs are useful in hemiplegic patients. Motorized wheelchairs should be used only in selected patients with significant neurologic disorders

6. Transferring (bed-wheelchair, wheelchair-toilet, tub transfers) requires adequate equipment to ensure safety (e.g., toilet seats should be 20 inches from floors, handrails should be on the hemiplegic's unaffected side, tub transfer benches will facilitate use of bathtub)

7. Various assistive devices for feeding, bathing, and dressing are easily

available and should be prescribed in collaboration with a physiatrist and therapists

| 9.4 |

POSTSTROKE REHABILITATION: ASSESSMENT, REFERRAL, AND PATIENT MANAGEMENT[4]

Purpose and scope

Each year in the United States, stroke occurs in approximately 550,000 persons, and about 3 million Americans are living with varying degrees of disability from stroke. Brain infarctions account for about 75% of all strokes, and intracerebral or subarachnoid hemorrhages account for about 15%. The remainder are due to other or unknown causes.

Stroke frequency increases dramatically with advancing age, doubling with every decade after 55 years. Men are more likely to have strokes than women, and African-Americans are more likely to have strokes than caucasians. Estimates of stroke mortality range from 17% to 34% in the first 30 days and from 25% to 40% in the first year. Mortality from stroke has declined in recent years because of a combination of factors, including reduced stroke severity, earlier and more accurate diagnosis, and better acute care. Modifiable or potentially modifiable risk factors for stroke include hypertension, diabetes mellitus, cigarette smoking, atrial fibrillation, left ventricular hypertrophy, transient ischemic attacks, high serum cholesterol levels, coronary heart disease, congestive heart failure, cocaine use, obesity, and heavy alcohol consumption. Fixed or nonmodifiable risk factors for stroke are gender, previous stroke, age, race, and family history.

Hemiparesis is a presenting finding in about 75% of patients. Acute neurologic impairment frequently resolves spontaneously, but persisting disabilities lead to partial or total dependence with regard to activities of daily living (ADLs) in 25% to 50% of stroke patients.

Most patients who have had a stroke are initially treated in a stroke unit or in the general medical service of an acute care hospital, where they receive rehabilitation services directed at preventing complications of stroke and, as medically feasible, encouraging mobilization and resumption of self-care activities. Figure 9-2 outlines the clinical algorithm for stroke rehabilitation. When the patient is medically stable, screening for postacute rehabilitation is performed. Patients with stroke who recover completely will not need rehabilitation, and those who remain severely incapacitated are not likely to benefit from rehabilitation, although some patients in this group may improve over a further period of recuperation and can be reevaluated at a later date. Between these extremes are patients with functional deficits who are candidates for either individual rehabilitation services or an interdisciplinary program. The key components of a rehabilitation program include the following factors

- Medical management
- Assessment, including use of selected standardized instruments
- Rehabilitation referrals, matching patient needs and program capabilities

Modified from Gresham GE, et al: *Post-stroke rehabilitation. Clinical practice guideline No. 16.* AHCPR Pub. No. 95-0662, Rockville, Md, May 1995, U.S. Department of Health and Human Services. Public Health Service, Agency for Health Care Policy and Research.

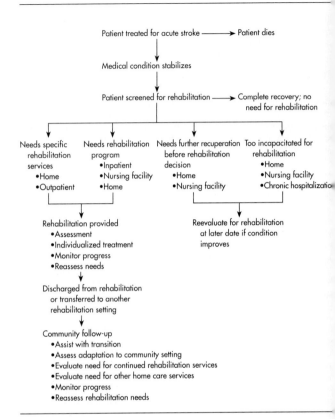

Figure 9-2
Clinical algorithm for stroke rehabilitation. (From Gresham GE et al: *Post-stroke rehabilitation. Clinical practice guideline No. 16.* AHCPR Pub. No. 95-0062, Rockville, Md, May 1995, U.S. Department of Health and Human Services. Public Health Service, Agency for Health Care Policy and Research).

- Provision of rehabilitation according to a well-defined management plan with explicit goals, measurement of progress, and adjustment of the plan or goals as needed
- Assistance in reintegrating the patient into the community

Medical management

1. *When possible, treat the patient with acute stroke in a setting that provides coordinated, multidisciplinary, stroke-related evaluation and services.*

Such settings include acute stroke units, well-staffed neurology or rehabilitation departments, or other acute hospital settings with coordinated stroke services. Studies have found improved rates of survival and greater likelihood of returning home when acute stroke care is coordinated and multidisciplinary. This improvement may be related to better organization of services, with an emphasis on early mobilization of the patient and early implementation of rehabilitation interventions.

2. *Fully document the patient's condition and clinical course in the medical record.*

Thorough documentation of clinical information during the acute hospitalization is essential to making appropriate rehabilitation decisions (Figure 9-3). The following information should be included in the patient's medical record

- Stroke etiology and areas of the brain involved
- Type(s), severity, and trajectory of neurologic deficits (The box on p. 438 describes perceptual deficits in CNS function.)
- Type(s) and severity of comorbid diseases
- Complications and abnormal health patterns
- Changes in clinical status that may occur over time
- Functional status before stroke

3. *Begin rehabilitation-oriented care immediately and increase the patient's activity as soon as medically feasible during the acute phase.*

Position changes to prevent skin breakdown and careful range-of-motion exercises to prevent contractures should be initiated shortly after admission. Further mobilization should begin when the patient is medically stable, preferably within the first 24 to 48 hours. Transfer techniques should be followed closely (Figures 9-4 and 9-5) and taught to the patient and family. As early as possible, the patient should be encouraged to participate in personal care activities and to communicate and interact with staff and other patients. Attention and gaze need to be directed away from the intact side to prevent unilateral neglect (Figure 9-6). The benefits of early mobilization include the following

- Prevention of deep venous thrombosis (DVT), skin breakdown, contracture formation, constipation, and pneumonia
- Better orthostatic tolerance
- Earlier return of mental and motor function and ability to perform ADLs
- Improved morale of both patient and family

Indications for delaying mobilization or approaching it with caution include the following:

- Coma or severe obtundation
- Progressing neurologic signs or symptoms
- Subarachnoid or intracerebral hemorrhage
- Severe orthostatic hypotension
- Acute myocardial infarction
- Acute DVT (until adequate anticoagulation has been achieved)

4. *Manage general health functions throughout all stages of treatment.*

Health functions that need to be monitored and managed during acute care and rehabilitation and after return to the community include the following

Clinical evaluation during acute care

<u>Purposes</u>
Determine etiology, pathology, and severity of stroke
Assess comorbidities
Document clinical course

<u>When</u>
On admission and during acute hospitalization

<u>By whom</u>
Acute care physician
Nursing staff
Rehabilitation consultants

Not referred
for rehabilitation

- No or minimal disability
- Too severely disabled
  to participate in
  rehabilitation. Provide
  supportive services;
  consider rescreening
  at a future date
  if condition improves

Screening for rehabilitation

<u>Purposes</u>
Identify patients who may benefit from rehabilitation
Determine appropriate setting for rehabilitation
Identify problems needing treatment

<u>When</u>
As soon as patient is medically stable

<u>By whom</u>
Rehabilitation clinicians

Referred for individual
rehabilitation services
(rehabilitation nurse,
occupational therapist,
physical therapist,
psychologist, speech-
language pathologist)

- Same assessment stages
  as for interdisciplinary
  program

Referred to interdisciplinary rehabilitation program
in outpatient facility, home, inpatient unit or facility,
or nursing facility

Assessment on admission to rehabilitation

<u>Purposes</u>
Validate referral decision
Develop management plan
Provide baseline for monitoring progress

<u>When</u>
Within 3 working days for an intense program;
1 week for a less intense inpatient program;
or three visits for an outpatient or home program

<u>By whom</u>
Rehabilitation clinicians/team

Assessment during rehabilitation

<u>Purposes</u>
Monitor progress
Adjust treatment regimen
Provide basis for discharge decision

<u>When</u>
Weekly for intense program
At least biweekly for less intense programs

<u>By whom</u>
Rehabilitation clinicians/team

Assessment after discharge from rehabilitation

<u>Purposes</u>
Evaluate adaptation to home environment
Determine need for continued rehabilitation services
Assess caregiver burden

<u>When</u>
Within 1 month of discharge
Regular intervals during first year

<u>By whom</u>
Rehabilitation clinicians
Principal physician

Figure 9-3

Stages of assessment for post–stroke rehabilitation. (Redrawn from *Post-stroke reha-bilitation. Clinical practice guideline*. Pub. No. 95-0662, 1995, U.S. Department of Health and Human Services.)

- *Dysphagia:* physicians should be alert to the possibility of dysphagia. If dysphagia is present, consultation should be obtained and an appropriate program initiated.
- *Nutrition and hydration:* the adequacy of food and fluid intake should be monitored regularly.
- *Bladder and bowel function:* persistent urinary incontinence should be evaluated to determine its etiology, and appropriate treatment should be provided. If possible, the use of indwelling urinary catheters should be avoided. Bowel management programs should be implemented in patients with persistent constipation or bowel incontinence.
- *Sleep and rest:* disturbances in sleep patterns should be evaluated to determine their cause. Interventions may include keeping the patient active during the day, teaching relaxation techniques, and changing medications.
- *Comorbid conditions:* symptoms and signs not clearly attributable to the stroke should be evaluated and treated as indicated.
- *Acute illnesses:* patients who develop an acute medical illness during rehabilitation should be evaluated promptly and, if necessary, transferred to an acute care facility.

5. *Take steps to prevent complications throughout all stages of treatment.*
    Preventive measures should be initiated during acute care and continued throughout rehabilitation and after the patient's return to the community. The following potential complications may occur

- *Deep venous thrombosis and pulmonary embolism:* preventive measures include early mobilization, low-dose heparin, or low-molecular-weight heparin. Warfarin, intermittent pneumatic compression, and elastic stockings are also effective.
- *Dysphagia and aspiration:* depending on the type of swallowing deficit, treatment may include training to relearn swallowing, compensatory approaches such as changes in food texture and, if necessary, a gastrostomy tube. Dysphagia frequently resolves spontaneously; however, the condition should be reassessed periodically during rehabilitation, and treatments should be continued or adjusted as necessary.
- *Skin breakdown:* preventive measures include daily skin inspection, gentle routine cleansing, minimizing exposure to moisture, avoidance of friction, reduction of pressure, upright sitting posture, proper nutrition and hydration, and early mobility.
- *Prevention of urinary tract infections:* if indwelling catheters are used, they should be removed as soon as is feasible.
- *Seizures:* anticonvulsant medications are recommended for preventing recurrent seizures in patients with stroke who have had one or more seizures but are not recommended for patients who have not had seizures.

Perceptual Deficits in CNS Dysfunction

Left Hemiparesis: Right Hemisphere—General Spatial-Global Deficits

Visual-perceptual deficits
  Hand-eye coordination
  Figure-ground discrimination
  Spatial relationships
  Position in space
  Form constancy
Behavioral and intellectual deficits
  Poor judgment, unrealistic behavior
  Denial of disability
  Inability to abstract
  Rigidity of thought
  Disturbances in body image and body scheme
  Impairment of ability to self-correct
  Difficulty retaining information
  Distortion of time concepts
  Tendency to see the whole and not individual steps
  Affect lability
  Feelings of persecution
  Irritability, confusion
  Distraction by verbalization
  Short attention span
  Appearance of lethargy
  Fluctuation in performance
  Disturbances in relative size and distance of objects

Right Hemiparesis: Left Hemisphere—General Language and Temporal Ordering Deficits

Apraxia
  Motor
  Ideational
Behavioral and intellectual deficits
  Difficulty initiating tasks
  Sequencing deficits
  Processing delays
  Directionality deficits
  Low frustration levels
  Verbal and manual perseveration
  Rapid performance of movement or activity
  Compulsive behavior
  Extreme distractability

From Umphred DA: *Neurological rehabilitation*, ed 2, St Louis, 1990, Mosby.

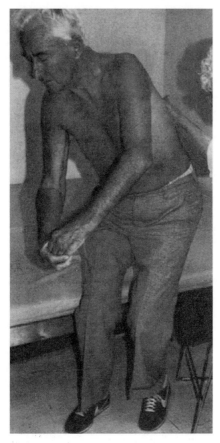

Figure 9-4
Transfers to the affected side encourage weight bearing onto the leg. This partial
stand is followed by pelvic and lower trunk rotation. (From Umphred DA: *Neurological rehabilitation,* ed 2, St Louis, 1990, Mosby.)

- *Falls:* patients who have had a stroke are at increased risk for falls.
  Risk factors include problems with perceptual deficits, visual impairments, impaired communication, confusion, drug side effects, environmental hazards, mobility, balance, and coordination. The risk is increased by rehabilitation treatments aimed at improving mobility. Risk
  prevention includes supervision of high-risk patients, proper seating
  and wheelchair modification, regular toileting, supervised transfer and
  ambulation, nurse call systems suited to a patient's abilities,

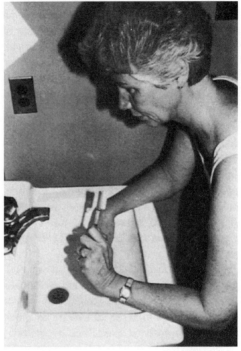

Figure 9-5
Weight bearing on the affected side during functional skills. (From Umphred DA: *Neurological rehabilitation,* ed 2, St Louis, 1990, Mosby.)

institution-wide fall prevention programs addressing both patient and environmental risk factors, and patient and family education for prevention of falls and proper ways to get up after a fall. Adequate supervision and environmental precautions should continue after the patient returns to the community.
- *Spasticity and contractures:* methods of prevention and treatment of spasticity and contracture include antispastic pattern positioning, range-of-motion exercises, stretching, splinting, and nerve blocks.
- *Shoulder injury:* this is a frequent cause of pain in stroke patients. Prevention emphasizes proper positioning and support as well as avoidance of overly vigorous range-of-motion exercises.
6. *Take steps to prevent recurrent stroke throughout all stages of treatment.*
  Persons who have had a stroke are at increased risk for another stroke. The following preventive measures should be taken throughout acute care and rehabilitation and after the patient returns to the community.
- Identification and control of modifiable risk factors such as hyperten-

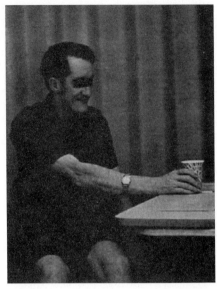

Figure 9-6
Patient is encouraged to reach for an object on the affected side of the body. Attention and gaze need to be directed away from intact side to prevent unilateral neglect. (From Duncan PW, Badke MB: *Stroke rehabilitation: the recovery of motor control,* Chicago, 1987, Year Book.)

sion, cigarette smoking, diabetes mellitus, high serum cholesterol, and heavy alcohol consumption
- Use of oral anticoagulants to prevent embolic strokes in patients with atrial fibrillation or prosthetic cardiac valves; these medications are not currently recommended for patients with ischemic stroke that is not attributed to embolism from the heart
- Use of aspirin or ticlopidine for prevention of recurrent stroke secondary to arterial diseases
- Use of carotid endarterectomy to prevent recurrent strokes following nondisabling strokes or transient ischemic attacks (TIAs) in selected patients with carotid artery stenosis greater than 70%; effectiveness of this procedure has been demonstrated to reduce the risk of stroke in patients who have not had previous stroke warning signs but who have greater than 60% stenosis of the carotid artery but has not been demonstrated for lesser degrees of stenosis
- Use of surgery to clip an intracranial aneurysm or resect an arteriovenous malformation

Patient assessment

7. *Systematically evaluate the patient at key stages throughout acute care and rehabilitation.*

A patient should be examined on admission to acute care and whenever questions arise concerning the person's condition. In addition, assessments should be performed at the following times

- When screening for rehabilitation
- On admission to a rehabilitation program
- During rehabilitation (to monitor progress)
- After discharge from rehabilitation and return to a community residence

8. *Use well-validated standardized measures.*

Use of standardized instruments is essential in evaluating stroke patients. For a listing of recommended standardized instruments refer to Table 9-1. Figure 9-7 describes the Functional Independence Measure (FIM) in more detail.

The rehabilitation referral

9. *Screen the patient for formal rehabilitation during the acute hospitalization.*

Screening for rehabilitation should be performed during the acute hospitalization, as soon as the patient's neurologic and medical conditions permit. The purposes of this screening are as follows

- To identify patients who may benefit from a formal rehabilitation program or from individual rehabilitation services
- To guide selection of the appropriate rehabilitation program

The types of information needed are listed in the box on p. 450. In addition to the patient's clinical status, information about the home environment, family circumstances, and patient and family preferences regarding rehabilitation have important influences on rehabilitation decisions. The use of standardized instruments is recommended to document the extent of impairment and disabilities. These instruments can also be used to detect subtle cognitive problems, which may be missed in the clinical examination.

The person performing the screening examination should be experienced in stroke rehabilitation and should have no direct financial interest in the referral decision. All screening information should be summarized in the medical record and provided to the rehabilitation setting at the time of referral.

10. *Recommend whether the patient should receive further rehabilitation and whether this should consist of individual services or an interdisciplinary program.*

The decision to recommend rehabilitation—and whether the choice should be individual services or an interdisciplinary program—is based on information obtained during the acute hospitalization and the rehabilitation screening examination. The most important patient considerations are as follows

- Medical stability
- Nature and extent of functional disabilities
- Ability to learn
- Physical activity endurance

Referral criteria for rehabilitation services are as follows

- Patients are potential candidates for formal rehabilitation if they have one or more significant disabilities, are at least moderately stable medi-

Text continued on p. 450.

Table 9-1 Standard instruments for assessment of stroke

Type	Name and Source	Approximate Time to Administer	Strengths	Weaknesses
Level-of-consciousness scale	Glasgow Coma Scale[a]	2 min	Simple, valid, reliable	None observed
Stroke deficit scales	NIH Stroke Scale[b]	5-10 min	Brief, reliable, can be administered by nonneurologists	Low sensitivity
	Canadian Neurological Scale[c]	5 min	Brief, valid, reliable	Some useful measures omitted
Global disability scale	Rankin Scale[d,e]	5 min	Good for overall assessment of disability	Walking is the only explicit assessment criterion; low sensitivity
Measures of disability/activities of daily living (ADLs)	Barthel Index[f]	5-10 min	Widely used for stroke; excellent validity and reliability	Low sensitivity for high-level functioning
	Functional Independence Measure (FIM)[g]	40 min	Widely used for stroke; measures mobility, ADLs, cognition, functional communication	"Ceiling" and "floor" effects
Mental status screening	Folstein Mini-Mental State Examination[h]	10 min	Widely used for screening	Several functions with summed score; may misclassify patients with aphasia

Continued

Table 9-1 Standard instruments for assessment of stroke—cont'd

Type	Name and Source	Approximate Time to Administer	Strengths	Weaknesses
	Neurobehavioral Cognition Status Exam (NCSE)[i]	30 min	Predicts gain in Barthel Index scores; unrelated to age	Does not distinguish right from left hemisphere; no reliability studies in stroke; no studies of factorial structure; correlates with education
Assessment of motor function	Fugl-Meyer[j]	30–40 min	Extensively evaluated measure; good validity and reliability for assessing sensorimotor function and balance	Considered too complex and time consuming by many
	Motor Assessment Scale[k]	15 min	Good, brief assessment of movement and physical mobility	Reliability assessed only in stable patients; sensitivity not tested
	Motricity Index[l]	5 min	Brief assessment of motor function of arm, leg, and trunk	Sensitivity not tested
Balance assessment	Berg Balance Assessment[m]	10 min	Simple, well established with stroke patients, sensitive to change	None observed
Mobility assessment	Rivermead Mobility Index[n]	5 min	Valid, brief, reliable test of physical mobility	Sensitivity not tested

| Assessment of speech and language functions | Boston Diagnostic Aphasia Examination[o] | 1-4 hr | Widely used, comprehensive, good standardization data; sound theoretic rationale | Time to administer long; half of patients cannot be classified |
| | Porch Index of Communicative Ability (PICA)[p] | ½-2 hr | Widely used, comprehensive, careful test development and standardization | Time to administer long; special training required to administer; inadequate sampling of language other than one word and single sentences |

From Gresham GE et al: *Post-stroke rehabilitation. Clinical practice guideline No. 16.* AHCPR Pub. No. 95-0062. Rockville, Md. May 1995. U.S. Department of Health and Human Services, Public Health Service, Agency for Health Care Policy and Research.

ADLs, Activities of daily living; *IADLs,* instrumental activities of daily living.

[a]Teasdale G, Jennett B: Assessment of coma and impaired consciousness: a practical scale, *Lancet* 2:81-83, 1974. Teasdale G et al: Adding up the Glasgow Coma Scale. *Acta Neurochir* 28:13-26, 1979.

[b]Brott T et al: Measurements of acute cerebral infarction: a clinical examination scale, *Stroke* 20:864-870, 1989.

[c]Cote R et al: The Canadian Neurological Scale: a preliminary study in acute stroke, *Stroke* 17:731-737, 1986.

[d]Rankin J: Cerebral vascular accidents in patients over the age of 60, *Scott Med J* 2:200-215, 1957.

Bonita R, Beaglehole R: Modification of Rankin Scale: recovery of motor function after stroke, *Stroke* 19(12):1497-1500, 1988. Van Swieten JC et al: Interobserver agreement for the assessment of handicap in stroke patients, *Stroke* 19(5):604-607, 1988.

[f]Mahoney FI, Barthel DW: Functional evaluation: the Barthel Index, *Md State Med J* 14:61-65, 1965. Wade DT, Collin C: The Barthel ADL Index: a standard measure of physical disability? *Int Disabil Stud* 10(2):64-67, 1988.

[g]Guide for the uniform data set for medical rehabilitation (Adult FIM), version 4.0 Buffalo, NY 14214: State University of New York at Buffalo; 1993. Granger CV et al: Advances in functional assessment for medical rehabilitation, *Top Geriatr Rehabil* 1(3):59-74, 1986. Granger CV, Hamilton BB, Sherwin FS: *Guide for the use of the uniform data set for medical rehabilitation,* 1986, Uniform Data System for Medical Rehabilitation Project Office, Buffalo General Hospital, NY. Keith RA et al: The functional independence measure: a new tool for rehabilitation. In Eisenberg MG, Grzesiak RC, editors: *Advances in clinical rehabilitation,* vol 1, New York, 1987, Springer-Verlag.

[h]Folstein MF, Folstein SE, McHugh PR: "Mini-mental state,": a practical method for grading the cognitive state of patients for the clinician, *J Psychiatr Res* 12(3):189-198, 1975.

Table 9-1 Standard instruments for assessment of stroke—cont'd

Type	Name and Source	Approximate Time to Administer	Strengths	Weaknesses
	Western Aphasia Battery[q]	1-4 hr	Widely used, comprehensive	Time to administer long; "aphasia quotients" and "taxonomy" of aphasia not well validated
Depression scales	Beck Depression Inventory (BDI)[r]	10 min	Widely used, easily administered; norms available; good with somatic symptoms	Less useful in elderly and in patients with aphasia or neglect; high rate of false positives; somatic items may not be due to depression
	Center for Epidemiologic Studies Depression (CES-D)[s]	<15 min	Brief, easily administered, useful in elderly, effective for screening in stroke population	Not appropriate for aphasic patients
	Geriatric Depression Scale (GDS)[t]	10 min	Brief, easy to use with elderly, cognitively impaired, and those with visual or physical problems or low motivation	High false-negative rates in minor depression
	Hamilton Depression Scale[u]	<30 min	Observer rated; frequently used in stroke patients	Multiple differing versions compromise interobserver reliability

Measures of instrumental ADLs	PGC Instrumental Activities of Daily Living[v]	5-10 min	Measures broad base of information necessary for independent living	Has not been tested in stroke patients
	Frenchay Activities Index[w]	10-15 min	Developed specifically for stroke patients; assesses broad array of activities	Sensitivity and interobserver reliability not tested; sensitivity probably limited
Family assessment	Family Assessment Device (FAD)[x]	30 min	Widely used in stroke; computer scoring available; excellent validity and reliability; available in multiple languages	Assessment subjective; sensitivity not tested; "ceiling" and "floor" effects

[i]Kiernan RJ et al: The Neurobehavioral Cognitive Status Examination: a brief but differentiated approach to cognitive assessment, *Ann Intern Med* 107:481-485, 1987.

[j]Fugl-Meyer AR et al: The post stroke hemiplegic patient. I. A method for evaluation of physical performance, *Scand J Rehabil Med* 7:13-31, 1975.

[k]Carr JH et al: Investigation of a new motor assessment scale for stroke patients, *Phys Ther* 65(2):175-180, 1985. Poole JL, Whitney SL: Motor assessment scale for stroke patients: concurrent validity and interrater reliability, *Arch Phys Med Rehabil* 69(3 Pt 1):195-197, 1988.

[l]Collin C, Wade D: Assessing motor impairment after stroke: a pilot reliability study, *J Neurol Neurosurg Psychiatry* 53(7):576-579, 1990. Demeurisse G, Demol O, Robaye E: Motor evaluation in vascular hemiplegia, *Eur Neurol* 19(6):382-389, 1980.

[m]Berg K et al: Clinical and laboratory measures of postural balance in an elderly population, *Arch Phys Med Rehabil* 73:1073-1083, 1992. Berg K et al: Measuring balance in the elderly: preliminary development of an instrument, *Physiother Can* 41:304-311, 1989.

[n]Collen FM et al: The Rivermead Mobility Index: a further development of the Rivermead Motor Assessment, *Int Disabil Stud* 13:50-54, 1991. Wade DT et al: Physiotherapy intervention late after stroke and mobility, *Br Med J* 304(6827):609-613, 1992.

[o]Goodglass H, Kaplan E: The assessment of aphasia and related disorders. In *Test procedures and rationale: manual for the BDAE*, Philadelphia, 1983, Lea & Febiger. Kaplan E: *Boston Diagnostic Aphasia Examination (BDAE)*, Philadelphia, 1972, Lea & Febiger. Goodglass H,

[p]Porch B: *Porch Index of Communicative Ability (PICA)*, Palo Alto, Calif, 1981, Consulting Psychologists Press.

[q]Kertesz A: *Western Aphasia Battery*, New York, 1982, Grune & Stratton.

[r]Beck AT et al: An inventory for measuring depression, *Arch Gen Psychiatry* 4:561-571, 1961. Beck AT, Steer RA: *Beck Depression Inventory: manual (revised edition)*, New York, 1987, Psychological Corporation.

[s]Radloff LS: The CES-D scale: a self-report depression scale for research in the general population, *J Appl Psychol Meas* 1:385-401, 1977.

Table 9-1 Standard instruments for assessment of stroke—cont'd

Type	Name and Source	Approximate Time to Administer	Strengths	Weaknesses
Health status/quality of life measures	Medical Outcomes Study (MOS) 36-Item Short-Form Health Survey[y]	10-15 min	Generic health status scale SF36 is improved version of SF20; brief, can be self-administered or administered by phone or interview; widely used in United States	Possible "floor" effect in seriously ill patients (especially for physical functioning) suggests it should be supplemented by an ADL scale in stroke patients
	Sickness Impact Profile (SIP)[z]	20-30 min	Comprehensive and well evaluated; broad range of items reduces "floor" or "ceiling" effects	Time to administer somewhat long; evaluates behavior rather than subjective health; needs questions on well-being, happiness, and satisfaction

[t]Yesavage JA et al: Development and validation of a geriatric depression screening scale: a preliminary report, *J Psychiatr Res* 17(1):37-49, 1982-83.

[u]Hamilton M: A rating scale for depression, *J Neurol Neurosurg Psychiatry* 23:56-62, 1960. Hamilton M: Development of a rating scale for primary depressive illness, *Br J Soc Clin Psychol* 6:278-296, 1967.

[v]Lawton MP: Assessing the competence of older people. In Kent D, Kastenbaum R, Sherwood S, editors: *Research planning and action for the elderly*, New York, 1972, Behavioral Publications.

[w]Holbrook M, Skilbeck CE: An activities index for use with stroke patients, *Age Ageing* 12(2):166-170, 1983.

[x]Epstein NB, Baldwin LM, Bishop DS: The McMaster Family Assessment Device, *J Marital Fam Ther* 9(2):171-180, 1983.

[y]Ware JE, Sherbourne CD: The MOS 36-Item short-form health survey (SF-36). I. Conceptual framework and item selection, *Med Care* 30(6):473-483, 1992.

[z]Bergner M et al: The Sickness Impact Profile: development and final revision of a health status measure, *Med Care* 19:787-805, 1981. Instrument is available from the Health Services Research and Development Center, The Johns Hopkins School of Hygiene and Public Health, 624 North Broadway, Baltimore, MD 21705

LEVELS	7 Complete Independence (Timely, Safely) 6 Modified Independence (Device)	NO HELPER
	Modified Dependence 5 Supervision 4 Minimal Assist (Subject = 75% +) 3 Moderate Assist (Subject = 50% +) Complete Dependence 2 Maximal Assist (Subject = 25% +) 1 Total Assist (Subject = 0% +)	HELPER

	ADMIT	DISCHG	FOL-UP
Self Care			
A. Feeding			
B. Grooming			
C. Bathing			
D. Dressing-Upper Body			
E. Dressing-Lower Body			
F. Toileting			
Sphincter Control			
G. Bladder Management			
H. Bowel Management			
Mobility			
Transfer:			
I. Bed, Chair, W/Chair			
J. Toilet			
K. Tub, Shower			
Locomotion			
L. Walk/wheel Chair	W/C	W/C	W/C
M. Stairs			
Communication			
N. Comprehension	a/v	a/v	a/v
O. Expression	v/n	v/n	v/n
Social Cognition			
P. Social Interaction			
Q. Problem Solving			
R. Memory			
Total			

Figure 9-7

Functional independence measure. Scoring is from 1 (total assistance) to 7 (full independence) for each functional measure. "Dependence" (1 or 2) and "Modified dependence" (3 to 5) both require a helper; no assistance is needed for a score of 6 but the patient uses adaptive equipment. (From Research Foundation, State University of New York, 1987.)

Screening for Rehabilitation

Current Clinical Status

Neurologic deficits

Comorbid diseases

Functional health patterns: nutrition and hydration, ability to swallow, bowel and bladder continence, skin integrity, activity tolerance, sleep patterns

Special Emphases

Functional status before stroke

Current functional deficits

Mental status and ability to learn

Emotional status and motivation to participate in rehabilitation

Functional communication

Physical activity endurance

Social and Environmental Factors

Presence of spouse or significant other

Previous living situation

Ethnicity and native language

Adjustment of patient and family to stroke

Patient and family preferences for and expectations of rehabilitation

Extent of support by family or others (relationships, number, health, availability)

Characteristics of potential postdischarge environments

Standardized instruments

Stroke deficit scale

Measure of disability (ADLs)

Mental status screening test

From Gresham GE et al: *Post-stroke rehabilitation. Clinical practice guideline No. 16.* AHCPR Pub. No. 95-0062, Rockville, Md, May 1995, U.S. Department of Health and Human Services. Public Health Service, Agency for Health Care Policy and Research.
ADLs, Activities of daily living.

cally, are able to learn, have enough physical endurance to sit supported for 1 hour, and are able to participate to at least some extent in active rehabilitation treatments.

- Patients are candidates for an interdisciplinary rehabilitation program if they meet the criteria listed above and also have significant disabilities in at least two of the following areas of function: mobility, basic ADLs, bowel or bladder control, cognition, emotional functioning, pain management, swallowing, or communication.
- Patients with only a single area of disability are candidates for individual rehabilitation services but do not require an interdisciplinary program.
- Patients who are too impaired to participate in rehabilitation should receive appropriate supportive services, and their families should receive thorough education regarding care of the patient.

Some patients may not be recommended for rehabilitation initially. With time, however, these patients may recover sufficiently to become candidates for rehabilitation. Providers should be alert to such opportunities.

11. *Be familiar with local rehabilitation programs and their capabilities.*

Rehabilitation programs should maintain and make available information on staffing patterns, services offered, and performance. Programs vary widely, and physicians and other medical personnel who refer patients for rehabilitation should be knowledgeable about the capabilities of programs in their community. Basic rehabilitation settings are as follows

- Hospital inpatient rehabilitation programs may be located in freestanding rehabilitation hospitals or may be distinct units in acute care hospitals. These programs are staffed by the full range of rehabilitation professionals, and an interdisciplinary team provides a comprehensive rehabilitation program for each patient. Hospital inpatient rehabilitation is generally more intense than rehabilitation in other settings and requires greater physical and mental effort from the patient.

- Rehabilitation programs in nursing facilities vary widely in the spectrum of services they provide. Hospital-based nursing facilities are located in or adjacent to acute care hospitals. Rehabilitation is designed primarily for patients who have the potential to improve enough during 2 to 3 weeks of treatment to become candidates for inpatient, home, or outpatient rehabilitation. Programs in community-based nursing facilities vary. Some are as comprehensive as hospital inpatient programs, although usually less intense, while others are very limited.

- Outpatient rehabilitation programs are offered by hospital outpatient departments and freestanding outpatient facilities. Outpatient programs can provide either a comprehensive rehabilitation program or individual rehabilitation services. An advantage of outpatient programs is that they enable the patient to live at home while still having access to an interdisciplinary program and to rehabilitation equipment. Opportunities are also available for the patient to make social contacts and obtain peer support. Although frequently more intense, day hospital programs are similar to outpatient programs. The patient spends several hours, 3 to 5 days each week, in a typical day hospital program. Availability of transportation is a prerequisite for both outpatient and day hospital programs.

- Home rehabilitation programs usually provide physical therapy, occupational therapy, and nursing services. Some of these programs can also provide speech therapy and social work services. Programs are expanding their capabilities, and some now provide comprehensive services, including home visits by physicians and intense rehabilitation. An advantage of home rehabilitation programs is that new skills are learned in the same environment where they will be applied. An additional advantage is that many patients function better in a familiar environment.

12. *If the patient is a candidate for interdisciplinary rehabilitation, choose an appropriate program in consultation with the patient and family.*

CRITERIA FOR PROGRAM CHOICE

Figure 9-8 shows the step-by-step process of arriving at rehabilitation recommendations on the basis of clinical and social/environmental factors. For patients who have been identified as candidates for interdisciplinary rehabilitation the most important patient characteristics in choosing a program are as follows

- Medical stability
- Nature and extent of functional disabilities

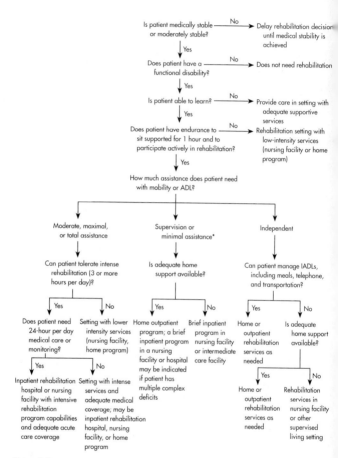

Figure 9-8

Selection of setting for rehabilitation program after hospitalization for acute stroke.
*Under special circumstances, inpatient programs may be appropriate for some pa-
tients with multiple, complex, functional deficits. (*ADL*, Activities of daily living;
IADL, instrumental activities of daily living.) (From Gresham GE et al: *Post-stroke
rehabilitation. Clinical practice guideline No. 16.* AHCPR Pub. No. 95-0062, Rockville, Md, May 1995, U.S. Department of Health and Human Services. Public Health
Service, Agency for Health Care Policy and Research).

Table 9-2   Resources for stroke survivors and families/caregivers

Corporation for National Service (formerly known as ACTION)
  1201 New York Avenue NW
  Washington, DC 20525
  Telephone: 202-606-5000
  Call for number of regional office

Administration on Aging
  330 Independence Avenue SW
  Washington, DC 20201
  Telephone (toll-free): 800-677-1116
  (Eldercare Locator Number)
  Call for list of community services for elders in local area

AHA Stroke Connection (formerly the Courage Stroke Network)
  American Heart Association
  7272 Greenville Avenue
  Dallas, TX 75231-4596
  Telephone (toll-free): 800-553-6321
  Or check telephone book for local AHA office

American Dietetic Association
National Center for Nutrition and Dietetics
  216 West Jackson Boulevard
  Suite 800
  Chicago, IL 60606-6995
  Telephone: 312-899-0040
  Telephone (toll-free): 800-366-1655
  (consumer nutrition hotline)

American Self Help Clearinghouse
  St. Clares Riverside Medical Center
  25 Pocono Road
  Denville, NJ 07834
  Telephone: 201-625-7101
  Call for name and number of state or local clearinghouse

National Aphasia Association
  P.O. Box 1887
  Murray Hill Station
  New York, NY 10156-0611
  Telephone (toll-free): 800-922-4622

National Easter Seal Society, Inc.
  230 West Monroe Street, Suite 1800
  Chicago, IL 60606-4802
  Telephone: 312-726-6200
  Or check telephone book for local Easter Seal Society

National Stroke Association
  8480 East Orchard Road, Suite 1000
  Englewood, CO 80111-5015
  Telephone: 303-771-1700
  Telephone (toll-free): 800-STROKES (787-6537)

Rosalynn Carter Institute
  Georgia Southwestern College
  600 Simmons Street
  Americus, GA 31709
  Telephone: 912-928-1234

Stroke Clubs International
  805 12th Street
  Galveston, TX 77550
  Telephone: 409-762-1022

The Well Spouse Foundation
  610 Lexington Avenue, Suite 814
  New York, NY 10022
  Telephone: 212-644-1241
  Telephone (toll-free): 800-838-0879
  FAX: 212-644-1338

From Gresham GE et al: *Post-stroke rehabilitation. Clinical practice guideline No. 16.* AHCPR Pub. No. 95-0062, Rockville, Md, May 1995, U.S. Department of Health and Human Services. Public Health Service, Agency for Health Care Policy and Research.

- Physical activity endurance
- Need for assistance
- Extent of support by family or caregivers
- Patient and family wishes

The following are criteria for program choice

- Patients who meet threshold criteria for an interdisciplinary program and need moderate to total assistance with mobility or basic ADLs are candidates for an intense rehabilitation program, if they can tolerate 3 or more hours of physically demanding rehabilitation activity each day. Otherwise, a less intense program is usually more appropriate.
- Patients who can benefit from intense rehabilitation but have complex medical problems should be treated in inpatient hospital programs that have 24-hour coverage by physicians and nurses skilled in acute medical care and rehabilitation.
- Patients who need only supervision or minimal assistance can usually be managed in home or outpatient rehabilitation programs if the home environment and support are adequate. If not, a nursing facility program should be considered.

NEED FOR CONSENSUS WITH PATIENT AND FAMILY

In order to succeed, rehabilitation must have the full support and active participation of the patient and family. Hence, rehabilitation decisions need to be agreed on by the patient, family, treating physician, and accepting rehabilitation program to the maximum extent possible. To this end, health care providers should carry out the following recommendations

- Explain clearly the reasons for their recommendations concerning rehabilitation.
- Listen carefully to any concerns of the patient or family that might dictate a different choice.
- Point out the possibility of transfer to a different program in the future (if the patient's condition changes).

Table 9-2 lists resources for stroke survivors and their families and caregivers.

| 9.5 | **GERIATRIC REHABILITATION FOLLOWING HIP FRACTURE[3]**

1. Good postoperative care begins preoperatively. A functional assessment involving physical, cognitive, and psychosocial aspects (in addition to a system-oriented medical assessment) should be performed preoperatively on all geriatric patients
2. Elderly are particularly susceptible to the adverse effects of medications
   a. Preoperative medications should be closely reviewed and unnecessary drugs should be discontinued
   b. Serum levels of selected drugs (e.g., digoxin, theophylline) should be measured preoperatively and frequently monitored postoperatively
   c. Codeine should be avoided for pain control (increased constipation and confusion). Acetaminophen 650 mg q4h around the clock is preferred
   d. Use of NSAIDs can result in GI bleeding, delirium, and renal failure
   e. Use of sedatives can cause delirium, urinary retention, and pulmonary or cardiac abnormalities

    f. Immediate resumption of antihypertensives postoperatively can result in hypotension

    g. Sudden discontinuation of antianginal medications (e.g., beta-blockers) can result in unstable angina and myocardial infarction

    h. Sulfonylureas must be temporarily discontinued. Glucose should be monitored every 6 hours and hyperglycemia should be treated with regular insulin in the immediate preoperative and postoperative period

    i. Patients receiving long-term steroids are at risk of developing relative hypoadrenalism if steroid doses are not augmented

    j. Antiseizure medications should be continued and the levels frequently monitored to avoid postoperative seizures or toxicity

    k. Antiparkinsonian drugs should be reinstituted as soon as possible postoperatively to avoid significant bradykinesia

    l. Vigorous bronchodilator therapy and monitoring of ABGs should be initiated preoperatively and postoperatively in all patients with asthma/COPD

3. The following medical complications should be rapidly identified and treated

    a. **Anemia:** hematocrit should be monitored daily in the immediate postoperative period. Transfusion is indicated only if there is significant blood loss and the patient is symptomatic. Patients with compromised cardiovascular status should receive a small dose of furosemide between units of blood to prevent fluid overload. If oral iron replacement is started, a laxative should be added to minimize its constipating effect

    b. **Urinary tract infections:** prolonged catheterization should be avoided. Intermittent postoperative catheterization is preferred if urinary retention develops. In the elderly, UTIs may have nonspecific symptoms such as delirium. Suspicion of incontinence should be investigated and situational factors (e.g., difficulty in gaining access to the toilet, slow staff response time to the patient's request to urinate) should be eliminated before labeling the patient incontinent

    c. **Constipation:** usually multifactorial (inactivity, poor fluid intake, opiates). Scrupulous bowel care must be instituted preoperatively with enemas, bulking agents, lactulose, glycerin suppositories, and other agents. Fecal impaction can result in urinary retention and spurious diarrhea (caused by intermittent bowel blockage with leakage of feces). Digital examination should be done in any cases of suspected constipation. Manual disimpaction may be required in severe cases of obstipation

    d. **Pressure ulcers:** skin care must be carefully addressed (see Section 5.8). Unnecessary pressure on heels and sacrum should be avoided. Frequent positioning and avoidance of incontinence are necessary to prevent decubitus ulcerations. Early postoperative mobilization is critical

    e. **Venous thromboembolism:** adequate prophylaxis of DVT in patients undergoing hip surgery involves external pneumatic compression of lower extremities (intermittent pneumatic compression [IPC] boots) plus low-dose warfarin started 1 to 2 days before surgery

Table 9-3 Sample post–hip fracture gait training

Fracture Type	Fixation Type	Gait Training Program
Stable intertrochanteric or subtrochanteric	Nail plate or medullary nail	Progressive weight bearing within first postoperative week initially, PWB in standing, then WBAT during ambulation
Femoral neck	Multiple pins	From day 1: OOB in wheelchair; day 5-7: begin standing, ambulation with walker—WBAT; continue walker until healed; cane later
	Screw plate; pin/plate combination, compression screw	From day 1: OOB in wheelchair; from day 3-4: begin bedside standing, then ambulation with walker, WBAT; from week 6-12; FWB with walker

Modified from Sisk DT: Fractures of the hip and pelvis. In Crenshaw AH, editor: *Campbell's operative orthopedics*, St Louis, 1992, Mosby.
PWB, Some (partial) weight bearing on affected limb allowed during standing or ambulation; *FWB*, full weight bearing allowed on affected limb during ambulation; *WBAT*, weight bearing allowed to tolerance of patient (usually limited by pain); may be partial or full; *OOB*, out of bed.

   f. **Fluid and electrolyte imbalance:** hypovolemia, CHF, and electrolyte abnormalities are very common in the postoperative period and can significantly alter cognitive function. Daily monitoring of electrolytes and renal function is recommended in the early postoperative period

4. Physical therapy varies with the postoperative period. Initially only isometric exercises of the involved hip should be allowed. This is followed by gradual mobilization, ambulatory exercises 1 to 10 days postoperatively, and stair climbing after 10 to 12 days. A sample of post–hip fracture gait training is described in Table 9-3

5. Functional outcome varies with the presence of comorbid illness, social support, and type of surgery performed

   a. Functional outcome is generally better with prosthetic hip replacement than nail-and-plate or pin-and-plate fixation

   b. Poor recovery is associated with older age, rehospitalization, longer hospital stays, presence of depressive symptoms, and cognitive deficits (acute or chronic)[6]

   c. Greater contact with a social network following discharge enhances the probability of a good recovery

   d. Most recovery occurs within the first 6 months

References

1. Beck JC: *Geriatric review syllabus,* New York, 1991, American Geriatric Society.
2. Brown PS: The geriatric amputee. In *Physical medicine and rehabilitation: the aging population,* Philadelphia, 1990, Hanley & Belfus.
3. Gordon M: Restoring functional independence in the older hip fracture patient, *Geriatrics* 44:48-58, 1989.
4. Gresham GE et al: *Post-stroke rehabilitation: assessment, referral, and patient management. Clinical Practice Guideline.* Quick Reference Guide for Clinicians No. 16. AHCPR Pub. No.95-0663, Rockville, Md, May 1995, U.S. Department of Health and Human Services, Public Health Service, Agency for Health Care Policy and Research.
5. Hunt TE: Geriatric rehabilitation. In Ham RJ, editor: *Primary care geriatrics,* St Louis, 1983, Mosby.
6. Magaziner J et al: Prediction of functional recovery one year following hospital discharge for hip fracture, *J Gerontol* 45:M101-M107, 1990.
7. Murphy JB: Post-operative care of the older patient; the geriatric rehabilitation perspective, *RI Med J* 74:211-219, 1991.
8. Scharfenberger JA, Ill KC: Financing of health care for elderly stroke patients. In *Physical medicine and rehabilitation: state of the art reviews,* Philadelphia, 1989, Hanley & Belfus.

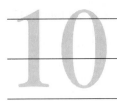

Socioeconomic and Legal Issues

Marsha D. Fretwell, MD

10.1 **COMPETENCE FOR SELF-CARE AND INFORMED CONSENT**

1. Issue of *competency* arises most frequently in two specific situations in the care of frail older patients
   a. It may be raised by family members or neighbors if there is a concern about an individual's capacity for *self-care* and making appropriate social and financial decisions
   b. It may be raised by the physician or another health care provider during an acute illness when *informed consent* for a treatment or procedure must be obtained
2. In both cases, there is the assumption that, at an earlier time, the older individual was able to care for self and/or make rational decisions about medical treatment

Evaluation of competence for self-care and informed consent

Step 1. What cognitive, emotional, or perceptive impairments underlie this change in capacity for self-care and/or medical decision making?

1. Evaluation of competence in older individuals should begin with an in-depth exploration of perceptive, cognitive, and emotional functions fundamental to the ability to make appropriate decisions
2. Consultation with a psychiatrist, neurologist, or psychologist is helpful if difficulties or inconsistencies are found in the evaluation of cognitive function
3. Cognitive functions that underlie competency (Figure 10-1)
   a. Attention
      (1) Ask the patient to perform tasks such as counting down from 10 to 1 or listing the days of the week backward
      (2) If the patient is unable to complete these tasks, evaluate for metabolic disorders, adverse drug reactions, or any other causes of acute confusional states or delirium (see Chapter 4)
      (3) The patient who cannot sustain adequate attention to take in or retain instructions and questions will not be able to complete fur-

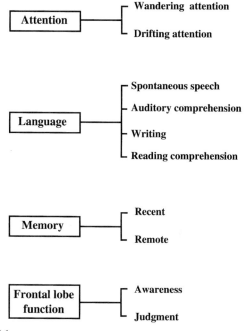

Figure 10-1
Cognitive functions underlying competency. (From Freedman M, Stuss DT, Gordon M: *Ann Intern Med* 115:203-207, 1991.)

ther elements of cognitive testing and, for the moment, must be considered incompetent

(4) Because most causes of isolated attention deficits are reversible, the incompetency should not be labeled permanent. After appropriate medical interventions, the patient's attention span should be frequently reevaluated

b. Language

(1) Disorders in language function (aphasia) are seen in patients with CVAs, severe head injury, or Alzheimer's disease

(2) Patients who are deaf, blind, or intubated have significant difficulty in communication

(3) When barriers to effective communication exist, physicians and families must make a concerted effort to overcome them before declaring a patient incompetent

c. Memory

(1) Loss of short-term memory is the most common impairment of cognition seen in older patients

(2) Depression must be ruled out as a cause of memory disorder

(3) If attention span is intact, a deficit in short-term memory will no[t] necessarily impair the ability to read and understand a consen[t] form for medical or surgical treatment

(4) A consistent response to the consent process on two separate oc[c]asions implies competency; an inconsistent response implies in[competency]

d. Frontal lobe dysfunction

(1) Frontal lobe dysfunctions are seen in frontal lobe dementia, Alz[heimer's] disease, Parkinson's disease, chronic alcoholism, an[d] CVAs

(2) Patient may have knowledge of appropriate facts but be unabl[e] to evaluate the impact of the facts or to respond appropri[ately]

(3) Frontal lobe assessment should include information and observa[tions] from both the patient and significant others

Step 2. Maximize the patient's residual capacity to make decisions by ad[dressing] the treatable causes underlying the change in capacity. Unless it i[s] an emergency situation, no statement about incompetency should be made until this process is completed.

Step 3. Examine for competency in each area of decision making.

1. Areas of decision making
   a. Place of residence
   b. Choice of guardian or caretaker
   c. Financial affairs
   d. Informed consent in medical treatments
2. An individual who is incompetent to manage financial affairs may be capable of making informed decisions about medical treatments; a person incapable of making a decision about medical treatment may be competent to choose the place of residence and caretakers
3. When an individual is declared incompetent, it should always be in the least restrictive manner and linked to a specific situation of decision making

10.2 PATIENT SELF-DETERMINATION ACT, HEALTH CARE PROXY, AND LIVING WILL

Patient Self-Determination Act

In December 1991 the Patient Self-Determination Act was implemented in all institutions reimbursed by Medicare, Medicaid, or both. This law was designed to increase patient involvement in decisions regarding life-sustaining treatment. Its purpose is to help implement a right that has been universally recognized: *the right to refuse any and all medical interventions, even life-sustaining interventions.* The act requires health care providers in hospitals, skilled nursing facilities, home care agencies, hospice programs, and HMOs to

1. Develop written policies concerning advance directives
2. Ask all new patients whether they have prepared an advance directive and include this information in the patient's chart
3. Give patients written materials regarding the facility's policies on advance directives and the patient's right to prepare such documents
4. Educate staff and the community about advance directives

Advance directives: living will and health care proxy

Before the Patient Self-Determination Act, the use of advance directives by patients was limited. Advance directives are legally binding documents that allow currently competent patients to document what medical treatments they would want should they become incompetent in the future. Two types of advance directives are currently in use

1. The living will is defined by statutes in about three quarters of the states. Statutes vary from state to state but usually allow a terminally ill individual to have life-sustaining treatments withheld or withdrawn should that individual be unable to direct the physician to do so. Typical statutes provide immunity to health care providers who execute the living will

2. The health care proxy or durable power of attorney for health care is a written document (see Appendix VII) that allows one to designate an individual to act on one's behalf if, in the future, one is unable to speak or act. It is based on the ethical principle of substituted judgment, which assumes that other individuals (the proxy) can make decisions that approximate the patient's values. It is referred to as durable because it is not invalidated (as is the traditional power of attorney) if and when the individual becomes incompetent. Currently, not all states specifically authorize the durable power of attorney for health care. With the impetus of the Self-Determination Act, it is likely that supporting statutes will soon follow

Steps in securing prior directives

1. Clarify what type of prior directive meets the legal requirements of the state
2. Initiate conversation with patients before the onset of acute illnesses and/or cognitive impairments
3. Include children and spouse of older patient in the discussion
4. Secure copy of prior directive for patient chart
5. Instruct patient to carry copy of directive

10.3 ELDERLY ABUSE

1. **Epidemiology:** each year, approximately 4% of individuals over the age of 65 (1 million individuals) experience abuse or neglect
2. **Types of abuse or neglect** (see the box on p. 462)
   a. Physical
   b. Psychologic
   c. Financial
3. **Risk factors for abuse:** although any older person may become a victim of abuse, certain characteristics or attributes appear to be associated with an increased risk (see the box on p. 462)
4. **Characteristics of abusers**
   a. Most (over 60%) abuse is committed by one spouse against another
   b. Approximately 25% of abuse is committed by an adult child of the victim who is living in the same home and is usually financially dependent on the victim
   c. Abuse occurs at all economic levels, in all age-groups, and to men as well as women

Types of Geriatric Abuse

Physical abuse
    Assault
    Rough handling
    Burns
    Sexual abuse
    Unreasonable physical confinement
Physical neglect
    Dehydration
    Malnutrition
    Poor hygiene
    Inappropriate or soiled clothing
    Medications given improperly
    Lack of medical care
Psychologic abuse
    Verbal or emotional abuse
    Threats
    Isolation/confinement
Material abuse
    Withholding finances
    Misuse of funds
    Theft
    Withholding means for daily living

From Bosker G et al: *Geriatric emergency medicine,* St Louis, 1990, Mosby, p. 534.

Characteristics of Abused Victims

- Age over 75 years
- Female
- White
- Widowed
- Severe cognitive and/or physical impairment
- Dependent on caretaker for most daily care needs
- Exhibits problematic behavior: incontinence, shouting, paranoia, nighttime shouting
- Socially isolated
- Psychosomatic or functional complaints

From Bosker G et al: *Geriatric emergency medicine,* St Louis, 1990, Mosby, p. 534.

5. **Assessment and treatment:** abuse is most often the result of interacting medical, psychologic, and social problems in both victim and abuser and therefore requires a comprehensive and functional orientation to diagnosis and treatment
   a. Have a low threshold for suspecting abuse, particularly when there is

unexplained physical trauma or unexplained loss of physical, cognitive, and emotional function. Create an opportunity to interview the patient in the presence of the caretaker

b. Complete a comprehensive geriatric assessment (see Chapter 2). Consider physical and psychologic neglect or abuse as a potential etiologic factor underlying problems or changes in each area of concern

  (1) Diagnosis

    (a) Falls, fractures

    (b) Absence of eyeglasses, hearing aids, dentures, prosthesis

    (c) Signs of physical restraints

    (d) Genital infections

    (e) Decubitus ulcers, skin lesions, or infections

  (2) Medications: evidence of noncompliance or misuse of medications (overdosing or underdosing)

  (3) Nutrition

    (a) Evidence of malnutrition or dehydration

    (b) Unexplained weight loss or gain

    (c) Increased alcohol intake

    (d) Loss of appetite

  (4) Continence: unexplained urinary incontinence

  (5) Defecation: unexplained fecal incontinence or impaction

  (6) Cognition

    (a) Unexplained confusion

    (b) New onset of disruptive behavior

  (7) Emotion

    (a) Unexplained insomnia or hypersomnia

    (b) Anxiety

    (c) Agitation

    (d) Paranoia

    (e) Depression

  (8) Mobility: unexplained change in social patterns and ambulatory activities out of home

  (9) Cooperation with care plan: unexplained or new onset of lack of cooperation with care plan

c. Establish competency of victim, inform a protective service agency, and decide whether emergency intervention is needed, indicated by

  (1) Urgent need for medical or psychiatric care

  (2) Life-threatening or permanently damaging abuse

  (3) Impairment of the abuser to the degree that he or she is unable to care for the victim

d. Reduce stresses in the care-taking situation

  (1) Treat all reversible medical disorders

  (2) Minimize or simplify medications

  (3) Reverse such functional impairments as urinary and fecal incontinence, immobility, confusion, and anxiety/depression/paranoia

  (4) Secure outside agencies to provide respite for housekeeping, personal care, or transportation needs

  (5) Assist abusing caretaker in seeking appropriate medical or psychologic support

e. If problem is likely to be ongoing and victim is not competent, con-

tact a protective services agency for consideration of guardianship and
a change in the living situation

 ## FINANCING OF HEALTH CARE

Medicare

Medicare is the U.S. government's health insurance. It is available to all
Americans age 65 and older who are eligible for Social Security and to
younger people who receive Social Security disability benefits. Medicare
benefits are divided into Part A (hospital and skilled nursing care benefits)
and Part B (physician and additional services) (Tables 10-1 and 10-2).

Medigap

Medigap, or Medicare supplement insurance, is designed to cover some of
the health care costs not paid by Medicare. Medigap policies are purchased

Table 10-1   Medicare Part A benefits

Benefits	Medicare Pays in 1990
Inpatient Hospital Services	
Includes semiprivate room and board and intensive care, drugs, operating room, and recovery room	
Inpatient deductible (first $628 of eligible hospital expenses per benefit period)	Nothing
Days 1 to 60	All but $628 deductible
Days 61 to 90	All but $157 per day
Days 91 to 150 (60 days of lifetime reserve)	All but $314 per day
Beyond 150 days	Nothing
Inpatient blood expenses	All but 3 pints
Private room (not medically necessary)	Nothing
Private duty nursing	Nothing
Skilled Nursing Care	
Care in a Medicare-certified facility for Medicare-approved acute skilled nursing care for medically necessary treatment following 3 days in hospital	
First 20 days	All covered expenses
Days 21 to 100	All but $78.50 per day
Beyond 100 days	Nothing
Intermediate nursing care	Nothing
Custodial nursing care	Nothing
Non–Medicare-certified skilled care	Nothing

Table 10-2   Medicare Part B benefits

Benefits	Medicare Pays in 1990
Medicare-approved expenses: physician services in and out of hospital, medical services and supplies, ER treatment, x-rays, diagnostic tests, laboratory tests, speech therapy, ambulance, limited chiropractor services	80% of Medicare-approved charges after $100 deductible
Calendar year deductible (first $100 of approved charges)	Nothing
Charges above Medicare-approved amounts	Nothing
Home health care—Parts A and B (visits limited to physician ordered, medically necessary care from certified HHC agencies)	Full cost of most services and 80% of durable medical equipment after $100 deductible
Outpatient drugs	Nothing
Care outside United States	Limited to U.S. territories and along the borders
Mammography screening (if not related to diagnosis)	80% up to a maximum of $55 every 2 yr
Outpatient psychiatric care	50% of approved charges
Hospice care (for terminally ill patients; physician certifies need)	All but limited costs for drugs and inpatient respite care

out of pocket, offer a variety of benefits, and range in price from $300 to $2000 per year. In 1992, the National Association of Insurance Commissioners created 10 standardized packages of coverage, designated by the letters A through J (Table 10-3).

Medicaid

Medicaid is a program that helps pay medical bills for very low-income individuals of any age. Eligibility requirements vary from state to state but can be established by contacting the Social Security Office or Office of Social Services. Starting in 1989, Medicare required state Medicaid programs to pay the care premiums, deductibles, and copayments for Medicare beneficiaries at or below 85% of the federal poverty level. Starting in 1992, states pay Medicare premiums, deductibles, and copayments for beneficiaries at or below 100% of the federal poverty level.

Services required by the federal government include inpatient and outpatient hospital care and services of physicians, laboratories, and skilled

Table 10-3 1992 Medigap Plans

This table shows the benefits each of the 10 plans provide. Medicare Part A covers hospital services; Part B, physician services. Medicare has an approved charge for each procedure, which varies from state to state and sometimes from region to region. Medicare pays 80 percent of that charge; beneficiaries pay the remaining 20 percent.

Benefits	A	B	C	D	E	F	G	H	I	J
Part A hospital coinsurance, days 61 to 90 ($174 per day)	✓	✓	✓	✓	✓	✓	✓	✓	✓	✓
Part A hospital coinsurance, days 91 to 150 ($348 per day)	✓	✓	✓	✓	✓	✓	✓	✓	✓	✓
All charges for extra 365 days in hospital	✓	✓	✓	✓	✓	✓	✓	✓	✓	✓
Part A blood deductible, 3 pints	✓	✓	✓	✓	✓	✓	✓	✓	✓	✓
Part B coinsurance (20% of approved charges)	✓	✓	✓	✓	✓	✓	✓	✓	✓	✓
Skilled-nursing facility coinsurance, days 21 to 100 ($87 per day)			✓	✓	✓	✓	✓	✓	✓	✓
Part A deductible ($696 per year)		✓	✓	✓	✓	✓	✓	✓	✓	✓
Emergency care in foreign countries			✓	✓	✓	✓	✓	✓	✓	✓
Part B deductible ($100 per year)			✓			✓				✓
Part B excess charges						✓	✓		✓	✓
At-home care needed after an injury, illness, or surgery				✓			✓		✓	✓
Prescription drugs								✓	✓	✓
Preventive medical care					✓					✓

The new Medigap plans, copyright 1991 by Consumers Union of US, Inc., Yonkers, NY 10703-1057. Reprinted by permission from *Consumer Reports*, September 1991.

ursing facilities for adults. States have the option to cover prescribed drugs, are in an intermediate care facility, physical therapy, and dental care.

Medicaid is the major public payer for long-term care, contributing close o 45% of the dollars spent for nursing home care. As more people live to ld age, Medicaid has become the de facto long-term care insurance for both he poor and the elderly. Some divest their assets to qualify for Medicaid vhen they enter a nursing home. Others enter nursing homes as private pa- ents but spend their savings down and thus qualify for Medicaid reimburse- nent for such services.

Veterans Administration (VA)

n the VA system, health care services are provided without charge on a pace-available basis, with priority going to veterans with service-connected lisabilities. Free from the restrictions of the Medicare fee-for-service struc- ure of reimbursement, the VA has launched several innovative geriatric pro- grams, including geriatric assessment units, interdisciplinary research and ducation centers, and hospital-based home health care programs. All of hese programs focus on continuity of services for older patients.

Crisis in health care financing

The United States spends approximately $1 trillion (14% of the gross na- ional product [GNP]) annually on health care. It is estimated that by the ear 2000 $1.5 trillion (15% to 17% of the GNP) will be spent annually. The United States spends more per person than any other nation in the world on health care, yet millions of Americans under the age of 65 years lack nsurance and go without needed care.

Medicare costs are rising faster than nearly all items in the federal bud- get. Despite this, Medicare beneficiaries are paying higher out-of-pocket ex- penses, such as increased coinsurance charges for hospital care and increased charges for medications. As a result, several proposals for significant changes n the Medicare program are currently being debated in the U.S. Congress:

- Reductions in benefits under Medicare
- Increases in deductions and copayments
- Increasing financial incentives for Medicare beneficiaries to join health maintenance organizations and other managed care programs

Suggested readings

Adelman RD, Breckman R: Mistreatment. In Abrams WB, Berkow R, editors: *The Merck manual of geriatrics,* Rahway, NJ, 1990, Merck Sharp & Dohme.
Annas GJ: The health care proxy and the living will, *N Engl J Med* 324:1210, 1991.
Freedman M, Stuss DT, Gordon M: Assessment of competency: the role of neurobe- havioral deficits, *Ann Intern Med* 115:203, 1991.
Greco PJ et al: The patient self-determination act and the future of advance directives, *Ann Intern Med* 115:639, 1991.
Jones JS: Geriatric abuse and neglect. In Bosker G et al, editors: *Geriatric emergency medicine,* St Louis, 1990, Mosby.

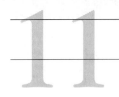

Alcohol Abuse
in the Elderly

Mark J. Fagan, MD

Definition

Alcoholism is a chronic disease with genetic, psychosocial, and environmental factors influencing its development and manifestations. It is characterized by impaired control over drinking, preoccupation with the drug alcohol, use of alcohol despite adverse consequences, and distortions in thinking, most notably denial. In the elderly the onset or continuation of drinking may become problematic because of physiologic and psychosocial changes that occur with aging, including increased sensitivity to the effects of alcohol.

Epidemiology

1. Estimated prevalence of alcohol abuse in community-dwelling elderly is 3% to 4%
2. Prevalence in hospitalized elderly is considerably higher, estimated at 20%
3. The rate of alcohol abuse is four times higher for elderly men than for elderly women
4. Some studies show that alcohol abuse in elderly women (compared to elderly men) is less likely to be detected by physicians
5. An estimated 5% to 10% of cases of dementia are related to alcohol abuse
6. An estimated one third of persons in Alcoholics Anonymous are over 50 years of age

DIAGNOSTIC APPROACH
SCREENING

Every geriatric patient should be screened for potential alcohol abuse by using an instrument such as the CAGE questionnaire

- Have you ever felt you should *cut* down on your drinking?
- Have people *annoyed* you by criticizing your drinking?
- Have you ever felt bad or *guilty* about your drinking?
- Have you ever had a drink first thing in the morning to steady your nerves or to get rid of a hangover *(eye-opener)?*

Any positive response to a CAGE question should prompt further inquiry (Figure 11-1).

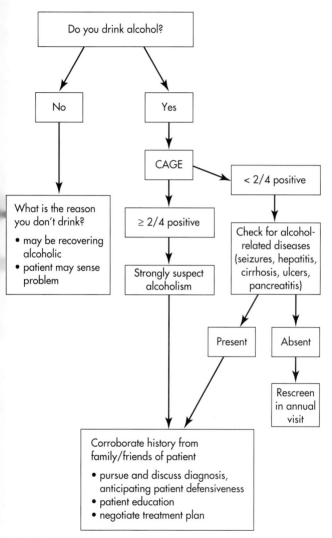

Figure 11-1
Interview for alcohol abuse.

Two or more positive responses should cause suspicion for current or past problem drinking and prompt the interviewer to obtain more information, such as additional history, interviews with family, physical examination, and laboratory tests.

GENERAL MEDICAL HISTORY

The following clues from the general medical history may signal the presence of alcoholism
1. Frequent falls and bruises
2. Insomnia
3. Malnutrition or weight loss
4. Incontinence
5. Change in behavior or social isolation
6. Memory loss
7. Symptoms of depression or anxiety
8. Prescription drug abuse
9. Evidence of drug/alcohol interactions

PHYSICAL EXAMINATION

The physical exam should include a search for signs of alcohol abuse such as
1. Systolic hypertension
2. Evidence of trauma
3. Evidence of chronic liver disease
4. Gastrointestinal bleeding
5. Peripheral neuropathy
6. Cardiomyopathy

LABORATORY TESTS

1. Often normal even in the presence of significant alcohol abuse
2. For a given amount of ingested alcohol, elderly patients have a higher blood alcohol level because of decreased total body water
3. For a given blood alcohol level, elderly patients show greater signs of intoxication because of increased CNS sensitivity to alcohol
4. Tests for hepatocellular injury (GGTP and AST) most sensitive laboratory tests
5. Anemia (often multifactorial and macrocytic) and thrombocytopenia

Treatment

1. Consider the possibility of a coexisting condition such as depression, anxiety, or dementia
2. Understand how to overcome denial
   a. Explain how alcohol is affecting the patient's health, interpersonal relationships, and family
   b. Enlist support of family members
   c. Express concern for the patient and eagerness to help
   d. Avoid hedging: state the data, conclusions, and opinion clearly but nonjudgmentally
3. Alcohol withdrawal delirium is associated with a higher mortality in older patients

e. Treat concomitant metabolic and nutritional problems
9. Plan for long-term treatment
   a. Residential
   b. Outpatient
   c. Self-help (Alcoholics Anonymous)
   d. Al-Anon for patient's family

Resources

1. Alcoholics Anonymous (listed in telephone directory under AA)
2. National Association of State Alcohol and Drug Abuse Directors: (202) 783-6868
3. National Association of Addiction Treatment Providers: (202) 371-6731

Prevention

1. Routinely screen for alcohol abuse
2. Inform patients of relationship between alcohol use and health problems
3. Be aware of potential drug/alcohol interactions
4. Before "approving" a patient's alcohol use, ensure that the patient has no drinking problem or any existing medical condition or drug therapy that could be adversely affected by a small amount of alcohol

Suggested readings

American Medical Association, Department of Geriatric Health: *Alcoholism in the elderly: diagnosis, treatment, prevention. Guidelines for primary care physicians,* Chicago, 1995, The Association.

Curtis JR et al: Characteristics, diagnosis, and treatment of alcoholism in elderly patients, *J Am Geriatr Soc* 37:310-316, 1989.

Kitchens JM: Does this patient have an alcohol problem? *JAMA* 272:1782-1787, 1994.

12

Formulary

Tom J. Wachtel, MD, and Lynn Wachtel, FNP, MSN

The following is a selected list of drugs that should treat the needs of most patients in a primary care setting. More dosage forms may exist than those described. "Elimination" of the drug is not intended to describe drug pharmacology but to indicate that an organ is involved in the metabolism or excretion of the drug and dysfunction of that organ may affect the pharmacology of a drug in a particular patient. The cost information is the average *wholesale* price range (¢: <$5; $: $5 to $10; $$: $10 to $20; $$$: $20 to $30; $$$$: $30 to $40; $$$$$: $40 to $50; actual figure above $50). Pharmacies neither purchase nor sell drugs at the wholesale price; therefore that price gives the clinician only a rough estimate (typically an underestimate) of what the patient will have to spend.

ANALGESICS

Acetaminophen (Tylenol)

Dosage forms: *cap* 325, 500 mg; *tab* 160, 325, 650 mg; *liq* 160 mg/5 ml, 500 mg/15 ml; *supp* 120, 325, 650 mg
Dosage: 325-1000 mg q4h (max, 4 g/day)
Half-life: 2-4 hr
Elimination: hepatic
Adverse effects: hepatotoxicity with overdosage
Drug interactions: ethanol
Cost: ¢ for 100 325-mg tablets

Codeine (e.g., Tylenol No. 3)

Dosage forms: *tab* 15, 30, 60 mg (often prescribed in combination with acetaminophen)
Dosage: 30-60 mg q4h prn
Half-life: 3-4 hr
Elimination: hepatic metabolism
Adverse effects: drowsiness, hypotension, nausea, constipation, respiratory depression, cough suppression, dependence
Drug interactions: barbiturates (additive CNS depression); cimetidine (increased narcotic effect); phenothiazines (possible hypotension and excess CNS depression)

Cost: $$ for 100 30-mg codeine tablets; $for 100 acetaminophen (325 mg) with codeine (30-mg) tablets

Hydrocodone (e.g., Vicodin)

Dosage forms: *tab* 5 mg with acetaminophen (500 mg)
Dosage: 5-10 mg q4-6h prn
Half-life: 4 hr
Elimination: hepatic metabolism
Adverse effects: drowsiness, hypotension, nausea, constipation, respiratory depression, cough suppression, dependence
Drug interactions: barbiturates (additive CNS depression); cimetidine (increased narcotic effect); phenothiazines (possible hypotension and excess CNS depression)
Cost: $ for 100 tablets hydrocodone (5 mg) with acetaminophen (500 mg)

Oxycodone (e.g., Percodan)

Dosage forms: *tab* 5 mg with acetaminophen (325 mg) or aspirin (325 mg)
Dosage: 5 mg q6h prn
Elimination: metabolized in liver, excreted primarily in urine
Adverse effects: drowsiness, hypotension, nausea, constipation, respiratory depression, cough suppression, dependence
Drug interactions: barbiturates (additive CNS depression); cimetidine (increased narcotic effect); phenothiazines (possible hypotension and excess CNS depression)
Cost: $$ for 100 tablets oxycodone (5 mg) with acetaminophen (325 mg)

Lidocaine (e.g., Xylocaine)

Dosage forms: *inj* (local) 0.5%, 1%, 1.5%, 2%; *top viscous* 2%; *ointment* 2.5%; 5%; *jelly* 2%; *oral spray* 10%
Dosage: *inj* 4.5 mg/kg (max, 300 mg) without epinephrine or 7 mg/kg (max, 500 mg) with epinephrine
Half-life: 1.5-2 hr
Elimination: hepatic
Cost: ¢ for 50 ml injectable solution, 1%; ¢ for 100 ml viscous, 2%; ¢ for 35 g ointment, 5%

ANTIBIOTICS

Penicillin V (V-cillin)

Dosage forms: *oral sol* 125, 250 mg/5 ml; *tab* 125, 250, 500 mg
Dosage: 250-500 mg qid
Half-life: 30-40 min
Elimination: renal
Cost: ¢ for 250 or 500 mg qid × 10 days

Amoxicillin (Amoxil)

Dosage forms: *cap* 250, 500 mg; *susp* 125, 250 mg/5 ml
Dosage: 250-500 mg tid
Half-life: 0.8-2 hr

Elimination: renal
Adverse effects: diarrhea (10%); rash (3%)
Drug interactions: allopurinol (increased risk of rash)
Cost: $ for 250 or 500 mg tid × 10 days

Azithromycin (Zithromax)

Dosage form: *cap* 250 mg
Dosage: 500 mg on day 1, then 250 mg qd for 4 days (to be taken at least 1 hr before or 2 hrs after a meal)
Half-life: 68 hr
Elimination: hepatic
Adverse effects
  1. Skin: rash, urticaria, photosensitivity
  2. GI: dyspepsia, flatulence, vomiting, hepatic dysfunction
  3. Neurologic: headache, vertigo
Drug interactions: none reported but see erythromycin (another macrolide)
Cost: $$$$/course

Dicloxacillin (Dynapen)

Dosage forms: *cap* 250, 500 mg; *susp* 62.5 mg/5 ml
Dosage: 250-500 mg qid
Half-life: 40-50 min
Elimination: renal
Cost: $$ for 250 mg qid × 10 days

Amoxicillin/clavulanic acid (Augmentin)

Dosage forms: *tab* 250 mg amoxicillin/125 mg clavulanic acid, 500 mg amoxicillin/125 mg clavulanic acid; *susp* 250 mg amoxicillin/62.5 mg clavulanic acid/5 ml
Dosage: 250 mg/125 mg to 500 mg/125 mg tid
Half-life: 1 hr
Elimination: renal
Adverse effects: nausea, vomiting, diarrhea, abdominal cramps
Cost: $$$ for 250 mg (amoxicillin component)/5 ml tid × 10 days; $52 for 500 mg (amoxicillin component) tid × 10 days

Cefadroxil (Duricef)

Dosage forms: *cap* 500 mg; *tab* 1 g; *susp* 250, 500 mg/5 ml
Dosage: 1-2 g per day in single or divided (bid) doses
Half-life: 1-2 hr
Elimination: renal
Cost: $$$$ for 500 mg bid × 10 days

Cefaclor (Ceclor)

Dosage forms: *cap* 250, 500 mg; *susp* 250 mg/5 ml
Dosage: oral—250-500 mg tid
Half-life: 0.5-1 hr
Elimination: renal
Cost: $75 for 500 mg tid × 10 days

Cefixime (Suprax)

Dosage forms: *tab* 200, 400 mg; *susp* 100 mg/5 ml
Dosage: 400 mg qd or 200 mg bid
Half-life: 3-4 hr
Elimination: renal and hepatic
Adverse effects: diarrhea, abdominal pain, nausea, vomiting, pseudomembranous colitis
Cost: $$$$$ for 400 mg qd for 10 days

Ceftriaxone (Rocephin)

Dosage forms: *inj* 500 mg, 1, 2 g
Dosage: 1-2 g q12-24h (max, 4 g/day); uncomplicated gonorrhea, 125-250 mg IM (single dose)
Half-life: 5-11 hr
Elimination: renal and hepatic
Adverse effects: diarrhea, nausea, vomiting, abnormal liver function test results
Cost: $$$ for 1 g (single IM); ¢ for 125 mg (single IM); $410 for 2 g/day × 7 days

Clarithromycin (Biaxin)

Dosage forms: *tab* 250, 500 mg; *susp* 125 mg/5 ml, 250 mg/5 ml
Dosage: 250-500 mg bid
Half-life: 6 hr
Elimination: mostly renal, hepatic hydroxylation
Adverse effects
1. GI: diarrhea, nausea, abnormal taste, dyspepsia, abdominal pain
2. Neurologic: headache
3. Renal: BUN elevation
4. Hematologic: neutropenia
5. Hepatic: transaminitis
Drug interactions: elevation of theophylline levels; elevation of carbamazepine levels; see erythromycin drug interactions (another macrolide)
Cost: $$$$$/7-day course; $91/14-day course

Erythromycin

Dosage forms: *cap* and *tab* 250, 500 mg; *susp* 100 mg/ml, 250 mg/5 ml
Dosage: 250-500 mg qid
Half-life: 1-1.5 hr
Elimination: hepatic
Adverse effects: epigastric pain, nausea, vomiting, hepatotoxicity (especially with Estolate)
Drug interactions: warfarin, carbamazepine, theophylline (increased serum levels)
Cost: $ for 250 mg qid × 10 days

Doxycycline (Vibramycin)

Dosage forms: *cap* 50, 100 mg; *tab* 50, 100 mg; *susp* 125 mg/5 ml
Dosage: 100 mg bid

Half-life: 14-17 hr
Elimination: renal
Adverse effects: nausea; deposition in teeth; skin photosensitivity
Drug interactions: antacids containing divalent or trivalent cations, milk, dairy products, iron preparations, and zinc; barbiturates, carbamazepine, phenytoin (reduced doxycycline concentrations)
Cost: ¢ for 100 mg bid × 10 days

Metronidazole (Flagyl)

Dosage forms: *tab* 250, 500 mg
Dosage
  1. Amebiasis: 750 mg tid × 5-10 days
  2. Antibiotic-induced colitis: 500 mg bid or tid × 10 days
  3. Bacterial vaginosis: 500 mg bid × 7 days or 2 g as single dose
  4. Trichomoniasis: 250 mg tid × 7 days or 2 g as single dose (patient and partner)

Half-life: 6-11 hr
Elimination: hepatic and renal
Adverse effects
  1. Blood: bone marrow aplasia
  2. CNS: peripheral neuropathy, seizures
  3. GI: anorexia, epigastric distress
  4. Other: disulfiram-like reaction

Drug interaction: warfarin (increased anticoagulant effect)
Cost: ¢ for 250 mg tid × 7 days

Nitrofurantoin (Macrodantin)

Dosage forms: *cap* 50, 100 mg; *tab* 50, 100 mg
Dosage (indicated only for UTIs)
  1. Acute UTI: 50-100 mg qid (with meals)
  2. Long-term suppressive therapy: 50-100 mg hs

Half-life: 20 min
Elimination: hepatic and renal
Adverse effects
  1. Blood: hemolytic anemia (rare)
  2. CNS: peripheral polyneuropathy, headache, dizziness
  3. GI: anorexia, vomiting, hepatotoxicity, cholestatic jaundice
  4. Respiratory: acute, subacute, and chronic pneumonitis

Cost: $ for 50 mg qid × 7 days

Cotrimoxazole (Bactrim, Septra)

Dosage forms: *tab* sulfamethoxazole/trimethoprim 400/80 mg, double strength (DS) 800/160 mg; *susp* sulfamethoxazole/trimethoprim 40/8 mg/ml
Dosage
  1. Acute UTI treatment, 800/160 mg bid or 1600/320 mg or 2400/480 mg as a single dose; prophylaxis, 200/40 mg qd
  2. *Pneumocystis carinii* pneumonia: sulfamethoxazole/trimethoprim 1600/320 mg qid × 14 days

Half-life: sulfamethoxazole, 8-11 hr; trimethoprim, 6-17 hr
Elimination: hepatic acetylation with 10% to 30% of sulfamethoxasole and 50% to 75% of trimethoprim excreted unchanged in urine
Adverse effects
1. Blood: pancytopenia, thrombocytopenia, megaloblastic anemia, hemolytic anemia
2. CNS: depression
3. Endocrine/metabolic: hypoglycemia
4. GI: nausea, vomiting, hepatotoxicity
5. Renal: nephrotoxicity
6. Respiratory: ARDS

Drug interactions: warfarin (increased anticoagulant effects); oral hypoglycemics (enhanced effects); phenytoin (increased phenytoin levels)
Cost: ¢ for 800/160 mg bid × 10 days

Ciprofloxacin (Cipro)

Dosage forms: *tab* 250, 500, 750 mg
Dosage
1. UTI: 250-500 mg bid
2. Respiratory tract infections: 500 mg bid; more severe and complicated infections, 750 mg bid
3. Infectious diarrhea: 500 mg bid

Half-life: 4 hr
Elimination: renal
Adverse effects
1. Blood: lowered platelet level and WBCs, eosinophilia
2. CNS: headache, dizziness, restlessness, insomnia, hallucinations, seizures
3. Cardiovascular (CV): palpitations, hypertension
4. GI: nausea, diarrhea, vomiting, abdominal discomfort, liver function test changes
5. Musculoskeletal: arthralgias, myalgias
6. Renal: elevated serum creatinine and BUN levels
7. Skin: phototoxicity

Drug interaction: theophylline (increased levels)
Cost: $65 for 500 mg bid × 10 days

Vancomycin (Vancocin)

Dosage forms: *cap* 125, 250 mg
Dosage: pseudomembranous colitis, 250 mg qid
Half-life: 5-11 hr
Elimination: renal
Adverse effects
1. Blood: neutropenia, thrombocytopenia
2. CNS: ototoxicity
3. Ocular: lacrimation
4. Renal: nephrotoxicity, interstitial nephritis

Cost: $275 for 500 mg qid for 10 days

ANTIFUNGALS

Fluconazole (Diflucan)

Dosage forms: *tab* 100, 150, 200 mg
Dosage
1. 100-400 mg/day qd for 2 wk (esophageal candidiasis) or 4 wk (systemic candidiasis) or for at least 2 wk after resolution of symptoms
2. Cryptococcal meningitis: 200-400 mg qd for 10-12 wk after CSF becomes culture negative
3. Suppression of relapse in patients with AIDS: 200 mg qd
4. Monilial vaginitis: 150 mg as single dose

Half-life: 30 hr
Elimination: renal
Adverse effects: headache, nausea, abdominal pain, vomiting
Drug interactions: warfarin (increased anticoagulant effect); oral antidiabetics (enhanced hypoglycemic effect)
Cost: $315 for 200 mg qd × 4 weeks; $$ for single dose

Ketoconazole (Nizoral)

Dosage form: *tab* 200 mg
Dosage: 200 mg qd
Elimination: hepatic
Adverse effects
1. CNS: headache, dizziness
2. GI: nausea, vomiting, abdominal pain, constipation, flatulence, diarrhea, hepatotoxicity
3. Endocrine: gynecomastia, inhibition of cortisol synthesis
4. Others: arthralgias, fever, chills, hemolytic anemia, tinnitus, impotence

Cost: $$$$$ for 200 mg qd × 4 weeks

Nystatin (e.g., Mycostatin)

Dosage forms: *susp* 100,000 U/ml; *tab* 500,000 U; *vaginal tab* 100,000 U
Dosage
1. Oral swish: 500,000-1 million U qid
2. Vaginal: 1-2 tablets hs for 2 wk

Elimination: entirely in feces
Adverse effects: mild nausea, vomiting, diarrhea with large doses
Cost: ¢ for 60-ml suspension; ¢ for 30 tablets

ANTITUBERCULOUS DRUGS

Ethambutol

Dosage forms: *tab* 100, 400 mg
Dosage: 25 mg/kg qd for 2 mo, then 15 mg/kg qd
Half-life: 3.3 hr
Elimination: hepatic and renal
Adverse effects
1. CNS: fever, malaise, headache, dizziness, mental confusion, disorientation, optic neuritis, peripheral neuropathy

2. GI: anorexia, nausea, vomiting, abdominal pain
3. Musculoskeletal: elevated uric acid levels

Cost: $$$$/mo for 800 mg/day

Isoniazid

Dosage forms: *tab* 50, 100, 300 mg
Dosage: 5-10 mg/kg (300 mg) qd; twice weekly dose, 15 mg/kg
Half-life: 0.5-1.5 hr (rapid acetylators) or 2-4 hr (slow acetylators)
Elimination: acetylation in liver
Adverse effects

1. CNS: peripheral neuropathy, convulsions, optic neuritis and atrophy, memory impairment, and psychosis
2. GI: nausea, vomiting, constipation, abnormal liver function test results (discontinue if transaminase levels are greater than three times normal), hepatitis
3. Musculoskeletal: positive antinuclear antibody (ANA)

Drug interactions: antacids (reduce peak INH levels); carbamazepine (increased carbamazepine levels); phenytoin (20% increase in phenytoin levels); corticosteroids (reduced INH levels)
Cost: ¢/mo for 300 mg qd

Pyrazinamide

Dosage form: *tab* 500 mg
Dosage: 20-35 mg/kg qd or divided (max, 3 g/day)
Half-life: 9-10 hr
Elimination: hepatic and renal
Adverse effects

1. Blood: sideroblastic anemia
2. GI: nausea, vomiting
3. Musculoskeletal: arthralgias, gout

Cost: $70/mo for 500 mg qid

Rifampin

Dosage forms: *cap* 150, 300 mg
Dosage

1. Tuberculosis: 600 mg qd
2. Meningococcal carrier: 600 mg qd × 4 days

Half-life: 1.5-5 hr
Elimination: mainly hepatic; 3% to 30% renal
Adverse effects

1. Blood: thrombocytopenia, hemolysis
2. CNS: headache, drowsiness, confusion, visual disturbances
3. GI: heartburn, epigastric distress, nausea, vomiting, diarrhea, sore mouth
4. Renal: hematuria, renal insufficiency

Drug interactions: warfarin, benzodiazepines, beta-adrenergic blockers, calcium channel blockers, contraceptives, corticosteroids, digoxin, narcotic analgesics, ketoconazole, quinidine, theophylline (all reduced serum concentrations); increased risk of INH hepatitis
Cost: $70/mo for 600 mg qd

ANTIVIRALS

Acyclovir (Zovirax)

Dosage forms: *cap* 200 mg; *tab* 400, 800 mg
Dosage
1. Primary genital and oral herpes simplex, 200 mg five times per day × 10 days
2. Recurrent genital: 200 mg five times per day × 5 days
3. Chronic suppression: 200-400 mg bid
4. Shingles: 800 mg five times per day × 5 days

Half-life: 3 hr
Elimination: renal
Adverse effects
1. CNS: lethargy, tremor, confusion, hallucinations, agitation, seizures, headache
2. GI: nausea and vomiting, diarrhea
3. Renal: nephrotoxicity

Cost: $64 for 100 200-mg capsules; $347 for 100 800-mg tablets

Amantadine (Symmetrel)

Dosage forms: *cap* 100 mg; *syrup* 50 mg/5 ml
Dosage
1. Influenza A: 100-200 mg/day
2. Parkinsonism: 100-200 mg bid

Half-life: 15 hr
Elimination: renal
Adverse effects
1. CV: hypotension
2. CNS: jitteriness, inability to concentrate, insomnia, tremors, confusion, depression
3. GI: nausea, constipation, dry mouth
4. GU: urinary retention

Cost: $$/mo for 200 mg qd

MUSCULOSKELETAL DRUGS

NONSTEROIDAL ANTIINFLAMMATORY DRUGS (NSAIDs)

Ibuprofen (Motrin)

Dosage forms: *tab* 200, 300, 400, 600, 800 mg; *susp* 200 mg/5 ml
Dosage: 1.2-3.2 g/day divided tid or qid (doses >400 mg do not provide greater analgesic activity but may be required for maximum antiinflammatory effect)
Half-life: 2-2.5 hr
Elimination: hepatic and renal
Adverse effects
1. Blood: reversible inhibition of platelet aggregation
2. CV: edema
3. CNS: headache, confusion, depression
4. GI: dyspepsia, gastritis, ulceration, bleeding, hepatoxicity

5. Renal: fluid retention, renal failure, interstitial nephritis, hyperkalemia

Drug interactions: antagonizes antihypertensives (e.g., ACE inhibitors, beta-blockers, hydralazine); potentiates anticoagulant effect

Cost: $/mo for 400 mg tid

Indomethacin (Indocin)

Dosage forms: *cap* 25, 50 mg; *susp* 25 mg/5 ml; *supp* 50 mg

Dosage
1. 25 mg bid or tid, increasing by 25 mg at weekly intervals until satisfactory response or a total dose of 150 to 200 mg/day is reached
2. Acute gouty arthritis: 50 mg tid

Half-life: 2-11 hr

Elimination: hepatic and renal

Adverse effects
1. Blood: reversible inhibition of platelet aggregation
2. CV: edema
3. CNS: headache, confusion, depression
4. GI: dyspepsia, gastritis, ulceration, bleeding, hepatoxicity
5. Renal: fluid retention, renal failure, interstitial nephritis, hyperkalemia

Drug interactions: antagonizes antihypertensives (e.g., ACE inhibitors, beta-blockers, hydralazine); potentiates anticoagulant effect

Cost: $/mo for 25 mg tid

Naproxen (Naprosyn, Anaprox)

Dosage forms: *tab* Naprosyn 250, 375, 500 mg, Anaprox 275, 550 mg; *susp* Naprosyn 125 mg/5 ml

Dosage: 250-500 mg bid to tid (max, 1.5 g/day)

Half-life: 12-15 hr

Elimination: hepatic and renal

Adverse effects
1. Blood: reversible inhibition of platelet aggregation
2. CV: edema
3. CNS: headache, confusion, depression
4. GI: dyspepsia, gastritis, ulceration, bleeding, hepatoxicity
5. Renal: fluid retention, renal failure, interstitial nephritis, hyperkalemia

Drug interactions: antagonizes antihypertensives (e.g., ACE inhibitors, beta-blockers, hydralazine); potentiates anticoagulant effect

Cost: $$$$/mo for 250 mg bid

Piroxicam (Feldene)

Dosage forms: *cap* 10, 20 mg

Dosage: 10-20 mg qd

Half-life: 50 hr

Elimination: hepatic and renal

Adverse effects
1. Blood: reversible inhibition of platelet aggregation
2. CV: edema
3. CNS: headache, confusion, depression
4. GI: dyspepsia, gastritis, ulceration, bleeding, hepatoxicity

5. Renal: fluid retention, renal failure, interstitial nephritis, hyperkalemia
Drug interactions: antagonizes antihypertensives (e.g., ACE inhibitors beta-blockers, hydralazine); potentiates anticoagulant effect
Cost: $$$$$/mo for 20 mg qd

Salicylates

Dosage forms: aspirin *tab* 325, 500, 650 mg; *chew tab* 65, 81 mg; *enteric-coated tab* 325, 500, 650, 975 mg; *buffered tab* 325, 500, 650 mg; *supp* 60, 120, 300, 600, 1200 mg
Dosage
1. Antipyretic-analgesic: 325-650 mg q4-6h (max, 4 g/day)
2. Antirheumatic: initial—2.4-3.6 g/day; increment—increase 0.325-1.2 g/day weekly; maintenance—3.6-5.4 g/day in four to six doses
3. Transient ischemic attacks: 30 mg qd to 650 mg bid
Half-life: dose dependent—2.4 hr with 0.25 g; 5 hr with 1 g; 19 hr with 10-20 g; significantly longer in elderly patients
Elimination: saturable metabolism of salicylate occurs as aspirin dosage is increased; salicylate and its metabolites are excreted in urine
Adverse effects
1. Blood: irreversible inhibition of platelet aggregation
2. CNS: delirium
3. CV: edema
4. GI: dyspepsia, gastritis, ulceration, bleeding, hepatotoxicity
5. Renal: nephrotoxicity
Drug interactions: warfarin (increases risk of bleeding by inhibition of platelet function and enhancement of anticoagulant effects); antacids (decreased serum salicylate concentrations); oral hypoglycemic agents (enhanced hypoglycemic response); corticosteroids (markedly increased salicylate elimination); probenecid (decreased uricosuric activity)
Cost: ¢/mo for 650 mg qid

GOUT DRUGS

Allopurinol (Zyloprim)

Dosage forms: *tab* 100, 300 mg
Dosage: 300 mg qd
Half-life: 1 hr
Elimination: metabolized to oxipurinol ($t_{1/2}$ = 12-30 hr); 10% of dose is excreted by the kidney as unchanged allopurinol (75% as oxipurinol)
Adverse effects
1. Blood dyscrasias
2. GI intolerance, hepatotoxicity (relatively rare)
3. Renal: nephrotoxicity
4. Skin: maculopapular rash, serum sickness
Drug interactions: warfarin (enhanced anticoagulant effect)
Cost: ¢/mo for 300 mg qd

Colchicine

Dosage forms: *tab* 0.5, 0.6 mg
Dosage
1. Acute gouty arthritis: initial—0.5-1.2 mg; follow with 0.5-1.2 mg

q1-2h until pain is relieved or until nausea, vomiting, or diarrhea occurs (max, 8 mg); wait 3 days before initiating a second course to minimize toxicity

2. Prophylaxis during intercritical periods: 0.5-1.2 mg qd

Half-life: 20 min

Elimination: hepatic and renal

Adverse effects

1. Blood: bone marrow depression with aplastic anemia
2. GI: vomiting, diarrhea, abdominal pain and nausea
3. Renal: hematuria, oliguria

Cost: $/mo for 0.6 mg bid

Probenecid

Dosage form: *tab* 500 mg

Dosage: 250-500 mg bid

Half-life: 4-17 hr

Elimination: hepatic

Adverse effects

1. CNS: headache
2. GI: anorexia, nausea, and vomiting

Cost: ¢/mo for 500 mg bid

OTHER

Quinine sulfate

Dosage forms: *cap* 200, 300 mg

Dosage: nocturnal recumbency leg cramps—200-300 mg hs prn

Half-life: 7-12 hr

Elimination: hepatic

Adverse effects

1. Blood: blood dyscrasias, hemolysis, increased anticoagulant effects
2. CNS: visual disturbances, deafness, confusion
3. CV: arrhythmias, hypotension (quinidine-like effects)
4. Renal: renal injury
5. Other: cinchonism (tinnitus, headache, nausea, abdominal pain, visual disturbance)

Cost: ¢/mo for 200 mg qd

ANTIHYPERTENSIVE DRUGS

DIURETICS

Hydrochlorothiazide (Hydrodiuril, Esidrix)

Dosage forms: *tab* 25, 50, 100 mg

Dosage: 25-100 mg/day qd (max, 200 mg/day); minimal additional antihypertensive effect at doses >25-50 mg/day

Half-life: 5-15 hr

Elimination: renal

Adverse effects

1. CV: orthostatic hypotension

2. Endocrine/metabolic: hyperglycemia, hypokalemia, hyperuricemia, hypercalcemia, hyponatremia, hypochloremic alkalosis, hypomagnesemia, elevated cholesterol and triglycerides
3. GI: pancreatitis, hepatitis

Drug interactions: cholestyramine and colestipol (decrease thiazide concentration; separate doses by 2 hours)

Cost: ¢/mo for 25 mg qd

Chlorthalidone (Hygroton)

Dosage forms: *tab* 25, 50 mg

Dosage: 25-100 mg qd; minimal antihypertensive effect at doses >25-50 mg/day

Half-life: 51-89 hr

Elimination: renal

Adverse effects

1. CV: orthostatic hypotension
2. Endocrine/metabolic: hyperglycemia, hypokalemia, hyperuricemia, hypercalcemia, hyponatremia, hypochloremic alkalosis, hypomagnesemia, elevated cholesterol and triglycerides
3. GI: pancreatitis, hepatitis

Drug interactions: cholestyramine and colestipol (decrease thiazide concentration; separate doses by 2 hours)

Cost: ¢/mo for 25 mg qd

Furosemide (Lasix)

Dosage forms: *tab* 20, 40, 80 mg; *oral sol* 10 mg/ml

Dosage: 20-120 mg qd or bid

Half-life: 2 hr but is prolonged in patients with renal failure and CHF

Elimination: 10% hepatic, 60% to 90% renal

Adverse effects

1. Blood: thrombocytopenia
2. CV: hypotension
3. Endocrine/metabolic: hypokalemia, alkalosis, hyperuricemia, hyperglycemia, hypocalcemia, hypomagnesemia
4. GI: pancreatitis
5. Others: photosensitivity, ototoxicity

Drug interactions: ACE inhibitors (a precipitous fall in BP may occur in some patients); corticosteroids (excessive potassium losses may occur); digoxin (hypokalemia increases risk of toxicity); indomethacin (reduction of diuretic effect)

Cost: ¢/mo for 40 mg qd

Triamterene (Dyrenium, Dyazide, Maxzide)

Dosage forms: *cap* 50, 100 mg; *combination cap* (Dyazide) triamterene 50 mg, hydrochlorothiazide 25 mg; *combination tab* (Maxzide) triamterene 37.5, 75 mg, hydrochlorothiazide 25, 50 mg

Dosage: triamterene alone, 50-100 bid; triamterene and hydrochlorothiazide, 1 or 2 capsules or tablets qd or bid

Half-life: 2-4 hr

Elimination: 80% hepatic, 10% renal

Adverse effects
1. Endocrine/metabolic: hyperkalemia
2. GI: nausea, vomiting, diarrhea
3. Renal: nephrotoxicity

Cost: ¢/mo for 1 cap qd (combination capsule)

ACE INHIBITORS

Captopril (Capoten)

Dosage forms: *tab* 12.5, 25, 37.5, 50, 100 mg
Dosage
1. Hypertension: 25-50 mg bid or tid
2. CHF: 6.25-50 mg tid (titrated depending on hypotensive response)

Half-life: 2 hr
Elimination: renal
Adverse effects
1. Blood; neutropenia
2. CV: hypotension
3. Endocrine/metabolic: hyperkalemia
4. GI: taste disorders, aphthous ulcers
5. Renal: proteinuria or nephrotic syndrome, nephrotoxicity
6. Respiratory: cough (15%)

Drug interactions: ethacrynic acid and furosemide—precipitous fall in blood pressure in some patients; NSAIDs—inhibit antihypertensive response, potassium—concurrent use may lead to hyperkalemia
Cost: $$$$/mo for 25 mg tid

Enalapril (Vasotec)

Dosage forms: *tab* 2.5, 5, 10, 20 mg
Dosage
1. Hypertension: 5-40 mg/day qd or bid
2. CHF: 2.5-20 mg/day qd or bid

Half-life: 1.3 hr
Elimination: hepatic metabolism to enalaprilat; renal excretion
Adverse effects
1. Blood; neutropenia
2. CV: hypotension
3. Endocrine/metabolic: hyperkalemia
4. GI: taste disorders, aphthous ulcers
5. Renal: proteinuria or nephrotic syndrome, nephrotoxicity
6. Respiratory: cough (15%)

Drug interactions: ethacrynic acid and furosemide—precipitous fall in blood pressure in some patients; NSAIDs—inhibit antihypertensive response, potassium—concurrent use may lead to hyperkalemia
Cost: $80/mo for 20 mg bid

Lisinopril (e.g., Zestril)

Dosage forms: *tab* 5, 10, 20, 40 mg
Dosage
1. Hypertension: 10-40 mg qd
2. CHF: 5-20 mg qd

Half-life: 12 hr
Elimination: renal
Adverse effects
1. Blood: neutropenia
2. CV: hypotension
3. Endocrine/metabolic: hyperkalemia
4. GI: taste disorders, aphthous ulcers
5. Renal: proteinuria or nephrotic syndrome, nephrotoxicity
6. Respiratory: cough (15%)

Drug interactions: ethacrynic acid and furosemide—precipitous fall in blood pressure in some patients; NSAIDs—inhibit antihypertensive response, potassium—concurrent use may lead to hyperkalemia
Cost: $$$/mo for 20 mg qd

BETA-BLOCKERS

Atenolol (Tenormin)

Dosage forms: *tab* 50, 100 mg
Dosage
1. Hypertension: 50-100 mg qd
2. Angina: 50-200 mg/day divided qd or bid

Half-life: 6-7 hr
Elimination: renal
Adverse effects
1. CNS: dizziness, confusion, insomnia, fatigue, depression
2. CV: bradycardia, intermittent claudication, orthostatic hypotension
3. Endocrine/metabolic: in patients with diabetes hypoglycemic response may be prolonged, exacerbated, or symptomatically altered; increased cholesterol
4. GU: impotence
5. Respiratory: bronchospasm
6. Other: positive ANA

Drug interactions
1. Antidiabetic agents (alters hypoglycemic response by causing hypertension and blocking tachycardia); calcium channel blocking agents (enhanced negative inotropic and chronotropic cardiac effects; nifedipine is less likely to interact); clonidine (exacerbation of hypertension with withdrawal of clonidine); NSAIDs (may alter antihypertensive or antianginal response to beta-blockers); phenothiazines (serum concentrations of both phenothiazines and beta-blockers may be increased)
2. The following drugs may increase beta-blocker concentrations: cimetidine, quinidine
3. Beta-blockers may increase serum concentrations of the following drugs: lidocaine, theophylline

Cost: $$/mo for 50 mg qd

Metoprolol (e.g., Lopressor, Toprol XL)

Dosage forms: *tab* 50, 100 mg
Dosage: angina and hypertension—50-200 mg bid

Half-life: 3-5 hr
Elimination: hepatic
Adverse effects
1. CNS: dizziness, confusion, insomnia, fatigue, depression
2. CV: bradycardia, intermittent claudication, orthostatic hypotension
3. Endocrine/metabolic: in patients with diabetes hypoglycemic response may be prolonged, exacerbated, or symptomatically altered; increased cholesterol
4. GU: impotence
5. Respiratory: bronchospasm
6. Other: positive ANA

Drug interactions
1. Antidiabetic agents (alter hypoglycemic response by causing hypertension and blocking tachycardia); calcium channel blocking agents (enhanced negative inotropic and chronotropic cardiac effects; nifedipine is less likely to interact); clonidine (exacerbation of hypertension with withdrawal of clonidine); NSAIDs (may alter antihypertensive or antianginal response to beta-blockers); phenothiazines (serum concentrations of both phenothiazines and beta-blockers may be increased)
2. The following drugs may increase beta-blocker concentrations: cimetidine, quinidine
3. Beta-blockers may increase serum concentrations of the following drugs: lidocaine, theophylline

Cost: $$$/mo for 50 mg PO bid

Propranolol (Inderal)

Dosage forms: *cap* (long-acting, LA) 60, 80, 120, 160 mg; *tab* 10, 20, 40, 60, 80 mg
Dosage
1. Angina: 10-80 mg tid or qid (LA preparations: 80-160 mg qd)
2. Arrhythmias: 10-80 mg tid or qid titrated upward (long-acting preparations not recommended for arrhythmias)
3. Essential tremor: 40-80 mg bid or tid
4. Hypertension: 40-80 mg bid or tid (LA preparations: 80-160 mg qd)
5. Migraine headache: 60-80 mg/day divided bid or tid
6. Thyrotoxicosis: dosage same as angina

Half-life: 3-4 hr (prolonged in liver disease)
Elimination: hepatic
Adverse effects
1. CNS: dizziness, confusion, insomnia, fatigue, depression
2. CV: bradycardia, intermittent claudication, orthostatic hypotension
3. Endocrine/metabolic: in patients with diabetes hypoglycemic response may be prolonged, exacerbated, or symptomatically altered; increased cholesterol
4. GU: impotence
5. Respiratory: bronchospasm
6. Other: positive ANA

Drug interactions
1. Antidiabetic agents (alters hypoglycemic response by causing hypertension and blocking tachycardia); calcium channel blocking agents

(enhanced negative inotropic and chronotropic cardiac effects; nifedipine is less likely to interact); clonidine (exacerbation of hypertension with withdrawal of clonidine); NSAIDs (may alter antihypertensive or antianginal response to beta-blockers); phenothiazines (serum concentrations of both phenothiazines and beta-blockers may be increased)

2. The following drugs may increase beta-blocker concentrations: cimetidine, quinidine
3. Beta-blockers may increase serum concentrations of the following drugs: lidocaine, theophylline

Cost: $/mo for 40 mg qid; $$/mo for 80 mg LA capsules qd

ALPHA-BETA BLOCKER

Labetalol (Normodyne, Trandate)

Dosage forms: *tab* 100, 200, 300 mg
Dosage: hypertension—100-800 mg bid
Half-life: 3.5-4.5 hr
Elimination: hepatic
Adverse effects

1. CNS: dizziness, confusion, insomnia, fatigue, depression
2. CV: bradycardia, intermittent claudication, orthostatic hypotension
3. Endocrine/metabolic: in patients with diabetes hypoglycemic response may be prolonged, exacerbated, or symptomatically altered
4. GU: impotence
5. Respiratory: bronchospasm
6. Other: positive ANA

Drug interactions

1. Antidiabetic agents (alters hypoglycemic response by causing hypertension and blocking tachycardia); calcium channel blocking agents (enhanced negative inotropic and chronotropic cardiac effects; nifedipine is less likely to interact); clonidine (exacerbation of hypertension with withdrawal of clonidine); NSAIDs (may alter antihypertensive or antianginal response to beta-blockers); phenothiazines (serum concentrations of both phenothiazines and beta-blockers may be increased)
2. The following drugs may increase beta-blocker concentrations: cimetidine, quinidine
3. Beta-blockers may increase serum concentrations of the following drugs: lidocaine, theophylline

Cost: $$$/mo for 200 mg bid

CALCIUM CHANNEL BLOCKERS

Diltiazem (Cardizem, Dilacor)

Dosage forms: *tab* 30, 60, 90, 120 mg; *cap* Cardizem SR 60, 90, 120 mg; Cardizem CD 120, 240, 300; Dilacor XR 120, 180, 240 mg
Dosage: tablets—30-90 mg tid; sustained-release capsules—60-180 mg bid; CD and XR prescribed qd
Half-life: 4-6 hr

Elimination: hepatic
Adverse effects
1. CNS: dizziness, headache
2. CV: bradycardia, AV block, peripheral edema, CHF, hypotension
3. Endocrine/metabolic: gynecomastia
4. GI: epigastric discomfort

Drug interactions: amiodarone; (addictive cardiotoxicity with bradycardia and decreased cardiac output) beta-blockers enhance effects; carbamazepine (increased anticonvulsant toxicity and/or reduced serum concentrations of calcium antagonists); cimetidine (increases serum concentrations of calcium blockers); digoxin (inconsistently increases digitalis concentration); quinidine (reduced blood concentrations of quinidine)
Cost: $$$$/mo for 60 mg tid

Nifedipine (Procardia, Adalat)

Dosage forms: *cap* 10, 20 mg; *sustained-release tab* 30, 60, 90 mg
Dosage: 10-30 mg tid or qid; hypertensive "urgencies"—10 mg sublingually or preferably "bite and swallow"
Half-life: 3-4 hr
Elimination: hepatic
Adverse effects
1. CNS: light-headedness, headache, dizziness
2. CV: peripheral edema not associated with left ventricular dysfunction, hypotension, CHF
3. Endocrine: gynecomastia
4. GI: constipation, flatulence

Drug interactions: beta-blockers (enhanced effects); cimetidine (increased serum concentrations of calcium blockers); quinidine (reduced blood concentrations of quinidine)
Note: Sustained release preferred (safer)
Cost: $$$/mo for Adalat cc 30 mg qd

Verapamil (Calan, Isoptin)

Dosage forms: *tab* 40, 80, 120, 160 mg; *sustained-release tab* 180, 240 mg
Dosage: 40-240 mg bid or tid (max, 720 mg/day)
Half-life: 2-7 hr
Elimination: hepatic and renal
Adverse effects
1. CNS: dizziness, headache, drowsiness, fatigue
2. CV: hypotension, bradycardia, asystole, CHF, AV block
3. Endocrine/metabolic: gynecomastia
4. GI: constipation

Drug interactions: amiodarone (additive cardiotoxicity with bradycardia and decreased cardiac output); beta-blockers (enhanced effects); carbamazepine (increased anticonvulsant toxicity and/or reduced serum concentrations of calcium antagonists); cimetidine (increases serum concentrations of calcium blockers); prazocin (enhanced hypotensive effects); quinidine (reduced blood concentrations of quinidine); theophylline(inhibition of theophylline metabolism and increased plasma concentrations)
Cost: $$/mo for 120 mg bid; $$$/mo for 240 mg SR qd

CENTRAL ALPHA-ADRENERGIC AGONISTS

Clonidine (Catapres)

Dosage forms: *tab* 0.1, 0.2, 0.3 mg; *transderm sys* 0.1, 0.2, 0.3 mg released per 24 hours

Dosage

1. Oral initial dose: 0.1 mg at bedtime, recumbent
2. Maintenance: 0.1-1.0 mg bid
3. Transdermal: 0.1-0.3 mg system changed weekly

Half-life: 12-16 hr; increase to 30-40 hr with impaired renal function

Elimination: hepatic and renal

Adverse effects

1. CNS: drowsiness, dizziness, sedation, headache
2. CV: orthostatic hypotension
3. GI: dry mouth, constipation
4. GU: impotence, sexual dysfunction

Drug interactions: tricyclic antidepressants (may inhibit the antihypertensive response); beta-blockers (hypertension occurring with withdrawal of clonidine may be exacerbated by beta-blockers)

Cost: ¢/mo for 0.1 mg bid; $$/mo for transdermal system therapy releasing 0.1 mg/24 hr

Hydralazine (Apresoline)

Dosage forms: *tab* 10, 25, 50, 100 mg

Dosage: 10-100 tid

Half-life: 3-7 hr

Elimination: renal

Adverse effects

1. CNS: headache, peripheral neuritis, dizziness, tremor
2. CV: palpitations, tachycardia, angina, edema
3. GI: anorexia, nausea, vomiting, diarrhea, SLE in "slow acetylators"

Cost: ¢/mo for 25 mg tid

PERIPHERAL ALPHA-ADRENERGIC BLOCKERS

Prazosin (Minipress)

Dosage forms: *cap* 1, 2, 5 mg

Dosage: 1-5 mg bid or tid (give the first dose of each increment at bedtime to reduce syncopal episodes)

Adverse effects

1. CNS: dizziness, drowsiness, asthenia, headache
2. CV: palpitations, tachycardia, postural hypotension, syncope; first-dose syncope incidence, 1%

Drug interactions: beta-blockers (first-dose response may be enhanced); calcium channel blockers (enhanced hypotensive effects)

Cost: $$$/mo for 2 mg bid

Terazosin (Hytrin)

Dosage forms: *tab* 1, 2, 5 mg

Dosage: 1-5 mg qd

Half-life: 9-12 hr

Elimination: renal
Adverse effects
1. CNS: dizziness, drowsiness, asthenia, headache
2. CV: palpitations, tachycardia, postural hypotension, syncope; first-dose syncope incidence, 1%

Drug interactions: beta-blockers (first-dose response may be enhanced); calcium channel blockers (enhanced hypotensive effects)
Cost: $$/mo for 2 mg qd

CARDIAC DRUGS

ANTIARRHYTHMIC AGENTS

Quinidine

Dosage forms: *tab* sulfate—100, 200, 300 mg, polygalacturonate—275 mg; *sustained-release tab* sulfate—300 mg, gluconate—330 mg
Dosage
1. Sulfate: 200-600 mg qid
2. SR products usually administered bid or tid, based on patient response

Half-life: 7.2 hr
Elimination: hepatic and renal
Adverse effects
1. Blood: thrombocytopenia, hemolytic anemia, agranulocytosis
2. CNS: psychosis, dementia, depression
3. CV: ECG effects (widening of QRS complex; lengthening of QT interval; PR interval prolongation possible), hypotension, syncope, torsades de pointes
4. GI: anorexia, nausea, vomiting, diarrhea, colic, hepatotoxicity
5. Musculoskeletal: SLE
6. Ocular: blurred vision

Drug interactions: amiodarone (increases quinidine concentrations); antacids (alkalinization of urine increases quinidine concentration); barbiturates (reduced quinidine concentration); beta-blockers (increased plasma concentrations of metoprolol and timolol); calcium channel blockers (verapamil may result in quinidine toxicity; nifedipine reduces quinidine concentrations; diltiazem has no effect); cholinergic drugs (quinidine may block therapeutic effects); cimetidine (elevates quinidine plasma concentration); digoxin (increased plasma level); phenytoin (may decrease quinidine level); sodium bicarbonate (alkalinization of urine increases quinidine level)
Cost: $/mo for 200 mg qid quinidine sulfate; $$$$/mo for 300 mg tid quinidine sulfate sustained release; $$/mo for 330 mg tid quinidine gluconate

Digoxin (Lanoxin)

Dosage forms: *tab* 0.125, 0.25, 0.5 mg
Dosage: 0.125-0.5 mg/day, guided by serum level monitoring
Half-life: 1.5-1.8 days
Elimination: hepatic (14%); major elimination route is renal; therapeutic concentration—0.8-2 ng/ml; best drawn 4-8 hours after dose to allow equilibration between serum and tissue

Drug interactions: amiodarone (interferes with digoxin elimination); calcium channel blockers (verapamil increased digoxin concentrations in nearly all patients; diltiazem is inconsistent in this effect); cholestyramine (reduced serum levels of digoxin); diuretics (diuretic-induced hypokalemia and hypomagnesemia may increase risk of digitalis toxicity); metoclopramide (reduces serum digoxin levels); phenytoin (small decreases in digoxin serum levels); quinidine (increases serum digoxin levels leading to increased toxicity)

Cost: ¢/mo for 0.25 mg qd

ANTIANGINALS

1. Beta-blockers (see "Antihypertensives")
2. Calcium channel blockers (see "Antihypertensives")
3. Nitrates

Isosorbide dinitrate (Isordil)

Dosage forms: *tab* (oral) 5, 10, 20, 30, 40 mg
Dosage: 5-40 mg tid or qid (8-hour daily drug-free interval to prevent tolerance)
Half-life: 30 min
Elimination: hepatic
Adverse effects
1. CNS: headache, apprehension, restlessness, vertigo, faintness
2. CV: tachycardia, palpitations, hypotension

Cost: ¢/mo for 30 mg tid

Nitroglycerin

Dosage forms: *sublingual* 0.15, 0.3, 0.4, 0.6 mg; *transderm sys* 2.5, 5, 7.5, 10, 15 mg released each 24 hr
Dosage
1. Sublingual: 0.4 mg STAT prn for acute anginal attack; repeat q5min until relief is obtained or maximum of 3 tablets in 15 minutes; if no relief, call physician immediately
2. Topical: transdermal systems—apply daily; remove at night for 8 hours to prevent development of tolerance

Half-life: 29 min
Elimination: hepatic
Adverse effects
1. CNS: headache, apprehension, restlessness, vertigo, faintness
2. CV: tachycardia, palpitations, hypotension
3. Other: tingling sensation in oral cavity

Cost: ¢ for 100 0.4-mg sublingual tablets; $$$/mo for 10 mg released/24 hr transdermal systems

LIPID-LOWERING AGENTS

Cholestyramine (e.g., Questran)

Dosage form: *powder* 4 g resin/9 g powder
Dosage: 12-16 g in one or two doses up to 16-32 g bid mixed with 60-180 ml of preferred beverage (water, milk, fruit juice); can be mixed with soups or pulpy fruits

Elimination: excreted in the feces as an insoluble complex with bile acids (not absorbed)

Adverse effects
1. Blood: vitamin K deficiency
2. GI: abdominal discomfort, nausea, flatulence, constipation, steator-rhea

Drug interactions: acetaminophen (markedly reduced plasma concentrations); warfarin (decreased anticoagulant effect by binding anticoagulants (reduced therapeutic effect); digoxin (reduced digoxin concentration): L-thyroxine (reduced thyroid hormone concentration)

Cost: $$$/mo for 8 g bid

Gemfibrozil (Lopid)

Dosage forms: *cap* 300, 600 mg
Dosage: 300-600 mg bid 30 minutes before morning and evening meals
Half-life: 1.5 hr
Elimination: renal
Adverse effects
1. GI: abdominal pain, cholelithiasis
2. Musculoskeletal: myopathy, arthralgia

Drug interactions: warfarin (increased anticoagulant effect); lovastatin (myositis)

Cost: $72/mo for 600 mg bid

Lovastatin (Mevacor)

Dosage forms: *tab* 20, 40 mg
Dosage: 20-80 mg qd administered with food in evening
Elimination: hepatic
Adverse effects
1. GI: hepatoxicity
2. Musculoskeletal: muscle cramps, elevated CPK, myositis, rhabdomyolysis

Drug interaction: warfarin (increased anticoagulant effect)
Cost: $65/mo for 20 mg qd

Niacin

Dosage forms: *tab* 20, 25, 50, 100, 500 mg; *cap, sustained release* 125, 250, 500 mg
Dosage: begin with 200 mg qd; titration to 500-1000 mg bid or tid
Half-life: 45 min
Elimination: renal
Adverse effects
1. CNS: headache
2. CV: cutaneous flush and pruritus (alleviated by aspirin 30 minutes before each dose until tolerance develops)
3. Endocrine/metabolic: hyperglycemia
4. GI: vomiting, diarrhea, hepatotoxicity

Cost: ¢/mo for 500-mg tablets tid

UPPER RESPIRATORY DRUGS

ANTIHISTAMINES

Astemizole (Hismanal)

Dosage form: *tab* 10 mg
Dosage: 10 mg qd or qod
Half-life: 19 days, with steady-state levels at 4-8 weeks
Elimination: hepatic
Adverse effects: GI—potential increased appetite and weight gain
Cost: $$$$/mo for 10 mg qd

Brompheniramine (e.g., Dimetane)

Dosage forms: *tab* 4, 8 mg; *sustained-release tab* 8, 12 mg; *elixir* 2 mg/5 ml; *combination tab* 2, 4 mg with pseudoephedrine (60 mg), phenylpropanolamine (25 mg), or phenylephrine (10 mg); *combination tab, sustained release* 6, 12 mg with pseudoephedrine (60, 120 mg) or phenylpropanolamine (75 mg); *combination syrup per 5 ml* 2 mg brompheniramine with phenylephrine, 5 mg, phenylpropanolamine, 12.5 mg, or pseudoephedrine, 30 mg
Dosage: 4-8 mg tid or qid; 8-12 mg (sustained release) bid
Half-life: 12-35 hr
Elimination: renal
Adverse effects
  1. CNS: drowsiness, dizziness, incoordination, agitation
  2. CV: postural hypotension
  3. GI: dry mouth, nausea, constipation
  4. GU: urinary retention
  5. Ocular: blurred vision
Cost: ¢ to $ per month

Diphenhydramine (e.g., Benadryl)

Dosage forms: *cap* 25, 50 mg; *tab* 25, 50 mg; *elixir* 12.5 mg/5 ml (14% alcohol); *syrup* 12.5 mg/5 ml
Dosage: 25-50 mg tid or qid (max dose, 300 mg/day)
Half-life 4-8 hr
Elimination: hepatic and renal
Adverse effects
  1. CNS: drowsiness, dizziness, incoordination, agitation
  2. CV: postural hypotension
  3. GI: dry mouth, nausea, constipation
  4. GU: urinary retention
  5. Ocular: blurred vision
Cost: ¢/mo

Hydroxyzine (e.g., Atarax, Vistaril)

Dosage forms: *cap* 25, 50, 100 mg; *tab* 10, 25, 50, 100 mg; *susp* 25 mg/5 ml; *sol* 10 mg/5 ml
Dosage: 25-100 mg tid or qid
Half-life: 3 hr
Elimination: hepatic

Adverse effects
1. CNS: drowsiness, dizziness, incoordination, agitation
2. CV: postural hypotension
3. GI: dry mouth, nausea, constipation
4. GU: urinary retention
5. Ocular: blurred vision

Cost: ¢/mo for 25 or 50 mg tid

Terfenadine (Seldane)

Dosage form: *tab* 60 mg
Dosage: 60 mg qd or bid
Half-life: 15-22 hr
Elimination: hepatic and renal
Adverse effects: CNS—sedation and motor coordination change much less than with conventional antihistamines
Cost: $$$$/mo for 60 mg bid

Antitussives

Benzonatate (Tessalon)

Dosage form: *perles* 100 mg
Dosage: 100 mg tid or qid
Adverse effects
1. CNS: dizziness, headache, drowsiness
2. GI: numbness of mouth if capsule is chewed, nausea

Cost: $$$$/mo

Guaifenesin (Robitussin)

Dosage forms: *syrup* 100 mg/5 ml, 67 mg/5 ml; *liquid* 200 mg/5 ml; *tab* 100, 200 mg; *sustained-release tab* 600 mg; *cap* 200 mg
Dosage: 100-400 mg qid (max, 2400 mg/day)
Adverse effects
1. CNS: drowsiness
2. GI: nausea and vomiting

Cost: ¢ for 120 ml, 100 mg/5 ml syrup

TOPICAL NASAL STEROIDS

Beclomethasone (Beconase, Vancenase)

Dosage form: 42 μg/inhalation
Dosage: one inhalation each nostril qd-qid
Adverse effects: adrenal suppression with large doses; nasal stinging and dryness; epistaxis
Cost: $$$for approximately 200 sprays

Flunisolide (Nasalide)

Dosage forms: *nasal inhaler* 0.025% solution, 25 μg/metered dose
Dosage: two sprays into each nostril bid or tid
Adverse effect: adrenal suppression with large doses; nasal stinging and dryness; epistaxis
Cost: $$ for approximately 200 sprays

DECONGESTANTS

Phenylpropanolamine

Dosage forms: *time-released cap* 37.5, 50, 75 mg; *tab* 25, 50 mg
Dosage: 25-50 mg tid or qid or 75-mg sustained-release capsules bid
Half-life: 5-6 hr
Elimination: hepatic
Adverse effects
1. CNS: headache, dizziness, insomnia, restlessness
2. CV: hypertension
3. Others: nasal dryness, dry mouth
Cost: ¢/mo for 50 mg tid

Pseudoephedrine (Sudafed)

Dosage forms: *tab* 30, 60 mg; *sustained-release cap* 120 mg; *liquid* 15 mg
or 30 mg/5 ml
Dosage: tablets 30-60 mg qid; sustained-release capsule 120 mg bid
Half-life: 9-16 hr
Elimination: renal
Adverse effects
1. CNS: stimulation, insomnia, restlessness, anxiety
2. CV: hypertension
Cost: ¢/mo for 60 mg qid

TOPICAL NASAL DECONGESTANT

Oxymetazoline (Afrin)

Dosage form: *nasal spray* 0.025%, 005%
Dosage: two or three sprays or drops bid; use only for 3-5 days to avoid
rebound congestion
Adverse effects
1. Burning, stinging, sneezing, dryness of nose and mouth, rebound congestion
2. Rhinitis medicamentosa treatment: withdraw topical medication and
substitute with oral decongestants; alternatively treat symptoms with
discontinued use in one nostril, then the other when clear; or add nasal corticosteroids
Cost: ¢ per 15-ml spray

ANTIVERTIGINOUS DRUG

Meclizine

Dosage forms: *tab* 12.5, 25 mg (available in chew tab)
Dosage: 12.5-25 mg tid or qid; for motion sickness, 25-50 mg 1 hour before departure
Half-life: 6 hr
Elimination: hepatic and renal
Adverse effects
1. CNS: drowsiness, dizziness, incoordination, agitation
2. CV: postural hypotension

3. GI: dry mouth, nausea, constipation
4. GU: urinary retention
5. Ocular: blurred vision

Cost: ¢/mo for 25 mg tid

DERMATOLOGICALS

TOPICAL ANTIBIOTICS

Mupirocin (Bactroban)

Dosage forms: 2% ointment
Dosage: tid × 5 days
Cost: $ for 15 g

Neomycin

Dosage form: *cream ointment* 0.5%
Dosage: qd-tid
Cost: ¢ for 15 g

TOPICAL ANTIFUNGALS

Clotrimazole (Lotrimin)

Dosage forms: *top cream, sol, lotion* 1%; *troches* 10 mg; *vaginal tab* 100, 200, and 500 mg; *cream* 1%
Dosage: oral troches—10 mg five times daily × 14 days; topical bid; vaginal tablets—100 mg hs × 7 days, 200 mg hs × 3 days, or 500 mg × 1 day; vaginal cream—one applicatorful (5 g) hs × 7 days
Adverse effects
 1. GI: nausea, vomiting, diarrhea, hepatoxocity
 2. GU: mild vaginal or vulvar erythema or irritation, urethritis
Cost: oral—$$$$ for 70 10-mg troches; topical—$$ for 30 g 1% cream, $$ for 30 ml 1% solution; vaginal—$$ for 45 g 1% cream with applicator; $$ for 7 100-mg tablets, 3 200-mg tablets, or 1 500-mg tablet

Ketoconazole (Nizoral)

Dosage form: *cream* 2%
Dosage: qd or bid
Cost: $$ for 30 g

Miconazole (Monistat)

Dosage forms: *cream, lotion, powder* 2%; *vaginal supp* 100, 200 mg
Dosage: topical—bid; vaginal—suppositories, 100 mg hs × 7 days or 200 mg hs × 3 days; cream—one applicatorful (5 g) hs × 7 days
Cost: $ for 30 g 1% cream; $$for 45 g 1% vaginal cream with applicators; $$ for 100-mg vaginal suppositories for 7 days

Nystatin (Mycostatin)

Dosage forms: *top cream, ointment, powder* 100,000 U/g
Dosage: qd or bid until healing complete
Cost: ¢ for 30-g cream

TOPICAL ANTIVIRAL

Acyclovir (Zovirax)

Dosage form: *top ointment* 5%
Dosage: genital herpes simplex—four to six times daily for 7-14 days
Cost: $$$ for 15 g

ANTISCABIES

Lindane (Kwell)

Dosage forms: *cream, lotion, shampoo* 1%
Dosage
  1. Pediculosis capitis: massage shampoo thoroughly into hair, ensuring coverage of the entire scalp, and leave in place 4-10 minutes before rinsing and drying; repeat treatment in 7 days if lice or nits are still present; treat all household contacts; disinfect clothing and bed linens by laundering in hot water and drying at high heat for at least 20 minutes
  2. Pediculosis pubis: lather the pubic area for 4 minutes, rinse, and dry; use clean underwear, nightwear, and bed linens after treatment; disinfect clothing as above
  3. Scabies: apply lotion or cream, taking care to cover hands, feet, web spaces, and intertriginous and subungual areas; bathing before applications is not recommended (skin should be cool and dry); wash off 8 to 12 hours after application; treat all family members; one application is usually curative although many patients exhibit persistent pruritus after treatment; dispense only the amount required for a single application with one refill only; 30 to 60 ml is sufficient for the average adult

Adverse effects
  1. CNS: seizures (usually from drug misuse)
  2. Skin: irritation, rash

Cost: $ for 60-g cream; ¢ for 60-ml lotion; ¢ for 60-ml shampoo

VITAMINS AND MINERALS

Calcium carbonate (Tums, OsCal)

Dosage forms: *tab* 250, 500 mg (OsCal available with vitamin D)
Dosage: 500 mg tid or qid
Adverse effect: hypercalcemia
Cost: ¢/mo

Potassium chloride

Dosage forms: *cap, sustained release* 8, 10 mEq; *tab, sustained release* 6.7, 8, 10, 20 mEq; *sol* 5%, 10%, 15%, 20%; *powders* 15, 20, 25 mEq/packet
Dosage: 10-100 mEq/day
Adverse effects: GI—nausea, vomiting diarrhea, abdominal discomfort, ulcer
Drug interactions: amiloride, spironolactone, triamterene, and ACE inhibitors can be associated with hyperkalemia
Cost: ¢/mo for 40 mEq/day liquid; $$/mo for 40 mEq/day sustained-release tablets

Vitamin B₁ (Thiamine)

Dosage forms: *tab* 50, 100, 250, 500 mg
Dosage: 5-30 mg/day for 1 month; for alcoholics begin with 100 mg/day ×
   3 days
Cost: ¢/mo

Vitamin B₆ (Pyridoxine)

Dosage forms: *tab* 10, 25, 50, 100, 200 mg
Dosage
   1. Drug-induced neuritis (caused by isoniazid or penicillamine): preven-
      tion, 10-50 mg/day; treatment, 100-200 mg/day × 3 weeks, then 25-
      100 mg/day
   2. Sideroblastic anemia: 200-600 mg/day (discontinue if no response by
      2 months)
Cost: ¢/mo

Vitamin D₂ (Calciferol)

Dosage forms: *cap* 50,000 IU; *tab* 50,000 IU
Dosage
   1. Rickets and osteomalacia: 50,000-500,000 IU/day
   2. Hypoparathyroidism: 50,000-200,000 IU/day plus calcium supple-
      mentation
Adverse effect: hypercalcemia
Cost: ¢/mo

GASTROINTESTINAL DRUGS

ANTIDIARRHEAL

Loperamide (Imodium)

Dosage forms: *cap* 2 mg; *liq* 1 mg/5 ml
Dosage
   1. Acute diarrhea: after failure of Kaopectate or PeptoBismol, 4 mg fol-
      lowed by 2 mg after each unformed stool (max dose, 16 mg/day);
      discontinue after 48 hours if no improvement
   2. Chronic diarrhea: initially use acute dosing until symptoms are con-
      trolled; then reduce dosage to meet patient's needs
Half-life: 11-14 hr
Elimination: hepatic
Adverse effects
   1. CNS: dizziness, fatigue
   2. GI: epigastric pain, nausea, dry mouth, vomiting, cramps, anorexia
Cost: ¢ for 10 2-mg capsules

PROKINETIC

Metoclopramide (Reglan)

Dosage forms: *tab* 5, 10 mg; *syrup* 5 mg/5 ml
Dosage: 5-15 mg qid (30 minutes before meals and hs)
Half-life: 3-6 hr

Elimination: renal
Adverse effects
1. CNS: drowsiness, extrapyramidal reactions
2. GI: diarrhea

Drug interaction: digoxin (reduced digoxin levels)
Cost: $$/mo for 10 mg qid

ANTIEMETIC

Prochlorperazine (Compazine)

Dosage forms: *tab* 5, 10, 25 mg; *syrup* 5 mg/5 ml; *supp* 25 mg
Dosage
1. Oral: 5-10 mg tid or qid
2. Rectal: 25 mg bid

Half-life: 7 hr
Elimination: hepatic
Adverse effects
1. Blood: neutropenia
2. CNS: extrapyramidal reactions
3. CV: hypotension, anticholinergic effects

Drug interactions: tricyclic antidepressants (increased antidepressant serum levels); anticholinergics (increased anticholinergic effects); beta-blockers (enhanced effect of both); meperidine (may cause excessive CNS depression, hypotension, or respiratory depression)
Cost: $63 for 100 5 mg tablets

ANTI–PEPTIC ULCER DRUGS

Cimetidine (Tagamet)

Dosage forms: *tab* 200, 300, 400, 800 mg
Dosage
1. Acute therapy: 800 mg hs, 400 mg bid, or 300 mg qid with meals and hs for 4-8 weeks
2. Maintenance therapy: 400 mg hs

Half-life: 1.5-2 hr
Elimination: hepatic and renal
Adverse effects
1. Blood: rarely neutropenia
2. CNS: headache, somnolence, fatigue, dizziness, confusion
3. GI: diarrhea, cholestatic hepatitis
4. Others: impotence and loss of libido, gynecomastia

Drug interactions: warfarin (increased anticoagulant effect); theophylline, tricyclic antidepressants, benzodiazepines, beta-blockers, calcium channel blockers, carbamazepine, ethanol, flecainide, lidocaine, narcotic analgesics, phenytoin, procainamide, quinidine (serum concentration increase)
Cost: $82/mo for 800 mg hs

Ranitidine (Zantac)

Dosage forms: *tab* 150, 300 mg; *syrup* 15 mg/ml
Dosage
1. Acute therapy: 150 mg bid or 300 mg hs for 4-8 weeks

2. Maintenance therapy: 150 mg hs
Half-life: 2-3 hr
Elimination: hepatic and renal
Adverse effects
1. Blood: rarely hematologic abnormalities
2. CNS: confusion, headache
3. GI: constipation, diarrhea, hepatotoxicity, nausea, vomiting
Cost: $90/mo for 300 mg hs

Omeprazole (Prilosec)

Dosage form: *cap* 20 mg
Dosage: 20 mg qd
Half-life: 0.5-1.5 hr
Elimination: hepatic and renal
Adverse effects
1. CNS: headache, dizziness
2. GI: diarrhea, abdominal pain, nausea, constipation, mild and transient liver function test elevations
Cost: $109/mo for 20 mg qd

Sucralfate (Carafate)

Dosage form: *tab* 1 g (may be crushed or mixed in suspension to facilitate swallowing)
Dosage and administration: 1 g qid on empty stomach (1 hour before meals and hs) for 4-8 weeks
Elimination: excreted unchanged in the feces
Adverse effects
1. CNS: dizziness, drowsiness
2. GI: constipation (most common), diarrhea, nausea, indigestion
Cost: $90/mo for 1 g qd

Antacids (Maalox, Mylanta, Riopan, Amphojel, Gaviscon)

Dosage forms: *tab* and *susp of variable acid-neutralizing capacity;* some also contain simethicone to bind gas
Dosage: adults—15-45 ml 1 hour and 3 hours after meals and hs; nonsystemic antacids (aluminum, magnesium, calcium) form compounds that are not absorbed to any significant extent and thus do not exert systemic effects
Adverse effects
1. Aluminum- and calcium carbonate-containing antacids: constipation
2. Magnesium-containing antacids: diarrhea
3. Sodium bicarbonate: sodium overload and metabolic alkalosis

LAXATIVES

Lactulose

Dosage form: *syrup* 10 g/15 ml
Dosage: 15-30 ml/day (max, 60 ml/day) as single daily dose, usually after breakfast; portal systemic encephalopathy—30-45 ml tid or qid adjusted every 2 to 3 days to achieve two or three soft stools per day

Absorption: poor
Elimination: in feces
Adverse effects: GI—diarrhea, gas distention, flatulence, abdominal discomfort
Cost: $$ for 240 ml

Bisacodyl suppositories (Dulcolax)

Dosage: 10-mg tablets or suppositories

Psyllium (Metamucil)

Dosage: usually 1 or 2 rounded tsp (6-7 g) qd to tid

Docusate sodium (Colace)

Dosage: 100 mg qd or bid

HEMATOLOGY

Vitamin K

Dosage forms: *tab* 5 mg; *inj* 10 mg/ml
Dosage: 5-10 mg PO, IM, or SQ
Elimination: hepatic and renal
Drug interactions: oral anticoagulants
Cost: ¢ per 10-mg injection

Warfarin (Coumadin) (Table 12-1)

Dosage forms: *tab* 1, 2, 2.5, 5, 7.5, 10 mg
Dosage: individualized based on prothrombin time (PT) and disease state
Half-life: 1.5-2.5 days
Elimination: hepatic
Drug interactions
  1. The following drugs may increase the anticoagulant effect of warfarin, possibly leading to bleeding (careful monitoring of PT is recom-

Table 12-1   Warfarin therapy

Indication	PT Ratio	INR*	Duration of Therapy
Treatment of venous thrombosis	1.3-1.5	2.0-3.0	3 mo
Treatment of pulmonary embolism	1.3-1.5	2.0-3.0	3 mo
Prevention of systemic embolism	1.3-1.5	2.0-3.0	3 mo
Acute myocardial infarction			
Atrial fibrillation	1.3-1.5	2.0-3.0	Lifetime
Mechanical prosthetic valves	1.5-2.0	3.0-4.5	Lifetime
Recurrent systemic embolism	1.5-2.0	3.0-4.5	Lifetime

INR, International normalized ratio.

mended): amiodarone, anabolic steroids, chloramphenicol, cimetidine (ranitidine or famotidine is less likely to interact), clofibrate, thyroxine, disulfiram, erythromycin, nalidixic acid, all NSAIDs, salicylates, sulfinpyrazone, sulfonamides
  2. The following drugs may decrease the anticoagulant response of warfarin (careful monitoring of PT is recommended): antithyroid drugs, barbiturates, carbamazepine, cholestyramine, colestipol, rifampin, vitamin K_1; phenytoin may initially increase warfarin's anticoagulant effect, then decrease it with chronic use

Cost: ¢/mo for 5 mg qd

Folic acid

Dosage form: *tab* 1 mg
Dosage: 1 mg qd
Elimination: hepatic
Adverse effects: irritability, nausea
Drug interaction: may decrease serum phenytoin
Cost: ¢/mo for 1 mg qd

Ferrous sulfate (Feosol), ferrous gluconate (Fergon)

Dosage forms: *tab* 200, 325 mg as the various salts
Dosage: 325 mg bid or tid
Adverse effects: GI—nausea, bloating, constipation or diarrhea, anorexia, stools may darken in color
Drug interactions: antacids (GI absorption of iron is decreased)
Cost: ¢ per milligram; 325-mg tablets ferrous sulfate

Vitamin B₁₂

Dosage forms: *tab* 1 mg; *inj* 1 mg/ml
Dosage: pernicious anemia—1 mg IM qod × 4 weeks, then 1 mg IM monthly (oral B_{12} is indicated only to correct a nutritional deficiency of B_{12} intake)
Elimination: renal
Cost: ¢/mo

ENDOCRINE AND METABOLISM

STEROID HORMONES

Glucocorticoids (Table 12-2)

Dexamethasone (Decadron)

Dosage forms: *tab* 0.5, 1, 2, 4, 6 mg
Dosage: variable
Half-life: 200 min
Elimination: hepatic metabolism with renal excretion
Adverse effects
  1. Dermatologic: ecchymoses, acneiform eruptions, striae, thinning of skin, bruising, poor wound healing
  2. Endocrine: hypercorticism, amenorrhea, hypothalamic-pituitary-adrenal axis suppression

Table 12-2   Glucocorticoids

Drug	Equivalent Glucocorticoid Activity (mg)	Mineralocorticoid Activity (mg)
Hydrocortisone	20.00	1.00
Prednisone	5.00	0.80
Dexamethasone	0.75	0.00

    3. Fluid and electrolyte: sodium retention, edema, hypokalemia, alkalo-
       sis, hypertension
    4. GI: increased risk of bleeding
    5. Immune deficiency: increased susceptibility to infections
    6. Musculoskeletal: muscle wasting, muscle pain, osteoporosis, aseptic
       necrosis
    7. Ophthalmologic: intraocular hypertension, cataracts, exophthalmos
    8. Psychologic: euphoria, depression, psychosis

Drug interactions: chlorthalidone, furosemide, thiazide diuretics (hypokalemia); antidiabetics (increased blood sugar); barbiturates, carbamazepine,
phenytoin, rifampin (reduced serum levels and corticosteroid effects); estrogens (enhanced corticosteroid effects); NSAIDs (increased incidence
and severity of GI ulceration); reduced isoniazid blood levels; salicylates
(enhanced elimination of salicylates, resulting in subtherapeutic salicylate
concentrations)

Cost: \$\$\$\$\$/mo for 4 mg PO q6h

Hydrocortisone (Cortef, Solu-Cortef)

Dosage forms: *tab* 5, 10, 20 mg; *susp* 10 mg/5 ml; *supp* 15, 25 mg; *inj*
100, 250, 500 mg

Dosage
    1. Antiinflammatory effect: 20-240 mg/day
    2. Chronic adrenocortical insufficiency: 20-30 mg/day (divided two
       thirds AM, one third PM)

Half-life: 90 min (biologic $t_{1/2}$—8-12 hr)

Elimination: metabolized by liver to inactive metabolites, which are
excreted in urine

Adverse effects
    1. Dermatologic: ecchymoses, acneiform eruptions, striae, thinning of
       skin, bruising, poor wound healing
    2. Endocrine: hypercorticism, amenorrhea, hypothalamic-pituitary-
       adrenal axis suppression
    3. Fluid and electrolyte: sodium retention, edema, hypokalemia, alkalo-
       sis, hypertension
    4. GI: increased risk of bleeding, increased susceptibility to infections
    5. Musculoskeletal: muscle wasting, muscle pain, osteoporosis, aseptic
       necrosis

6. Ophthalmologic: intraocular hypertension, cataracts, exophthalmos
7. Psychologic: euphoria, depression, psychosis

Drug interactions: chlorthalidone, furosemide, thiazide diuretics (hypokalemia); antidiabetics (increased blood sugar); barbiturates, carbamazepine, phenytoin, rifampin (reduced serum levels and corticosteroid effects); estrogens (enhanced corticosteroid effects); NSAIDs (increased incidence and severity of GI ulceration); reduced isoniazid blood levels; salicylates (enhanced elimination of salicylates, resulting in subtherapeutic salicylate concentrations)

Cost: ¢/mo for 30 mg/day; ¢ for 100-mg injection

Prednisone

Dosage forms: *tab* 1, 2.5, 5, 10, 20, 25, 50 mg: *sol* 5 mg/5 ml
Dosage
1. Oral: physiologic replacement: 5-7.5 mg qd (e.g., 5 mg in AM; 2.5 mg in PM)
2. Antiinflammatory or immunosuppression: 10-60 mg/day

Half-life: 3 hr (biologic $t_{1/2}$—18-36 hr)
Elimination: hepatic conversion to active form, prednisolone; renal excretion

Adverse effects
1. Dermatologic: ecchymoses, acneiform eruptions, striae, thinning of skin, bruising, poor wound healing
2. Endocrine: hypercorticism, amenorrhea, hypothalamic-pituitary-adrenal axis suppression
3. Fluid and electrolyte: sodium retention, edema, hypokalemia, alkalosis, hypertension
4. GI: increased risk of bleeding, increased susceptibility to infections
5. Musculoskeletal: muscle wasting, muscle pain, osteoporosis, aseptic necrosis
6. Ophthalmologic: intraocular hypertension, cataracts, exophthalmos
7. Psychologic: euphoria, depression, psychosis

Drug interactions: chlorthalidone, furosemide, thiazide diuretics (hypokalemia); antidiabetics (increased blood sugar); barbiturates, carbamazepine, phenytoin, rifampin (reduced serum levels and corticosteroid effects); estrogens (enhanced corticosteroid effects); NSAIDs (increased incidence and severity of GI ulceration); reduced isoniazid blood levels; salicylates (enhanced elimination of salicylates, resulting in subtherapeutic salicylate concentrations)

Cost: ¢/mo

Mineralocorticoid

Fludrocortisone (Florinef)

Dosage form: *tab* 0.1 mg
Dosage: 0.1-0.2 mg qd
Half-life: 35 min
Adverse effects: headache, edema, hypertension, hypokalemia, hypernatremia, adrenal suppression, alkalosis
Cost: $/mo

Sex hormones

Conjugated estrogens (Premarin)

Dosage forms: *tab* 0.3, 0.625, 0.9, 1.25, 2.5 mg
Dosage: menopausal symptoms, osteoporosis prevention—0.3-1.25 mg cyclically qd
Elimination: hepatic metabolism followed by renal excretion
Adverse effects
1. CNS: mental depression, dizziness, changes in libido, chorea, headache
2. CV: increased BP, thromboembolic disorders, edema
3. Endocrine/metabolic: breast tenderness and enlargement; decreased glucose tolerance, increased serum triglyceride concentrations, hypercalcemia, folic acid deficiency
4. GI: nausea, vomiting, abdominal cramps, bloating, diarrhea, cholestatic jaundice, hepatic adenomas
5. GYN: breakthrough bleeding, spotting, changes in menstrual flow, amenorrhea, cystitis, candidal vaginitis, endometrial carcinoma
6. Ocular: keratoconus, intolerance to contact lenses
7. Renal: fluid retention
8. Skin: chloasma, erythema multiforme, erythema nodosum

Drug interactions: anticonvulsants, barbiturates, carbamazepine, phenytoin, primidone, rifampin, and smoking (may reduce the effect of estrogens); corticosteroids (estrogens may enhance the effect of corticosteroids)
Cost: ¢/mo for 0.625-mg tablets qd

Estradiol transdermal system (Estraderm)

Dosage forms: *top* release rate, 0.05, 0.1 mg/24 hr
Dosage: start with 0.05-mg system applied twice weekly; adjust dose prn to control symptoms; apply system on clean, dry area of the skin on the trunk of the body (not breasts); rotate application sites
Adverse effects
1. CNS: mental depression, dizziness, changes in libido, chorea, headache
2. CV: increased BP, thromboembolic disorders, edema
3. Endocrine/metabolic: breast tenderness and enlargement; decreased glucose tolerance, increased serum triglyceride concentrations, hypercalcemia, folic acid deficiency
4. GI: nausea, vomiting, abdominal cramps, bloating, diarrhea, cholestatic jaundice, hepatic adenomas
5. GYN: breakthrough bleeding, spotting, changes in menstrual flow, amenorrhea, cystitis, candidal vaginitis, endometrial carcinoma
6. Ocular: keratoconus, intolerance to contact lenses
7. Renal: fluid retention
8. Skin: chloasma, erythema multiforme, erythema nodosum; also irritation at application site

Drug interactions: anticonvulsants, barbiturates, carbamazepine, phenytoin, primidone, rifampin, and smoking (may reduce the effect of estrogens); corticosteroids (estrogens may enhance the effect of corticosteroids)
Cost: $$/mo for 0.1 mg/24 hr

Finasteride (Proscar)

Dosage form: *tab* 5 mg

Dosage: 5 mg qd
Half-life: 6 hr
Elimination: renal and hepatic
Adverse effects
1. Sexual: decreased libido, impotence, decreased ejaculatory volume
2. Skin: rash
3. Gynecomastia
4. Not to be used if the female sexual partner might be or become pregnant; pregnant women should not handle broken tablets

Drug interactions: none of clinical significance. NOTE: finasteride reduces PSA levels by approximately 50%
Cost: $59/mo

Vaginal estrogens (Premarin cream)

Dosage form: 0.625 mg/g
Dosage: topical, vaginally—2-4 g qd × 2 weeks; then taper gradually and maintain with 1 g one to three times per week
Cost: $$ for 42.5-g tube

Medroxyprogesterone (Provera)

Dosage forms: *tab* 2.5, 5, 10 mg
Dosage
1. Secondary amenorrhea: 5-10 mg qd × 5-10 days
2. Abnormal uterine bleeding caused by hormonal imbalance in the absence of organic pathology: 5-10 mg qd × 5-10 days
3. Estrogen replacement therapy (prevention of endometrial hyperplasia): 10 mg qd, days 16-25 of menstrual cycle

Elimination: hepatic
Adverse effects
1. Blood: thromboembolic phenomena
2. CNS: depression
3. CV: edema
4. Endocrine/metabolic: breakthrough vaginal spotting and bleeding, changes in menstrual flow, amenorrhea, breast changes, masculinization, weight gain, glucose intolerance
5. GI: cholestatic jaundice
6. Skin: rash, acne, melasma, alopecia

Cost: ¢ for 10 mg qd × 10 days

Drugs for diabetes

INSULIN (Iletin, Humulin, Novolin) (Table 12-3)
Dosage forms: *SQ inj*—short acting, regular; intermediate acting, NPH
Dosage: must be adjusted in response to blood glucose levels

Table 12-3   Pharmacology of insulin

	Onset (hr)	Peak (hr)	Duration (hr)
Regular	½-1	2-4	5-7
NPH	1-2	6-14	24+

Adverse effects: hypoglycemia, lipoatrophy
Drug interactions: beta-blockers (alter the response to hypoglycemia by prolonging the recovery of normoglycemia and blocking tachycardia); ethanol (excessive ethanol intake may lead to altered glycemic control, most commonly hypoglycemia)
Cost: $$ per 1000 U

ORAL HYPOGLYCEMIC AGENTS

Acarbose (Precose)

Dosage form: *tab* 50, 100 mg
Dosage: 50 mg tid with first bite of each meal for people ≤60-kg weight; 100 mg tid for people >60-kg weight
Pharmacology: the drug is active only within the intestine (interferes with the digestion of complex and 2-ring carbohydrates) but some is absorbed
Elimination: renal (what is absorbed)
Adverse effects
  1. GI: abdominal pain (21%), flatulence (77%), diarrhea (33%); all diminish after 8 weeks of drug use
  2. Hepatic: transaminitis
  3. NOTE: acarbose does not cause hypoglycemia but a patient on acarbose who becomes hypoglycemic from another cause must be treated with glucagon or glucose and *not* sucrose (cane sugar)
Cost: $$$$$/mo

Metformin (Glucophage)

Dosage form: *tab* 500, 850 mg
Dosage: 500 mg bid to 850 mg tid
Half-life: 18 hr
Elimination: renal
Adverse effects
  1. GI: nausea, vomiting, anorexia, diarrhea, flatulence, metallic taste
  2. Hematologic: low vitamin B_{12} levels
  3. Lactic acidosis
Contraindications: renal failure with creatinine >1.5 mg/dl; hepatic dysfunction; alcohol use; any metabolic acidosis; hypoxia
Drug interactions: iodinated contrast materials; nifedipine and furosemide increase metformin levels
Cost: $$$/mo for 500 mg bid; $71/mo for 850 mg tid

Glipizide (Glucotrol)

Dosage forms: *tab* 5, 10 mg
Dosage: 5-20 mg qd or bid (before breakfast to achieve the greatest reduction in postprandial hyperglycemia); adjust by 2.5- to 5-mg increments; several days should elapse between titration steps (max recommended total daily dose, 40 mg)
Half-life: 2-4 hr
Elimination: hepatic and renal
Adverse effects
  1. Blood: dyscrasias

2. CNS: weakness, fatigue, lethargy, dizziness, vertigo, malaise, headache
3. Endocrine/metabolic: hypoglycemia
4. GI: nausea, vomiting, anorexia, intestinal gas, diarrhea, constipation, cramps, cholestatic jaundice, and alterations in liver function test results
5. Skin: photosensitivity reactions

Drug interactions: decreased hypoglycemic effects with beta-blockers, corticosteroids, thyroxine, ethanol, rifampin, sympathomimetics, thiazide diuretics; increased hypoglycemic effects with warfarin, aspirin

Cost: $$/mo for 10 mg qd

Glyburide (Diabeta, Micronase)

Dosage forms: *tab* 1.25, 2.5, 5 mg
Dosage
1. Initial: 2.5-5 mg qd (before breakfast)
2. Maintenance: 1.25-20 mg qd; give as a single dose or in divided doses (doses >10 mg should be divided); increase in 2.5-mg increments at weekly intervals (max, 20 mg/day)

Half-life: 10 hr
Elimination: hepatic and renal
Adverse effects
1. Blood: dyscrasias
2. CNS: weakness, fatigue, lethargy, dizziness, vertigo, malaise, headache
3. Endocrine/metabolic: hypoglycemia
4. GI: nausea, vomiting, anorexia, intestinal gas, diarrhea, constipation, cramps, cholestatic jaundice, and alterations in liver function test results
5. Skin: photosensitivity reactions

Drug interactions: decreased hypoglycemic effects: beta-blockers, corticosteroids, thyroxine, ethanol, rifampin, sympathomimetics, thiazide diuretics; increased hypoglycemic effects with warfarin, aspirin

Cost: $$/mo for 5 mg qd

DRUGS FOR OSTEOPOROSIS AND PAGET'S DISEASE OF BONE

Alendronate (Fosamax)

Dosage form: *tab* 10 mg
Dosage: 10 mg qd to be taken fasting in the morning with water; patient must remain upright and not eat or drink anything for 30 minutes
Half-life: 10 yr
Elimination: only 0.7% of an oral dose is absorbed and all of that is distributed to bone; alendronate is not metabolized
Adverse effects
1. GI: esophageal irritation/ulcer, heartburn, dyspepsia, constipation, diarrhea, flatulence

2. Musculoskeletal pain
3. Headache
4. Rash/urticaria

Drug interactions: none except that nothing should be taken by mouth within 30 minutes of taking alendronate

Cost: $$$$$/mo

Calcitonin (Calcimar, Cibacalcin, Miacalcin)

Dosage forms: *inj* 100, 200 IU/ml (salmon); 0.5 mg/vial (human); inhalation by metered-dose inhaler (2 ml) 200 IU (0.09 ml) per puff (approximately 22 sprays per metered-dose inhaler)

Dosage
1. Paget's disease: 0.25-0.5 mg (human) SQ two or three times weekly to qd; 50-100 IU (salmon) IM or SQ two or three times weekly to qd
2. Postmenopausal osteoporosis: 100 IU (salmon) IM or SQ qd; 1 spray/day (alternating nostrils)

Half-life: 45 min

Elimination: renal

Adverse reactions
1. GI: dyspepsia, nausea, vomiting, diarrhea, abdominal pain, hepatitis
2. Skin: rash, urticaria
3. Musculoskeletal: myalgias
4. Respiratory: rhinitis/sinusitis, cough, asthma
5. Cardiovascular: hypertension, tachycardia, flushing
6. Neurologic: headache, vertigo
7. Hematologic: anemia

Cost: SQ use—$$$ per 400 IU (salmon) and $$$$per 0.5 mg (human); inhaler use—$$$$ per month ($25 for metered-dose inhaler)

Etidronate (Didronel)

Dosage form: *tab* 200 mg

Dosage
1. Paget's disease: 400 mg qd for 6 months
2. Postmenopausal osteoporosis: intermittent cyclical therapy, 400 mg qd × 2 weeks, followed by 13 weeks without drug

Half-life: 12 days after multiple oral dosing

Elimination: renal

Adverse effects
1. Endocrine/metabolic: hyperphosphatemia
2. GI: diarrhea, abdominal discomfort, nausea, loss of taste
3. Renal: nephrotoxicity

Cost: $60/month for 400 mg qd (Paget's disease); $$$ per 15-week cycle (postmenopausal osteoporosis)

THYROID MEDICATIONS

Levothyroxine (Synthroid)

Dosage forms: *tab* 25, 50, 75, 100, 125, 150, 175, 200, 300 μg

Dosage
1. Initial, 25-50 µg qd
2. Titrate 25-50 µg/day at monthly intervals to optimal dosage determined by clinical response and laboratory studies

Half-life: 6 or 7 days

Elimination: extensive hepatic metabolism converts T_4 to T_3 (majority of activity from T_3); renal excretion

Adverse effects
1. Endocrine: iatrogenic hyperthyroidism
2. CNS: tremors, headache, nervousness, insomnia
3. CV: angina, MI
4. Others: changes in appetite, nausea, diarrhea, weight loss, menstrual irregularities, sweating, heat intolerance, fever, osteoporosis

Drug interactions: warfarin (anticoagulant effect altered by changes in thyroid status); carbamazepine (increases the elimination and may increase requirements for thyroid hormone); cholestyramine (reduced serum thyroid hormone concentrations); phenytoin (may increase thyroid replacement dosage requirements)

Cost: ¢/mo

NEUROLOGY

INCONTINENCE DRUGS

Oxybutynin (Ditropan)

Dosage form: *tab* 5 mg
Dosage: oral—5 mg bid to qid
Half-life: 1-2 hr
Elimination: hepatic
Adverse effects
1. CNS: somnolence
2. CV: arrhythmias
3. GI: dry mouth, constipation
4. GU: urinary retention or hesitancy, impotence
5. Ocular: blurred vision

Cost: $$$/mo for 5 mg tid

Bethanecol (Urecholine)

Dosage forms: *tab* 5, 10, 25, 50 mg
Dosage: 10-50 mg bid to qid
Adverse effects
1. CNS: headache
2. CV: hypotension
3. GI: abdominal cramps, diarrhea

Cost: ¢/mo for 10 mg qid

Phenytoin (Dilantin)

Dosage forms: *extended-release cap* (Dilantin) 100 mg (qd dosing); *susp* 125 mg/5 ml; *generic cap* 100 mg (tid dosing)

Dosage: 300-400 mg/day divided qd or tid; monitor serum levels
Half-life: range 7-42+ hr (average, 22 hr)
Elimination: hepatic (nonlinear kinetics can cause substantial increases in
serum levels from small increases in dosage)
Adverse effects
1. Blood: various dyscrasias, lymphadenopathy
2. CNS: nystagmus, vertigo, mental changes, dysarthria, lethargy, peripheral neuropathy
3. CV: hypotension and arrhythmias, hypocalcemia
4. GI: nausea, vomiting, constipation, gingival hyperplasia; hepatotoxicity (25% to 30% of patients develop elevated liver function tests
   results without any other symptoms); lymphadenopathy; interference
   with vitamin D and folate metabolism
Drug interactions
1. The following drugs may increase serum phenytoin concentrations: cimetidine, isoniazid, sulfonamides, trimethoprim, valproic
   acid
2. The following drugs may decrease serum phenytoin concentrations:
   diatoxide, chronic ethanol abuse, folic acid, rifampin
3. Phenytoin may decrease the pharmacologic effects of the following
   drugs: oral contraceptives, corticosteroids, digoxin, doxycycline,
   levodopa, quinidine, theophylline, thyroid hormones, warfarin
Cost: $/mo for 300 mg qd

Valproic acid (Depakene; divalproex [Depakotel])

Dosage forms: *cap* 250 mg (valproic acid); *enteric-coated tab* 125, 250,
500 mg (divalproex)
Dosage: 250 mg bid, increased by 250 mg/day at weekly intervals, guided
by serum levels
Half-life: 5-20 hr
Elimination: hepatic
Adverse effects
1. Blood: thrombocytopenia
2. CNS: sedation, headache, ataxia
3. GI: abdominal cramps, hepatotoxicity
Drug interactions: barbiturates and primidone (increased serum concentrations; phenytoin (increased or decreased phenytoin levels)
Cost: $$$$/mo for 250 mg tid (capsules)

MUSCLE RELAXANT

Carisoprodol (Soma)

Dosage form: *tab* 350 mg (also in combination with aspirin and codeine)
Dosage: 350 mg tid or qid
Half-life: 8 hr
Elimination: hepatic and renal
Adverse effects: drowsiness, dizziness, headache, nausea, vomiting, head-
ache
Cost: ¢ for 350 mg tid × 10 days

ANTIPARKINSONIAN DRUGS

Benztropine (Cogentin)

Dosage forms: *tab* 0.5, 1, 2 mg
Dosage: 0.5-2 mg qd or bid
Adverse effects
1. CNS: confusion, drowsiness, nervousness, hallucinations
2. CV: tachycardia, hypotension
3. GI: constipation, dry mouth
4. GU: urinary retention
5. Ocular: blurred vision

Drug interactions: amantadine (potentiates CNS side effects); digoxin (increased serum concentration); phenothiazines (excessive anticholinergic effects)

Cost: ¢ per month for 1 mg bid

Trihexyphenidyl (Artane)

Dosage forms: *tab* 2, 5 mg; *elixir* 2 mg/5 ml
Dosage: 2-5 mg qd to tid
Half-life: 3-4 hr
Adverse effects
1. CNS: confusion, drowsiness, nervousness, hallucinations
2. CV: tachycardia, hypotension
3. GI: constipation, dry mouth
4. GU: urinary retention
5. Ocular: blurred vision

Drug interactions: amantadine (potentiates CNS side effects); digoxin (increased serum concentration); phenothiazines (excessive anticholinergic effects)

Cost: ¢/month for 2 mg tid

Amantadine (Symmetrel) (see "Antivirals")

Bromocriptine (Parlodel)

Dosage forms: *tab* 2.5 mg; *cap* 5 mg
Dosage
1. Acromegaly: 1.25-2.5 mg qd or bid × 3 days, then increase by 1.25-2.5 mg weekly as tolerated; dosage range—20-30 mg/day divided bid or tid (max dose, 100 mg/day)
2. Hyperprolactinemic states: same but only up to 15 mg/day
3. Parkinsonism: 1.25 mg bid initially; increase by 2.5 mg q14d prn; careful titration and dosage individualization necessary (max, 100 mg/day)

Half-life: 6-8 hr
Elimination: hepatic
Adverse effects: headache, dizziness, fatigue, hypotension, nausea, constipation, dry mouth
Cost: $52 per month for 2.5 mg bid

Carbidopa/levodopa (Sinemet)

Dosage forms: *tab* carbidopa (mg)/levodopa (mg)—10/100, 25/100, 25/250

Dosage: 10 mg/100 mg tid, increasing by 1 tablet qd or qod (max, 8 tablets/day); or 25 mg/100 mg tablet tid, increasing by 1 tablet qd or qod (max, 6 tablets/day); if a higher dosage is needed, 25 mg/250 mg tid or qid, increasing by 0.5-1 tablet qd or qod (max, 6 tablets/day)

Half-life: levodopa, 2 hr when given with carbidopa

Elimination: 95% of levodopa is decarboxylated to dopamine peripherally (carbidopa inhibits this); metabolites and unchanged drugs are then excreted in the urine

Adverse effects: dyskinesias, bradykinesia and on-off phenomenon, depression, agitation, anxiety, hallucinations, orthostatic hypotension, nausea, vomiting, anorexia, elevation in liver function test results

Drug interaction: phenytoin (may inhibit effect of carbidopa/levodopa)

Cost: $$$$$/mo for 25/100 tid

Selegiline (Eldepryl)

Dosage form: *tab* 5 mg

Dosage: 5-10 mg bid at breakfast and lunch

Half-life: parent compound, 10 min (metabolites, 2-20 hr)

Elimination: metabolized in the liver to desmethyldeprenyl, amphetamine, and methamphetamine

Adverse effects

1. CNS: confusion, dyskinesias, sleep disturbances
2. CV: hypotension
3. GI: nausea, anorexia

Cost: $68/mo for 5 mg bid

PSYCHOTROPIC DRUGS

BENZODIAZEPINES

Alprazolam (Xanax)

Dosage forms: *tab* 0.25, 0.5, 1 mg

Dosage: 0.25-1 mg tid

Half-life: 12-15 hr

Elimination: renal

Adverse effects: depression, drowsiness, dizziness, headache, confusion, dependency

Drug interactions: cimetidine (increased bendiazepine level, confusion); alcohol (increased CNS depressant effect); levodopa (exacerbates parkinsonism symptoms)

Cost: $$$$/mo for 0.5 mg tid

Chlordiazepoxide (Librium)

Dosage forms: *cap* 5, 10, 25 mg; *tab* 5, 10, 25 mg

Dosage: 5-25 mg tid or qid

Half-life: 24-48 hr

Elimination: renal

Adverse effects: depression, drowsiness, dizziness, headache, confusion, dependency
Drug interactions: cimetidine (increased bendiazepine level, confusion); alcohol (increased CNS depressant effect); levodopa (exacerbates parkinsonism symptoms)
Cost: ¢/mo

Temazepam (Restoril)

Dosage forms: *cap* 15, 30 mg
Dosage: 15-30 mg hs prn (used mostly as a hypnotic)
Half-life: 16 hr in women, 12 hr in men; metabolites, 2 hr
Elimination: renal
Adverse effects: depression, drowsiness, dizziness, headache, confusion, dependency
Drug interactions: cimetidine (increased benzodiazepine level, confusion); alcohol (increased CNS depressant effect); levodopa (exacerbates parkinsonism symptoms)
Cost: $$/mo

Clonazepam (Klonopin)

Dosage forms: *tab* 0.5, 1, 2 mg
Dosage: 1-10 mg qd or bid
Half-life: 18-50 hr
Elimination: hepatic
Adverse effects: depression, drowsiness, dizziness, headache, confusion, dependency
Drug interactions: cimetidine (increased benzodiazepine level, confusion); alcohol (increased CNS depressant effect), levodopa (exacerbates parkinsonism symptoms)
Cost: $$$ per month for 1 mg bid

Diazepam (Valium)

Dosage forms: *tab* 2, 5, 10 mg
Dosage: 2-10 mg bid to qid
Half-life: 20-50 hr (metabolites, up to 200 hr)
Elimination: extensive hepatic metabolism to active metabolites, which are then excreted in the urine as the glucuronic acid forms
Adverse effects: depression, drowsiness, dizziness, headache, confusion, dependency
Drug interactions: cimetidine (increased benzodiazepine level, confusion); alcohol (increased CNS depressant effect); levodopa (exacerbates parkinsonism symptoms)
Cost: ¢/mo for 5 mg tid

Lorazepam (Ativan)

Dosage forms: *tab* 0.5, 1, 2 mg
Dosage: 1-3 mg bid or tid
Half-life: 10-20 hr
Elimination: hepatic and renal

Adverse effects: depression, drowsiness, dizziness, headache, confusion, dependency

Drug interactions: cimetidine (increased benzodiazepine level, confusion); alcohol (increased CNS depressant effect); levodopa (exacerbates parkinsonism symptoms)

Cost: $/mo for 1 mg bid

ANTIDEPRESSANTS

Amitriptyline (Elavil)

Dosage forms: *tab* 10, 25, 50, 75, 100, 150 mg

Dosage
1. Initial: 25-50 mg qd in late afternoon or qhs; increase 25-50 mg q1-7d prn
2. Maintenance: 100-300 mg qhs

Half-life: 10-50 hr

Elimination: hepatic and renal

Adverse effects
1. CNS: sedation, confusion, agitation, psychosis, tremor, incoordination
2. CV: orthostatic hypotension, tachycardia
3. Endocrine: weight changes, gynecomastia
4. GI: dry mouth, constipation
5. GU: impotence, sexual dysfunction, urinary retention
6. Ocular: blurred vision

Drug interactions: barbiturates (decreased serum levels of both); clonidine (decreased effect); cimetidine (increased level of amitriptyline); phenylephrine (increased pressor effect)

Cost: ¢/mo

Desipramine (Norpramin, Pertofrane)

Dosage: *cap* 25, 50 mg; *tab* 10, 25, 50, 75, 100, 150 mg

Dosage
1. Initial: 50 mg qhs
2. Maintenance: 100-200 mg qd

Half-life: 7-60 hr

Elimination: hepatic and renal

Adverse effects
1. CNS: sedation, confusion, agitation, psychosis, tremor, incoordination
2. CV: orthostatic hypotension, tachycardia
3. Endocrine: weight changes, gynecomastia
4. GI: dry mouth, constipation
5. GU: impotence, sexual dysfunction, urinary retention
6. Ocular: blurred vision

Drug interactions: barbiturates (decreased serum levels of both); clonidine (decreased effect); cimetidine (increased level of desipramine); phenylephrine (increased pressor effect)

Cost: $$$/mo

Fluoxetine (Prozac)

Dosage forms: *cap* 10, 20 mg

Dosage: 10-40 mg qd
Half-life: fluoxetine, 2-3 days; norfluoxetine, 7-9 days
Elimination: hepatic and renal
Adverse effects
   1. Blood: anemia
   2. CNS: headache, nervousness, insomnia, agitation, hypomania, palpitations
   3. Endocrine: weight loss
   4. GI: nausea, diarrhea, dry mouth, anorexia
   5. GU: sexual dysfunction
   6. Others: various aches, muscle twitching, nasal congestion
Cost: $$$$/mo for 20 mg qd

Imipramine (Tofranil)

Dosage forms: *tab* 10, 25, 50 mg; *cap* 75, 100, 125, 150 mg
Dosage
   1. Initial: 50 mg qhs; increase gradually
   2. Maintenance: 150-300 mg qhs
Half-life: 8-16 hr
Elimination: hepatic and renal
Adverse effects
   1. CNS: sedation, confusion, agitation, psychosis, tremor, incoordination
   2. CV: orthostatic hypotension, tachycardia
   3. Endocrine: weight changes, gynecomastia
   4. GI: dry mouth, constipation
   5. GU: impotence, sexual dysfunction, urinary retention
   6. Ocular: blurred vision
Drug interactions: barbiturates (decreased serum levels of both); clonidine (decreased effect); cimetidine (increased level of imipramine); phenylephrine (increased pressor effect)
Cost: ¢/mo

Trazodone (Desyrel)

Dosage forms: *tab* 50, 100, 150 mg
Dosage: initial—150 mg qhs; increase by 50 mg every 3-4 days (max dose [outpatients], 400 mg/day)
Half-life: 5-9 hr
Elimination: hepatic and renal
Adverse effects
   1. Blood: dyscrasias
   2. CNS: sedation, dizziness
   3. CV: hypotension, tachycardia
   4. GI: nausea, dry mouth, constipation
   5. GU: priapism, impotence
   6. Musculoskeletal: twitches
Cost: $/mo for 150 mg qd

Lithium carbonate

Dosage forms: *cap* 150, 300, 600 mg
Dosage: 300-1800 mg bid

Half-life: 14-24 hr
Elimination: renal
Adverse effects
1. Blood: transient leukocytosis
2. CNS: lethargy, confusion
3. CV: hypotension
4. Endocrine: hypothyroidism, nephrogenic diabetes insipidus
5. GI: anorexia, dry mouth

Drug interactions: calcium channel blockers (decrease calcium transport into cells, neurotoxicity); carbamazepine (possible neurotoxicity); haloperidol (possible neurotoxicity, extrapyramidal symptoms); indomethacin, piroxicam (reduce lithium excretion, increase lithium concentration); phenothiazines (lithium-induced reductions in plasma chlorpromazine); potassium iodide (lithium and iodide may have synergistic hypothyroid activity); theophylline (enhances renal excretion of lithium; reduced plasma level); thiazide diuretics (reduce lithium clearance)
Cost: $/mo

NEUROLEPTICS (ANTIPSYCHOTICS)

Chlorpromazine (Thorazine)

Dosage forms: *tab* 10, 25, 50, 100, 200 mg
Dosage: 25-200 mg bid
Half-life: 10-20 hr
Elimination: metabolized in liver; 50% excreted through kidney, 50% through enterohepatic circulation
Adverse effects
1. Blood: agranulocytosis
2. CNS: depression, headache, tremor
3. Extrapyramidal: dystonic reactions, akathisia, tardive dyskinesia, neuroleptic malignant syndrome
4. CV: hypotension, tachycardia
5. Endocrine: galactorrhea, menstrual irregularities, SIADH
6. GI: dry mouth, constipation
7. GU: sexual dysfunction, urinary retention
8. Ocular: blurred vision

Drug interactions: tricyclic antidepressants (increased serum levels of both drugs); levodopa (inhibits antiparkinsonian effect); lithium (may lower concentration of both drugs); narcotic analgesics (hypotension and extreme CNS depression)
Cost: ¢/mo

Haloperidol (Haldol)

Dosage forms: *tab* 0.5, 1, 2, 5, 10, 20 mg
Dosage: 0.5-20 mg bid
Half-life: 13-35 hr
Elimination: renal and hepatic
Adverse effects: same as chlorpromazine, but less anticholinergic, less sedating, and with more extrapyramidal side effects (pseudoparkinsonism)
Drug interactions: carbamazepine (increased metabolism of haloperidol, de-

creased antipsychotic response); lithium carbonate (severe neurotoxic and extrapyramidal side effects possible)

Cost: $$/mo for 5 mg bid

Buspirone (Buspar)

Dosage forms: *tab* 5, 10 mg
Dosage: 5-10 mg bid or tid
Half-life: 2-11 hr
Elimination: hepatic
Adverse effects
1. CNS: dizziness, drowsiness, headache, insomnia
2. GI: nausea, dry mouth

Cost: $66/mo for 10 mg tid

Risperidone (Risperdal)

Dosage forms: *tab* 1, 2, 3, 4 mg
Dosage: 0.5-3 mg bid
Half-life: 20-30 hr
Elimination: renal and hepatic
Adverse effects
1. Neurologic: neuroleptic malignant syndrome, tardive dyskinesia, extrapyramidal symptoms, cognitive impairment, seizure, headache
2. Cardiovascular: orthostatic hypotension, proarrhythmic effect at high dose (QT interval lengthening on ECG)
3. Endocrine: hyperprolactinemia, gynecomastia, male erectile dysfunction
4. Skin: rash, photosensitivity
5. Respiratory: rhinitis/sinusitis, cough
6. GI: constipation, dyspepsia, nausea, vomiting, abdominal pain, dry mouth, hepatic transaminitis

Drug interactions: all drugs that are metabolized through the cytochrome P 450 pathway (e.g., benzodiazepines, H_2 blockers, quinidine)
Cost: $190/10, 1-mg tablets; $316/100, 2-mg tablets; $395/100, 3-mg tablets; $526/100, 4-mg tablets

PULMONARY DRUGS

BRONCHODILATORS

Albuterol (Proventil, Ventolin)

Dosage forms: *tab* 2, 4 mg; *inhalation metered-dose inhaler (MDI) aerosol* 90 mg/metered spray (approximately 200 inhalations)
Dosage
1. Oral: 2-4 mg tid or qid; increase to maximum of 32 mg/day (8 mg qid)
2. Inhalation MDI: 2 puffs q4-6h
3. Prophylaxis of exercise-induced bronchospasm: 2 puffs 15 minutes before exercise

Adverse effects: tremor, nervousness, headache, insomnia, tachycardia, palpitations, nausea, vomiting, unusual taste
Cost: $$for one MDI unit (200 puffs)

Theophylline (Slophyllin, Theodur)

Dosage forms: *tab* or *cap* 100, 200, 300 mg
Dosage: 100-200 mg tid or qid (Slophyllin), 100-300 mg qd or bid (Theo dur)
Half-life: highly variable because of age, disease states, and conditions (e.g. in healthy, nonsmoking adults, $t_{1/2}$ 7-9 hr)
Elimination: hepatic and renal
Adverse effects
   1. CNS: seizures, nervousness, headache, insomnia
   2. CV: tachycardia, cardiac arrhythmias
   3. GI: anorexia, nausea, vomiting, diarrhea, gastroesophageal reflux
Drug interactions
   1. The following drugs may increase serum theophylline concentrations: beta-blockers, calcium channel blockers, erythromycin, quinolones
   2. The following drugs reduce serum theophylline: tobacco use, barbiturates, phenytoin, rifampin
Cost: $/mo for 200 mg tid

Ipratropium (Atrovent)

Dosage form: *inhalation (MDI)* 0.018 mg spray (approximately 200 inhalations)
Dosage: 2 puffs qid
Half-life: 2-3 hr
Elimination: hepatic metabolism, fecal excretion greater than urinary excretion
Adverse reactions
   1. CV: palpitations
   2. GI: dry mouth, bitter taste
   3. Ocular: glaucoma
Cost: $$ per MDI (approximately 200 doses)

INHALED CORTICOSTEROIDS

Beclomethasone (Beclovent, Vanceril)

Dosage form: *inhalation (MDI)* 42 μg/metered spray
Dosage: 2 puffs tid or qid
Half-life: 15 hr
Elimination: hepatic
Adverse effects: adrenal suppression with large doses; oral candidiasis
Cost: $$$ per MDI (approximately 200 inhalations)

Flunisolide (Aerobid)

Dosage form: *inhalation (MDI)* 250 μg/metered spray
Dosage: 2-4 puffs bid
Half-life: 1-2 hr
Elimination: hepatic
Cost: $$ per MDI (approximately 200 inhalations)

Suggested readings

Ellsworth AJ et al: *The family practice drug handbook,* St Louis, 1991, Mosby.
Red book, 1993, Montvale, NJ, 1993, Medical Economics Data, Inc.

Comparison Tables

13

Fred F. Ferri, MD

Table 13-1 ACE inhibitors

Agent	Preparations	Initial Dosage (PO)	Onset of Action (min)	Time of Peak Effect on BP Levels (hr)	Effective Half-life (hr)	Cost
Benazepril (Lotensin)	Tab: 5, 10, 20, 40 mg	HTN: 10 mg qd	60	1-2	10-11	$$
Captopril (Capoten)	Tab: 12.5, 25, 50, 100 mg	HTN: 25 mg bid CHF: 12.5 mg tid	15-30	1-2	2	$$$$
Enalapril (Vasotec)	Tab: 2.5, 5, 10, 20 mg Inj: 125 mg/ml	HTN: 5 mg qd CHF: 2.5 mg bid	60-120	4-8	11	$$$
Fosinopril (Monopril)	Tab: 10, 20 mg	HTN: 10 mg qd	60	2-4	12	$
Lisinopril (Prinivil, Zestril)	Tab: 5, 10, 20, 40 mg	HTN: 10 mg qd CHF: 5 mg qd	60	2-7	12	$$
Moexipril (Univasc)	Tab: 7.5, 15 mg	7.5 mg qd	120	1-2	2-9	$
Quinapril (Accupril)	Tab: 5, 10, 20, 40 mg	HTN: 10 mg qd CHF: 5 mg bid	60	1-2	3	$
Ramipril (Altace)	Cap: 1.25, 2.5, 5, 10 mg	HTN: 2.5 mg qd	60-120	2-4	13-17	$
Trandolapril (Mavik)	Tab: 1, 2, 4 mg	HTN: 1-2 mg qd	60	4-10	6-10	$

HTN, Hypertension; *CHF,* congestive heart failure; $, least expensive; $$$$, most expensive.

Table 13-2 Adrenergic antagonists

Agent	Preparations	Initial Dosage	Comments
Clonidine (Catapres)	Tab: 0.1, 0.2, 0.3 mg Transdermal therapeutic system (TTS): 1 (2.5 mg), 2 (5 mg), 3 (7.5 mg)	PO: 0.1 mg bid Patch: TTS-1, apply one every 7 days	Centrally acting alpha-blocker
Doxazosin (Cardura)	Tab: 1, 2, 4, 8 mg	1 mg qd	Selective alpha-adrenergic blocker
Guanabenz (Wytensin)	Tab: 4, 8 mg	4 mg bid	Centrally acting alpha-blocker
Guanadrel (Hylorel)	Tab: 10, 25 mg	5-10 mg bid	Peripherally acting alpha-blocker
Guanethidine (Ismelin)	Tab: 10, 25 mg	10-25 mg qd	Peripherally acting alpha-blocker
Guanfacine (Tenex)	Tab: 1, 2 mg	1 mg qd at hs	Centrally acting alpha-blocker
Labetalol (Normodyne, Trandate)	Tab: 100, 200, 300 mg Inj: 5 mg/ml	PO: 100 mg bid IV: 20 mg by slow injection over 2 min	Combined alpha- and beta-adrenergic blocker
Methyldopa (Aldomet)	Tab: 125, 250, 500 mg Susp: 250 mg/5 ml Inj: 250 mg/5 ml	PO: 250 mg bid or tid IM/IV: 125-250 mg q6h	Centrally acting alpha-blocker
Prazosin (Minipress)	Cap: 1, 2, 5 mg	1 mg hs (first dose), then 1 mg bid or tid	Alpha$_1$-adrenergic blocker
Reserpine (Serpasil)	Tab: 0.1, 0.25 mg	0.5 mg daily for 1-2 wk, then reduce dosage to 0.1-0.25 mg qd	Peripherally acting alpha-blocker
Terazosin (Hytrin)	Tab: 1, 2, 5, 10 mg	1 mg hs (first dose), then increase to 2 mg qd after 3 days	Alpha$_1$-adrenergic blocker

Table 13-3 Antidepressants

Agent	Preparations	Initial Dosage (PO)	Class	Sedating Effect	Anticholinergic Effect	Orthostatic Effect	Effect on Cardiac Function	Average Elimination Half-life (hr)
Amitriptyline (Elavil)	Tab: 10, 25, 50, 75, 100, 150 mg; Inj: 10 mg/ml	10-75 mg qhs	Tricyclic	++++	++++	++++	++++	24
Amoxapine (Asendin)	Tab: 25, 50, 100, 150 mg	25-50 mg bid or tid	Dibenzoxazepine	++	+	+++	++	10
Bupropion (Wellbutrin)	Tab: 75, 100 mg	100 mg bid	Aminoketone	+	+	+	+	14
Clomipramine* (Anafranil)	Cap: 25, 50, 75 mg	25 mg qd	Tricyclic	+++	+++	++	++	24
Desipramine (Norpramin)	Tab: 10, 25, 50, 75, 100, 150 mg	10-50 mg qd	Tricyclic	+	+	++	+	18
Doxepin (Adapin, Sinequan)	Cap: 10, 25, 50, 75, 100, 150 mg	10-25 mg tid	Tricyclic	++++	+++	+++	+++	17
Fluoxetine* (Prozac)	Cap: 10, 20 mg; Oral soln: 20 mg/5 ml	20 mg qd	Serotonin reuptake inhibitor	0	+	0	0	70

Imipramine (Tofranil)	Tab: 10, 25, 50 mg; Cap (Tofranil-PM): 75, 100, 125, 150 mg; Inj: 25 mg/2 ml	75 mg qd	Tricyclic	+++	+++	+++	++	22
Maprotiline (Ludiomil)	Tab: 25, 50, 75 mg	50-75 mg qd	Tetracyclic	++	++	+++	++	43
Nefazodone (Serzone)	Tab: 100, 150, 200, 250 mg	100 mg bid	Phenylpiperazine	+++	+	++	+	2-4
Nortriptyline (Pamelor)	Cap: 10, 25, 50, 75 mg; Liq: 10 mg/5 ml	10 mg qd	Tricyclic	+++	++	+	++	26
Paroxetine (Paxil)	Tab: 20, 30 mg	10-20 mg qd	Serotonin reuptake inhibitor	0	+	0	0	24
Protriptyline (Vivactil)	Tab: 5, 10 mg	5 mg tid	Tricyclic	+	+++	++	++	76
Sertraline (Zoloft)	Tab: 50, 100 mg	50 mg qd	Serotonin reuptake inhibitor	+	0	0	0	24
Trazodone (Desyrel)	Tab: 50, 100, 150, 300 mg	50 mg tid	Triazolopyridine	+++	+	++	+	8
Venlafaxine (Effexor)	Tab: 25, 37.5, 50, 75 mg	25 mg tid or 37.5 mg bid	Serotonin and norepinephrine reuptake inhibitor	++	++	0	0	—

0, None; +, weak; ++, mild; +++, moderate; ++++, strong.
*Indicated for obsessive-compulsive disorder.

Table 13-4 Antipsychotics

Agent	Preparations	Dosage	Class/Frequent Adverse Effects
Chlorpromazine (Thorazine)	Tab: 10, 25, 50, 100, 200 mg Cap: 30, 75, 150, 200, 300 mg Syrup: 10 mg/5 ml Inj: 25 mg/ml Supp: 25, 100 mg	Initial: 10-25 mg PO tid Acute agitation: 25 mg IM; repeat in 1 hr if necessary	Phenothiazine, aliphatic Drowsiness, anticholinergic effects, postural hypotension
Clozapine (Clozaril)	Tab: 25, 100 mg	Initial: 25 mg qd or bid	Tricyclic dibenzodiazepine Agranulocytosis
Fluphenazine (Prolixin)	Tab: 1, 2.5, 5, 10 mg Conc: 5 mg/ml Inj: 2.5 mg/ml	Initial: 0.5-1 mg tid IM: 1.25 mg	Phenothiazine, piperazine Extrapyramidal effects, akathisia, dystonia
Haloperidol (Haldol)	Tab: 0.5, 1, 2, 5, 10, 20 mg Conc: 2 mg/ml Inj: 5 mg/ml	Initial: 0.5 mg bid or tid Acute agitation: 2-5 mg IM	Butyrophenone Extrapyramidal effects, dystonia, akathisia
Lithium	Cap: 150, 300, 600 mg Tab: 150, 300 mg	300 mg tid	Thirst, fine tremor, GI irritation, mild diarrhea, leukocytosis, polyuria
Mesoridazine (Serentil)	Tab: 10, 25, 50, 100 mg Conc: 25 mg/ml Inj: 25 mg/ml	PO: psychosis, 50 mg tid initially; psychoneurosis, 10 mg tid initially IM: 25 mg, may repeat in 30-60 min	Piperidine phenothiazine Tardive dyskinesia, anticholinergic and extrapyramidal effects

Drug	Preparations	Dosage	Class / Adverse effects
		Initial: 4-8 mg tid	Phenothiazine, piperazine
Perphenazine (Trilafon)	Tab: 2, 4, 8, 16 mg Conc: 16 mg/5 ml Inj: 5 mg/ml		Extrapyramidal effects, akathisia, dystonia
Risperidone (Risperdal)	Tab: 2, 3, 4 mg	Initial: 1 mg bid on day 1, then 2 mg bid on day 2, then 3 mg bid; usual range: 4-6 mg/day, max 16 mg/day	Benzisoxazole derivative Anxiety, somnolence, extrapyramidal and anticholinergic effects, orthostatic hypotension
Thioridazine (Mellaril)	Tab: 10, 15, 25, 50, 100, 150, 200 mg Conc: 30, 100 mg/ml Susp: 25 mg/5 ml	10-100 mg tid	Phenothiazine, piperidine Drowsiness, anticholinergic effects, postural hypotension
Thiothixene (Navane)	Cap: 1, 2, 5, 10, 20 mg Conc: 5 mg/ml Inj: 2, 5 mg/ml	Initial: 2 mg tid Acute agitation: 4 mg IM	Thioxanthene Extrapyramidal effects, akathisia, dystonia, anticholinergic effects
Trifluoperazine (Stelazine)	Tab: 1, 2, 5, 10 mg Conc: 10 mg/ml	Initial: 2-5 mg bid Acute agitation: 1-2 mg IM	Phenothiazine, piperazine Extrapyramidal effects, akathisia, dystonia

Modified from Drugs for psychotic disorders, *Med Lett Drugs Ther* 31:13, 1989.

Table 13-5   Benzodiazepines

Agent	Preparations	Equivalent Dose	Dosage	Half-life (hr)	Main Indication	Cost
Alprazolam (Xanax)	Tab: 0.25, 0.5, 1 mg	0.5	0.25-0.5 mg tid	14	Anxiety	$$$$
Chlordiazepoxide (Librium)	Cap: 5, 10, 25 mg Amp: 100 mg/5 ml	10	5-25 mg qid	48-96	Anxiety	$ (generic)
Clorazepate (Tranxene)	Tab: 3.75, 7.5, 15 mg; long-acting (Tranxene SD): 11.25, 22.5 mg	7.5	Tab: 3.75-15 mg tid Tranxene SD: 11.25-22.5 qd	48-96	Anxiety	$ (generic)
Diazepam (Valium)	Tab: 2, 5, 10 mg Amp: 5 mg/ml	5	2-10 mg bid to qid	48-96	Anxiety	$ (generic)
Flurazepam (Dalmane)	Cap: 15, 30 mg	15	15-30 mg hs	48-72	Insomnia	$$ (generic)
Lorazepam (Ativan)	Tab: 0.5, 1, 2 mg Inj: 2, 4 mg/ml	1	1 mg bid or tid	10-20	Anxiety	$ (generic)
Oxazepam (Serax)	Tab: 15 mg Cap: 10, 15, 30 mg	15	10-15 mg tid or qid	8-12	Anxiety	$$ (generic)
Prazepam (Centrax)	Tab: 10 mg Cap: 5, 10, 20 mg	10	10 mg bid or tid	30-60	Anxiety	$$$$
Quazepam (Doral)	Tab: 7.5, 15 mg	7.5	7.5-15 mg hs	15-35	Insomnia	$$$$
Temazepam (Restoril)	Cap: 7.5, 15, 30 mg	15	7.5-15 mg hs	10-20	Insomnia	$$ (generic)
Triazolam (Halcion)	Tab: 0.125, 0.25 mg	0.25	0.125-0.25 mg hs	2-5	Insomnia	$$$$

$, Least expensive; $$$$, most expensive.

Table 13-6 Beta-adrenergic blocking agents

Drug	Oral Preparations	Initial Dosage	Maintenance Dosage	Cardio-selectivity	ISA	Lipid Solubility	Elimination Half-life (hr)	Primary Excretion Route
Acebutolol (Sectral)	Cap: 200, 400 qd	400 mg qd	200-800 mg	Yes	Yes	+	6-12	Renal
Atenolol (Tenormin)	Tab: 50, 100 mg	50 mg qd	50-100 mg qd	Yes	No	+	6-9	Renal
Betaxolol (Kerlone)	Tab: 10, 20 mg	10 mg qd	20 mg qd	Yes	No	++	16	Hepatic
Bisoprolol (Zebeta)	Tab: 5, 10 mg	2.5 mg qd	5 mg qd	Yes	No	+	9-12	Renal
Carteolol (Cartrol)	Tab: 2.5, 5 mg	2.5 mg qd	2.5-5 mg qd	No	Yes	+	6-12	Renal
Esmolol (Brevibloc)	No oral preparation	500 μg/kg/min over 1 min	—	Yes	No	+	0.15	RBC esterase metabolism
Labetalol (Normodyne, Trandate)	Tab: 100, 200, 300 mg	100 mg bid	200-400 mg bid	No	No	++	3-4	Hepatic
Metoprolol (Lopressor, Toprol XL)	Tab: 50, 100, 200 mg	100 mg qd	50-200 mg/day	Yes	No	++	3-4	Hepatic
Nadolol (Corgard)	Tab: 20, 40, 80 mg	40 mg qd	40-80 mg qd	No	No	+	14-24	Renal
Penbutolol (Levatol)	Tab: 20 mg	20 mg qd	20 mg qd	No	Yes	++	5	Renal
Pindolol (Visken)	Tab: 5, 10 mg	5 mg bid	5-10 mg bid	No	Yes	++	3-4	Hepatic/renal
Propranolol (Inderal)	Tab: 10, 20, 60, 80, 90 mg	10-20 mg bid	40-320 mg bid	No	No	+++	3-4	Hepatic
Sotalol (Betapace)	Tab: 80, 160, 240 mg	80 mg bid	160-320 mg/day	—	No	+	12	Renal
Timolol (Blocadren)	Tab: 5, 10	10 mg	10-20 mg bid	No	No	+	4-5	Hepatic

+, Low; ++, medium; +++, high; *ISA*, intrinsic sympathomimetic activity.

Table 13-7 Calcium channel blockers

Agent	Oral Preparations	Initial Dosage	Myocardial Contractility	Chemical Class	AV Nodal Conduction	Cardiac Output	Peripheral Vasodilation	Safe for Concomitant Use With Beta-Blocker	Cost
Amlodipine (Norvasc)	Tab: 2.5, 5, 10 mg	HTN: 5 mg qd Angina: 5-10 mg qd	↑	Dihydropyridine	N	↑	++	++	$$$$
Diltiazem (Cardizem, Dilacor)	Tab: 30, 60, 90, 120 mg Cap, SR: 120, 180, 240, 300 mg qd	Angina: 30 mg qid HTN: 120-300 mg/day	↓	Benzothiazepine	↓	N/↑	+	+	$$ (generic) $$$$
Felodipine (Plendil)	Tab: 5, 10 mg	HTN: 5 mg qd	↑	Dihydropyridine	N	↑	++	++	$$$
Isradipine (DynaCirc)	Cap: 2.5, 5 mg	HTN: 2.5 mg bid	N	Dihydropyridine	N	↑	++	++	$$$

Nicardipine (Cardene)	Cap: 20, 30 mg Cap, SR: 30, 45 mg bid	Angina: 20 mg tid HTN: 40-120 mg/day	N	Dihydropyridine	N/↑	−	++	++	$$$
Nifedipine (Procardia, Adalat)	Cap: 10, 20 mg Tab, XR: 30, 60, 90 mg	Angina: 10 mg tid HTN: 30-90 mg/day	→	Dihydropyridine	N	↑	++	++	$$ (generic)
Nisoldipine (Sular)	Tab (ext. rel.): 10, 20, 30, 40 mg	HTN: 10-60 mg/day	N/↓	Dihydropyridine	N	↑	++	++	$$
Verapamil (Calan, Isoptin, Verelan)	Tab: 40, 80, 120 mg Caplet, SR: 120 mg Cap: 120, 180, 240 mg	Angina: 40 mg tid HTN: 120-240 mg/day	↓↓	Diphenylalkylamine	↓↓	↓↑	+	0	$ (generic) $$$

SR, XR, Extended release preparation; ↑, increase; ↓, decrease; *N*, no significant effect; 0, least; + +, most; *HTN*, hypertension; $, least expensive, $$$$, most expensive.

Table 13-8 Diuretics

Class	Agent	Preparations	Dosage (mg/day)	Site of Action
Thiazide	Chlorothiazide (Diuril)	Tab: 250, 500 mg; Susp: 250 mg/5 ml	125–500	Distal tubule
	Hydrochlorothiazide (Esidrix)	Tab: 25, 50, 100 mg	12.5–50	Distal tubule
	Methyclothiazide (Enduron)	Tab: 2.5, 5 mg	2.5–5	Distal tubule
	Quinethazone (Hydromox)	Tab: 50 mg	50–100	Distal tubule
Phthalimidine derivative	Chlorthalidone (Hygroton)	Tab: 25, 50, 100 mg	12.5–50	Distal tubule
Quinazoline	Metolazone (Diulo, Zaroxolyn, Mykrox)	Tab: 2.5, 5, 10 mg; Tab: 0.5 mg (Mykrox)	2.5–10; 0.5 (Mykrox)	Cortical diluting site and proximal convoluted tubule
Indoline	Indapamide (Lozol)	Tab: 1.25, 2.5 mg	2.5–5	Distal tubule
Loop	Bumetanide (Bumex)	Tab: 0.5, 1, 2 mg; Inj: 0.25 mg/ml	0.5–5; PO/IV/IM	Ascending limb of loop of Henle
	Ethacrynic acid (Edecrin)	Tab: 25, 50 mg	25–100	Ascending limb of loop of Henle
	Furosemide (Lasix)	Tab: 20, 40, 80 mg; Oral sol: 10 mg/ml; Inj: 10 mg/ml	20–160; PO/IV/IM	Ascending limb of loop of Henle
	Torsemide (Demadex)	Tab: 5, 10, 20, 100 mg; Inj: amp 20, 50 mg	10–20 mg PO/IV	Ascending limb of loop of Henle
Carbonic anhydrase inhibitors	Acetazolamide (Diamox)	Tab: 125, 250 mg	250 mg–1 g	Carbonic anhydrase inhibitor
	Methazolamide (Neptazane)	Tab: 25, 50 mg	100–300 mg	Carbonic anhydrase inhibitor
Potassium-sparing	Amiloride (Midamor)	Tab: 5 mg	5–10	Distal tubule
	Spironolactone (Aldactone)	Tab: 25, 50, 100 mg	25–100	Distal tubule
	Triamterene (Dyrenium)	Cap: 50, 100 mg	50–150	Distal tubule

Table 13-9 Nonsteroidal antiinflammatory drugs (NSAIDs)

Agents	Preparations	Dosage	Plasma Half-life (hr)	Chemical Class	Cost
Aspirin	Tab: 325, 500, 650, 800, 975 mg Supp: 325, 650 mg	325-650 mg q4h	9-16	Salicylate	$
Diclofenac (Voltaren, Cataflam)	Tab: 25, 50, 75 mg	50-75 mg bid	2	Phenylacetic	$$$$
Diflunisal (Dolobid)	Tab: 250, 500 mg	250-500 mg q8-12h	8-12	Salicylate	$$$
Etodolac (Lodine)	Cap: 200, 300, 400 mg	200-400 mg q6-8h	7.3	Pyranocarboxylic acid	$$$$$
Fenopren (Nalfon)	Tab: 600 mg	200-600 mg tid or qid	3	Propionic acid	$$$$
Flurbiprofen (Ansaid)	Tab: 50, 100 mg	100 mg bid or tid	5	Propionic acid	$$$$
Ibuprofen (Motrin)	Tab: 200, 300, 400, 600, 800 mg	200-800 mg tid or qid	2	Propionic acid	$ (generic)
Indomethacin (Indocin)	Cap: 25, 50, 75 mg (SR) Supp: 50 mg Susp: 25 mg/5 ml	PO: 25-50 mg tid (SR qd or bid) PR: 50 mg qd	5-6	Indoleacetic acid	$ (generic)
Ketoprofen (Orudis, Oruvail)	Cap: 25, 50, 75 mg Controlled release cap (Oru-vail): 200 mg	50-75 mg tid 200 mg qd	2 1-4	Propionic acid	$$$$$

Continued

Table 13-9 Nonsteroidal antiinflammatory drugs (NSAIDs)—cont'd

Agents	Preparations	Dosage	Plasma Half-life (hr)	Chemical Class	Cost
Ketorolac (Toradol)	Prefilled syringe: 15, 30, 60 mg Tab: 10 mg	30-60 mg IM initially followed by 15-30 mg IM q6h PO: 10 mg q6h	4-6	Propionic acid	$$$$$
Meclofenamate (Meclomen)	Cap: 50, 100 mg	50 mg q4-6h	4	Fenamic acid	$$$$
Nabumetone (Relafen)	Tab: 500, 750 mg	1000 mg as single dose qd	20-30	Naphthylkanone	$$$$
Naproxen (Naprosyn, Anaprox)	Tab: 250, 375, 500 mg Susp: 125 mg/5 ml Anaprox tabs: 275, 550 mg	250-500 mg bid 275-550 mg bid	12-15	Propionic acid	$$$ $$ (generic)
Oxaprosin (Daypro)	Tab: 600 mg	1200 mg as single dose qd	42-50	Propionic acid	$$$$$
Piroxicam (Feldene)	10, 20 mg	20 mg qd	40	Oxicam	$$$$
Salsalate (Disalcid)	Tab: 500, 750 mg Cap: 500 mg	1500 mg bid	3-16	Salicylate	$$$$
Sulindac (Clinoril)	Tab: 150, 200 mg	150-200 mg bid	16	Indoleacetic acid	$$ (generic)
Tolmetin (Tolectin)	Tab: 200, 400, 600 mg	200-600 mg tid	2	Indoleacetic acid	$$$$$

$, Least expensive; $$$$$, most expensive.

Table 13-10 Sulfonylureas

Drug	Starting Dose (mg)	Maximum Daily Dose	Frequency	Duration of Action (hr)	Half-life $t_{1/2}$ (hr)	Excretion	Cost
First generation							
Tolbutamide (Orinase)	500	3 g	qd, bid	6-12	6	Urine	$ (generic)
Tolazamide (Tolinase)	100	1.0 g	qd, bid	12-14	7	Urine	$ (generic)
Chlorpropamide (Diabinese)	100	750 mg	qd	≥36	35	Urine	$ (generic)
Second generation							
Glyburide* (DiaBeta, Micronase)	2.5	20 mg	qd, bid	Up to 24	4-10	Urine 50%; feces 50%	$$
Glipizide (Glucotrol)	5.0	40 mg	qd, bid	12-24	3-7	Urine 88%; feces 12%	$$$
Glyburide, micronized (Glynase Prestab)	1.5-3	12 mg	qd, bid	Up to 24	4-10	Urine 50%; feces 50%	$$$$
Glimepiride (Amaryl)	1-2 mg	8 mg	qd	>24	9	Urine and feces	$$$$

$, Least expensive; $$$$, most expensive.
*Useful in patients with renal disease because of dual excretion routes (urine and bile).

Appendices

Fred F. Ferri, MD

I

Frequently Used
Clinical Formulas

1. Calculation of creatinine clearance (CCr)

$$CCr\ (male) = \frac{(140 - age) \times wt\ (in\ kg)}{Serum\ creatinine \times 72}$$

$$CCr\ (female) = 0.85 \times CCr\ (male)$$

2. Alveolar-arterial oxygen gradient (Aa gradient)

$$Aa\ gradient = \left[(713)\ (Fio_2) - \left(\frac{Paco_2}{0.8} \right) \right] - Pao_2$$

Normal Aa gradient = 5-15 mm
Fio_2 = Fraction of inspired oxygen (normal = 0.21-1.0)
$Paco_2$ = Arterial carbon dioxide tension (normal = 35-45 mm Hg)
Pao_2 = Arterial partial pressure oxygen (normal = 70-100 mm Hg)
Differential diagnosis of Aa gradient:

Abnormality	15% O_2	100% O_2
Diffusion defect	Increased gradient	Correction of gradient
Ventilation/perfusion mismatch	Increased gradient	Partial or complete correction of gradient
Right-to-left shunt (intracardiac or pulmonary)	Increased gradient	Increased gradient (no correction)

3. Anion gap (AG)

$$AG = Na^+ - (Cl^- + HCO_3^-)$$

4. Fractional excretion of sodium (FE_{Na})

$$FE_{Na} = \frac{U_{Na}/P_{Na}}{U_{Cr}/P_{Cr}} \times 100$$

5. Serum osmolality (Osm)

$$Osm = 2(Na' + K') + \frac{Glucose}{18} + \frac{BUN}{2.8}$$

6. Corrected sodium in hyperglycemic patients

$$Corrected\ Na^+ = Measured\ Na^+ + 1.6 \times \frac{Glucose - 140}{100}$$

7. Water deficit in hypernatremic patients

$$Water\ deficit\ (in\ liters) = 0.6 \times body\ weight\ (kg) \times$$

$$\left(\frac{Measured\ serum\ sodium}{Normal\ serum\ sodium} - 1 \right)$$

II

Toxic and Therapeutic Serum Values of Commonly Used Drugs

Drug	Therapeutic Level	Toxic Level
Acetaminophen	5-20 μg/ml	>70 μg/ml
Amikacin	Peak: 15-30 μg/ml	Peak: >35 μg/ml
	Trough: 5-10 μg	Trough: >10 μg/ml
Amitriptyline	125-250 ng/ml	>500 ng/ml
Barbiturates		
Short acting	1-5 μg/ml	>8 μg/ml
Long acting	15-40 μg/ml	>40 μg/ml
Carbamazepine	2-10 μg/ml	>12 μg/ml
Clonazepam	15-60 ng/ml	>100 ng/ml
Diazepam	100-1500 ng/ml	>3000 mg/ml
Digitoxin	10-30 ng/ml	>35 ng/nl
Digoxin	0.9-2 ng/ml	>2 ng/ml
Ethanol	—	Fatal: >450 mg/dl
Ethosuximide	40-100 μg/ml	>150 μg/ml
Gentamicin	Peak: 5-8 μg/ml	Peak: >10 μg/ml
	Trough: 1-2 μg/ml	Trough: >2 μg/ml
Glutethimide	2-6 μg/ml	>10 μg/ml
Kanamycin	Peak: 20-30 μg/ml	Peak: >35 μg/ml
	Trough: 5-10 μg/ml	Trough: >10 μg/ml
Lidocaine	2-5 μg/ml	>6 μg/ml
Lithium	0.5-1.5 mEq/L	>1.5 mEq/L
Nortriptyline	50-150 ng/ml	>500 ng/ml
Phenobarbital	15-35 μg/ml	>60 μg/ml
Phenytoin	10-20 μg/ml	>30 μg/ml
Primidone	5-10 μg/ml	>12 μg/ml
Procainamide and NAPA	10-30 μg/ml	>30 μg/ml
Quinidine	2-5 μg/ml	>6 μg/ml
Salicylate	2-29 mg/dl	>30 μg/dl
Streptomycin	Peak: 15-20 μg/ml	Peak: >30 μg/ml
	Trough: 5 μg/ml	Trough: >5 μg/ml

Drug	Therapeutic Level	Toxic Level
Theophylline	10-20 μg/ml	>20 μg/ml
Thiocyanate (nitroprusside)	4-10 μg/ml	>10 μg/ml
Tobramycin	Peak: 5-8 μg/ml	Peak: >10 μg/ml
	Trough: 1-2 μg/ml	Trough: >2 μg/ml
Valproic acid	50-100 μg/ml	>200 μg/ml
Vancomycin	Peak: 25-40 μg/ml	Peak: >40 μg/ml
	Trough: 5-10 μg/ml	Trough: >10 μg/ml

From Ferri FF: *Practical guide to the care of the medical patient,* ed 3, St Louis, 1995, Mosby.

III

Parameters of Nutritional Assessment

Test	Degree of Malnutrition			Na/K Correlation	Reflects
	Mild	Moderate	Severe		
Ideal body weight (%)	80-90	70-80	<70	—	Total body change
Usual body weight (%)	85-95	75-85	<75	—	Total body change
Creatinine height index	—	60%-80%	<60%	0.37	Lean body mass change
Skinfold thickness (%)*	35-40	25-35	<25	0.79	Fat mass status
Midarm circumference (%)*	35-40	25-35	<25	0.68	Lean body mass change
Albumin (g/dl)	2.8-3.5	2.1-2.7	<2.1	0.67	Visceral protein status
Transferrin (mg/dl)	150-200	100-150	<100	—	Visceral protein status
Absolute lymphocyte count (thousands of cells/mm^3)	1.2-2.0	0.8-1.2	<0.8	—	Visceral protein status and immunocompetence

From Cerra FB: *Manual of critical care*, St Louis, 1987, Mosby.
*Measured against a percentile table of norms.

Determination of Caloric Needs

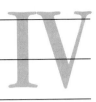

Basal energy expenditure (BEE) can be determined by the Harris-Benedict formulas*

BEE for male: 66 + (13.7 × wt [in kg]) + (5 × ht [in cm]) − (6.8 × age [in yr])

BEE for female: 655 + (9.6 × wt [in kg]) + (1.7 × ht [in cm]) − (4.7 × age [in yr])

For states other than basal, the BEE is multiplied by a correction factor
  Low stress: 1.3 × BEE
  Moderate stress: 1.5 × BEE
  Cancer: 1.6 × BEE
  Sepsis (normotensive): 1.7 × BEE
  Severe stress: 2 × BEE
  Severe burn (>40% of body surface area, normotensive patient): 2.5 × BEE

From Ferri FF: *Practical guide to the care of the medical patient,* ed 3, St Louis, 1995, Mosby.
*From Rutten P et al: Determination of optimal hyperalimentation infusion rate, *J Surg Res* 18:477, 1975.

Nomogram for Calculation of Body Surface Area

Place a straight edge from the patient's height in the left column to his weight in the right column. The point of intersection on the body surface area column indicates the body surface area (BSA). (Reproduced from Behrman RE, Vaughn VC, editors: *Nelson's textbook of pediatrics,* ed 12, Philadelphia, 1983, Saunders.)

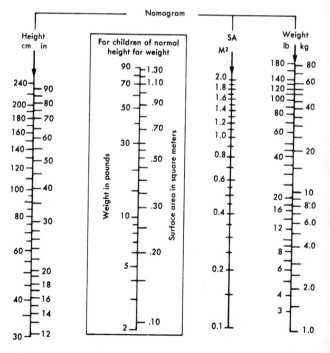

Functional
Assessment
Instruments

VI

Table VI-A Procedure for functional assessment screening in the elderly

Target Area	Assessment Procedure	Abnormal Result
Vision	Test each eye with Jaeger card while patient wears corrective lenses (if applicable).	Inability to read better than 20/40
Hearing	Whisper a short, easily answered question such as "What is your name?" in each ear while the examiner's face is out of direct view.	Inability to answer question
Arm	Proximal: "Touch the back of your head with both hands." Distal: "Pick up the spoon."	Inability to do task
Leg	Observe the patient after asking: "Rise from your chair, walk 10 feet, return, sit down."	Inability to walk to or transfer out of chair
Urinary incontinence	Ask: "Do you ever lose your urine and get wet?"	Yes
Nutrition	Weigh the patient. Measure height.	Weight is below acceptable range for height
Mental status	Instruct: "I am going to name three objects (pencil, truck, book). I will ask you to repeat their names now and then again in a few minutes from now."	Inability to recall all three objects after 1 min

Continued

Table VI-A Procedure for functional assessment screening
in the elderly—cont'd

Target Area	Assessment Procedure	Abnormal Result
Depression	Ask: "Do you often feel sad or depressed?"	Yes
ADL-IADL*	Ask: "Can you get out of bed yourself?" "Can you make your own meals?" "Can you do your own shopping?	No to any question
Home environment	Ask: "Do you have trouble with stairs inside or outside of your home?" Ask about potential hazards inside the home with bathtubs, rugs, or lighting.	Yes
Social support	Ask: "Who would be able to help you in case of illness or emergency?"	Not applicable

From Lachs MS et al: *Ann Intern Med* 112:699, 1990.
*Activities of daily living–instrumental activities of daily living.

Table VI-B Instruments used to assess physical function*

Instrument	Function Assessed	Range of Sensitivity	Administration	Strengths	Weaknesses
ADL Scale	Basic self-care	Limited to basic activities; not sensitive to small changes	By patient or interviewer; based on judgments	Simple assessment of basic skills; useful in rehabilitational setting	Limited range of activities assessed; ratings subjective
Barthel Index	Self-care and ambulation	Slightly broader range than ADL Scale; includes stair climbing, wheelchair use	By interviewer; based on judgment or observation	Range of activities in rehabilitational setting	Range not useful for small impairments; ratings subjective
Kenny Self-Care Scale	Self-care and ambulation	Similar to Barthel Index	By interviewer; based on judgment or observation	Range useful in rehabilitational setting	Range narrow for small impairments; ratings subjective
Instrumental ADL Scale	More complex activities: food preparation, shopping, housekeeping	Higher range of performance than ADL Scale, not sensitive to small changes	By interviewer or patient based on judgment	Assessed functions important for independent living	Ratings subjective

Continued

Modified from Applegate WB, Blass JP, Williams TF: *N Engl J Med* 322:1211, 1990; from Bock JC: *Geriatric review syllabus,* New York, 1991, American Geriatric Society.

ADL, Activities of daily living.

*All these instruments can be used to establish a baseline, screen for risk factors or undetected problems, set rehabilitational goals, and monitor progress.

Table VI-B Instruments used to assess physical function*—cont'd

Instrument	Function Assessed	Range of Sensitivity	Administration	Strengths	Weaknesses
Timed Manual Performance	Timed assessment of performance of structured manual tasks	Broad range, from signing name to lifting latches	By interviewer; based on observation; requires special props	Assesses actual performance; sensitive to small changes	Difficult to use in patients who are seriously ill or cognitively impaired
Performance Test of ADL	Self-care, mobility, and transfers	Ranges from ADL and instrumental ADL to mobility and transfers	By professional or trained interviewer; requires observation of patient performing specific activities; requires props	Direct observation of range of functions; useful in variety of clinical settings	Time-consuming; difficult to use in seriously ill patients

				...	*...* summary scores may hide important problems observed in performance of individual tasks
		Assesses broad range of activities; detects persons with less serious disabilities			Difficult to use in seriously ill patients
Framingham Disability Scale	Self-care and physical activities	Broad range of activities, from self-care to lifting objects; not sensitive to small changes	By interviewer	Assesses broad range of activities; detects persons with less serious disabilities	
Physical Performance Test	Physical function	Broad range from writing to stair climbing	By trained interviewer; requires observation of patient performing specific activities; requires props	Assesses actual performance of range of functions	

Table VI-C Instruments used to assess cognitive function

Instrument	Function Assessed	Range of Sensitivity	Administration	Strengths	Weaknesses
Short Portable Mental Status Questionnaire	Memory, attention, orientation	Basic 10-item questionnaire, only capable of detecting gross cognitive dysfunction	By interviewer	Quick screen of basic function	Insensitive to small changes
Mini-Mental State Examination	Memory, orientation, attention, constructional ability	Fairly broad range; detects moderate but not mild or subtle impairment	By interviewer	Fairly quick and sensitive	Does not detect mild disability
Wechsler Memory Scale	Broader categories of memory	In-depth assessment of fairly broad range of memory functions; more sensitive to subtle change	By interviewer	In-depth assessment of memory	Takes a long time to administer; inadequate norms for older persons

			By interviewer or informant	Practical, clinically useful range	Quality of information dependent on informant
Dementia Rating Scale	Memory and behavior	Broad range of functions, including ability to manage money and find way indoors and outdoors	By interviewer or informant		
Short Care Scale*	Cognitive impairments	Short, multicomponent instrument; includes questions on basic mental status	By interviewer	Most useful as short combined screen of physical, emotional, and cognitive function	Scoring requires training; diagnostic index for dementia of doubtful validity
CERAD battery of tests	Dementia	Broad range of functions: memory, praxis, language; may be sensitive to disease progression	By interviewer	Assesses a number of functions often impaired in dementia; associated structured clinical evaluation available	Validity and reliability still being tested; requires training

Modified from Applegate WB, Blass JP, Williams TF: *N Engl J Med* 322:1211, 1990; from Bock JC: *Geriatric review syllabus*, New York, 1991, American Geriatric Society.

All these instruments can be used to establish a baseline description, screen for risk factors or undetected problems, and monitor progress.

*This instrument can be used to assist in diagnosis.

Table VI-D Instruments used to assess emotional state

Instrument	Function Assessed	Range of Sensitivity	Administration	Strengths	Weaknesses
Beck Depression Inventory*	Symptoms of depression	Questions range from assessment of mood to vegetative symptoms	By patient	Validated in older patients; brief	Relies too heavily on somatic symptoms
Zung Self-Rating Depression Scale*	Symptoms of depression	Range of questions about mood, vegetative symptoms, hopefulness	By patient or interviewer	Short and simple	Relies too heavily on somatic symptoms; not reliable in older patients
Hamilton Depression Inventory*	Symptoms of depression	Range of questions about mood; can estimate severity of depression	By interviewer	Provides an estimation of severity	Requires interviewer; reliance on somatic symptoms makes it less useful in ill older patients
Center for Epidemiologic Studies Depression Scale*	Symptoms of depression	Broad range of questions about mood; responsive to mood changes	By patient	Good measure of symptoms of depression	Does not distinguish between emotional effect of illness and overt depression; data on validity in older patients lacking

					Lacks normative data on older patients
Profile of Mood States*	Broad array of mood states	Range of mood states; particularly useful for psychiatric patients	By interviewer	Assesses wide spectrum of mood states	Lacks normative data on older patients
Geriatric Depression Scale*	Symptoms of depression	Broad range of questions about mood; designed for older patients	By patient	Quick; reliable, avoids an excess of somatic questions	Not evaluated for specificity among medically ill patients
Short Care Scale*	Symptoms of depression	Part of a short multi-component instrument; includes standard range of questions about symptoms of depression; responsive to mood changes	By interviewer	Useful when a short screen of physical, emotional, and cognitive function is needed	Requires asking other questions related to physical and cognitive function; scoring to assist in clinical diagnosis of depression is suspect

Modified from Applegate WB, Blass JP, Williams TF: *N Engl J Med* 322:1212, 1990; from Bock JC: *Geriatric review syllabus*, New York, 1991, American Geriatric Society.
*This instrument can be used to establish a baseline description, screen for risk factors or undetected problems, and monitor progress.

Continued

Table VI-D Instruments used to assess emotional state—cont'd

Instrument	Function Assessed	Range of Sensitivity	Administration	Strengths	Weaknesses
Hopkins Symptom Checklist†	Psychiatric symptoms commonly encountered in medical outpatients	Scored on five underlying symptom dimensions—somatization, obsessive-compulsive behavior, interpersonal sensitivity, anxiety, and depression	By patient	Easy to administer; broad range of symptoms; symptoms assessed often respond to pharmacotherapeutic agents; each scale is reliable; instrument has been demonstrated to be sensitive to those symptoms that are likely to respond to psychotropic medications, especially antianxiety and antidepressive agents	Not widely tested in older persons; not specific for psychiatric disorders

†This instrument can be used to assist in diagnosis.

Health Care Proxy and Durable Power of Attorney

VII

POWER OF ATTORNEY FOR HEALTH CARE INSTRUCTIONS

CAUTION:

THE ATTACHED POWER OF ATTORNEY FOR HEALTH CARE IS PRO-
VIDED FOR YOUR CONVENIENCE. IT MAY OR MAY NOT FIT THE RE-
QUIREMENTS OF YOUR PARTICULAR STATE. A GROWING NUMBER OF
STATES HAVE SPECIAL FORMS OR SPECIAL PROCEDURES FOR CRE-
ATING HEALTH CARE POWERS OF ATTORNEY. IF POSSIBLE, SEEK LE-
GAL ADVICE BEFORE SIGNING ANY POWER OF ATTORNEY. IF NOT
CLEARLY RECOGNIZED BY LAW IN YOUR STATE, THE DOCUMENT
MAY STILL PROVIDE THE BEST EVIDENCE OF YOUR WISHES IF YOU
SHOULD BECOME UNABLE TO SPEAK FOR YOURSELF.

Page 1 Instructions

Section 1—Designation of Health Care Agent: Print your full name
here as the "principal" or creator of the power of attorney.

Print the full name, address and telephone number of the person
(over age 18) you appoint as your health care "attorney-in-fact" or
"agent." Appoint *only* a person whom you trust to understand and
carry out your values and wishes. Do not name any of your health
care providers as your agent, since some states prohibit them acting as your agent.

Section 2—Effective Date and Durability: The sample document is
effective if and when you become unable to make health care decisions. That point in time is determined by your agent and your
doctor. You can, if you wish, specify other effective dates or other
criteria for incapacity (such as requiring two physicians to evaluate your capacity). You can also specify that the power will end at
some later date or event before death. In any case, you have the
right to revoke the agent's authority at any time by notifying your
agent or health care provider orally or in writing. If you revoke, it
is best to notify both your agent and physician in writing and to
destroy the power of attorney document itself.

Section 3—Agent's Powers: This grant of power is intended to be as
broad as possible so that your agent will have authority to make any
decision you could make to obtain or terminate any type of health
care.

(continued on next instruction page)

POWER OF ATTORNEY FOR HEALTH CARE

1. Designation of Health Care Agent.

I, _____ hereby appoint:
(principal)

_____
(Attorney-in-fact's name)

_____
(Address)

_____
Home:_____ Work:_____

as my attorney-in-fact (or "Agent") to make health and personal care decisions for me as authorized in this document.

2. Effective Date and Durability.

By this document I intend to create a durable power of attorney effective upon, and only during, any period of incapacity in which, in the opinion of my agent and attending physician, I am unable to make or communicate a choice regarding a particular health care decision.

3. Agent's Powers.

I grant to my Agent full authority to make decisions for me regarding my health care. In exercising this authority, my Agent shall follow my desires as stated in this document or otherwise known to my Agent. In making any decision, my Agent shall attempt to discuss the proposed decision with me to determine my desires if I am able to communicate in any way. If my Agent cannot determine the choice I would want made, then my Agent shall make a choice for me based upon what my Agent believes to be in my best interests. My Agent's authority to interpret my desires is intended to be as broad as possible, except for any limitations I may state below. Accordingly, unless specifically limited by Section 4, below, my Agent is authorized as follows:

A. To consent, refuse, or withdraw consent to any and all types of medical care, treatment, surgical procedures, diagnostic procedures, medication, and the use of mechanical or other procedures that affect any bodily function, including (but not limited to) artificial respiration, nutritional support and hydration, and cardiopulmonary resuscitation;

Page 1 of 5.

Page 2 Instructions

Section 3—Agent's Powers, continues on this page

Even under this broad grant of authority, your agent still must follow your desires and directions, communicated by you in any manner now or in the future. You can specifically limit or direct your agent's power, if you wish, in Section 4.

Section 4—Statement of Desires, Special Provisions, and Limitations:

Paragraph A. Here you may include any limitations you think are appropriate, such as instructions to refuse any specific types of treatment that are against your religious beliefs or unacceptable to you for any other reasons, such as blood transfusion, electro-convulsive therapy, sterilization, abortion, amputation, psychosurgery, admission to a mental institution, etc. State law may not allow your agent to consent to some of these procedures, regardless of your health care power of attorney. Be very careful about stating limitations, because the specific circumstances surrounding a future health care decision are impossible to predict. If you do not want any limitations, simply write in "No limitations."

B. To have access to medical records and information to the same extent that I am entitled to, including the right to disclose the contents to others;

C. To authorize my admission to or discharge (even against medical advice) from any hospital, nursing home, residential care, assisted living or similar facility or service;

D. To contract on my behalf for any health care related service or facility on my behalf, without my Agent incurring personal financial liability for such contracts;

E. To hire and fire medical, social service, and other support personnel responsible for my care;

F. To authorize, or refuse to authorize, any medication or procedure intended to relieve pain, even though such use may lead to physical damage, addiction, or hasten the moment of (but not intentionally cause) my death;

G. To make anatomical gifts of part or all of my body for medical purposes, authorize an autopsy, and direct the disposition of my remains, to the extent permitted by law;

H. To take any other action necessary to do what I authorize here, including (but not limited to) granting any waiver or release from liability required by any hospital, physician, or other health care provider; signing any documents relating to refusals of treatment or the leaving of a facility against medical advice, and pursuing any legal action in my name, at the expense of my estate to force compliance with my wishes as determined by my Agent, or to seek actual or punitive damages for the failure to comply.

1. **Statement of Desires, Special Provisions, and Limitations.**

A. The powers granted above do not include the following powers or are subject to the following rules of limitations:

_____
_____
_____
_____
_____
_____

Page 3 Instructions

Section 4—Statement of Desires, Special Provisions, and Limitations continues on this page.

Paragraph B: Because the subject of "life-sustaining treatment" is particularly important to many people, this paragraph provides a place for you to give general or specific directions on the subject, if you want to do so. The different paragraphs are options— choose only *one,* or write your desires or instructions in your own words (in the last option). If you already have a "Living Will", you can simply refer to it by choosing the first option. Or, the instructions you provide here can do what a Living Will would do.

Paragraph C: Because people differ widely on whether nutrition and hydration is something that ought to be refused or stopped under certain circumstances, it is important to make your wishes clear on this topic. Nutrition and hydration means food and fluids provided by a nasogastric tube or tube into the stomach, intestines, or veins. This paragraph allows you to include or not include these procedures among those that may be withheld or withdrawn under the circumstances described in the preceding paragraph. Either choice still permits non-intrusive efforts such as spoon feeding or moistening of lips and mouth.

B. With respect to any *Life-Sustaining Treatment*, I direct the following:

(Initial Only One of the Following Paragraphs)

☐ REFERENCE TO LIVING WILL. I specifically direct my Agent to follow any health care declaration or "living will" executed by me.

☐ GRANT OF DISCRETION TO AGENT. I do not want my life to be prolonged nor do I want life-sustaining treatment to be provided or continued if my Agent believes the burdens of the treatment outweigh the expected benefits. I want my Agent to consider the relief of suffering, the expense involved and the quality as well as the possible extension of my life in making decisions concerning life-sustaining treatment.

☐ DIRECTIVE TO WITHHOLD OR WITHDRAW TREATMENT. I do not want my life to be prolonged and I do not want life-sustaining treatment:
a. if I have a condition that is incurable or irreversible and, without the administration of life-sustaining treatment, expected to result in death within a relatively short time; or
b. if I am in a coma or persistent vegetative state which is reasonably concluded to be irreversible.

☐ DIRECTIVE FOR MAXIMUM TREATMENT. I want my life to be prolonged to the greatest extent possible without regard to my condition, the chances I have for recovery, or the cost of the procedures.

☐ DIRECTIVE IN MY OWN WORDS: _____
_____
_____
_____
_____

C. With respect to *Nutrition and Hydration* provided by means of a nasogastric tube or tube into the stomach, intestines, or veins, I wish to make clear that . . .

(Initial Only One)

☐ I <u>intend</u> to include these procedures among the "life-sustaining procedures" that may be withheld or withdrawn under the conditions given above.

☐ I <u>do not intend</u> to include these procedures among the "life-sustaining procedures" that may be withheld or withdrawn.

Page 3 of 5.

Page 4 Instructions

Section 5—Successors: If you wish to name alternate agents in case your first agent becomes unavailable, print the appropriate information in this paragraph. You can name as many successors in the order you wish.

Section 6—Protection of Third Parties Who Rely on My Agent: In most states, health care providers cannot be compelled to follow the directions of your agent, although in some states, they may be obligated to transfer your care to another provider who is willing to comply. This paragraph is intended to encourage compliance with the power of attorney by waiving potential civil liability for good faith reliance on the agent's statements and decisions.

Section 7—Nomination of Guardian: The use of a health care power of attorney is intended to *prevent* the need for a court-appointed guardian for health care decision-making. However, if for any reason, court involvement becomes necessary, this paragraph expressly names your Agent to serve as guardian. A court does not have to follow your nomination, but it will normally comply with your wishes unless there is good reason not to.

Section 8—Administration Provisions: These items address miscellaneous matters that could affect the implementation of your power of attorney.

5. **Successors**

   If any Agent named by me shall die, become legally disabled, resign, refuse to act, be unavailable, or (if any Agent is my spouse) be legally separated or divorced from me, I name the following (each to act alone and successively, in the order named) as successors to my Agent:

   A. First Alternate Agent _____
      Address: _____
      Telephone: _____

   B. Second Alternate Agent _____
      Address: _____
      Telephone: _____

6. **Protection of Third Parties Who Rely on My Agent.**
   No person who relies in good faith upon any representations by my Agent or Successor Agent shall be liable to me, my estate, my heirs or assigns, for recognizing the Agent's authority.

7. **Nomination of Guardian.**
   If a guardian of my person should for any reason be appointed, I nominate my Agent (or his or her successor), named above.

8. **Administrative Provisions.**

   A. I revoke any prior power of attorney for health care.

   B. This power of attorney is intended to be valid in any jurisdiction in which it is presented.

   C. My Agent shall not be entitled to compensation for services performed under this power of attorney, but he or she shall be entitled to reimbursement for all reasonable expenses incurred as a result of carrying out any provision of this power of attorney.

   D. The powers delegated under this power of attorney are separable, so that the invalidity of one or more powers shall not affect any others.

Page 5 Instructions

Signing the Document: Required procedures for signing this kind of document vary from signature only to very detailed witnessing requirements, or, in some states, simply notarization. The suggested procedure here is intended to meet most of the various state requirements for signing by non-institutionalized persons. The procedure here is likely to be more detailed than is required under your own state's law, but it will help ensure that your Health Care Power is recognized in other states, too. First, sign and date the document in front of *two witnesses*. Your witnesses should know your identity personally and be able to declare that you appear to be of sound mind and under no duress or undue influence. Further, your witnesses should not be:

- Your treating physician, health care provider, or health facility operator, nor an employee of any of these.
- Anyone related to you by blood, marriage, or adoption.
- Anyone entitled to any part of your estate under an existing will or by operation of law. Even a creditor of yours should not be used under these guidelines.

If you are in a nursing home or other institution, be sure to consult state law, because a few states require that an ombudsman or patient advocate be one of your witnesses.

Second, have your signature *notarized*. Some states permit notarization as an alternative to witnessing. Others may simply apply the rules for signing ordinary durable powers of attorney. Ordinary durable powers of attorney are usually notarized. This form includes a relatively typical notary statement, but here again, it is wise to check state law in case a special form of notary acknowledgement is required.

BY SIGNING HERE I INDICATE THAT I UNDERSTAND THE CONTENTS OF THIS DOCUMENT AND THE EFFECT OF THIS GRANT OF POWERS TO MY AGENT.

I sign my name to this Health Care Power of Attorney on this
_____ day of _____, 19_____
My current home address is: _____
_____

    Signature: _____
    Name: _____

Witness Statement

I declare that the person who signed or acknowledged this document is personally known to me, that he/she signed or acknowledged this durable power of attorney in my presence, and that he/she appears to be of sound mind and under no duress, fraud, or undue influence. I am not the person appointed as agent by this document, nor am I the patient's health care provider, or an employee of the patient's health care provider. I further declare that I am not related to the principal by blood, marriage, or adoption, and, to the best of my knowledge, I am not a creditor of the principal nor entitled to any part of his/her estate under a will now existing or by operation of law.

Witness #1:

Signature: _____ Date: _____
Print Name: _____ Telephone: _____
Residence Address: _____
_____

Witness #2:

Signature: _____ Date: _____
Print Name: _____ Telephone: _____
Residence Address: _____
_____

Notarization

STATE OF _____)
) ss.
COUNTY OF _____)

On this ____ day of _____, 19___, the said _____, known to me (or satisfactorily proven) to be the person named in the foregoing instrument, personally appeared before me, a Notary Public, within and for the State and County aforesaid, and acknowledged that he or she freely and voluntarily executed the same for the purposes stated therein.

My Commission Expires: _____
_____   *NOTARY PUBLIC*

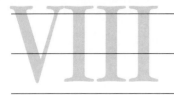

Enteral Nutritional Products

Routine oral or tube supplemental feeding (Ensure)

Intact protein, protein isolates, lactose-free product; each 100 ml contains

Protein	3.65 g	Calcium	2.7 mEq
Carbohydrate	14.24 g	Chloride	3.0 mEq
Fat	3.65 g	Calories	106
Potassium	3.2 mEq	mOsm = 450	
Sodium	3.3 mEq		

This product also contains all known essential vitamins and minerals for adults and for children 4 years or older.

Routine tube feeding (Isocal)

Lactose-free and low in sodium; each 100 ml contains

Protein	3.25 g	Calcium	3.00 mEq
Carbohydrate	12.50 g	Chloride	2.80 mEq
Fat	4.20 g	Calories	100
Potassium	3.20 mEq	mOsm = 300	
Sodium	2.20 mEq		

This product also contains all known essential vitamins and minerals for adults and for children 4 years or older.

Routine tube feeding (Osmolite HN)

Lactose-free and low in sodium; each 100 ml contains

Protein	4.4 g	Calcium	76 mg
Carbohydrate	13.9 g	Chloride	4.1 mEq
Fat	3.6 g	Calories	106
Potassium	4.0 mEq	mOsm = 310	
Sodium	4.0 mEq		

This product also contains all known essential vitamins and minerals for adults and for children 4 years or older.

High-calorie supplemental feeding (Magnacal)

Lactose-free product; each 100 ml contains

Protein	7.0 g	Calcium	5.0 mEq
Carbohydrate	25.0 g	Chloride	2.7 mEq
Fat	8.0 g	Calories	200

Potassium	3.2 mEq	mOsm = 590
Sodium	4.3 mEq	

This product also contains all known essential vitamins and minerals for adults and for children 4 years or older.

Low-residue oral or tube feeding (Criticare)

High-nitrogen elemental diet; each 100 ml contains

Protein	3.80 g
Carbohydrate	22.20 g
Fat	0.03 g
Calories	106

mOsm = 650

This product also contains all known essential vitamins and minerals for adults and for children 4 years or older.

Essential amino acid formulation (Amin-Aid)

Nutritional product for management of uremic patients; each 100 ml contains

Protein	1.94 g
Carbohydrate	36.54 g
Fat	4.62 g
Calories	195.5

mOsm = 850

This product is low in electrolytes and contains no vitamins.

Branched-chain amino acid formulation (Hepatic-Aid)

Nutritional management of liver disease; each 100 ml contains

Protein	4.26 g
Carbohydrate	28.80 g
Fat	3.62 g
Calories	164.7

mOsm = 900

This product contains negligible electrolytes and no vitamins or minerals.

Oral supplemental feeding (Citrotein)

Lactose-free, cholesterol-free, gluten-free; each 100 ml contains

Protein	4.29 g
Carbohydrate	13.0 g
Fat	0.18 g
Potassium	1.9 mEq
Sodium	3.2 mEq
Calcium	5.6 mEq
Chloride	2.9 mEq
Calories	71

mOsm = 496

Routine oral supplemental feeding (Forta Pudding)

Each 150 g contains

Protein	6.8 g
Carbohydrate	34.0 g

Fat	9.7 g
Potassium	7.7 mEq
Sodium	9.6 mEq
Calcium	10.0 mEq
Chloride	6.0 mEq
Calories	250

This product also contains all known essential vitamins and minerals for adults and for children 4 years or older.

Caloric additive product (Polycose)

Each 100 ml contains

Carbohydrate	50.0 g
Potassium	0.5 mEq
Sodium	2.5 mEq
Calcium	1.5 mEq
Chloride	3.1 mEq
Calories	200

mOsm = 850

Routine oral supplemental feeding (Instant Breakfast)

Each 100 ml contains

Protein	6.25 g
Carbohydrate	12.10 g
Fat	3.40 g
Potassium	5.90 mEq
Sodium	4.70 mEq
Calcium	7.30 mEq
Chloride	n/a
Calories	103.6

Nutritionally complete supplement when mixed with 8 oz. whole milk.

High-protein clear liquid product (high-protein gelatin)

Each 150 ml contains

Protein	17.0 g
Carbohydrate	18.0 g
Fat	0.0 g
Potassium	5.3 mEq
Sodium	10.8 mEq
Calories	140

This product may be used as a supplement on clear liquid diets.

Geriatric Depression Scale (GDS)

IX

Y/N Choice

1. Are you basically satisfied with your life?   N = 1
2. Have you dropped any of your activities or interests?   Y = 1
3. Do you feel that your life is empty?   Y = 1
4. Do you often get bored?   Y = 1
5. Are you hopeful about the future?   N = 1
6. Are you bothered by thoughts you can't get out of your head?   Y = 1
7. Are you in good spirits most of the time?   N = 1
8. Are you afraid that something bad is going to happen to you?   Y = 1
9. Do you feel happy most of the time?   N = 1
10. Do you often feel helpless?   Y = 1
11. Do you often get restless and fidgety?   Y = 1
12. Do you prefer to stay at home, rather than going out and doing new things?   Y = 1
13. Do you frequently worry about the future?   Y = 1
14. Do you feel you have more problems with memory than most?   Y = 1
15. Do you think it is wonderful to be alive now?   N = 1
16. Do you often feel downhearted and blue?   Y = 1
17. Do you feel pretty worthless the way you are now?   Y = 1
18. Do you worry a lot about the past?   Y = 1
19. Do you find life very exciting?   N = 1
20. Is it hard for you to get started on new projects?   Y = 1
21. Do you feel full of energy?   N = 1
22. Do you feel that your situation is hopeless?   Y = 1
23. Do you think that most people are better off than you are?   Y = 1
24. Do you frequently get upset over little things?   Y = 1
25. Do you frequently feel like crying?   Y = 1
26. Do you have trouble concentrating?   Y = 1
27. Do you enjoy getting up in the morning?   N = 1
28. Do you prefer to avoid social gatherings?   Y = 1
29. Is it easy for you to make decisions?   N = 1
30. Is your mind as clear as it used to be?   N = 1

A score of 11 has been shown to be useful in the diagnosis of depression.

Modified from Yesavage JA et al: *J Psychiatr Res* 17:37, 1982.

X

Cancer Screening for Persons 65 Years and Older

Cancer Screening Modality	Recommendations		
	U.S. Preventive Services Task Force	American Cancer Society	Canadian Task Force
Breast Cancer			
Self-examination	No evidence	No evidence	No evidence
Clinical examination	Every 1-2 yr until 75	Yearly	Yearly
Mammogram	Every 1-2 yr until 75	Yearly	Yearly
Colon Cancer			
Fecal occult blood	No evidence*	Yearly	No evidence*
Sigmoidoscopy	No evidence*	Every 3-5 yr according to physician	No evidence*
Cervical Cancer			
Pap smear	NR‡ if consistently normal up to age 65	Yearly; less frequently if consistently normal 3 times or more	Every 5 yr; more or less depending on clinical judgment
Prostate Cancer			
Digital rectal examination	No evidence	Yearly	No evidence
Prostate-specific antigen	NR	No evidence	NE‡
Skin Cancer			
Self-examination	No evidence	NE	NE
Clinical examination	If high risk	Yearly	If high risk

Continued

Cancer Screening Modality	Recommendations		
	U.S. Preventive Services Task Force	American Cancer Society	Canadian Task Force
Ovarian Cancer			
Pelvic examination	NR	Yearly above 40	NE
Oral Cancer			
Clinical examination	NR except if high risk	Yearly	No evidence
Thyroid Cancer			
Clinical examination	Regularly if exposed to upper body radiation	Yearly	NE
Testicular Cancer			
Clinical examination	NE	Yearly	No evidence

From Yoshikawa TT, Cobbs EL, Brummel-Smith K, editors: *Ambulatory geriatric care*, 1993, Mosby.

*No evidence; there is insufficient evidence for or against the use of a test in asymptomatic persons aged 65 and older without risk factors; further data are needed (*for low-risk groups only).

†*NR*, Not recommended.

‡*NE*, Not evaluated.

The Hebrew Rehabilitation Center for the Aged Vulnerability Index

1. Now I will ask you about your meals. Do you prepare them yourself?
   _____Yes   _____No
   If Yes, ask: Do you have great difficulty doing it yourself?
   If No, ask: Do you need this help?
   _____Yes   (P)   _____No

2. Do you take out the garbage yourself?
   _____Yes   _____No
   If Yes, ask: Do you have great difficulty doing it yourself?
   If No, ask: Do you need this help?
   _____Yes   (P)   _____No

3. Are you healthy enough to do the ordinary work around the house without help?
   _____Yes   _____No

4. Are you healthy enough to walk up and down stairs without help?
   _____Yes   _____No

5. Do you use a walker or four-pronged cane at least some of the time to get around?
   _____Yes   (P)   _____No

6. Do you use a wheelchair at least some of the time to get around?
   _____Yes   _____No

7. Could you please tell me what year it is?
   _____Correct   _____Incorrect (P)
   A. Record number of (P) boxes checked for questions 1.
   to 7.   A.( )

8. In the last month, how many days a week have you usually gone out of the building in which you live?
   _____2 or more days a week
   _____1 day a week or less (P)

From Yoshikawa TT, Cobbs EL, Brummel-Smith K, editors: *Ambulatory geriatric care*, St Louis, 1993, Mosby.

Continued

9. Are you able to dress yourself (including shoes and socks) without help?

_____Seldom, sometimes, or never

_____Frequently or most of the time (P)

B. Record number of (P) boxes checked for questions 8. to 11.   B.( )

C. Person is functionally vulnerable if

   A. box is greater than 1 or

   A. box equals 1 and B. box is greater than 0.   C.( )

   Check ( ) if vulnerable

Functional

Dementia

Scale

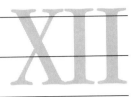

Circle one rating for each item:	Date:_____
1 = None or little of the time	Patient:_____
2 = Some of the time	Observer:_____
3 = Good part of the time	Relation to patient:_____
4 = Most or all of the time	

1 2 3 4   1. Has difficulty in completing simple tasks on own (e.g., dressing, bathing, doing arithmetic)

1 2 3 4   2. Spends time either sitting or in apparently purposeless activity

1 2 3 4   3. Wanders at night or needs to be restrained to prevent wandering

1 2 3 4   4. Hears things that are not there

1 2 3 4   5. Requires supervision or assistance in eating

1 2 3 4   6. Loses things

1 2 3 4   7. Has disorderly appearance if left to own devices

1 2 3 4   8. Moans

1 2 3 4   9. Cannot control bowel function

1 2 3 4   10. Threatens to harm others

1 2 3 4   11. Cannot control bladder function

1 2 3 4   12. Needs to be watched so doesn't injure self (e.g., by careless smoking, leaving the stove on, falling)

1 2 3 4   13. Destroys materials around him or her (e.g., breaks furniture, throws food trays, tears up magazines)

1 2 3 4   14. Shouts or yells

1 2 3 4   15. Accuses others of doing him or her bodily harm or stealing his or her possessions when you are sure the accusations are not true

1 2 3 4   16. Is unaware of limitations imposed by illness

1 2 3 4   17. Becomes confused and does not know where he or she is

1 2 3 4   18. Has trouble remembering

1 2 3 4   19. Has sudden changes of mood (e.g., gets upset, gets angry, or cries easily)

1 2 3 4   20. Wanders aimlessly during the day or needs to be restrained to prevent wandering, if left alone

From Yoshikawa TT, Cobbs EL, Brummel-Smith K, editors: *Ambulatory geriatric care,* St Louis, 1993, Mosby.

1. My daily life is not interesting .... T or F
2. It is hard for me to get started on my daily chores and activities .... T or F
3. I have been more unhappy than usual for at least a month .... T or F
4. I have been sleeping poorly for at least the last month .... T or F
5. I gain little pleasure from anything .... T or F
6. I feel listless, tired, or fatigued a lot of the time .... T or F
7. I have felt sad, down in the dumps, or blue much of the time during the last month .... T or F
8. My memory or thinking is not as good as usual .... T or F
9. I have been more easily irritated or frustrated lately .... T or F
10. I feel worse in the morning than in the afternoon .... T or F
11. I have cried or felt like crying more than twice during the last month .... T or F
12. I am definitely slowed down compared to my usual way of feeling .... T or F
13. The things that used to make me happy don't do so anymore .... T or F
14. My appetite or digestion of food is worse than usual ...... T or F
15. I frequently feel like I don't care about anything anymore .... T or F
16. Life is really not worth living most of the time .... T or F
17. My outlook is more gloomy than usual .... T or F
18. I have stopped several of my usual activities .... T or F
19. I cry or feel saddened more easily than a few months ago .... T or F
20. I feel pretty hopeless about improving my life .... T or F
21. I seem to have lost the ability to have any fun .... T or F
22. I have regrets about the past that I think about often .... T or F

From Yoshikawa TT, Cobbs EL, Brummel-Smith K, editors: *Ambulatory geriatric care,* St Louis, 1993, Mosby.

*If patient has 0-5 true answers, no major depression; 6-11 true answers, intermediate or borderline; 12 or more true answers, probable major depression.

Katz Index of Activities of Daily Living*

1. **Bathing (either sponge bath, tub bath, or shower)**
   a. Receives no assistance (gets in and out of tub by self if tub is usual means of bathing)
   b. Receives assistance in bathing only one part of body such as the back or a leg
   c. Receives assistance in bathing more than one part of body or is not bathed
2. **Continence**
   a. Controls urination and bowel movement completely by self
   b. Has occasional "accidents"
   c. Needs supervision to keep urine or bowel control, uses catheter, or is incontinent
3. **Dressing (gets clothes from closets and drawers, including underclothes, outer garments; uses fasteners, including braces, if worn)**
   a. Gets clothes and gets completely dressed without assistance
   b. Gets clothes and gets dressed without assistance except in tieing shoes
   c. Receives assistance in getting clothes or getting dressed or stays partly or completely undressed
4. **Eating**
   a. Feeds self without assistance
   b. Feeds self except for assistance in cutting meat or buttering bread
   c. Receives assistance in feeding or is fed partly or completely by using tubes or intravenous fluids
5. **Toileting (going to the "toilet room" for bowel and urine elimination; cleaning self after elimination and arranging clothes)**
   a. Goes to "toilet room," cleans self, and arranges clothes without assistance (may use object for support such as cane, walker, or wheelchair and may manage night bedpan or commode and emptying same in morning)
   b. Receives assistance in going to "toilet room," cleaning self, or arranging clothes after elimination or receives assistance in using night bedpan or commode
   c. Does not go to "toilet room" for the elimination process

From Yoshikawa TT, Cobbs EL, Brummel-Smith K, editors: *Ambulatory geriatric care*, St Louis, 1993, Mosby.

*Response a., 3 points; b., 2 points; c., 1 point; maximum score, 18 points.

Continued

6. **Transferring**
   a. Moves in and out of bed or chair without assistance (may use object for support such as cane or walker)
   b. Moves in and out of bed or chair with assistance
   c. Does not get out of bed

Folstein Mini–Mental State Examination

XV

Mini–Mental State Inpatient Consultation Form

Maximum Score	Score	
		Orientation
5	( )	What is the (year) (season) (date) (day) (month)?
5	( )	Where are we: (state) (county) (town) (hospital) (floor)?
		Registration
3	( )	Name 3 objects: 1 second to say each. Then ask the patient all 3 after you have said them. Give 1 point for each correct answer. Then repeat them until he learns all 3. Count trials and record.
		Trials
		Attention and calculation
5	( )	Serial 7s. 1 point for each correct answer. Stop after 5 answers. Alternatively, spell "world" backwards.
		Recall
3	( )	Ask for 3 objects repeated above. Give 1 point for each correct answer.
		Language
9	( )	Name a pencil and watch. (2 points) Repeat the following: "No Ifs, and, or buts." (1 point) Follow a 3-stage command: "Take a paper in your right hand, fold it in half, and put it on the floor." (3 points)

Continued

Mini–Mental State Inpatient Consultation Form—cont'd

Read and obey the following: "Close your
eyes." (1 point)
Write a sentence. (1 point)
Copy design. (1 point)

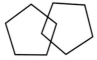

Total Score   ASSESS level Alert Drowsy Stupor Coma
                     of conscious-
                     ness along
                     a continuum.

From Folstein MF, Folstein SE, McHugh P: Mini–mental state: a practical method for grading the cognitive state of patients for the clinician, *J Psychiatr Res* 12, 1975.

Index

Page numbers in italics indicate illustrations; *t* indicates tables.